Treating Mental Illness and Behavior Disorders in Children and Adults With Mental Retardation

Treating Mental Illness and Behavior Disorders in Children and Adults With Mental Retardation

Edited by

Anton Došen, M.D., Ph.D.
Kenneth Day, M.B., Ch.B., F.R.C.Psych., D.P.M.

American Psychiatric Press, Inc.

Washington, DC
London, England

Note: The authors have worked to ensure that all information in this book concerning drug dosages, schedules, and routes of administration is accurate as of the time of publication and consistent with standards set by the U.S. Food and Drug Administration and the general medical community. As medical research and practice advance, however, therapeutic standards may change. For this reason and because human and mechanical errors sometimes occur, we recommend that readers follow the advice of a physician who is directly involved in their care or the care of a member of their family.

Books published by the American Psychiatric Press, Inc., represent the views and opinions of the individual authors and do not necessarily represent the policies and opinions of the Press or the American Psychiatric Association.

Manufactured in the United States of America on acid-free paper
First Edition
04   03   02   01   4   3   2   1

American Psychiatric Press, Inc.
1400 K Street, NW
Washington, DC   20005
www.appi.org

Library of Congress Cataloging-in-Publication Data
Treating mental illness and behavior disorders in children and adults
with mental retardation / edited by Anton Dosen, Kenneth Day.— 1st ed.
      p. ; cm.
   Includes bibliographical references and index.
   ISBN 0-88048-850-6 (alk. paper)
   1. Mentally handicapped—Mental health—Handbooks, manuals, etc. 2. Mentally
   handicapped—Mental health services—Handbooks, manuals, etc. 3. Mental
   illness—Treatment—Handbooks, manuals, etc. I. Dosen, Anton. II. Day, Kenneth, D.P.M.
   [DNLM: 1. Mental Retardation—psychology. 2. Behavior Therapy. 3. Mental
   Disorders—therapy. 4. Mentally Disabled Persons—psychology. 5.
   Psychotherapy—methods. WM 307.M5 H2365 2001]
   RC451.4.M47 H366 2001
   616.85'8806—dc21
                                                                    00-032793

British Library Cataloguing in Publication Data
A CIP record is available from the British Library.

To our wives
Renata and Ruth

Contents

I

Introduction

Anton Došen, M.D., Ph.D.
Kenneth Day, M.B., Ch.B., F.R.C.Psych., D.P.M.

II

Treatment Methods

Sheila Hollins, M.B., B.S., F.R.C.Psych.

Stephen Tyrer, M.A., M.B., B.Chir.L.M.C.C., F.R.C.Psych.
Sarah Hill, B.Sc.

William I. Gardner, Ph.D.
Janice L. Graeber-Whalen, Ph.D.
Debby R. Ford, Ph.D.

III
Psychotherapeutic Methods

IV
Treatment of Mental Illness

V

Treatment of Behavior Disorders

VI

Treatment Methods With Children

VII

Mental Health Services for the
Mentally Retarded and Staff Training

VIII

Integrative Treatment

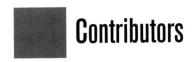
Contributors

Betsey A. Benson, Ph.D.
Psychologist, Nosing Center, Ohio State University, Columbus, Ohio

Thomas P. Berney, M.B., Ch.B., D.P.M., F.R.C.Psych., F.R.C.P.C.H.
Consultant Psychiatrist, Prudhoe Hospital, Northumberland; Clinical Lecturer, Department of Psychiatry, University of Newcastle Upon Tyne, United Kingdom

Nick Bouras, M.B., Ph.D., F.R.C.Psych.
Professor of Psychiatry, Division of Psychological Medicine, Guy's, King's, and St. Thomas's Medical School, York Clinic, Guy's Hospital, London, United Kingdom

David J. Clarke, M.B., Ch.B., M.R.C.Psych.
Senior Lecturer, Department of Psychiatry, University of Birmingham, Birmingham, United Kingdom

John Corbett, F.R.C.P., F.R.C.Psych., D.P.M.
Professor of Developmental Psychiatry, University of Birmingham, Birmingham, United Kingdom

Diane Cox-Lindenbaum, A.C.S.W.
Clinical Consultant, Clinical Supervisor, Ridgefield, Connecticut

Henry F. Crabbe, M.D., Ph.D.
Medical Director, Psychiatric Medicine Center, New London, Connecticut

Kenneth Day, M.B., Ch.B., F.R.C.Psych., D.P.M.
Lately Medical Director and Honorary Consultant Psychiatrist, Northgate and Prudoe NHS Trust, Northumberland; Senior Lecturer, Department of Psychiatry, University of Newcastle Upon Tyne, United Kingdom

Anne Des Noyers-Hurley, Ph.D.
Director of Psychology, Department of Psychiatry, New England Medical Center; Assistant Professor of Psychiatry, Tufts University School of Medicine, Boston, Massachusetts

Anton Došen, M.D., Ph.D.
Professor of Psychiatric Aspects of Mental Retardation, University of Nijmegen; Medical Director, Clinic for Behavioral and Psychiatric Disorders in the Mentally Retarded, Nieuw Spraeland, Oostrum, The Netherlands

Earl H. Faulkner, M.A.
Mental Health Coordinator, Medical Center, University of Nebraska, Omaha, Nebraska

Mark Fleisher, M.D.
Director, Dual Diagnosis Clinic, Medical Center, University of Nebraska, Omaha, Nebraska

Larry Folk, B.A.
Mental Health Coordinator, Medical Center, University of Nebraska, Omaha, Nebraska

Debby R. Ford, Ph.D.
Psychologist, Bethesda Lutheran Home, Watertown, Wisconsin

Christian Gaedt, M.D.
Medical Director, Institute for the Mentally Retarded, Neuerkerode, Germany

William I. Gardner, Ph.D.
Professor of Department of Rehabilitation Psychology and Special Education, University of Wisconsin, Madison, Wisconsin

Ann Gath, M.D., F.R.C.Psych., D.P.M., D.C.H.
Lately Professor of Developmental Psychiatry, University of London; Honorary Consultant Psychiatrist, Essex and Harts Health Services, London, United Kingdom

Gijs van Gemert, Ph.D.
Professor of Special Education, University of Groningen, The Netherlands

Janice L. Graeber-Whalen, Ph.D.[†]
Psychologist, Waismen Center on Mental Retardation and Human Development, University of Wisconsin, Madison, Wisconsin

Dorothy Griffiths, Ph.D.
Psychologist, Brock University, St. Catharines, Ontario, Canada

Sarah Hill, B.Sc.
Assistant Psychologist, Department of Psychiatry, University of Newcastle-Upon-Tyne, United Kingdom

Sheila Hollins, M.B., B.S., F.R.C.Psych.
Professor of Psychiatry of Learning Disability, St. George's Hospital Medical School, University of London, United Kingdom

Geraldine Holt, M.B., B.S., M.R.C.Psych.
Consultant Psychiatrist, Division of Psychological Medicine, Guy's, King's, and St. Thomas's Medical School, York Clinic, Guy's Hospital, London, United Kingdom

Michael Lowry, Ph.D.
Psychologist, Department of Mental Retardation, Holyoke, Massachusetts

Garry Prouty, Ph.D.
Faculty Associate, Nisonger Center, Ohio State University, Columbus, Ohio

Wilhelm Rotthaus, M.D.
Consultant Psychiatrist, Rheinische Landesklinik, Viersen, Germany

Stephen Ruedrich, M.D.
Associate Professor of Psychiatry, Case Western Reserve University, School of Medicine, Cleveland, Ohio

Richard Ruth, Ph.D.
Chief Psychologist, Community Psychiatric Clinic, Montgomery County, Wheaton, Maryland

Robert L. Schalock, Ph.D.
Psychologist, Medical Center, University of Nebraska, Omaha, Nebraska

---

[†]Deceased

Nefeli Schneider, Ph.D.
Psychologist, Joseph County Community Center, Lakewood, Colorado

Robert Sovner, M.D.[†]
Associate Professor, The Habilitive Psychiatry Service, Department of Psychiatry, New England Medical Center, Boston, Massachusetts

Sigfried Tuinier, M.D., Ph.D.
Senior Lecturer of Psychiatry, Vincent van Gogh Institute, Venray, The Netherlands

Stephen Tyrer, M.A., M.B., B.Chir.L.M.C.C., F.R.C.Psych.
Consultant Psychiatrist, Prudhoe Hospital, Northumberland; Clinical Lecturer, Department of Psychiatry, University of Newcastle Upon Tyne, United Kingdom

Denise Valenti-Hein, Ph.D.
Psychologist, Institute on Disability and Human Development, University of Illinois at Chicago, Chicago, Illinois

Willem M.A. Verhoeven, M.D., Ph.D.
Professor of Psychiatry Erasmus, University of Rotterdam and Vincent van Gogh Institute, Venray, The Netherlands

[†]Deceased.

Preface

Since the 1970s, and in parallel with the introduction of normalization philosophy and care in community policies, the nature and treatment of psychiatric and behavior disorders in people with mental retardation have become a major area of concern to professionals working in psychiatry. Scientific interest and knowledge have increased during this period, and there is now a substantial body of research on the phenomenology of mental illness and behavior disorders in mentally retarded persons. This has been accompanied by an increasing interest in treatment approaches and service provision.

In this book, we aim to provide a comprehensive account of the current theory and practice of mental health treatment and care in mentally retarded children and adults. All forms of disorder and treatment are covered. The book begins with an introductory chapter on the epidemiology and presentation of psychiatric and behavior problems in the mentally retarded. Section 2 overviews all the major treatment methods: drug therapy, psychotherapy, behavior therapy, cognitive and social learning therapies, and family therapy. Sections 3, 4, 5, and 6 discuss in detail the application of these treatment approaches to specific mental health problems in mentally retarded children and adults. The book concludes with chapters on service provision and staff training.

Our primary objective has been to provide a source for all disciplines working in the field of mental health care for mentally retarded people, including psychiatrists, general medical practitioners, nurses, psychologists, educationalists, teachers, social workers, and other medical specialists. It is our hope that it will also act as a stimulus to practitioners and investigators in the field to further develop and research treatment approaches for this patient group and provide a useful source of information for education, training, and research.

We are indebted to all the contributors to this book and to our secretaries, Willa Coulthard and Nelly Lemmens, for typing and compiling the final manuscript.

Anton Došen
Kenneth Day

Introduction

1 Epidemiology, Etiology, and Presentation of Mental Illness and Behavior Disorders in Persons With Mental Retardation

Anton Došen, M.D., Ph.D.
Kenneth Day, M.B., Ch.B., F.R.C.Psych., D.P.M.

A distinction between mental retardation and mental illness was first made in medieval times principally for legal purposes and the protection of property. That mentally retarded people might also suffer from mental illness was first noted in the mid-nineteenth century (Berrios 1994; Reid 1989), and by the turn of the century surprisingly accurate clinical descriptions of the main forms of mental disorder occurring in mental retardation were appearing in text books (see Tredgold 1908, for example). It is evident that earlier physicians experienced the same difficulties in categorizing certain disorders as we do today.

During the first half of the twentieth century, interest in psychiatric disorder in mental retardation gradually waned as the focus shifted from the neuropathological basis of mental illness to neurotic disorders and psychotherapy. Psychiatric input into large mental retardation institutions was variable, and, with some notable exceptions, the psychiatric problems of the mentally retarded became progressively neglected.

The development of normalization philosophy and the implementation of community care policies during the past three decades have once again highlighted the psychiatric problems of mentally retarded people and rekindled the interest of scientists, practitioners, and service providers. There is now a substantial body of new information on epidemiology, classification, and clinical features. In this chapter, we aim to provide an overview of the current state of knowledge, research trends, questions, and problems concerning treatment of psychiatric disorders in the mentally retarded.

■ EPIDEMIOLOGY

Overall Prevalence

Psychiatric disorder appears to be more common in mentally retarded populations than in the general population. Overall prevalence rates range from 20% to 74% (Bregman and Harris 1996; Campbell and Malone 1991; Corbett 1979; Eaton and Menolascino 1982; Einfeld and Tonge 1996; Lund 1985; Szymanski 1994) depending on the diagnostic criteria employed; the type of disorder screened (whether behavior disorders are included, for example); the nature of the sample (community or institution); the type of data collected (case note studies or new data); and the level of mental retardation, ages, and gender of the populations studied (Jacobson 1990). Surveys of representative population samples indicate an overall prevalence of 30%–40% in adults (Corbett 1979; Gostason 1985; Lund 1985; Reiss 1990) and 40%–60% in children (Gillberg et al. 1986; Koller et al. 1983; Rutter et al. 1976). Overall prevalence declines with age, falling to around 20% in those age 65 and older (Corbett 1979; Day 1985; Kiernan and Moss 1990). Higher rates of psychiatric disorder have been reported in severely mentally retarded people compared with mildly retarded people in some studies (Gillberg et al. 1986; Gostason 1985; Koller et al. 1983), whereas others have found lower rates (Jacobson 1982a, 1982b).

Mental Illness

Major depressive disorder and bipolar disorders occur with the same frequency as in the general population. Despite methodological differences, all studies give remarkable consistent prevalence rates of between 1.2% and 1.9% (Day 1990). Psychotic disorders and particularly schizophrenia appear to be more common in people with mental retardation. Most studies give a point prevalence of 3%–3.5% (Turner 1989) for schizophrenia, the exception being Lund (1985), who found an overall prevalence of 1.3% but, interestingly, found rates of 2.6% and 3.3% in the mild and borderline mentally retarded patients in his sample. Specific factors such as organic brain damage and brain dysfunction, which occur more commonly in mental retardation, may explain this increased prevalence (Turner 1989; Tyrer and Dunstan 1997). Neurotic disorders (now separated as anxiety disorders, somatoform disorders, and dissociative disorders) were rarely reported in early prevalence studies (Ballinger and Reid 1977; Corbett 1979), suggested explanations being protection from external and internal stress, the greater likelihood of behavioral or psychotic responses to stress, and diagnostic overshadowing (Reiss and Szyszko 1983). Recent studies, however, have shown that these disorders are at least as common in the mildly mentally retarded as they are in the general population and are a common reason for their hospitalization (Day 1983, 1985; Gostason 1985; Lund 1985; Ollendick et al. 1993; Richardson et al. 1979). Dysthymic disorder is apparently more common among this population than in the general population. The prevalence has been estimated at 15%–33% of clinic samples (Benson 1985; Bregman and Harris 1996; Day 1990; Došen 1996). Depressive reactions to life events are particularly common (Day 1985), whereas panic disorders and obsessive-compulsive disorders are comparatively rare (Day 1985; Ghaziuddin 1988; Vitiello and Behar 1992; Vitiello et al. 1989).

The prevalence rate of around 12% for both mild and severe dementia in mentally retarded people ages 65 years and older is similar to that in the general population (Day and Jancar 1994). Both senile dementia and cerebral arteriosclerotic dementia occur (Harper 1993; Reid and Aungle 1974; Reid et al. 1978b; Tait 1983). The predisposition of people with Down's syndrome to develop Alzheimer's type dementia in middle age is well known (Day and Jancar 1994; Harper 1993; Holland 1994). Prevalence rates for clinical dementia range from 6% to 45%, although Alzheimer's type neuropathology is virtually universally present in the brains of Down's individuals after age 35 and increases in magnitude with age (Wisniewski et al. 1994). The lack of correlation between clinical symptoms and neuropathology is unexplained, but recent studies suggest that male sex (Raghavan et al. 1994) and the presence of apolipoprotein E type 2 allele (Royston et al. 1994) might be protective.

Personality Disorders

In Corbett's (1979) total population study of over 400 adults, 25% showed evidence of a personality disorder mainly of the impulsive, immature, and anxiety prone types, and these tended to be more common in patients with a history of epilepsy. Reid and Ballinger (1987), using a standardized assessment of personality, found significant personality disorders in 56% and disabling personality disorders in 22% of 100 moderately and mildly mentally retarded hospitalized adults. These disorders were mostly of the explosive and hysterical types, the former being more common in males and the latter more common in females. Zigler and Burack (1989) identified several personality characteristics in persons with mental retardation, such as overdependency, low ideal self-image, limited levels of aspiration, and an outer directed style of problem solving. A recent study by Goldberg et al. (1995) has provided further confirmation of the high prevalence of personality disorders in the mildly and moderately mentally retarded, postulating a link between certain traits and the onset of mental illness in later life. The relationship between personality disorder and mental illness and behavioral problems has yet to be established, but studies have shown that severe personality disorder is a significant factor leading to hospitalization (Ballinger et al. 1991) or preventing discharge from the hospital (Ballinger and Reid 1998; Deb and Hunter 1991). However, the relevance of the concept of personality disorder in the severely mentally retarded has been questioned by some investigators (Dana 1993; Došen 1993a, 1996; Gostason 1985).

Autism Spectrum Disorders

Current thinking conceptualizes the autism spectrum disorders (Kanner's syndrome, Rett's syndrome, Asperger's syndrome, and other subgroups as yet unidentified) as a clinical syndrome of brain dysfunction with many underlying etiologies (Andersson et al. 1990; Volkmar 1996). Mental retardation is present in 65%–85% of cases (Rutter 1983), it is more common in males (Wing 1981), and epilepsy is a frequent complication (Gillberg 1990). Prevalence rates are around 1 per 1,000 children for severe autism (Gillberg and Steffenburg 1989), and 2–3 per 1,000 for Asperger's syndrome (Gillberg and Gillberg 1989). Autism spectrum disorders persist into adult life (Lotter 1978; Rutter 1970). Up to one-half of severely mentally retarded people have a disorder in the autism continuum, and they account for a large proportion of those presenting behavior disorders (Wing 1989). It appears that onset of mental illness as a secondary disorder among these individuals is a relatively frequent feature (Došen and Petry 1994).

Behavior Disorders

Behavior disorders, including aggression, self-injury, destructiveness, restless and disruptive behavior, and maladaptive and antisocial behavior, occur commonly in persons with mental retardation, and prevalence rates of between 20% and 44% are consistently reported (Jacobson 1982a; Kiernan and Moss 1990; Lund 1986; Rojahn et al. 1993). They are particularly associated with severe mental retardation and other psychiatric symptoms (Jacobson 1982a; Nihira et al. 1988; Reiss and Rojahn 1994) and can be remarkably persistent (Reid et al. 1984), although different forms of behavior disorder exhibit different kinds of longitudinal stability with aggression being the most persistent (Leudar et al. 1984). The evidence from many studies indicates that behavior disorders are related to a range of psychological, neurobiological, neuropsychiatric, and sociocommunicative factors (Berg and Gosse 1990; Cole 1988; Fraser and Rao 1991; Holt 1994; Hucker et al. 1979; Hunt and Cohen 1988; Lund 1985; Reid 1972, 1985). In recent years the concept of the behavioral phenotypes associated with specific genetic or chromosomal abnormalities has been gaining ground undergirded by advances in molecular genetics (O'Brien and Yule 1995).

Many attempts have been made without success to distinguish between behavior disorders and psychiatric illness in the mentally retarded. The descriptive terminology currently in use does not help. For example, the same type of maladaptive behavior may reflect deficits in interpersonal skill development without underlying psychopathology in one patient but be a symptom of underlying mental illness in another. There is a need for a broader taxonomy covering both behavioral characteristics and etiology to facilitate more accurate diagnosis and treatment (MacLean 1990). Menolascino (1977) differentiated three types of behavior disorder in persons with mental retardation—primitive behavior, atypical behavior, and abnormal behavior—each specific to a particular level of mental retardation and a particular type of emotional disorder. This work has been taken forward by Reid et al. (1978a, 1984), who, using cluster analysis, identified eight behavioral syndromes and traced their natural history, and Leudar et al. (1984), who identified six behavioral dimensions and followed up their longitudinal stability. Gardner and Cole (1990) have proposed a biopsychosocial diagnostic approach that takes account of the multiple factors underlying and maintaining behavior disturbance in a particular individual. They point out that behavior disorders with a neuropsychiatric and organic basis can still acquire a functional component if they are being reinforced by the environment or are of value to the individual and stress the need for multidimensional treatment programs.

Etiology

Higher prevalence rates of psychiatric disorder in the mentally retarded are associated with a range of neurological, social, psychological, and personality risk factors including impaired cognition, organic brain damage, communication problems, physical disabilities, family psychopathology, and psychosocial factors (Fraser and Nolan 1994; Gualtieri 1988; Reid 1985; Szymanski 1980). Singly or in combination, these factors increase the vulnerability of mentally retarded people to psychiatric or behavior disorders. Specific chromosomal abnormalities may also predispose to psychiatric illness or behavior disorder (Crow 1988; Day 1993; Holland and Gosden 1990).

Achenbach and Zigler (1968) have pointed to the importance of social incompetence as a factor in interactional and intrapsychic problems, and this theoretical prospective has received support from studies in which discrepancies between self-image and the expectations of others have been shown to provide fertile ground for the onset of psychopathology (Reiss 1994; Reiss and Benson 1985; Reiss et al. 1982; Zigler and Spitz 1978). Menolascino (1970, 1977) emphasized the importance of neurophysiological and sociological developmental processes that may have a different timing and take a different direction in the mentally retarded individual, causing deviations from normal development, the so-called biodevelopmental theory (Matson and Frame 1986). Matson (1985) has proposed the so-called biosocial theory, which hypothesizes that due to specific biological factors (e.g., neurological, biochemical, genetic), together with specific social factors (family interactions, culture and other environmental variables) and specific psychological processes (cognitive development, personality variables), the psychopathology of mentally retarded people differs in numerous aspects from that of the nonretarded.

Others (Došen 1989, 1990a; Gaedt and Gärtner 1990; Gilson and Levitas 1987; Tanguay 1984) favor a developmental theoretical approach. Tanguay (1984) has suggested applying a developmental model based on Piaget's stages of cognitive development to achieve a better understanding of psychopathology in childhood. Gilson and Levitas (1987) stressed the importance of crisis periods during the process of personality development of mentally retarded people and related psychosocial problems. Došen (1989, 1990a) and Gaedt and Gärtner (1990) have applied psychodynamic theory to make a link between psychopathology and disturbances in psychosocial development.

Behavioral Phenotypes

There have been numerous reports of particular behavior profiles linked to specific mental retardation symptoms (Berg and Gosse 1990; O'Brien 1992; O'Brien and Yule 1995). Autism and hyperkinetic conditions have been described in association with fragile X syndrome (Turk 1994). Psychotic states, autism, and disruptive behavior have been reported in patients with tuberose sclerosis (Hunt and Dennis 1987; Parsons et al. 1984; Reid 1985). Depressive conditions including depression associated with anorexia nervosa and autistic features have been described in people with Down's syndrome (Lund 1988; Prasher and Hall 1996; Szymanski and Biederman 1984). Self-injurious behavior and aggression toward others dominate the picture in Lesch-Nyhan syndrome (Berg and Gosse 1990). A repertoire of behavior disturbances has been reported in Rett's syndrome (Berg and Gosse 1990), and hyperphagia and other behavior and psychiatric problems such as obsessive-compulsive disorder are prominent features of Prader-Willi syndrome (Clarke et al. 1996; Došen and Petry 1994; Greenswag 1987; Whitman and Accardo 1987). An association among sex chromosome abnormalities, mental retardation, and antisocial behavior problems has been reported but is far from proven (Day 1993). The precise nature of all of these associations is unexplained and the subject of continued research.

■ CLINICAL FEATURES AND PRESENTATION

Factors Affecting Presentation

The presentation of mental illness in people with mild and borderline mental retardation is similar to that in the general population, although it requires skill, experience, and patience to elicit symptoms in the face of communication problems and the general lack of subjective complaints. In moderately and severely retarded people the clinical picture becomes less and less typical, and it is generally agreed that with our present level of knowledge and clinical skills it is difficult to make a confident diagnosis of mental illness in the severely mentally retarded (Reid 1972).

Sovner (1986) has categorized the following three factors that influence the presentation of mental illness in people with mental retardation and that may create diagnostic difficulties.

Intellectual Distortion

Concrete thinking and limited communication skills impair a mentally retarded person's ability to conceptualize his or her feelings and to describe them to others. This leads to a general lack of subjective complaints, although the classic symptoms of mental illness can usually be obtained by means of a careful history and examination in mildly and moderately mentally retarded people. There is an associated failure to make links with major life events or other possible precipitating factors so that careful inquiry into these areas is required. Intellectual distortion increases as the intellectual level decreases.

Psychological Masking

The impoverished social skills and life experiences of mentally retarded people result in a lack of the usual richness of symptomatology found in the general population. Delusions may be so bland in content that they are easily missed and hallucinatory experiences so simple, unelaborated, unconnected, and fleeting that they can be mistaken for manipulative behavior. Mentally retarded patients rarely attempt to question or interpret what is happening to them, and secondary elaboration and systematization of delusions are unusual; the same delusion often reappears unchanged in successive illnesses.

Baseline Exaggeration

Emotional stress or mental illness in people with mental retardation may cause an increase in preexisting maladaptive behavior, which may be mistakenly regarded as a further deterioration in the latter rather than the onset of a mental illness. All mentally retarded people presenting with a newly arising behavioral problem or a sudden increase in behavioral problems should have a full psychiatric examination to exclude the possibility of an underlying mental illness before the assumption is made that the condition is primarily functional in origin.

Psychiatric Disorders in Childhood and Adolescence

Studies using standardized methods of assessment reveal similar rates of attention-deficit/hyperactivity disorders (ADHD), conduct disorders, and anxiety disorders among mentally retarded and nonretarded children. Self-injurious behavior (SIB), depressive conditions, and pervasive developmental disorders are, however, more common among children with mental retardation.

SIB is reported among 8%–14% of residents of institutions for the mentally retarded (Farber 1987; Oliver et al. 1987). This behavior occurs more often among persons with moderate and severe mental retardation (IQ < 50) and most frequently between the ages 10 and 30 years, with a peak between 15 and 20 years (Oliver et al. 1987; Rojahn 1986). The occurrence of SIB is related to genetic and organic disturbances and adverse environmental and developmental conditions. Also, particular psychiatric disorders such as depression may elicit SIB (Došen 1993b; Reiss 1994).

Recent investigations suggest that ADHD children with mental retardation show significant behavioral and emotional problems in their early adolescence, which may mean that there are some qualitative differences in the outcome of these children as compared with nonretarded children with ADHD (Aman et al. 1996). Other relatively frequent psychiatric disorders among children and adolescents with mental retardation, such as depression, separation anxiety, oppositional defiant disorder, reactive attachment disorder, conduct disorder, and disturbance of personality forming, have been related by some authors to disturbances of early emotional development (Došen 1993a, 1996, 1998; Gaedt 1995; Gaedt and Gärtner 1990). Some investigators have suggested that serious problems during attachment forming may occur among infants with mental retardation, hindering the process of normal personality development and increasing proneness to psychiatric disorders (Clegg and Lansdall-Welfare 1995; Gaedt 1995; Levitas and Gilson 1990; Rogers et al. 1993). In general it must be stressed that despite a growing body of evidence that particular types of mental retardation show particular problems of emotional development and thus are probably associated with specific psychiatric disorders, there are still few comprehensive studies of psychosocial development of children with mental handicap.

Psychoses and Major Mood Disorders

The psychoses are the best studied of all psychiatric disorders in the mentally retarded. Classical clinical features are present in both major mood disorders and schizophrenia (Hucker et al. 1979; Meadows et al. 1991; Reid 1972; Sovner and Hurley 1983). Symptoms tend to be florid but banal with, for example, a higher incidence of stupor and mutism in depression and acting out of delusions in schizophrenia. Visual hallucinations are common in both conditions. Affective psychoses tend to occur at an earlier age than in the general population, and bipolar disorders appear more common. Depressed mood and vegetative symptoms are prominent, but symptomatic complaints of depression are not invariable, mood disturbance is poorly sustained, and an elevation of mood is usually not expressed in mania (Day 1990; Došen and Gielen 1993; Hucker et al. 1979; Meins 1995; Reid 1972). In schizophrenia, delusions and hallucinations tend to reflect the limited personal experience, interest, and social horizons of the patient (Reid 1993). There is little attempt to interpret the strange phenomena experienced, and secondary elaboration rarely occurs. Catatonic features are common (Hucker et al. 1979; Reid 1972). Thought disorder is difficult to detect, but it is more obvious in written material and drawings than in conversation; computer-assisted language analysis can be of help (Fraser and Nolan 1994).

Atypical features such as regression to childlike dependency, incontinence, and loss of social skills in depression and hysterical symptoms like overbreathing, pseudo-fits, paralysis, gait disturbance, and Ganser states in schizophrenia are common and may mask classical symptomatology and cause diagnostic confusion (Hucker et al. 1979; Reid 1972). Mixed states with features of both mania and depression, schizoaffective psychoses, psychotic responses to acute stress, and rapid-cycling bipolar disorder all appear to be more common in mentally retarded people than in the nonretarded (Day 1990; Glue 1989; Reid 1972; Sovner and Pary 1993).

Dysthymic Disorder

Mild depression is a relatively common disorder among mildly and moderately retarded individuals (Day 1985) and may become chronic (Jancar and Gunaratne 1994). The symptomatology includes loss of energy and interest, negative self-image, feeling of helplessness, and significant behavior problems such as irritability, anger, destructibility, and aggressivity (Day 1990). Often the disorder is related to a specific stressor such as loss of an effective relationship, change of the surroundings, or hospitalization. Of particular importance, especially in the middle-aged and elderly, is the loss of the last caring relative and its catastrophic consequences (Day 1985, 1990). Social interactional problems, poor social skills, and difficulties of emotional development have been considered to be predisposing factors (Day 1990; Reiss 1994). Chronic states, possibly caused by chronic, overdemanding social deprivation or repeated abuse, may surface early in adolescence or even in childhood and may cause a dysthymic state lasting into adulthood. These states may be interrupted by episodes of a major depression, usually elicited by an acute stress (Došen 1990b).

Anxiety Disorders

The most commonly reported anxiety disorders are simple phobia, social phobia, and generalized anxiety disorder. Obsessive-compulsive disorder and panic disorders are little studied. It seems that adults with mental retardation have fears similar to those of children matched for mental age: fear of separation, fear of natural events, fear of injury, and fear of animals (Reiss 1994).

Probably the anxiety and fear are related to traumatic events and the accumulated failure experience of these persons (Ollendick et al. 1993). These disorders usually present with typical clinical features found in the general population.

Aggression

Aggressive behavior is a common problem among people with mental retardation. Gardner and Graeber (1993) developed a model that suggests that aggressive behavior in this population is determined by a number of factors, including operant conditioning, genetic disorders, personality traits, and psychopathology. Situational factors may also be important. Aggression is often a feature of the psychoses, conduct disorder, depression, and antisocial personality disorder and is often described in genetic disorders such as fragile X, Prader-Willi, and Klinefelter syndromes. Learned aggression through the imitation of aggressive models or as a function of communication is also found relatively often among people with mental retardation (Reiss 1994).

Dementia

The typical features of memory impairment, personality change, loss of social skills, and deterioration in habits are always present. Behavioral problems may be the most obvious manifestation, and nocturnal confusion, transient psychotic episodes, and late onset of epilepsy should always alert one to the possibility of a dementing illness in the aging mentally retarded person. Memory loss is generally difficult to identify in the early stages but becomes more obvious as the illness progresses (Day and Jancar 1994; Reid and Aungle 1974). Medical risk factors include a history of hypertension, ischemic episodes, neurological symptoms, organic brain damage, and a family history of dementia (Harper 1993). Dementia in individuals with Down's syndrome presents a similar picture and is usually associated with a generalized premature aging process (Day and Jancar 1994).

■ ASSESSMENT, CLASSIFICATION, AND DIAGNOSIS

An accurate diagnosis is essential before embarking on treatment. The difficulties attendant on this process have already been discussed. Accurate diagnosis requires a full and detailed history, careful examination and observation of the patient, and a knowledge of the natural history of the illness (see also Chapter 29 in this book). Support for the diagnosis may be provided by the use of rating scales or investigatory means, such as the dexamethasone suppression test in the case of depression. In complex cases, a period of inpatient observation may be required, and sometimes the diagnosis may only be finally established with certainty after a prolonged observation period or by the treatment response. There is a danger of overdiagnosis as well as underdiagnosis, and extreme caution should be exercised in the interpretation of symptoms in the more severely retarded in whom additional disorder and impairments can result in behavior that resembles psychosis.

History and Examination

The value and importance of the skilled clinical interview and examination cannot be overstressed. The standardized format for psychiatric history taking should be followed, albeit modified, to include additional information such as developmental history, associated physical disabilities such as epilepsy, current social functioning, social circumstances, and level of mental retardation and its etiology. The aim is to provide as complete a picture of the patient as possible to facilitate treatment and rehabilitation. As full a history of the current illness as is possible should be obtained from the patient together with corroborative histories from the patient's relatives and caregivers.

Assessment should never rely on a single informant. Inquiries should focus on behavioral changes such as sleep disturbance, loss of appetite, weight loss, lack of interest, deterioration of social skills, bizarre behavior, and any other deviations from usual behavior. Possible predisposing or precipitating factors should be fully explored. Information should also be sought on premorbid personality and functioning. Full details about any previous psychiatric illness experienced by the patient, including the medical notes relating to a hospital referral or admission, should be obtained. Any family history of mental illness should be thoroughly explored.

Mental examination should follow the standard approach modified as necessary to take account of the level of mental retardation. Leading questions should be avoided. The general paucity of subjective complaints means that much greater reliance has to be placed on objective data, and careful attention should be paid to patient's appearance and evidence of hallucinations such as the adoption of listening poses or talking to him- or herself. Direct observation should be made in as wide a range of settings as possible. Care is needed when one interprets unusual mannerisms and postures, particularly with the severely mentally retarded. A full physical examination should always be carried out to rule out other possible physical causes of the aberrations, such as toothache or earache.

Investigations

EEG studies will be necessary if organic brain damage or dementia is suspected or if it becomes necessary to unravel disturbed behavior from epilepsy. The dexamethasone suppression test and other biological markers may be helpful in establishing a diagnosis of psychotic depression (Pirodsky et al. 1985; Ruedrich et al. 1987, 1990). IQ assessment, personality tests, and measurement of adaptive behavior can provide useful background information for the treatment program and future care. Specific tests, for thought disorder in schizophrenia, for example, may be helpful in establishing the diagnosis but are so far not standardized for mentally retarded populations. For the future, noninvasive neuroimaging techniques promise to be potentially a most valuable diagnostic tool, particularly in nonverbal profoundly and severely retarded individuals. Structured interview schedules and rating scales are increasingly being used in an attempt to improve diagnostic accuracy. Instruments developed for use with nonretarded populations rely heavily on the ability of the patient to describe subjective feelings and are of limited value (Ballinger et al. 1975). Diagnostic rating scales for the mentally retarded should, as far as possible, reflect behavioral rather than subjective components. An early attempt at this was made by Day and colleagues (Hucker et al. 1979), who published diagnostic criteria for mania, depression, and schizophrenia for use with mentally retarded people. These criteria have been further refined by Sovner (1986) and Menolascino and Weiler (1990). A number of scales have been developed specifically for use with mentally retarded people. These include the Psychopathology Inventory for Mentally Retarded Adults (PIMRA) (Senatore et al. 1985), which includes self report and informant versions; the Reiss Screen for Maladaptive Behavior (Reiss 1988); the Diagnostic Assessment for the Severely Handicapped Scale (DASH) (Matson 1991); and, most recently, the Psychiatric Assessment of Adults With Developmental Disability (PAS-ADD), a semistructured interview (Moss et al. 1993, 1996), and the Developmental Behavior Checklist (Einfeld and Tonge 1995). The use and limitations of rating scales in diagnoses have been usefully discussed by Aman (1991). These scales have been developed primarily as research instruments; although they play an invaluable role in epidemiological studies and population screening and can be useful in the monitoring response to treatment, they are of limited value in clinical practice and rarely, if ever, solve a diagnostic problem.

■ CLASSIFICATION

Numerous attempts have been made to apply the traditional psychiatric diagnostic categories of the ICD-9/10 and DSM-III/IV to the psychopathology of persons with mental retardation (Ballinger et al. 1991; Corbett 1979; Day 1985; Menolascino 1990; Reid 1980). Their applicability to the mentally retarded has, however, been questioned (Hucker et al. 1979; Jacobson 1990; Levitas and Gilson 1990; Sturmey 1995; Szymanski 1988). Whereas the ICD and DSM criteria may be applied to people functioning in the mild to borderline mental retardation ranges without alteration or with little modification, they become increasingly unreliable as the severity of mental retardation increases. The limited communication skills of these persons make it very difficult to ascertain the presence of certain symptoms such as delusions and hallucinations. As the role of underlying organic brain damage increases, the phenomenology is increasingly characterized by a range of atypical symptoms (Reid 1982). The nonspecific nature of behavioral disturbances further confounds diagnostic endeavors. Szymanski (1994), among others, has pointed out that behavior disturbance is not a psychiatric condition but a symptom, and Reid (1982) has noted that behaviors that would be deemed abnormal in people functioning in the average intellectual range may be developmentally appropriate to the mental age of a severely mentally retarded person.

Other authors (Bregman and Harris 1996; Došen 1989, 1993a) suggest a developmental approach in the understanding and diagnosis of psychiatric and behavioral disorders among persons with mental retardation. On the one hand, there are findings that suggest a link between certain developmental syndromes and specific neuropsychiatric disorders. On the other hand, it is likely that as the developmental level lowers, the symptoms of a particular disorder may change. Furthermore, there are disorders that are more common among persons of low developmental levels, such those with autistic disorder or SIB.

Not surprisingly there have been calls for the development of a broader taxonomy that takes account of the atypical presentation of mental illness in people with mental retardation, thereby allowing for objective behavioral measurements and incorporating a more sophisticated approach to the measurement and classification of behavior disturbances (MacLean 1990; Sovner and Hurley 1990; Tuinier and Verhoeven 1993). Some movement in this direction has been made in the latest revisions of the traditional diagnostic classifications systems. Both DSM-III/IV and ICD-9/10 allow for the substitution of caregivers' observations in the absence of patients' subjective reports. The 10th revision of the ICD includes a special volume, titled "Describing Developmental Disability," which discusses the difficulties of diagnosis, particularly in the severely mentally retarded, and gives guidance on interviewing people with mental retardation and assessing and diagnosing specific illnesses as they occur in mentally retarded people.

■ CONCLUSIONS

Mentally retarded people are more prone to psychiatric disorder than the general population. Predisposing factors include organic brain damage, epilepsy, sensory deficits, communication problems, and a range of psychosocial factors. The full scale of mental disorders is encountered. Mentally retarded people appear to be at a higher risk for certain disorders, and some disorders, such as autism, are specifically associated with mental retardation. The phenomenology is influenced by the underlying mental retardation, and assessment and diagnosis require skill and experience because of the high frequency of atypical features that may dominate the clinical picture particularly in the severely mentally retarded. Traditional nosological classifications do not adequately accommodate the phenomenology of psychiatric and behavior disorder in mentally retarded people. The challenge for the future is to develop techniques to improve diagnostic accuracy and to establish a diagnostic and classification system that takes account of the special nature and presentation of psychiatric and behavior disorder in persons with mental retardation.

■ REFERENCES

Achenbach TM, Zigler EF: Cue-learning and problem-learning strategies in normal and retarded children. Child Dev 39:827–848, 1968

Aman MG: Review and evaluation of instruments for assessing emotional and behavioral disorders. Australia and New Zealand Journal of Developmental Disabilities 17:127–145, 1991

Aman MG, Pejean C, Osborne P, et al: Four-year follow-up of children with low intelligence and ADHD. Res Dev Disabil 17:417–432, 1996

Andersson L, Bohman M, Campbell M, et al: Autism: diagnosis and treatment: the state of the art, in Diagnosis and Treatment of Autism. Edited by Gillberg C. New York, Plenum, 1990, pp 50–68

Ballinger BR, Reid AH: Psychiatric disorders in an adult training centre and a hospital for the mentally handicapped. Psychol Med 7:525–528, 1977

Ballinger BR, Reid AH: Standardised assessment of personality disorder in mental handicap. Br J Psychiatry 152:577–585, 1988

Ballinger BR, Armstrong J, Presly AS, et al: Use of standardised psychiatric interview in mentally handicapped patients. Br J Psychiatry 127:540–544, 1975

Ballinger BR, Ballinger CB, Reid AH, et al: The psychiatric symptoms, diagnosis, and care needs of 100 mentally handicapped patients. Br J Psychiatry 158:251–254, 1991

Benson BA: Behavior disorder and metnal retardation: association with age, sex and level of functioning in an outpatient clinic sample. Applied Research in Mental Retardation 6:79–88, 1985

Berg JM, Gosse GC: Specific mental retardation disorders and behavior problems. International Review of Psychiatry 2:53–60, 1990

Berrios GE: Mental illness and mental retardation: history and concepts in mental health, in Mental Retardation. Edited by Bouras N. Cambridge, UK, Cambridge University Press, 1994, pp 5–18

Bregman JD, Harris JC: Mental retardation, in Comprehensive Textbook of Psychiatry, Vol VI. Edited by Kaplan HL, Sadock BJ. Baltimore, MD, Williams & Wilkins, 1996, pp 2207–2242

Campbell M, Malone RP: Mental retardation and psychiatric disorders. Hospital and Community Psychiatry 42:379, 1991

Clarke DJ, Boer H, Chung MC: Maladaptive behavior in Prader-Willi syndrome in adult life. J Intellect Disabil Res 40:159–165, 1996

Clegg JA, Lansdall-Welfare R: Attachment and learning disability, a theoretical review informing three clinical interventions. J Intellect Disabil Res 39:295–305, 1995

Cole JT: Psychiatry, neuroscience and the double disabilities, in Mental Retardation and Mental Health: Classification, Diagnoses, Treatment, Services. Edited by Stark JA, Menolascino FJ, Alberelli MH, et al. New York, Springer-Verlag, 1988, pp 81–89

Corbett JA: Psychiatric morbidity and mental retardation, in Psychiatric Illness and Mental Handicap. Edited by James FE, Snaith RP. London, Gaskell Press, 1979, pp 11–25

Crow TJ: Sex chromosomes and psychoses: a pseudoautosomal locus. Br J Psychiatry 153:675–683, 1988

Dana L: Personality disorders, in Mental Health Aspects of Mental Retardation. Edited by Fletcher R, Došen A. New York, Lexington Books, 1993, pp 130–140

Day K: A hospital based psychiatric unit for mentally handicapped adults. Mental Handicap 11:137–140, 1983

Day K: Psychiatric disorder in the middle aged and elderly mentally handicapped. Br J Psychiatry 147:660–667, 1985

Day K: Depression in mildly and moderately retarded adults, in Depression in Mentally Retarded Children and Adults. Edited by Došen A, Menolascino FL. Leiden, Netherlands, Logon Publications, 1990, pp 129–154

Day K: Crime and mental retardation: a review, in Clinical Approaches to the Mentally Disordered Offender. Edited by Howells K, Hollin CR. Chichester, UK, Wiley, 1993, pp 111–144

Day K, Jancar J: Mental and physical health and aging in mental handicapped: a review. J Intellect Disabil Res 38:241–256, 1994

Deb S, Hunter D: Psychopathology of people with mental handicap and epilepsy; III: personality disorder. Br J Psychiatry 159:830–834, 1991

Došen A: Diagnostics and treatment of mental illness in mentally retarded children: a developmental model. Child Psychiatry Hum Dev 20:73–84, 1989

Došen A: Psychische en Gedragsstoornissen bij Zwakzinnigen. Amsterdam, Netherlands, Boom, 1990a

Došen A: Depression in mentally retarded children, in Depression in Mentally Retarded Children and Adults. Edited by Došen A, Menolascino FJ. Leiden, Netherlands, Logon Publications, 1990b, pp 113–128

Došen A: A Developmental-Psychiatric Approach in the Diagnosis of Psychiatric Disorders of Persons With Mental Retardation. Venray, Netherlands, Nieuw Spraeland, 1993a

Došen A: Self-injurious behavior in persons with mental retardation: a developmental psychiatric approach, in Mental Health Aspects of Mental Retardation. Edited by Fletcher R, Došen A. New York, Lexington Books, 1993b, pp 141–168

Došen A: Persoonlijkheidsstoornissen en-trekken bij verstandelijke handicap, in Verstandelijke Handicap en Persoonlijkheidsstoornissen. Edited by van Osch G, den Besten L, Došen A, et al. Assen, Netherlands, van Gorcum, 1996, pp 29–41

Došen A, Gielen J: Depression in persons with mental retardation: assessment and diagnosis, in Mental Health Aspects of Mental Retardation. Edited by Fletcher R, Došen A. New York, Lexington Books, 1993, pp 70–77

Došen A, Petry D: Psychiatric and emotional adjustment of individuals with mental retardation. Current Opinion in Psychiatry 7:387–391, 1994

Eaton LF, Menolascino FJ: Psychiatric disorders in the mentally retarded: types, problems, and challenges. Am J Psychiatry 139:1297–1303, 1982

Einfeld SL, Tonge BJ: The developmental behavior checklist. J Autism Dev Disord 25:1–4, 1995

Einfeld SL, Tonge BJ: Population prevalence of psychopathology in children and adolescents with intellectual disability; II: epidemiological findings. J Intellect Disabil Res 40:99–109, 1996

Farber JM: Psychopharmacology of self injurious behavior in the mentally retarded. J Am Acad Child Adolescent Psychiatry 26:296–302, 1987

Fraser WI, Nolan M: Psychiatric disorders in mental retardation, in Mental Health in Mental Retardation. Edited by Bouras N. Cambridge, UK, Cambridge University Press 1994, pp 79–92

Fraser WI, Rao JM: Recent studies of mentally handicapped young people's behavior. J Child Psychol Psychiatry 23:79–108, 1991

Gaedt C: Psychotherapeutic approaches in the treatment of mental illness and behavioral disorders in mentally retarded people: the significance of a psychoanalytic perspective. J Intellect Disabil Res 39:233–239, 1995

Gaedt C, Gärtner D: Depressive grundprozesse-reinzeniering der selbstentwertung. Neuerkerode, Germany, Neuerkeroder Forum 4, 1990

Gardner WJ, Cole CL: Aggression and related difficulties, in Handbook of Behavior Modification With the Mentally Retarded. Edited by Matson JL. New York, Plenum, 1990, pp 225–251

Gardner WI, Graeber JL: Treatment of severe behavioral disorders in persons with mental retardation, in Mental Health Aspects of Mental Retardation. Edited by Fletcher R, Došen A. New York, Lexington Books, 1993, pp 45–69

Ghaziuddin M: Behavioral disorder in mentally handicapped: the role of life events. Br J Psychiatry 152:683–686, 1988

Gillberg C: What is autism? International Review of Psychiatry 2:61–66, 1990

Gillberg JC, Gillberg C: Asperger syndrome: some epidemiological considerations. J Child Psychol Psychiatry 30:631–638, 1989

Gillberg C, Steffenburg S: Outcome and prognostic factors in infantile autism and similar conditions. Journal of Autism and Developmental Disorders 17:273–287, 1989

Gillberg C, Persson E, Grufman E, et al: Psychiatric disorders in mildly and severely retarded urban children and adolescents: epidemiological aspects. Br J Psychiatry 149:68–74, 1986

Gilson SF, Levitas AS: Psychosocial crisis in the lives of mentally retarded people. Psychiatric Aspects of Mental Retardation Reviews 6:27–32, 1987

Glue P: Rapid cycling affective disorders in the mentally retarded. Biol Psychiatry 26:250–256, 1989

Goldberg B, Gitta MZ, Puddephatt A: Personality and trait disturbances in adult mental retardation population: significance for psychiatric management. J Intellect Disabil Res 39:284–294, 1995

Gostason R: Psychiatric illness among the mentally retarded: a Swedish population study. Acta Psychiatrica Scandinavica Suppl 318:1–117, 1985

Greenswag LR: Adults with Prader-Willi syndrome: a survey of 232 cases. Dev Med Child Neurol 29:145–152, 1987

Gualtieri CT: Mental health of persons with mental retardation, a solution obstacles to the solution and a resolution for the problem, in Mental Retardation and Mental Health. Edited by Stark JA, Menolascino FJ, Albarelli MH, et al. New York, Springer-Verlag, 1988, pp 173–188

Harper DC: A primer on dementia in persons with mental retardation: conclusions and current findings, in Mental Health Aspects of Mental Retardation. Edited by Fletcher R, Došen A. New York, Lexington Books, 1993, pp 169–198

Holland A: Down's syndrome and Alzheimer's disease, in Mental Health in Mental Retardation. Edited by Bouras N. Cambridge, UK, Cambridge University Press, 1994, pp 154–167

Holland AJ, Gosden C: A balanced chromosomal transfication partially co-segregating with psychotic illness in a family. Psychiatric Res 32:1–8, 1990

Holt G: Challenging behavior, in Mental Health in Mental Retardation. Edited by Bouras N. Cambridge, UK, Cambridge University Press, 1994, pp 126–132

Hucker SJ, Day KA, George S, et al: Psychoses in mentally handicapped adults, in Psychiatric Illness and Mental Handicap. Edited by James FE, Snaith RP. London, Gaskell Press, 1979, pp 27–35

Hunt RD, Cohen DJ: Attentional and neurochemical components of mental retardation: new methods and old problems, in Mental Retardation and Mental Health. Edited by Stark JA, Menolascino FJ, Albarelli MH, et al. New York, Springer-Verlag, 1988, pp 90–97

Hunt A, Dennis J: Psychiatric disorder among children with turberous sclerosis. Dev Med Child Neurol 29:190–198, 1987

Jacobson JW: Problem behavior and psychiatric impairment in a developmentally disabled population. Applied Research in Mental Retardation 3:121–139, 1982a

Jacobson JW: Problem behavior and psychiatric impairment in a developmentally disabled population; II: behavior severity. Applied Research in Mental Retardation 3:369–381, 1982b

Jacobson JW: Assessing the prevalence of psychiatric disorders in a developmentally disabled population, in Assessment of Behavioral Problems in Persons with Mental Retardation Living in the Community (DHHS Publ No ADM-90-1642). Rockville, MD, National Institute of Mental Health, 1990, pp 19–70

Jancar J, Gunaratne IJ: Dysthymia and mental handicap. Br J Psychiatry 164:691–693, 1994

Kiernan C, Moss SC: Behavioral and other characteristics of the population of a mentally handicapped hospital. Mental Handicap Research 3:3–20, 1990

Koller H, Richardson S, Catz M, et al: Behavior disturbance since childhood among a five year birth cohort of all mentally retarded young adults inner city. American Journal of Mental Deficiency 97:386–395, 1983

Leudar I, Fraser WI, Jeeves MA: Behavior disturbance in mental handicap: typology and longitudinal trends. Psychol Med 14: 923–935, 1984

Levitas A, Gilson S: Towards the Developmental Understanding of the Impact of Mental Retardation on Assessment and Psychopathology in Assessment of Behavioral Problems in Persons With Mental Retardation Living in the Community (DHHS Publ No ADM-90-1642). Rockville, MD, National Institute of Mental Health 1990, pp 71–106

Lotter V: Follow-up studies, in Autism: A Reappraisal of Concepts and Treatment. Edited by Rutter M, Schopler B. New York, Plenum, 1978, pp 475–496

Lund J: The prevalence of psychiatric morbidity in mentally retarded adults. Acta Psychiatrica Scandinavica 72:563–570, 1985

Lund J: Behavioral symptoms and autistic psychosis in the mentally retarded adult. Acta Psychiatrica Scandinavica 73:420–428, 1986

Lund J: Psychiatric aspects of Down's syndrome. Acta Psychiatrica Scandinavica 78:369–374, 1988

MacLean WE: Issues in the assessment of aberrant behavior among persons with mental retardation, in Assessment of Behavioral Problems in Persons With Mental Retardation Living in the Community (DHHS Publ No ADM-90-1642). Rockville, MD, National Institute of Mental Health, 1990, pp 135–146

Matson JL: Bio-social theory of psychopathology: a three by three factor model. Applied Research in Mental Retardation 6:199–227, 1985

Matson JL, Frame C: Psychopathology Among Mentally Retarded Children and Adolescents. Beverly Hills, CA, Sage, 1986

Matson JL, Gardner WI, Coe DA, et al: A scale for evaluating emotional disorders in severely and profoundly mentally retarded persons. Br J Psychiatry 159:404–409, 1991

Meadows G, Turner L, Campbell SW, et al: Assessing schizophrenia in adults with mental retardation: a comparative study. Br J Psychiatry 158:103–105, 1991

Meins W: Symptoms of major depression in mentally retarded adults. J Intellect Disabil Res 39:41–45, 1995

Menolascino FJ: Challenges in Mental Retardation: Progressive Ideologies and Services. New York, Human Sciences Press, 1977

Menolascino FJ: Mental retardation and the risk, nature and types of mental illness, in Depression in Mentally Retarded Children and Adults. Edited by Došen A, Menolascino FJ. Leiden, Netherlands, Logon Publications, 1990, pp 11–34

Menolascino FJ, Weiler MA: The challenge of depression and suicide in severely mentally retarded adults, in Depression in Mentally Retarded Children and Adults. Edited by Došen A, Menolascino FJ. Leiden, Netherlands, Logon Publications, 1990, pp 155–174

Moss S, Patel P, Prosser H, et al: Psychiatric morbidity in older people with moderate to severe learning disability; 1: development and reliability of the patient interview (PAS-ADD). Br J Psychiatry 163:471–480, 1993

Moss S, Prosser H, Goldberg D: Validity of the schizophrenia diagnosis of the psychiatric assessment schedule for adults with developmental diability (PAS-ADD). Br J Psychiatry 168:359–367, 1996

Nihira K, Price-Williams DR, Wyatt JF: Social competence and maladapted behavior of people with dual diagnoses. Journal of Multi-Handicapped Person 1:185–199, 1988

O'Brien G: Behavioral phenotypes and their measurement. Dev Med Child Neurol 34:379–381, 1992

O'Brien G, Yule W: Behavioral Phenotypes. London, Myceith Press, 1995

Oliver C, Murphy GH, Corbett JA: People with mental handicap: a total population study. Joural of Mental Deficiency Research 31:146–162, 1987

Ollendick T, Oswald D, Ollendick D: Anxiety disorders in mentally retarded persons, in Psychopathology in the Mentally Retarded. Edited by Matson JL, Barret RP. Boston, MA, Allyn & Bacon, 1993, pp 41–86

Parsons JA, May JG, Menolascino FJ: The nature and incidence of mental illness in mentally retarded individuals, in Handbook of Mental Illness in the Mentally Retarded. Edited by Menolascino FJ, Stark JA. New York, Plenum, 1984, pp 3–44

Pirodsky DM, Gibbs JW, Hesse RA, et al: Use of the dexamethasone suppression test to detect depressive disorders of mentally retarded individuals. American Journal of Mental Deficiency 90:245–252, 1985

Prasher VP, Hall W: Short-term prognosis of depression in adults with Down's syndrome: association with thyroid status and effects on adaptive behavior. J Intellect Disabil Res 40:32–38, 1996

Raghavan R, Khin-nu C, Brown AG, et al: Gender differences in the phenotypic expression of Alzheimer's disease in Down's syndrome (trisomy 21). Clinical Neuroscience and Neuropathology: Neuro Report 5:1393–1396, 1994

Reid AH: Psychoses in adult mental defectives. Br J Psychiatry 120:205–218, 1972

Reid AH: Diagnosis of psychiatric disorder in the severely and profoundly retarded patient. J R Soc Med 73:607–609, 1980

Reid AH: The Psychiatry of Mental Handicap. Oxford, UK, Blackwell Scientific Publications, 1982

Reid AH: Psychiatry and mental handicap, in Mental Handicap: A Multi-Disciplinary Approach. Edited by Craft M, Bicknell J, Hollins S. London, Balliere Tindall, 1985, pp 317–332

Reid AH: Psychiatry and mental handicap: a historical perspective. Journal of Mental Deficiency Research 33; 363–368, 1989

Reid A: Schizophrenic and paranoid syndromes in persons with mental retardation, in Mental Health Aspects of Mental Retardation. Edited by Fletcher R, Došen A. New York, Lexington Books, 1993, pp 98–110

Reid AH, Aungle BG: Dementia in aging mental defectives: a clinical psychiatric study. Journal of Mental Deficiency Research 18:15–23, 1974

Reid AH, Ballinger BR: Personality disorder in mental handicap. Psychol Med 17:983–987, 1987

Reid AH, Ballinger BR: Behavioral symptoms among severely and profoundly mentally retarded patients: a 16 to 18 year follow up study. Br J Psychiatry 167:452–455, 1995

Reid AH, Ballinger BR, Heather BB: Behavioral systems identified by cluster analysis in a sample of 100 severely and profoundly retarded adults. Psychol Med 8:399–412, 1978a

Reid AH, Maloney AF, Aungle B: Dementia in aging mental defectives: a clinical and neuropathological study. Journal of Mental Deficiency Research 22:233–241, 1978b

Reid AH, Ballinger BR, Heather B, et al: The natural history of behavioral symptoms amongst severely and profoundly mentally retarded patients. Br J Psychiatry 145:289–291, 1984

Reiss S: Test Manual for the Reiss Screen for Maladapted Behavior. Worthington, OH, IDS Publications, 1988

Reiss S: The prevalence of dual diagnosis in community based day programmes in the Chicago metropolitan area. Am J Ment Retard 94:578–585, 1990

Reiss S: Handbook of challenging behavior: mental health aspects of mental retardation. Worthington, OH, IDS Publications, 1994

Reiss S, Benson BA: Psychosocial correlates of depression in mentally retarded adults: minimal social support and stigmatisation. American Journal of Mental Deficiency 89:331–337, 1985

Reiss S, Rojahn J: Joint occurrence of depression and aggression in children and adults with mental retardation. J Intellect Disabil Res 37:287–294, 1994

Reiss S, Szyszko J: Diagnostic overshadowing and professional experience with mentally retarded persons. American Journal of Mental Deficiency 87:396–402, 1983

Reiss S, Levitan GW, McNallly RJ: Emotionally disturbed mentally retarded people: an undeserved population. Am Psychol 37:361–367, 1982

Richardson SA, Katz M, Koller H, et al: Some characteristics of a population of mentally retarded young adults in a British city: a basis for estimating some service needs. Journal of Mental Deficiency Research 23:275–286, 1979

Rogers S, Ozonoff S, Maslin-Cole C: Developmental aspects of attachment behavior in young children with pervasive developmental disorders. J Am Acad Adolesc Psychiatry 32:1274–1282, 1993

Rojahn J: Self-injurious and steroptype behavior of noninstitutionalised mentally retarded people: prevalance and classification. American Journal of Mental Deficiency 91(3):268–276, 1986

Rojahn J, Borthwick-Duffy SA, Jacobsen JW: The association between psychiatric diagnoses and severe behavior problems in mental retardation. Ann Clin Psychiatry
5:163–170, 1993

Royston MC, Mann D, Pickering-Brown S, et al: Apolipoprotein E e 2 allele promotes
longevity and protects patients with Down's syndrome from dementia. Clinical
Neuroscience and Neuropathology: Neuroreport 5:2583–2585, 1994

Ruedrich SL: Biochemical findings in depressed mentally retarded individuals, in Depression in Mentally Retarded Children and Adults. Edited by Došen A, Menolascino FJ. Leiden, Netherlands, Logon Publications, 1990, pp 219–233

Ruedrich SL, Wadle CV, Sallach HS, et al: Adrenocortical function and depressive illness in mentally retarded patients. Am J Psychiatry 144:597–602, 1987

Rutter M: Autistic children: infancy to adulthood. Seminars in Psychiatry 2:435–450,
1970

Rutter M: Cognitive deficits in the pathogenesis of autism. J Child Psychol Psychiatry
24:513–531, 1983

Rutter M, Tizard J, Yule W, et al: Isle of Wight Studies: 1964–1974. Psychol Med 7:
13–332, 1976

Senatore V, Matson JL, Kazdin AE: An inventory to assess psychopathology of mentally retarded adults. American Journal of Mental Deficiency 89:459–466, 1985

Sovner R: Limiting factors in the use of DSM III criteria with mentally ill/mentally retarded persons. Psychopharmacol Bull 22:1055–1058, 1986

Sovner R, DeNoyes Hurley A: Do the mentally retarded suffer from affective illness?
Arch Gen Psychiatry 40:61–67, 1983

Sovner R, Hurley A: Assessment tools which facilitate psychiatric evaluation of treatment. The Habilitative Mental Health Care Newsletter 9:11, 1990

Sovner R, Pary R: Affective disorders in developmentally disabled persons, in Psychopathology in the Mentally Retarded, 2nd Edition. Edited by Matson J, Barrett R.
Boston, MA, Longwood Professional Book, 1993, pp 87–148

Sturmey P: DSM-III-R and persons with dual diagnosis: conceptual issues and strategies for future research. J Intellect Disabil Res 39:357–364, 1995

Szymanski LS: Psychiatric diagnoses of mentally retarded persons, in Emotional Disorders of Mentally Retarded Persons. Edited by Szymanski LS, Tanguay PE. Baltimore, MD, University Park Press, 1980, pp 19–35

Szymanski LS: Integrative approach to diagnosis of mental disorders in retarded persons, in Mental Retardation and Mental Health. Edited by Stark J, Menolascino
FJ, Albarelli N, et al. New York, Springer, 1988, pp 124–139

Szymanski L: Mental retardation and mental health: concepts, aetiology and incidence,
in Mental Health in Mental Retardation. Edited by Bouras N. Cambridge, UK,
Cambridge University Press, 1994, pp 19–33

Szymanski LS, Biederman J: Depression and anorexia nervosa of persons with Down's
syndrome. American Journal of Mental Deficiency 89:246–251, 1984

Tait D: Mortality and dementia among aging defectives. Journal of Mental Deficiency Research 27:133–142, 1983

Tanguay PE: Towards a new classification of serious psychopathology in children. J Am Acad Child Psychiatry 32:373–384, 1984

Tredgold AF: Mental Deficiency (Amentia). London, Balliere Tindall, 1908

Tuinier S, Verhoeven WMA: Psychiatry and mental retardation: towards a pharmacological concept. J Intellect Disabil Res 37 (suppl 1):16–25, 1993

Turk J, Hagerman RJ, Barnicoat A, et al: The Fragile X syndrome, in Mental Health in Mental Retardation. Edited by Bouras N. Cambridge, UK, Cambridge University Press, 1994, pp 135–153

Turner TH: Schizophrenia and mental handicap: a historical review with implications for further research. Psychol Med 19:301–314, 1989

Tyrer SP, Dunstan JA: Schizophrenia, in Psychiatry in Learning Disability. Edited by Read SG. London, WB Saunders, 1997, pp 185–215

Vitiello B, Behar D: Mental retardation and psychiatric illness. Hospital and Community Psychiatry 43:494–499, 1992

Vitiello B, Spreat S, Behar D: Obsessive compulsive disorder in mentally retarded patients. J Nerv Ment Dis 17:232–236, 1989

Volkmar FR: Autism and the pervasive developmental disorders, in Child and Adolescent Psychiatry. Edited by Lewis M. Baltimore, MD, Williams & Wilkins, 1996, pp 489–497

Whitman BY, Accardo P: Emotional symptoms in Prader-Willi syndrome adolescents. Am J Med Genet 28:897–905, 1987

Wing K: Hospital Closure and the Effects on the Residents. Aldershot, UK, Avebury, 1989

Wing L: Sex ratios in early childhood autism and related conditions. Psychiatry Res 5:129–137, 1981

Wisniewski HM, Silverman W, Wegiel J: Aging, Alzheimer disease and mental retardation. J Intellect Disabil Res 38: 233–239, 1994

Zigler E, Burack JA: Personality development and the dually diagnosed person. Res Dev Disabil 10:225–240, 1989

Zigler EF, Spitz V: Changing trends in socialisation theory and research. American Behavioral Scientists 21:731–756, 1978

Treatment Methods

2 Psychotherapeutic Methods

Sheila Hollins, M.B., B.S., F.R.C.Psych.

Psychotherapy can be an effective psychological method of treating disorders of emotion, behavior, or mental health in children and adults with mental retardation. It includes a variety of highly specific therapeutic methods, each with its own theoretical and clinical basis, and its own extended training, and it is not synonymous with counseling. Although the traditional vehicle for communication between therapist and patient is language, other media may need to be used when working with people with mental retardation, for example, art, music, or drama. This approach can lead to new ways of working for traditional psychoanalytic psychotherapists and group analysts who may derive useful ideas from play, art, or music therapy. In the scientific literature, a number of articles discuss the pros and cons of a psychotherapeutic approach with people with mental retardation (e.g., Coffman and Harris 1980; Hollins and Sinason 2000; Matson 1984; Stavrakaki and Klein 1986; Woody and Billy 1966) and the use of play, music, or drama therapy or techniques such as role play (Weinstock 1979). The authors of published case reports are modest in their claims, although enthusiastic and optimistic about the value of their work. In this chapter, I explore some of these psychotherapeutic methods, including an introduction to individual psychoanalytic psychotherapy and to group and family therapy. More detailed accounts are available in the book *Psychotherapy and Mental Handicap*, by Waitman and Conboy-Hill (1992), in which music, art, and drama therapy are also discussed.

■ MENTAL RETARDATION: A CONCEPTUAL FRAMEWORK FOR PSYCHOTHERAPEUTIC APPROACHES

A person does not exist in a vacuum but as part of a social group, and his or her interactions with other members of the group will affect his or her development. The overused phrase, "A handicapped child is a handicapped family," may have originally referred to the practical and social consequences of having a child with a disability. For example, in the United Kingdom the burden of caring fell largely on the parents with little help from statutory or voluntary agencies. The 1971 Education Act and the enlightened white paper, "Better Services for the Mentally Handicapped," recognized the need for education for all and the development of community support. The ideology of normalization began to influence policy makers and service planners during the 1970s and 1980s, culminating in the speech by Dorell (1991), Parliamentary Undersecretary of State for Health, in June 1991 acclaiming that people with learning disabilities (the official U.K. term for mental retardation) ". . . are citizens; they are full members of our society"; ". . . are people whose own views and wishes—as well as their relationships and friendships—must be taken seriously and respected"; and ". . . should have their health and social care needs assessed on an individual basis." Now, 30 years after "better services for the mentally handicapped," the department of health in London is launching a new strategy for services for this patient group with a strong focus on social inclusion.

The emergence of the individual with mental retardation as someone whose own wishes should be taken into account challenges service providers to facilitate access to the full range of health provision, including mental health services. A reinterpretation in this first decade of the twenty-first century of the degree of burden experienced by the family might extend the disabling effect of mental retardation to the wider network or social milieu of the individual. McCormack (1991) takes a more individually oriented view and suggests it is the discourse that is impaired, with one person having difficulty making him- or herself understood and the other person having difficulty understanding. Leudar (1989) and others have looked at the communicative competence of people with mental retardation and the implications of this. Pragmatic communicative competence is more useful than formal linguistic competence, and opportunities for communication are normally more frequent in community than institutional settings.

■ INDICATIONS AND CONTRAINDICATIONS FOR REFERRAL

The presence of either psychosis, severe personality disorder, or pervasive developmental disorder is usually considered a contraindication for psychodynamic psychotherapy, depending on the therapeutic aims and experience of the therapist. The problems presented by the prospective patient are most likely to reflect developmental, personality, or relationship difficulties, or represent an adjustment reaction to a life event. Presenting problems may be framed in behavioral terms (e.g., wandering, attention-seeking behavior) or may be attributed to an event, such as a loss or other significant change. The presence of spoken language is not a prerequisite, and there is no clear cutoff point for intellectual level.

Realistic requests for therapy may arise from a wish for the individual to come to terms with the internal and external experiences of his or her disability. To understand it further demands that the therapist know which features are often seen in the psychological adjustments of disabled people and their families. Bicknell (1983) described the reaction of parents to the news of disability in their child as akin to bereavement. The stages of grief described include shock, panic, denial, anger experienced as guilt or blame, depression, and finally acceptance and adjustment. Disabled people, regardless of the nature of their disability, are usually themselves only too conscious of their own difference from the other members of their family or social group, with each person having feelings and attitudes about his or her own limitations and the effect of these on the family (Selwa 1971).

The primary impairment may indeed be a biological insult of some kind to the developing brain leading to cognitive or intellectual disability. An emotional disability appears to be quite separate and to present as a secondary impairment that may obscure painful memories of personal history (Sinason 1986). An important focus for psychotherapeutic work is to enable patients to recognize the contribution of their past experiences to their current relationships.

The Therapeutic Alliance and Confidentiality

There is a technical problem that must be considered before working with people who have a level of mental retardation that requires special services to lead an ordinary life: the therapist's relationship with the caregivers (whether they are natural parents or professional caregivers). When we think of the traditional psychoanalytic model of therapist and patient or patients, we think particularly of intimate relationships that are bound by the confidentiality of the treatment setting. Psychotherapeutic treatments are usually offered in outpatient clinic or office settings, or in an interview (or group) room in an inpatient setting. But to offer treatment to people living in long-stay hospital wards or group homes provokes considerable curiosity. It is rare in such a setting that anything is totally private, and explanations about the reasons for the desired privacy may be misunderstood. If therapy is such an important part of the treatment program, why are the caregivers being excluded from it? The more the maintenance of privacy is insisted on, the more suspicious and uncooperative the caregivers may become. In addition, the therapists may be party to information about the client between sessions with pressure exerted on them to take day-to-day issues up in the therapy. In some instances therapists will need to play a more active role to ensure the safety of their patient (for example, suspected sexual abuse) or to enable access to treatment in a convenient venue. One practical way to address these possible threats to confidentiality is to share any outside communication with the patient in the therapy session and to agree to the form of any reply.

Similar problems can be expected in work with adults who still live with their family of origin. For the parents of an adult "child" who functions in many ways like a 4- or 5-year-old, there is little they do not already know about him, and they will expect to know the details of anything new that happens. The child psychiatry model of someone working with a mentally retarded person and someone else working with the parents, with an occasional meeting together, may be appropriate for patients in group or individual therapy. The confidentiality of both therapeutic alliances must be respected and the effect of the involvement of the caregivers on the therapeutic process borne in mind.

■ ASSESSMENT

In assessing an individual for a psychotherapeutic treatment, the therapist must judge the willingness and ability of the patient to engage in a therapeutic relationship (see also Chapter 7 of this book).

Insight-oriented therapists will look for an emotional response, such as tearfulness or a further revelation, following an interpretation or confrontation made in an assessment interview. Art and music therapists will look for a response in their medium. The patient him- or herself may recognize the relevance of this initial encounter and ask to meet the therapist again. It is unrealistic to expect the patient to understand any theoretical explanation of what therapy is about. The patient's willingness to engage will depend on the relevance of the therapists' interventions during the first two or three meetings. It follows that the therapist should start the way he or she means to go on.

■ INDIVIDUAL PSYCHOANALYTIC PSYCHOTHERAPY

The main requirement of candidates for psychotherapy is that they be capable of making an emotional relationship (see also Chapters 7, 22, and 23 of this book). One misconception about people with mental retardation is that their limited intellect will preclude them from a treatment mode that seeks to increase effective understanding. But all that is required to engage in therapy is emotional contact between patient and therapist, and the belief that the patient has even a limited ability to make object relationships. In psychodynamic work, therapeutic use is made of the transference and countertransference feelings in the relationship between therapist and patient. Transference interpretations can be made in a straightforward way.

The main tool of the therapist is his or her own reaction to the patient (countertransference) with which he or she can choose to confront the patient or simply to inform his or her own therapeutic response. The patient's expression of emotion is encouraged rather than forbidden. Such a professional relationship is a long way from the ordinary businesslike and scientific doctor-patient encounter (see also Chapter 7). The patient and his family are to be valued and respected, with the successful end point of therapy being the resolution of disordered relationships or the initiation of healthy ones. This may require the therapist to enter and share in the patient's or family's dysfunction. Skynner (1976) is not alone in recognizing that therapists who feel uncomfortable and threatened by what the situation arouses in their own psychology tend to do more harm than good through their need to protect themselves by defining the problem fully and by keeping it in view and safely outside themselves.

It is appropriate for the therapists to be able to share the reality of the disability to be able to feel the hopelessness and the sense of disappointment and even panic that the disabled individual, with some insight, may have about him- or herself. However, the level of psychotherapy offered will take into account the assessed need of the individual for either supportive psychotherapy, which aims to restore the status quo without disturbing fragile psychological defenses (Cawley 1977), or the possibility of working at deeper levels, clarifying problems within a deepening relationship (Bird and Harrison 1984).

Training

Psychoanalytic psychotherapy is best learned by attending clinical seminars and treating patients under intensive supervision. Most therapists do not begin with patients who have mental retardation but train as psychotherapists first and then later learn to apply their well-practiced skills with this patient group. Other therapists have professional skills as social workers, nurses, psychologists, or psychiatrists and are familiar with people with mental retardation before becoming interested in psychotherapeutic approaches. There is a danger that such prospective therapists will neglect their own training and will fail to obtain adequate supervision. Supervision from a fully trained psychoanalytic psychotherapist is important even if the supervisor has little experience in mental retardation. In the United Kingdom, seminars and supervision are available from therapists experienced in both mental retardation and psychoanalytic psychotherapy. Membership criteria for the newly formed Institute of Psychotherapy and Disability stipulates a number of supervised cases (disabled patients), even for experienced therapists, and evidence that people with mental retardation are treated with respect (Sinason 2000). The trainee therapist is taught to write detailed notes after each session, paying attention to the behavior and mood of the patient, the content, and the trainee's own change of feelings during the session.

The Content and Process of Sessions

The boundaries of the therapeutic session are rigidly adhered to. This enables attempts to manipulate the boundaries to be addressed in patients who always want more than the therapist is able to offer. Regular holiday breaks are taken to explore feelings of dependence and anxieties about the eventual termination of therapy. The experience of a trusting relationship with someone who will not always be available can be an invaluable way of facing up to loss. There may be clear objectives at the start of therapy, such as relief of symptoms or an increase in self-esteem, but the actual outcome of therapy is often difficult to evaluate (Beail 1998; Symington 1981).

A failure to face the attacks of the past may lead to a fear to face the challenges of the present. Vanier (1985) writes about the "wounded heart" or the common experience of being a disappointment to parents because of the inevitable difference from parents' idealized expectations.

The three secrets of death or loss, impairment and dependence, and sexuality (Hollins and Grimer 1988) are the secrets of each person's life, but the denial of them, in a forgotten or expurgated version of an individual life story, brings confusion and mistrust to adult life. Such denial is often compounded by the failure of communication between a succession of caregivers, who may leave the disabled person as the lone historian of his or her own experiences and relationships. These secrets are commonly brought to sessions by the patient in one way or another.

■ FAMILY THERAPY

There are two elements that are central to the practice of family therapy: first, the family must take responsibility for itself, and second, change must arise from within the family (Skynner 1976). The approach used may derive from a number of theoretical models, including structural, strategic, and systemic approaches. Within treatment, therapists may employ a variety of techniques such as the use of the genogram (or family tree), sculpting, or paradox (Bloch 1973; Minuchin and Fishman 1981).

Boundaries and Rules

Somewhat in contrast to the nondirective approach used in individual psychoanalytic psychotherapy, family therapists seek to change rules so that new ways

of behaving emerge within the dysfunctional system presented by the family. Such family rules that have become habitual and rigid, and that lead families to "dance the safe dance" all the time, require the therapist to problem-solve at a number of different levels. The members of the family must relearn how to relate to each other and to transfer their learning to new situations (Gorell-Barnes 1982). Even when the identified patient is admitted to an inpatient setting, a family approach is still possible, with treatment being conducted either by the inpatient multidisciplinary team or by the referring community team, as in the following example:

> G had been known to a multidisciplinary specialist health care team (for people with mental retardation) since he left school at 17. He was the only son of elderly parents whose family life was exceptionally well ordered and controlled. G failed to engage in the activities of a local day center, but his parents were not unduly perturbed as he was good company and helpful around the house. He had no friends, and no social activities outside his home. His own obsessive behavior increased over the years until by his mid-20s he was spending 3–4 hours each day engaged in ritualistic behavior, such as reading food packet labels and rearranging the contents of the kitchen cupboards. He had always been slightly built, but at the time of re-referral to the team his weight had dropped to below 98 lbs. Anorexia nervosa was suspected, but the possibility of inpatient treatment was remote, given his parents' reluctance to share his care. Outpatient family therapy was offered and accepted, and after six sessions at monthly intervals hospital admission was achieved. His weight had fallen to below 84 lbs., and he was often too frail to attend the family therapy clinic. His parents cooperated with his intensive inpatient treatment regime until his weight had increased to 126 lbs., and he had begun to demonstrate a sexual drive. After an aggressive outburst on the ward, his parents took him home against advice and found that G was more assertive and more "difficult" to live with. Family therapy continued with disagreement between the parents about G's longer term needs gradually emerging. His mother had enjoyed life without him and had begun to recognize G's own need for a separate existence. His father was still struggling with his fear of his son being rejected by the wider community. The treatment setting provided a safe place for these disagreements to emerge and for plans for G's own future to be discussed.

◼ GRIEF THERAPY

Death and mental retardation are both taboo subjects in our society. We are all affected by loss and death, yet often people with mental retardation are not given the chance to grieve nor to grow as a result of grief. The greater the degree of impairment, the less likely it is that the individual's grief will be recognized: caregivers tend to ignore or misunderstand the effects of such losses. Furthermore, the shorter life expectancy of people with mental retardation is

not widely known or understood and the secret of an individual's own morbidity and mortality not shared with him or her. Normal and pathological grief are fully described elsewhere (Ainsworth-Smith and Speck 1982; Kubler-Ross 1981; Murray-Parkes 1986), but the variations in the expression of grief in this special population are still being explored (Bonell-Pascual et al. 1999; Hollins and Esterhuyzen 1997; Kloeppel and Hollins 1989; Oswin 1985).

There is one concern that parents of people with mental retardation all share: what will happen to their child when they die. This concern encompasses several aspects including where their child will live and who will care for him or her. Concern may also extend to other areas such as the feelings of grief their child might experience and how the child's expression of grief might affect his or her behavior and subsequent care. The provision of respite care to families is a commonly available contribution to planning for later permanent separation, but the flexibility required of service providers to meet individual needs at a time of bereavement is largely missing.

Sensitive bereavement care is also needed for people already resident in long-term institutional or community residences. This includes the death of relatives, friends, or staff and also the losses experienced when friends or staff move on. The diagnosis of depression following a bereavement is frequently missed, perhaps because it is often masked with aggressive behavior.

Guided mourning approaches are useful either individually or in groups (Hollins and Sireling 1991, 1994), and mainstream bereavement counseling services are a valuable source of expertise. Bereavement counselors who are not familiar with the needs of people with mental retardation should look to specialist nurses, doctors, psychologists, or social workers to support them in adapting their skills appropriately. Communicating about feelings must not rely on language alone but must encompass the use of gesture, color, and other nonverbal communication to express emotion (Hollins and Roth 1994).

■ GROUP THERAPY

The reader must examine his or her own images of group work and see if they are flexible enough to allow for the possibility of a group of individuals with mental retardation being able to do useful work together. In reality the medium of therapy is never exclusively verbal, and part of the therapist's task is to increase the group's awareness of nonverbal communication and their experience of emotionally charged self-discovery. The leaders may concentrate their efforts on the functioning of the group, mobilizing the members' ability to help each other. They may do this by being concerned with the social matrix (Yalom 1970) and with the way groups try to avoid functioning as a group (Bion 1961). This has been described as therapy *of* the group. Alternatively,

doing therapy with the group involves the leaders in clarifying unconscious group and individual processes (Foulkes 1965). With people with mental retardation, although therapy is likely to be complicated by conceptual and communication difficulties, and by an impaired sense of self, both styles of therapy are possible (see Chapter 7 of this book).

Aims of Group Therapy

The main aims of group therapy are to enable individuals to accept their own limitations and to improve their personal relationships. Groups can be offered at different levels, for example, supportive to restore or maintain the status quo or dynamic to effect change in the individual. Yalom (1970) described 10 curative factors in groups, which included imparting of information, instillation of hope, interpersonal learning, and catharsis.

Group therapy may also have clearly focused goals, for example, related to individual maturation or to adjusting to the loss of a parent. Throughout our lives we belong to natural groups, and our behavior is influenced by interaction with the other members and by their expectations. Therapeutic groups are artificially constructed to create a peer group of people experiencing similar difficulties. Such groups may be small with a membership of between 5 and 10 people or large with a membership of 20 or more. Groups may be open with members free to join and leave when they choose or closed with an expected commitment from members to attend regularly throughout the life of the group. The work described in this chapter includes small groups of both the open and closed kinds.

Stavrakaki and Klein (1986) argued that group psychotherapy in this field should focus clearly on the need to comprehend and alter disordered personality functioning, and to improve communication and social interaction. Given that social style and temperament contribute more to adjustment as an adult than intellectual levels, such aims are valuable.

Several published articles describe work with groups of adolescents or adults living in institutional care (e.g., Cogan et al. 1966; Miezio 1967; Pantlin 1985; Slivkin and Bernstein 1968), but there are few references to outpatient group work in the literature (Hollins and Evered 1990; Hollins and Sinason 2000). It seems there has been very little confidence in the past in the use of group analytic approaches with people who have mental retardation.

Therapists and Supervision

Therapists may be fully trained group analysts or members of a health or social care profession such as psychiatry, social work, psychology, occupational therapy, or nursing.

Regular supervision throughout the life of the group is invaluable, particularly when the leaders' expertise lies more in the field of mental retardation than in that of psychotherapy even if the supervisor has no direct experience of working with people with mental retardation. The supervisor will question, challenge, and support the leaders throughout the group and will enable an exploration of their different perceptions and experiences of the group.

It is inadvisable for therapists to have any other regular contact with group members outside the group sessions, and for this reason, a named person or *keyworker* should be available to assist with any practical problems in each group member's life.

A year is usually too short for a useful group experience for the members, and the departure of one of the therapists is not a reason to end the group. The feelings aroused in the group by events such as the departure of a member or leader will provide an additional focus for work.

Assessment for a Small Group

The important aspects to address at a first meeting are related to the issues and behavior the person presents. The ability of an individual to engage with the therapists on an emotional level is paramount. It may be necessary to see someone more than once to determine his or her commitment to therapy and understanding of what it might involve.

The unmet or partially met dependency needs of some people may cause anxiety about their potential ability to share the leaders with the group. This may cause the leaders to minimize the amount of preliminary contact they have with any individual or to reject people who show very demanding or dependent behavior. In practice, engagement on an individual level does appear to lead to a smoother transition to group functioning. Acceptance for group therapy is likely to be on a "try it and see" basis for both therapists and patients. The intellectual and verbal ability of the group can vary between group members, but care should be taken to choose people who are peers. The one person who is 20 years older, or the only wheelchair user, or the only woman, or the only person with Down's syndrome is unlikely to remain a member for very long.

Rules, Boundaries, and Practical Considerations

The same time and space boundaries should be observed as with any analytic group. Some people have difficulties with time, and it is not uncommon for someone to arrive an hour or more early. A suitable waiting area is essential so that the members can foregather and for any escorts to sit during the session. The group members are asked to telephone their apologies in advance if they are unable to come. It will be important to use a telephone number that is regularly staffed by the same person and whose only role with the group is that of message taker. Leaders will not normally accept calls from members or caregivers between groups and will avoid being drawn into clinical involvement in other areas to do with an individual's life. I have found it helpful to give the group written reminders of the date of the next meeting at the last session before a break. Group members are told that things that are shared in the group are confidential to the group. Their understanding of the meaning of confidentiality may be in doubt. Keeping secrets is discouraged for obvious reasons in vulnerable people who might be exploited. In addition, confidentiality is less easily sustained when group members are likely to have histories and experiences in common with some other members through attending the same day center, respite hostel, or club or having been to school together in the past. My experience is that confidentiality is learned during group sessions. However, the need for confidentiality and other boundaries may not be understood or respected by parents or caregivers. To illustrate this, I will describe a young woman who attended an outpatient group in a district general hospital:

> J was 19 and had lived in residential care since her early teens when her mother died. Her father visited her about once a year, and she had developed a rich fantasy life to compensate for her painful feelings of abandonment. She used a manic defense as a thin disguise for her depression. J was one of only two members who had to be escorted to the group, and the escort was unreliable, obviously having no idea of the nature of the treatment and the need for confidentiality. Although time boundaries were adhered to strictly, it was not unusual for a new escort to walk in before the end and to stand and wait for the group to finish. Needless to say, the escort would be asked to wait outside until "time," but these few occasions showed the change that took place in J after the intrusion, as she reverted to the "giggly little girl" known in the hostel, her depression once again hidden.

Transference and Countertransference

The main work of therapy with the group will be done through interpreting the transference and countertransference in the relationship between the leaders and the group and between members (see earlier section on individual therapy).

In a report of one of my groups (Hollins 1991), I wrote,

> The therapists sometimes experienced profound feelings of boredom leading to difficulty staying awake. In supervision it became clear that these heavy feelings were in the countertransference—it was not boredom: we were being challenged. We were in touch with some of the pain for our clients of being damaged, and some of our own pain and intolerance of their disabilities. (p. 137)

These feelings were usefully shared with the group. The problem of the idealization of the leaders and of an individual's caretakers can be addressed, the group members can give up their expectation of being "cured," and the therapists can drop the burden of being expected to "cure" the members' impairments (Menolascino et al. 1986).

The Content of Group Sessions

The three secrets of death, dependence or disability, and sexuality are usually exposed and explored in psychoanalytic psychotherapy (Hollins and Grimer 1988). Experiences of major loss appear to be more common in this patient group and are quickly shared in small groups, although mourning is often discouraged by caregivers. In one group, J, the young woman referred to earlier, chatted happily about hairdos and the comings and goings of various members of the royal family. A second woman showed her own operation scar and then talked about her mother's terminal illness. J dropped her manic defense and blurted "I haven't got a mother." She appeared depressed and was suddenly in touch with some very painful feelings. The group listened to J and allowed her to be sad. Nobody told her to cheer up or to forget about her unhappy experiences. Instead the group asked her about her mother and acknowledged that she was upset. Her feelings were accepted and respected.

The experience of being different, the second secret, is often described as "hurting inside" and is seldom shared until later sessions. Therapists may have difficulty in confronting the group's initial denial of their disabilities. It is not socially acceptable to point to someone's disability. Group members may be reticent to talk about impairment and disability for similar reasons, not wanting to upset others. Their perceptions of what constitutes a disability may be surprising. For example, B admitted to three kinds of disabled people. The first was wheelchair users, the second kind had epilepsy, and the third had speech difficulties. None of these were characteristics of her own, but three members had marked speech and/or language problems, which B took responsibility for interpreting. "Because I can understand them," she said. G had severe expressive dysphasia but was able to express his frustration about B's insensitivity very eloquently (for us all to understand) with the first syllable of each of two swear words. Throughout the first few months our perception of B was that her thinking was impaired. She was articulate and had plenty to say, but the content of her speech was borrowed from her mother. Her own independent thought emerged only very slowly.

The third secret, of sexuality, provokes a range of responses in groups from curiosity to disgust and from embarrassment to naivete. For example, after meeting weekly for 3 months, the members of one group began to joke and talk in an awkward and embarrassed way about a group home that would include two men and two women. There was some uncertainty about what sort of relationship might be possible among these four people.

The widespread lack of suitable sex education and personal relationship education in special schools inevitably compounds the difficult adjustments that face all adolescents. The changes of puberty are not well or easily explained, and if the main source of information is a largely illiterate peer group, one can imagine that considerable misinformation is the norm. Television programs supplement this with "soaps" providing stimulating material for discussion in the group. "Why did she have a baby when she wasn't married?" "Why did he leave his wife?" These explorations may lead members to share their own worries or confusions in this area: "My social worker says I can't have babies and I'm very lucky."

Termination of Therapy

As each group moves through different phases of initial rejection to partial acceptance and hopefully to sharing, the reality of the short life of the group is held in mind. Regular holiday breaks three or four times a year serve to remind everyone about the temporary nature of the group. Each break is a rehearsal for the final ending of the group and is a painful reminder of other separations. Rejoining after a break is also difficult, with some members taking several weeks to learn to trust the group again. Such struggles may lead inexperienced leaders to minimize breaks in an attempt to avoid the anger of the group. In an open group that lasted for 3 years, one man returned time and again to the theme of the insincerity of "normal" people who welcomed him one day and rejected him the next. Toward the end of the group he became very quiet and eventually owned up to the sad insight he had gained that his idealized image of other people was false. His disappointment was real, but he accepted it and felt better able to face life on his own without the group's help.

In the final session of a closed 1-year group that I was supervising, the members shared their bewilderment—they still could not understand why the group was ending. Their fantasies about the leaders, which they had vividly spelled out in earlier groups, persisted with the assumption that they must be going on to better things, whereas the members would once more be left behind.

As the last session approaches, individual members and/or their caregivers or keyworkers may seek out alternative activities or a replacement therapy to fill the gap. But feelings about the group and about its ending will be important for some time afterwards and should not be a cause of apprehension. It is usually advisable to delay any further assessment for some months to allow time for the effects of the therapeutic experience to be seen.

Focused Therapy: Bereavement Work in Groups

More focused work will rely less on traditional group analytic techniques, although the group will remain important. The guided mourning approach described by Hollins and Sireling (1991) uses more active techniques drawn from education, art, and drama. Death education and counseling resources should be prepared in advance so that the group can be systematically led through the stories of their own losses. Sharing each person's own story and listening to other members' stories may be easier if the leaders also have a story to tell. For this purpose the story of the death of a parent has been told in simple pictures, with color and mime emphasizing the feelings experienced at each stage (Hollins and Sireling 1994). Asking members to bring a photo or other memento of their deceased relative or friend will provide a guide for the leaders about the extent of avoidance of painful cues. The presence of such objects also helps to make each person's loss more real for the other members.

A group visit to a cemetery or crematorium may be an important practical lesson in how to say good-bye. Such a group might meet weekly for 4–6 months and would avoid other themes that threatened to divert the members from the declared purpose. The ending of the group has its own purpose and poignancy as the members face a new loss, which the group works toward together.

Outcome

Attitude and personality assessments are very difficult with this patient group. Many of the concepts used in psychotherapy are notoriously difficult to measure. Repertory grids have been used to study personality and behavioral difficulties in individuals with mental retardation (Spindler-Barton et al. 1976) and to compare individuals in resettlement groups (Hulbert and Atkinson 1987). I used repertory grid analysis as an assessment and evaluation tool before and after a 1-year closed outpatient group. It seemed likely that people with very similar life experiences might show some similar changes in their grids over time. The grid is rated by putting a set of elements—in this case, important people in the life of each person—against a set of bipolar constructs. The persons themselves are rated twice as an element, once as their real selves and again as their ideal selves. One of the analyses that proved interesting was the discrepancy between real self and ideal self as rated against each of the constructs and as they changed over time.

In my study (S. Hollins, unpublished observations, 1996), the constructs were fixed by the researchers and included upsetting, caring, happy, handicapped, exciting, and so on. The results are complex to interpret, but an example may be illustrative:

> Before the group began, M saw himself as the most disabled person out of 12 elements (or important people in his life), and this was where his biggest self/ ideal-self discrepancy was found. His ideal self would be only the seventh most disabled. This seemed a reasonable ambition and he did achieve it. However, he also wanted to be the most happy, having seen himself as the sixth "most happy at the beginning." This he did not achieve.
>
> His other self-ratings had changed very little except that he saw himself as more respecting of other people. In addition, the therapists' clinical observations provide ample rich evidence of a reduction in distressing symptoms and of emotional maturation for M and for other members of the group.

Rigorous documentation of clinical experience and an extension of the range of outcome measures used in studies would add to our knowledge and understanding (Hollins 2000).

■ CONCLUSIONS

Psychoanalytic psychotherapies are effective but are not easy options for the therapists, who must be prepared to tolerate the fact that there is no cure for their patients' impairments. Without training and supervision, psychodynamic insights are evasive. Group approaches to treatment are an economical way of working and require little more than an accessible and comfortable room with enough chairs for the members, a guarantee of no outside interruptions, and a commitment to training and supervision for the leaders.

The necessary expertise can be brought into settings where people live and work in order to meet their emotional needs in a preventive way rather than by expensive hospital admission at a point of crisis and breakdown. Individual, group, and family therapy have fallen within my role as a developmental psychiatrist. This includes an understanding of the emotional and social development of the disabled person in the context of his or her family or caregivers, teachers, and peers. We know that psychological distress, low self-esteem, and depression are much more common in young people with mental retardation and those with physical disability (with or without intellectual disability) (Offer et al. 1984; Rutter et al. 1974). We know that problem behavior that challenges the resources of caregivers is much increased in people with mental retardation. Psychoanalytic therapies are not either/or treatments but can be offered in conjunction with other treatment approaches.

A wide range of psychotherapeutic approaches is both possible and desirable. Skilled assessment is an essential precursor of an offer of treatment, and referrers must not assume that a request for therapy equates with a decision to offer therapy. Supervision by a qualified therapist is essential for trainees and may be advisable for qualified and experienced professionals engaged in long-term work. Psychotherapeutic approaches have not been exploited to the fullest in work with people with mental retardation. In the future we should expect to see the full range of available treatments being developed and researched for use with this patient group. The training needs of staff will need to be addressed to achieve these developments.

■ REFERENCES

Ainsworth-Smith I, Speck P: Letting Go: Caring for the Dying and Bereaved. London, Society for Promoting Christian Knowledge, 1982

Beail N: Psychoanalytic psychotherapy with men with intellectual disabilities: a preliminary outcome study. British Journal of Medical Psychology 71:1–11, 1998

Bicknell J: Inaugural lecture: the psychopathology of handicap. Br J Med Psychol 56:167–178, 1983

Bion WR: Experiences in Groups. London, Tavistock Publication, 1961

Bird J, Harrison G: Examination Notes in Psychiatry. Bristol, UK, Wright, 1984

Bloch DA: Techniques of Family Psychotherapy: A Primer Pub. New York and London, Grune & Stratton, 1973

Bonell-Pascual E, Huline-Dickens S, Hollins S, et al: Bereavement and grief in adults with learning disabilities: A follow up study. Br J Psychiatry 175:348–350, 1999

Cawley RH: The teaching of psychotherapy. Association of University of Teachers of Psychiatry Newsletter, January 19–36, 1977

Coffman TL, Harris M: Transition shock and adjustments of mentally retarded persons. Ment Retard 18:3–7, 1980

Cogan F, Monson L, Bruggeman W: Concurrent group and individual treatment of the mentally retarded. Social Psychiatry Journal 12:404–409, 1966

Dorell S: Text of Speech to Mencap on Services for People With Learning Disabilities. London, Department of Health, Alexander Fleming House, 1991

Education Act. Department of Education and Science, HMSO Publications Center, PO Box 276, London SW8 5DT, 1971

Foulkes SR, Anthony EJ: Group Psychotherapy. Harmondsworth, UK, Penguin, 1965

Gorell-Barnes G: Pattern and intervention in family therapy, in Complementary Frameworks of Theory and Practice. Edited by Bentovim A, Gorell-Barnes G, Cooklin A. London, Academic Press, 1982, pp 22–45

Hollins S: Group analytic therapy, in Psychotherapy and Mental Handicap. Edited by Waitman A, Conboy-Hill S. London, Sage, 1991, pp 129–139

Hollins S: Treating with respect: the growth of therapeutic approaches in the community. The Psychoanalytic Review 2(8):374–375, 2000

Hollins S, Esterhuyzen A: Bereavement and grief in adults with learning disabilities. Br J Psychiatry 170:497–501, 1997

Hollins S, Evered C: Group process and content: the challenge of mental handicap. Group Analysis 23:55–67, 1990

Hollins S, Grimer M: Going Somewhere: Pastoral Care for People With Learning Disability. London, Society for Promoting Christian Knowledge, 1988

Hollins S, Roth T: Hug me, touch me, in Beyond Words. London, Department of Mental Health Sciences, St. George's Hospital Medical School, Pranmer Terrace, 1994

Hollins S, Sinason V: New perspectives: Psychotherapy, learning disabilities and trauma. Br J Psychiatry 176:32–36, 2000

Hollins S, Sireling L: "When Dad Died": Working Through Loss With People Who Have Learning Disabilities. Windsor, UK, Nfer Nelson, 1991

Hollins S, Sireling L: "When Dad Died and When Mum Died": The Sovereign Series, 2nd Edition. St. George's Hospital Medical School, 1994

Hollins S, Sireling L: Understanding Grief: Working with grief and people who have learning disabilities. London, Pavilion, 1999

Hulbert C, Atkinson D: On the way out, and after. British Journal of Mental Subnormality 33: 109–116, 1987

Kloeppel DA, Hollins SC: Double handicap: mental retardation and death in the family. Death Studies 13:31–38, 1989

Kubler-Ross E: Living With Death and Dying. London, Souvenir Press, 1981

Leudar I: Communicative environments for mentally handicapped people, in Language and Communication in Mentally Handicapped People. Edited by Beveridge M, Cont-Ramsden G, Leudar I. London, Chapman & Hall, 1989, pp 274–300

Matson JL: Psychotherapy with persons who are mentally retarded. Ment Retard 22:170–175, 1984

McCormack B: Thinking, discourse and the denial of history; psychodynamic aspects of mental handicap. Irish Journal of Psychological Medicine 8:59–64, 1991

Menolascino FJ, Gilson SF, Levitas AS: Issues in the treatment of mentally retarded patients in the community mental health system. Community Ment Health J 22:314–327, 1986

Miezio S: Group therapy with mentally retarded adolescents in institutional settings. Journal of Group Psychotherapy 17:321–327, 1967

Minuchin S, Fishman HC: Family Therapy Techniques. Cambridge, MA, Harvard University Press, 1981

Murray-Parkes C: Bereavement: Studies of Grief in Adult Life. London, UK, Penguin, 1986

Offer D, Ostrov E, Howard KI: Body image, self perception and chronic illness in adolescents, in Chronic Illness and Disabilities in Childhood and Adolescence. Edited by Blum RW. Orlando, FL, Grune & Stratton, 1984, pp 59–83

Oswin M: Bereavement, in Mental Handicap: A Multi-Disciplinary Approach. Edited by Craft M, Bicknell DJ, Hollins S. London, Bailliere Tindall, 1985

Pantlin AW: Group-analytic psychotherapy with mentally handicapped patients. Group Analysis 18: 44–53, 1985

Rutter M, Tizard J, Yule P, et al: Isle of Wight studies. Psychol Med 6:313–332, 1974

Selwa BI: Preliminary considerations in psychotherapy with retarded children. Journal of School Psychology 9:12–15, 1971

Sinason V: Secondary Mental Handicap and its Relationship to Trauma. Psychoanalytical Psychotherapy 2:131–154, 1986

Sinason V: Psychotherapeutic work with disabled individuals: The past is alive in the present. Psychotherapy Review 2(7):325–382, 2000

Skynner ACR: One Flesh, Separate Persons. London, Constable, 1976

Slivkin SE, Bernstein NR: Goal-directed group psychotherapy for retarded adolescents. Am J Psychother 22:35–45, 1968

Spindler-Barton E, Walton T, Rowe D: Using grid techniques with the handicapped, in The Measurement of Interpersonal Space by Grid Techniques. Edited by Slater P. Chichester, Sussex, UK, Wiley, 1976, pp 125–139

Stavrakaki O, Klein J: Psychotherapies with the mentally retarded. Psychiatric Clin North Am 9:733–743, 1986

Symington N: The psychotherapy of a subnormal patient. Br J Med Psychol 54:187–199, 1981

Vanier J: Man and Woman: He Made Them. London, Darton, Longman, & Todd, 1985

Waitman A, Conboy-Hill S: Psychotherapy and Mental Handicap. London, Sage Publications, 1992

Weinstock A: Group treatment of characterologically damaged developmentally disabled adolescents in a residential treatment center. Int J Group Psychother 29:369–381, 1979

Woody RH, Billy JJ: Counselling Psychotherapy for the Mentally Retarded: A Survey of Opinions and Practices. Ment Retard 12:20–23, 1966

Yalom ID: Theory and Practice of Group Psychotherapy. New York, Basic Books, 1970

3 Psychopharmacological Approaches

Stephen Tyrer, M.A., M.B., B.Chir.L.M.C.C., F.R.C.Psych.
Sarah Hill, B.Sc.

Psychopharmacological agents are widely used to treat people with mental retardation, and often the indications are meager. These drugs are used in five main areas:

1. For treatment of psychiatric illness
2. For the control of behavior disorder
3. To reduce aberrant or uncontrolled sexual drive
4. For the treatment of epilepsy and associated disturbances
5. For other conditions

In this chapter, I discuss the principles of the drug treatment of the mentally retarded. The subject is covered in more detail in Part 4, and the treatment of epilepsy is dealt with in Chapter 14 of this book.

The rationale for giving psychotropic drugs to patients with unequivocal signs of mental illness is much stronger than for the control of disturbed behavior. Nevertheless, these drugs are still widely employed in the control of behavioral disturbances in this population (Baumeister et al. 1993). In this chapter, I provide a general survey of the use of these drugs in mentally retarded individuals with particular reference to the differences that are found in the response to these agents in mentally retarded people versus people of normal intelligence. The treatment of patients with characteristic syndromes will also be described briefly.

■ PREVALENCE OF PSYCHOTROPIC DRUG USE

Until 1952 there were few drugs that were available and even less that were used for the treatment of people with mental retardation. The drugs that were employed were used primarily to "keep the patient quiet." Agents such as the barbiturates, in particular phenobarbitone, and bromide salts were used for this purpose. Little attempt was made to try and determine if the person with mental retardation also had a mental illness and whether specific treatment was implicated for this. Even when the neuroleptic drugs were developed in the 1950s, there was simply a substitution of these drugs for the previous older agents. Specific psychopharmacological treatment for a particular mental illness was not raised, as it was a rare event for the physician to even make a diagnostic formulation along the standard psychiatric lines.

Because the neuroleptics were safer than the drugs that previously had been prescribed for this group, they were used in high doses, and it is of interest to note that the people who were admitted to hospitals for the mentally retarded in the 1940s and 1950s as children were found, by means of a survey conducted many years later, to be taking higher doses of these drugs than those people admitted to the hospital later (Wressell et al. 1990).

Neuroleptic agents and other psychotropic drugs are widely prescribed for people with mental retardation, often on poor indicative basis. Between 20% and 50% of the residents in institutions for the mentally retarded receive psychotropic drugs, not including those required for the control of epilepsy (Brooke 1998; Rinck et al. 1989). A similar number receive anti-epileptic drugs (Fischbacher 1987). Although surveys in the past have suggested that a similar frequency of drug use is found in community settings (Hemming 1984), more recent surveys have shown a lower frequency of drug use there (Clarke et al. 1990). The most frequently employed drugs are the neuroleptics, but antidepressants, anticonvulsants for use other than the control of epilepsy, lithium, β-blockers, benzodiazepines, antimuscarinic drugs, and hypnotics are also prescribed. Occasionally, CNS stimulants, opiate antagonists, and neurotransmitter-depleting agents such as the benzoquinolizine drug tetrabenazine are used. Many of the patients receive more than one psychotropic drug. In a study of group homes in North Dakota, almost 50% of the patients received more than one psychotropic drug, with 4% of them receiving more than four of these agents at any one time (Burd et al. 1991).

The reasons for the widespread use of these agents is not readily apparent. Although the incidence of psychiatric illness, in particular schizophrenia, is higher in people with mental retardation than in those of normal intelligence (Lund 1985), the majority of people taking psychotropic drugs do not have clear psychiatric illnesses and most would be described as having a behavioral disturbance (Baumeister et al. 1993; Wressell et al. 1990).

■ WHEN SHOULD ANTIPSYCHOTIC DRUGS BE USED?

The indications for the use of these agents depend on the condition for which treatment is being given. The treatment suggestions given below are only an outline of the therapeutic options that are available for the specific disorders described. For further information about defining criteria and details of drug treatment, the reader is directed to the appropriate illness or condition covered in more detail in subsequent chapters of this book.

Psychiatric Illness

Psychoses

If the patient has a psychiatric illness that fulfills ICD-10 or DSM-IV criteria for a clearly defined illness for which drug treatment is effective, then it is usual to give drugs in the first instance. Unequivocal symptoms of schizophrenia and mania are normally treated with drugs, although the automatic prescription of drugs for patients with depression in this group is not advised. As shown by Ruedrich and colleagues in Chapter 12 of this book, alternative nondrug treatments for depression can be effective in mentally retarded people. In practice, many patients with mental retardation do not fulfill sufficient criteria to confidently indicate that they have a psychotic illness. In particular, it is not possible to make a confident diagnosis of schizophrenia in those functioning in the severe mental retardation range (Reid 1985). However, even in this population if there is evidence of affective flattening, incongruous behavior, self-preoccupation, and catatonic posturing, the exhibition of neuroleptic medication can have dramatic effects, suggesting that such symptoms in those of lower intelligence are of schizophrenic origin (Tyrer and Dunstan 1997).

A diagnosis of affective disorder can be made more confidently in mentally retarded people even if they have major communicative difficulties. The symptom triad of recent insomnia, loss of weight, and reduced activity, in the absence of a physical cause, usually indicates depression. Conversely, increasing activity accompanied by euphoria and/or irritability is suggestive of mania in the absence of other factors. The treatment of schizophrenia and affective disorder in mentally retarded persons is not essentially different from the treatment of these illnesses in people of normal intelligence.

The treatment of schizophrenia is covered in Chapter 11, which details the drugs and dosages indicated. There is an increased usage of the newer antipsychotic drugs in people with mental retardation because of the dangers of tardive dyskinesia (Shriqui et al. 1990). A recent study showed that 34% of the mentally retarded adults who were living in the hospital and who had received neuroleptic drugs had tardive dyskinesia (Sachdev 1992). There have been lawsuits in the United States in which mentally retarded patients who had received neuroleptic drugs for long periods of time obtained compensation for the side effects that resulted (Intagliata and Rinck 1985). Akathisia, a syndrome involving a subjective feeling of restlessness associated with a compulsion to move about, is frequently found in patients treated with the older neuroleptic agents (Gross et al. 1993) and is another reason for using the newer antipsychotic agents.

The substitute benzamide derivative, sulpiride, differs from other antipsychotic agents in that it acts on the presynaptic dopamine receptor. It is reputed to cause less extrapyramidal side effects and tardive dyskinesia than the older drugs, although until this drug has been used for a longer period of time this claim cannot be definitely substantiated. A valuable new drug that rarely causes tardive dyskinesia or extrapyramidal side effects is clozapine, a tricyclic drug of the dibenzodiazepine family. Its successful use with mentally retarded people has recently been reported (Boachie and McGinnity 1997; Thuresson and Farnstrand 1999). However, clozapine causes agranulocytosis in 1%–2% of patients (Tschen et al. 1999), and its use must be strictly monitored. Weekly blood counts must be taken, and the drug stopped immediately if there is a fall in the total white cell count of less than 3×10^9/L, a total neutrophil count of less than 1.5×10^9/L, or a platelet count below 100×10^9/L. In the United Kingdom it is only licensed for the treatment of resistant schizophrenia.

Risperidone is a new neuroleptic drug that blocks dopamine D_2 receptors but also has antagonist actions at the 5-HT_2 receptor. There are pharmacological reasons for supposing that this drug is also less prone to cause movement disorders (Wirshing et al. 1999), and studies suggest that it is particularly advantageous to use it with patients who have negative symptoms (Gutierrez-Estinon and Grebb 1997).

A further hazard of neuroleptic drugs is the occurrence of the potentially fatal neuroleptic malignant syndrome. This disorder, which is reported frequently nowadays, is characterized by excessive muscular rigidity, hyperpyrexia, fluctuating blood pressure, and excessive sweating. The diagnosis is confirmed when very high serum creatine kinase levels, usually over 1,000 IU/L, are found. It has been estimated that the approximate incidence of neuroleptic malignant syndrome is 1% overall and that individuals with mental retardation are thought to be at a greater risk of contracting this syndrome (Boyd 1992). Neuroleptic malignant syndrome has also been reported following treatment with atypical neuroleptics such as clozapine and risperidone (Hasan and Buckley 1998). There has also been a recent report of neuroleptic-induced dementia in four adults with mental retardation (Gedye 1998).

Treatment strategies for mentally retarded people who have affective disorder are not dissimilar from the treatment of these conditions in patients with normal intelligence (Tyrer 1989). Antidepressants are the mainstay of treatment as there is some suggestion that drugs such as carbamazepine, which have mood-stabilizing effects in those of normal intelligence, may be less effective in the mentally retarded (this issue is discussed further in Chapter 12 of this book). Langee and Conlon (1992) have shown that mentally re-tarded patients who respond to antidepressants are more likely to present symptoms of depression, psychosis, or tantrums, whereas those with self-injurious behavior are less likely to have beneficial effects.

If antidepressants fail to relieve depressive symptoms in a mentally retarded patient with a major depressive disorder, the prescription of lithium may yield improvement within a 4-week period (Austin et al. 1991). This strategy is not widely reported in patients with mental retardation. For an extensive review of the treatment of unipolar depression, the reader is referred to Lund (1990).

The treatment of bipolar affective disorder in the mentally retarded is cov-ered in Chapter 12 of this book. Lithium is normally the drug of choice for patients with a clearly determined bipolar disorder and who have had at least three episodes of illness, including one manic and one depressive episode, within a period of 3–4 years (Ferrier et al. 1995). However, lithium may well be less effective for mentally retarded patients with bipolar affective disorder, probably partly because more individuals with mental retardation have a rap-id-cycling bipolar disorder (i.e., more than four episodes in 1 year) compared with those of normal intelligence. A certain degree of brain damage is often present among mentally retarded people, and it is known that organic cerebral injury is a factor that is associated with rapid-cycling disorder. The advantages of the combination of lithium and carbamazepine in the treatment of bipolar disorder in the mentally retarded have been shown by Glue (1989), but of all the mood stabilizers used, sodium valproate may be the most effective (Van-straelen and Tyrer 1999).

Neuroses (Anxiety Disorders, Somatoform Disorders, Dissociative Disorders)

In general, psychotropic drugs are not widely used for the treatment of neu-roses in the mentally retarded. In many cases the neurotic symptoms exhibited in this population are the result of environmental changes (Day 1985), and supportive psychotherapy and restoration of previous activities and relation-ships are the treatments of choice.

The use of drugs to control anxiety should be largely confined to the con-trol of acute anxiety reactions. Even in these situations drug treatment is usu-ally not required—reassurance and provision of a calm environment may be sufficient. The shorter-acting benzodiazepines such as lorazepam and mid-azolam are to be preferred above the longer acting drugs such as diazepam. If more rapid action is required, 2–4 mg of lorazepam can be given intramuscu-larly, or if immediate response is necessary, diazepam 10 mg in the nonirritant form, Diazemuls. This is not normally necessary unless the patient is aggres-sive or is in danger of harming him- or herself.

Prolonged treatment for anxiety is not likely to be necessary. If long-term treatment is envisaged, benzodiazepines should not be given. Buspirone, an azaspirodecanodione, is a new anti-anxiety drug that has been used successfully in people with mental retardation to reduce anxiety and behavioral disturbance (Neppe 1999; Ratey et al. 1991; Verhoven and Tuinier 1996). The usual starting dose is 5 mg bd with a maximum of 30 mg daily. Propranolol and β-blocking agents that do not cross the blood-brain barrier, such as atenolol and nadolol, may be useful in patients who show sympathetic overactivity when emotionally aroused. (Other treatments in anxiety are reviewed in Chapter 13 of this book.)

Sleep Disorders

Nondrug treatment should be used as much as possible with those complaining of poor sleep. The benefits of exercise, avoidance of caffeine-containing drinks, a hot milk drink at night, and prevention of sleeping during the day may render a previously poor sleeper somnolent at night. If drugs are to be given, they should be given for short periods only or intermittently. Short-acting drugs such as zolpidem 5–10 mg or zopiclone 3.75–7.5 mg are preferred to the benzodiazepines because there is less likelihood of causing dependence. However, lormetazepam 1 mg or flunitrazepam 1 mg are suitable for short-term use. Promethazine 25–50 mg or trimeprazine 20–30 mg nocte are alternatives if benzodiazepines are contraindicated or if there is a danger of dependence. The sedative antidepressants such as trimeprazine and trazodone are helpful in sleep disorders because of their sedative side effects, but their use for long periods of time in patients without affective disturbance should be avoided.

Personality Disorders

There have been no controlled trials carried out on the treatment of personality disorders in the mentally retarded. Studies carried out on persons with a personality disorder who have normal intelligence indicate that people with an emotionally unstable personality disorder, a category that includes those with borderline personality disorder, may benefit from small doses of neuroleptic drugs (Stein 1992). The treatment of organic personality disorder, as defined in ICD-10, is covered in Chapter 15 of this book.

Behavior Disorder

The category of behavior in the field of mental retardation is a difficult one to define. It includes persistent episodes of stealing carried out by a mildly disabled youth, temper tantrums in those with all levels of a disability who are frustrated by not receiving what they regard as their just desserts, and self-injurious behavior in the severely retarded. The category of behavior disorder in this population includes conditions such as organic personality disorder; adjustment disorders; reactions to severe stress including posttraumatic stress disorder; antisocial (or dissocial) and emotionally unstable personality disorders (the latter being further divided into impulsive and borderline types); the catastrophic behavior of those with pervasive development disorders who are faced with acceptable levels of stimulus; conduct disorder that starts in childhood or adolescence; and psychological and behavioral disorders associated with sexual development and orientation. In practice, it is difficult to accurately define such behavior disorders because of a lack of precise information but particularly because of the inability of the retarded person to be able to give a clear account of why he or she has behaved in the fashion observed. It is also important to note that many people with mental retardation behave in an impulsive fashion without thinking about the consequences, whereas others have been poorly trained in acceptable social behavior. On many occasions when behavioral disturbances occur in these individuals, it is not possible to make a diagnosis following the guidelines described in DSM-IV or ICD-10. Indeed, behavior disorder without definite evidence of psychiatric illness is the most common reason why those with mental retardation are referred to a psychiatrist (Bouras and Drummond 1992). The remarks below apply to these individuals, although there is an overlap between such patients and those with antisocial personality disorder, conduct disorder, and organic personality disorder due to early cerebral damage.

Even though drugs are commonly employed, before prescribing them it is instructive to determine the antecedents of the behaviors, what actually happens at the time of the disturbed act, and what the consequences are. Some individuals carry out aggressive acts or are behaviorally disturbed because they are bored and understimulated, whereas others may attack people because they feel threatened. The former type of aggression is referred to as *predatory* or *instrumental aggression*, and the latter is termed *defensive* or *frustrative aggression*. Reduction in the undesirable outbursts is associated with different treatment approaches on the psychological and behavioral fronts. There is also evidence that drug treatment in instrumental aggression differs from that in defensive aggression (Tyrer 1998). This issue is discussed more fully in Chapter 15 of this book.

Behavioral and psychological techniques should be used whenever possible when mentally retarded people are behaviorally disturbed without there being evidence of underlying psychiatric illness. Only if these techniques are not effective, or if the environment involved cannot be altered in any major way, should pharmacological treatment be employed. Even when drug treatment is recommended, there should be a continual search for the factors precipitating aggression. For instance, many mentally retarded people who are unable to communicate are aggressive or self-injurious when they are in pain. Toothache, recurrent otitis media, and dysmenorrhea are examples of conditions in which aggressive or self-injurious behavior may be manifest and that can effectively be treated by addressing the underlying medical cause.

Treatment of Acute Behavioral Disturbance

It may be necessary to use drugs to control an acutely aggressive individual. The drugs most widely employed for this purpose are the antipsychotics and the benzodiazepines. A suggested flow chart to identify the most appropriate drug is shown in Figure 3–1.

Chlorpromazine has been used for many years for this purpose but has the disadvantage of causing prolonged sedation and hypotension. A quicker acting drug with a shorter duration of action is droperidol, a butyrophenone. This can be given in tablet form or by intramuscular injection. The onset of action when administered parenterally is between 3 and 10 minutes after administration (Thomas 1992). The sedative effects last for 2–4 hours. A dose of 10–20 mg is usually given depending on the body weight, and this may be given intramuscularly with acute disturbance. The main problems with this drug are its extrapyramidal side effects for which a muscarinic antiparkinson drug like procyclidine 5 mg may be needed.

Alternatively, quick-acting benzodiazepine drugs can be used. Lorazepam and midazolam administered by the buccal route are the preferred agents because of their relatively short half-lives and lack of respiratory depression. Suitable dosages are 4 mg for lorazepam and 10–30 mg for midazolam. Midazolam is quicker acting. Lorazepam may be given by intramuscular injection although oral treatment usually achieves adequate blood levels effective within 30–45 minutes.

The paradoxical proaggressive effects of benzodiazepines have been overemphasized. However, these drugs can sometimes cause an increase in aggression, and alternative agents should be sought. Paraldehyde is an effective drug although its smell and difficulty in administration are a major problem. A large part of the drug is excreted through the breath and so even if the liver function is impaired, the drug can still be excreted adequately. It has to be given by glass syringe if an injection is given because it dissolves plastic. Lactic acidosis has also been reported (Linter and Linter 1986).

Drug Treatment in Chronic Behavioral Disturbance

Drug treatment of chronic behavior disturbance should only be undertaken if the behavior is frequent, it reduces the capacity of the individual to undertake activities that would otherwise be of benefit to him or her, it is not possible to

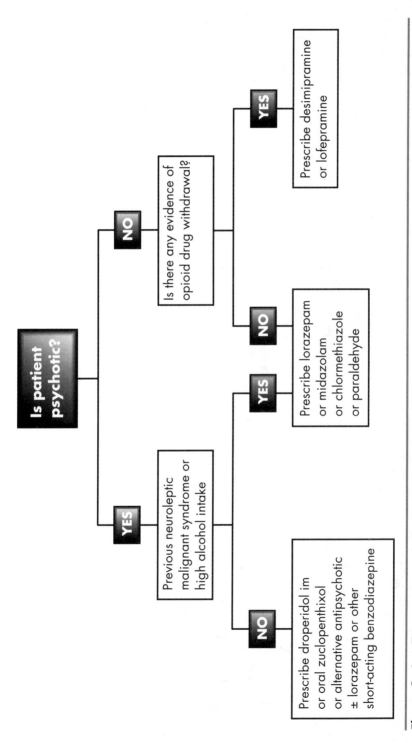

Figure 3–1. Drug treatment in acute aggressive episode.

change environmental contingencies, and behavioral and psychological therapies have proved unsuccessful. It is important to exclude physical and psychiatric illness as a cause of the aggressive behavior. Patients with manic or paranoid illnesses are often hostile, and those with pervasive developmental disorder often react with aggression when their territorial space is invaded. Confusional states and drug abuse are also associated with aggression although the latter is unusual in mental retardation. If there is evidence of a psychiatric illness, this should be treated in its own right with the appropriate pharmacological agents.

Classification of Chronic Behavioral Disturbance

The delineation of different syndromes in mentally retarded people with different behavioral abnormalities is still in its infancy. Although it is well recognized that many people with severe mental retardation have behavioral disturbances, the relationship of pathology to such disturbances has not been shown clearly. The most promising line of inquiry would seem to be the examination of the relationship between organic brain damage and the manifestation of behavior disturbance. Sovner and Lowry (see Chapter 15 of this book) have attempted to classify organic mental syndromes according to psychobiological dysfunctions and behavioral presentations. They posit four major psychobiological dysfunctions in this group: excitement, irritability, overarousal, and rage; they suggest different pharmacological options for the treatment of each. If this classification was shown to be associated with specific pathological damage to the brain or to be clearly associated with biochemical abnormalities, there would be a sound basis for classifying behavioral disturbance in this population according to the parameters proposed. No such relationship has been definitely shown to date. Nevertheless, the schema proposed in Chapter 15 is a useful working model and provides guidance for the clinician dealing with such patients.

Choice of Drug Treatment

The choice of drug depends not only on the clinical presentation of the disturbance at the time of the interview but also on the past history, family history, and the previous course of illness. Information obtained from reliable sources may suggest a well-recognized psychiatric illness. In the absence of such information or when it is noncontributory, it may be appropriate to treat according to the symptoms and type of behavior exhibited. A flow chart that attempts to identify the most appropriate drug for the treatment of persistent behavioral abnormalities is presented in Figure 3–2. This chart should be used in conjunction with Table 15–2 in Chapter 15. More precise details of the drug regimen employed will be found in other chapters later in this book.

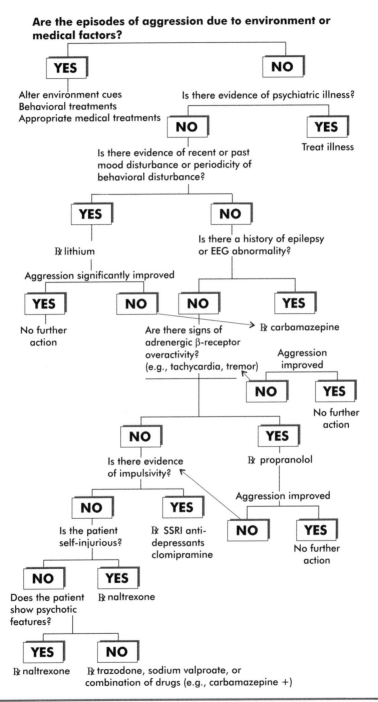

Figure 3–2. Drug treatment in chronic behavior disturbance.

If there is evidence of recent or past mood disturbance, or if there is a periodic cycle of disturbed behavior with affective manifestations, then lithium and carbamazepine are the drugs of choice. Lithium is effective in patients with mental retardation who show aggression toward others (Craft et al. 1987; Tyrer et al. 1984) and is the clear treatment of choice in those individuals with a bipolar affective illness (Carlson 1979). Those who show physical aggression toward others respond best to it (Tyrer et al. 1993).

Lithium is a potentially dangerous drug, and blood levels should be monitored carefully (Tyrer 1996). Toxicity frequently occurs if serum lithium levels are above 1.5 mmol/L, but it can occur at much lower serum levels (Bell et al. 1993). Toxic symptoms include ataxia, tremor, a feeling of being drugged, and a gray and ill appearance. Lithium should be stopped immediately if toxicity is suspected—there is no disadvantage to terminating administration of the drug for a 24-hour period.

There is no firm evidence that carbamazepine is valuable in treating similar syndromes in mental retardation unless there is an affective component, although this drug has been shown to be of value to patients with normal intelligence who have a rapid-cycling affective disorder (i.e., more than four episodes per year). Retrospective studies have shown that carbamazepine is more effective in reducing behavioral disturbance if there is evidence of any electroencephalographic abnormality (Langee 1989).

If there are signs of adrenergic β-receptor overactivity (e.g., tachycardia, tremor, palpitations, or other somatic signs of overarousal), then β-blocking drugs may be of value (see Chapter 15 of this book). Propranolol has been the most widely used drug of this group and can be effective at a dosage of 120 mg daily, although the dose may need to be raised to three times this value (Ratey and Lindem 1992). Nadolol at dosages of 80–160 mg has also been used with this population, and β-blocking agents that do not cross the blood-brain barrier such as atenolol and oxprenolol may also be useful in this regard. All β-blocking drugs slow down the heart rate and reduce myocardial contraction. They should not be given if the pulse falls below 48 beats per minute or if there are signs of heart failure or myocardial depression. They should *never* be used with patients who have a recent history of obstructive airway disease or asthma.

Naltrexone, an opioid antagonist, although widely canvassed as a useful agent in reducing self-injurious behavior in severely and profoundly mentally retarded individuals, has recently been shown in double-blind trials to be ineffective (Willemsen-Swinkels et al. 1995).The use of opioid antagonists is covered more fully in Chapter 16 of this book.

Antidepressant drugs that increase the synaptic availability of 5-HT are valuable in the control of impulsive behavior in those of normal intelligence

(Linnoila et al. 1993). These drugs may reduce persistent aggressive behavior (see Chapter 16 of this book). The selective serotonin reuptake inhibitor agents (e.g., fluoxetine, fluvoxamine) are the most frequently used drugs, although trazodone and the tricyclic antidepressant drugs (e.g., clomipramine) have been used to good effect. L-tryptophan, a precursor drug in the synthesis of 5-HT, is also helpful although it is now not generally available because of the occasional occurrence of the eosinophil-myalgia syndrome accompanying use of this drug. There have been encouraging reports of a new class of 5-HT$_{1A}$ agonists, called serenics, in reducing aggression in the mentally retarded, the best known example of which is eltoprazine (De Koning et al. 1994). This drug is valuable on a short-term basis but loses potency after a few weeks. Other agents, including buspirone (Ratey et al. 1991; Verhoeven and Tuinier 1996) and amantadine (Chandler et al. 1991), have been successful in open trials.

In practice, the drugs used most frequently for mentally retarded patients with a history of chronic behavioral disturbance are the neuroleptic drugs (Clarke et al. 1990; Wressell et al. 1990). These have the advantage of having an immediate sedative effect and have been used for over 30 years before the newer agents described above were available—this despite the fact that no well-controlled trial had been conducted that would seem to indicate that antipsychotic drugs are more effective alone than other agents in the treatment of disturbed behavior in this population, or even more effective than placebo (Manchester 1993).

One of the reasons why, once started, neuroleptic drug treatment is frequently continued is because withdrawal of treatment is often associated with an increase in aggressive behavior (Lynch et al. 1985). It is not generally realized that sudden withdrawal of antipsychotic drugs, particularly those with pronounced anticholinergic effects, is associated with withdrawal symptoms of nausea, anorexia, restlessness, and muscle pain (Dilsaver 1994; Keks et al. 1995), which may contribute to aggressive behavior in patients who cannot communicate in other ways.

As neuroleptic drugs are known to cause tardive dyskinesia when administered for long periods of time, particularly when there is evidence of brain damage, their long-term use with the mentally retarded patients who exhibit behavioral disturbance without psychosis should be avoided (Gualtieri 1991). However there have been encouraging reports of the benifits of a newer neuroleptic drug, risperidone, in treating behavior disorders in mentally retarded people (Van den Borre et al. 1993), and recent double-blind trials have confirmed its value in children and adolescents (Aman et al. 2000) and adults (Gagiano et al. 2000). Zuclopenthixol has also been shown to be effective in this population (Malt et al. 1995).

Aberrant Sexual Behavior

Sexual offenses committed by mentally retarded people are not infrequent and often lead to a request for psychiatric help (Day 1994). Many of those who perpetuate sexual offenses are not fully aware of what constitutes acceptable sexual practice. Sex education instruction packages are available and are valuable in determining gaps in the knowledge of the patients and may, indirectly, help to assess the degree of motivation. Psychological and behavioral treatment have a greater part to play than drug therapy (see Chapter 20 of this book). However, drugs may assist patients in avoiding sexual temptation. Before prescribing these drugs, it is important to seek the consent of the patient or, if this is not possible, to consult a close relative to expound on the likely effects of the drug being administered. In some countries it is not possible to give some of these agents without legal sanction.

The drug that is the most widely used in North America for this purpose is medroxyprogesterone acetate (MPA). In the United Kingdom and Europe this progestogen is hardly ever used for this purpose; instead cyproterone acetate, an anti-androgen drug, is preferred.

MPA is most commonly prescribed for hypersexual pedophiles of normal intelligence, but the drug is also used for people with mental retardation as well as those with normal intelligence when recurrent exhibitionism, incest, transvestism, and other sexual disorders are manifest (Glasser 1990).

Cyproterone decreases serum testosterone, and open studies have reported its efficacy in reducing masturbation, indecent exposure, and sexual offenses in mentally retarded men (Clarke 1989). Sexual interest and sexual activity were reduced in sexual offenders receiving this drug in a controlled trial (Bancroft et al. 1974). Cyproterone has been reported to be hepatotoxic if given in a dosage of more than 200 mg daily (Lewis 1995), and regular liver function tests should be carried out.

Benperidol, which is an antipsychotic from the butyrophenone group, is also licensed for the control of deviant and antisocial sexual behavior. Its use is supported by a wealth of uncontrolled trials, but the few double-blind investigations that have been performed do not suggest that it is an effective drug in reducing sexual desire (Clarke 1989). Because benperidol does not affect the concentration of testosterone or luteinizing hormone, these results are not surprising.

Day (1994) has pointed out that in many individuals with mental retardation the offenses are committed by persons who have a normal sexual drive but a poor understanding of sexual manners. It is not appropriate to state that these individuals have a sexual perversion. Effective training and supervision would be more beneficial than giving drugs that do not help the individual solve the problem by using his or her own resources.

Another drug that has rarely been used in Europe is goserelin. Goserelin is a luteinizing-releasing hormone analogue that effectively reduces testosterone. Although it is not licensed for the reduction of male sexual drive, it has been used effectively for this purpose (Delle Chiaie and Picardi 1994).

Other Conditions

Hyperactivity and stereotypy occasionally require treatment with drugs. Carbamazepine (Reid et al. 1981) and the central nervous stimulants (e.g., pemoline, dexamphetamine, and methylphenidate) (Barkley 1990) have been found to be more effective than placebo. Carbamazepine is probably the best first-line drug.

There is good evidence that the antipsychotic drugs reduce stereotypy, and their effects are greatest in the most severely affected individuals (Aman et al. 1984). Clomipramine may be beneficial (Garber et al. 1992). There is a suggestion that lithium may be helpful in this condition (Tyrer et al. 1993).

■ USE OF PSYCHOPHARMACOLOGICAL AGENTS IN THE TREATMENT OF SPECIFIC MENTAL RETARDATION SYNDROMES

The treatment strategies applied within the field of mental retardation are often directed toward controlling the symptoms or aberrant behavior rather than treating specific syndromes. This is not always the best policy. For instance, the self-injurious behavior manifest by sufferers of Lesch-Nyhan syndrome is treated in a very different way from self-mutilatory behavior manifest by a bored, understimulated person confined to the back wards of an institution.

An account of pharmacological treatments that are recommended in specific mental retardation syndromes follows.

Autism

Between 4 and 5 people in every 10,000 have autism, and twice as many have pervasive developmental disorder (Mauk 1993). Although there is a good deal of overlap between autism and other diagnostic groups in mental retardation, this group is sufficiently distinct and warrants attention in its own right. There is also evidence suggesting that treatment in this group is different than for other individuals with mental retardation.

Before treating an autistic patient with psychotropic drugs, it is important to decide which particular symptom or feature is being addressed. Is the aim of treatment to improve social interaction and communication or to reduce stereotypic behavior, secondary aggression, or self-injury? The drugs indicated below are included on the basis of their effects on core autistic symptoms. The treatment of secondary disturbance is covered in the first part of this chapter.

Fenfluramine, a fluorinated amphetamine that does not have the stimulant properties of its parent drug and blocks serotonin receptors, was enthusiastically promoted for the treatment of autism following a report of its use in three autistic boys (Geller et al. 1982). There was an improvement in fundamental autistic features and behavior. However, a later multicenter trial from California did not show major benefits, and treatment successes were mainly related to the reduction of hyperactivity and stereotypy (Ritvo et al. 1987) and it is no longer available for this purpose (Santosh and Baird 1999). More promising results have been obtained using the selective serotonin reuptake inhibitor (SSRI) fluoxetine (Cook et al. 1992) and an experimental 5-HT1A agonist, eltoprazine (Tyrer and Moore 1993). Recent suggestions that the neuropeptide secretin may be helpful have not been supported in a multicenter study in the United States (Sandler et al. 1999).

The opiate antagonist drugs have been used in the treatment of autism since Gillberg et al. (1985) showed high levels of endorphins in the CSF of autistic children. Since then, studies have shown increased physical and eye contact, improved communication, and reduction of aggression and negativism in children and adults treated with naltrexone (Panksepp and Lensing 1991). However, recent studies have been inconclusive (Feldman et al. 1999; Kolmen et al. 1997).

Stereotypic behavior improves with the aid of neuroleptic drugs, which may also decrease the amount of withdrawal, hyperactivity, and negativism. However, the long-term side effects of these drugs make it difficult to recommend them (Sloman 1991). Drugs that decrease sympathetic arousal such as the β-adrenergic blocking drugs and buspirone amend the autistic symptoms (see Chapter 16 of this book) but do not improve sociability and communication.

Pyridoxine, magnesium, and tetrahydrobiopterin have all been used in the treatment of autism in uncontrolled studies, but no consistent benefits have been shown.

There is no drug of choice in autism. The SSRI drugs, β-blockers, and naltrexone may all be used. The specific serotonin reuptake blocking drugs may be of most benefit.

Fragile X Syndrome

There is no convincing evidence that specific drug treatment is useful in fragile X syndrome. However, patients with fragile X often have high levels of arousal (Hagerman and Sobesky 1989), and clonidine and β-blocking drugs may be valuable in reducing these. As the fragile X site is only apparent on chromosomal examination in a folate-deficient medium, folic acid treatment has been proposed for this condition. Barthélémy et al. (1987) found no overall improvement in the behavior of 18 children with fragile X syndrome who were treated with folic acid at a dose of 0.5 mg/kg/day for 8 weeks, but a subgroup of patients with reduced urinary homovanillic acid reduction did have some benefit. Although these results suggest that patients with fragile X syndrome with reduced noradrenergic turnover may benefit from the administration of folic acid, this treatment is not recommended for all patients with this disorder. When fragile X is associated with pervasive developmental disorder, the drugs suggested for the treatment of autism should be considered.

Down's Syndrome

Individuals with Down's syndrome have reduced serotonergic turnover (Tu and Partington 1972). It is therefore not surprising that depression occurs more frequently in Down's syndrome individuals than in other people with mental retardation. The literature suggests that these patients respond well to tricyclic antidepressants (see Chapter 12 of this book). Although mania is not widely reported in Down's syndrome (Sovner et al. 1985), it does occur and lithium and sodium valproate are effective drugs in controlling this.

Lesch-Nyhan Syndrome

In Lesch-Nyhan syndrome there is reduction of dopamine production, leading to dopamine D_2 receptor supersensitivity. It has been shown that the neuroleptic drug fluphenazine is valuable in reducing the self-mutilatory behavior exhibited by Lesch-Nyhan syndrome subjects (Gualtieri and Schroeder 1989). There is evidence that it is the D_2 receptors that are supersensitive (see Chapter 16 of this book), and drugs such as sulpiride and pimozide may be of particular advantage in this condition.

Cornelia de Lange Syndrome

Cornelia de Lange syndrome is another syndrome in which self-injurious behavior has frequently been reported. Isolated patients with low blood serotonin levels have been treated with serotonergic-enhancing drugs, in particular trazodone combined with L-tryptophan (O'Neil et al. 1986). Drugs that reduce arousal may help in this condition.

Prader-Willi Syndrome

Manifest in Prader-Willi syndrome are excessive eating, obesity, and severe aggressive episodes. It has now been recognized that there is a disorder of satiety in these individuals, and drug treatment has been given in an attempt to correct this. Fenfluramine, an appetite suppressant, was used in early studies, and a recent case report suggests that fluoxetine, an antidepressant that marginally reduces weight, is effective in this condition (Benjamin and Buot-Smith 1993). Naltrexone, carbamazepine, and testosterone have also been used in this syndrome (Tu et al. 1992).

■ CONCLUSIONS

The use of psychotropic drugs in mental retardation should be based on accurate diagnoses and sound pharmacological principles. Guidelines encouraging rational prescribing practices are helpful (Deb and Fraser 1994). If success is achieved with the prescribed agent, the decision should then be made as to how long treatment with the drug should be continued and if or when the dose should be reduced. One must keep in mind that patients who demonstrate intermittent behavioral disturbance are likely to improve following a severe behavioral outburst and that the drug which has been given to control the behavior may not be the agent responsible for the improvement. Above all, symptoms and signs that are observed should be assessed so as to determine to what degree these are exhibited due to the drugs or due to psychiatric or behavioral factors. The psychiatrist prescribing psychotropic drugs has to be much more aware of the side effects of these drugs when treating a population who, in the main, are not able to accurately report side effects (Singh et al. 1996).

Once a decision has been made to treat a specific condition with drugs, it may be advantageous to use combination treatments after a single agent has been used for a sufficient length of time with the adequate dosage. In particular, the benefits of lithium and carbamazepine should be more widely utilized.

■ REFERENCES

Aman MG, White AG, Field C: Chlorpromazine effects on stereotypic and conditioned behavior of severely retarded patients: a pilot study. Journal of Mental Deficiency Research 28:253–260, 1984

Aman MG: Risperidone versus placebo for severe conduct disorder in children with mental retardation. Paper presented at the 22nd Collegium Internationale Neuro-Psychopharmacologicum Congress, Brussels, Belgium, July 9–13, 2000

Austin MPV, Souza FGM, Goodwin GM: Lithium augmentation in antidepressant-resistant patients: a quantitative analysis. Br J Psychiatry 159:510–514, 1991

Bancroft J, Tennent G, Loucas K, et al: The control of deviant sexual behavior by drugs. Br J Psychiatry 125:310–315, 1974

Barkley RA: Attention-Deficit Hyperactivity Disorder. New York, Guilford, 1990, pp 34–36

Barthélémy C, Garreau B, Bruneau N, et al: Biological and behavioral effects of magnesium plus vitamin B6, folates, and fenfluramine in autistic children, in Aspects of Autism: Biological Research. Edited by Wing L. Oxford, UK, Gaskell, 1987, pp 59–73

Baumeister AA, Todd ME, Sevin JA: Efficacy and specificity of pharmacological therapies for behavioral disorders in persons with mental retardation. Clin Neuropharmacol 16:271–294, 1993

Bell AJ, Cole A, Eccleston D, et al: Lithium neurotoxicity at normal therapeutic levels. Br J Psychiatry 162:689–692, 1993

Benjamin E, Buot-Smith T: Naltrexone and fluoxetine in Prader-Willi Syndrome. J Am Acad Child Adolesc Psychiatry 32:870–873, 1993

Boachie A, McGinnity MGA: Use of Clozapine in a mental handicap hospital: report of the first 17 patients. Irish Journal of Psychological Medicine 4:16–19, 1997

Bouras N, Drummond C: Behavior and psychiatric disorders of people with mental handicaps living in the community. J Intellect Disabil Res 36:349–357, 1992

Boyd RD: Recurrence of neuroleptic malignant syndrome via an inadvertent rechallenge in a woman with mental retardation. Ment Retard 30:77–79, 1992

Brooke D: Patients with learning disability at Kneesworth House Hospital: the first five years. Psychiatric Bulletin 22:29–32, 1998

Burd L, Fisher W, Vesely BN, et al: Prevalence of psychoactive drug use among North Dakota group home residents. Am J Ment Retard 96:119–126, 1991

Carlson G: Affective psychoses in mental retardates. Psychiatr Clin North Am 2(3):499–510, 1979

Chandler M, Burnhill LJ, Gualtieri CT: Amantadine: profile of use in the developmentally disabled, in Mental Retardation: Developing Pharmacotherapies. Edited by Ratey JJ. Washington, DC, American Psychiatric Press, 1991, pp 139–162

Clarke DJ: Antilibidinal drugs and mental retardation: a review. Med Sci Law 29:136–146, 1989

Clarke DJ, Kelley S, Thinn K, et al: Psychotropic drugs and mental retardation; 1: disabilities and the prescription of drugs for behavior and for epilepsy in three residential settings. Journal of Mental Deficiency Research 34:385–395, 1990

Cook EH, Rowlatt R, Jaselskis C, et al: Fluoxetine treatment of children and adults with autistic disorder and mental retardation. J Am Acad Child Adolesc Psychiatry 31:739–745, 1992

Craft M, Ismail IA, Krishnamurty D, et al: Lithium in the treatment of aggression in mentally handicapped patients: a double-blind trial. Br J Psychiatry 150:685–689, 1987

Day K: Psychiatric disorder in middle aged and elderly mentally handicapped. Br J Psychiatry 147:660–667, 1985

Day K: Male mentally handicapped sex offenders. Br J Psychiatry 165:630–639, 1994

Deb S, Fraser W: The use of psychotropic medication in people with learning disability: towards rational prescribing. Human Psychopharmacology 9:259–272, 1994

De Koning P, Mak M, de Vries MH, et al: Eltoprazine in aggressive mentally handicapped patients: a double-blind placebo and baseline-controlled multi-centre study. Int Clin Psychopharmacol 9:187–194, 1994

Delle Chiaie R, Picardi A: Supra-hypophyseal block in gonad function in treatment of paraphelia: administration of goserelin in five case reports. Rivistia di Psichiatrica 29(suppl):39–46, 1994

Dilsaver SC: Withdrawal phenomena associated with antidepressant and antipsychotic agents. Drug Safety 10:103–114, 1994

Feldman HM, Kolmen BK, Gonzaga AM: Natrexone and communication skills in young children with autism. J Am Acad Child Adolesc Psychiatry 38:587–593, 1999

Ferrier IN, Tyrer SP, Bell A: Lithium therapy. Advances in Psychiatric Treatment 1:102–110, 1995

Fischbacher E: Prescribing in a hospital for the mentally retarded. Journal of Mental Deficiency Research 31:17–19, 1987

Gagiano CA, Read S, Thorpe L: A double-blind study of risperidone versus placebo for behavioural disturbances in adults with conduct spectrum disorders and subaverage IQs (abstract). International Journal of Neuropsychopharmacy 3:164, 2000

Garber HJ, McGonigle JJ, Slumke GT, et al: Clomipramine treatment of stereotypic behaviors and self-injury in patients with developmental disabilities. J Am Acad Child Adolesc Psychiatry 31:1157–1160, 1992

Gedye A: Neuroleptic-induced dementia documented in four patients with mental retardation. Ment Retard 36:182–186, 1998

Geller E, Ritvo E, Freeman BJ, et al: Preliminary observations on the effect of fenfluramine on blood serotonin and symptoms in three autistic boys. N Engl J Med 307:165–168, 1982

Gillberg C, Terenius L, Lonnerholm G: Endorphin activity in childhood psychosis. Arch Gen Psychiatry 42:780–783, 1985

Glasser M: Paedophilia, in Principles and Practice of Forensic Psychiatry. Edited by Bluglass R, Bowden P. Edinburgh, UK, Churchill Livingstone, 1990, pp 739–748

Glue P: Rapid-cycling affective disorders in the mentally retarded. Biol Psychiatry 26:250–256, 1989

Gross EJ, Hull HG, Lytton GJ, et al: Case study of neuroleptic-induced akathisia: important implications for individuals with mental retardation. Am J Ment Retard 98:164–156, 1993

Gualtieri CT: TMS: a system for prevention and control, in Mental Retardation: Developing Pharmacotherapies. Edited by Ratey JJ. Washington, DC, American Psychiatric Press, 1991

Gualtieri CT, Schroeder SR: Pharmacotherapy for self-injurious behavior: preliminary tests of the D1 hypothesis. Psychopharmacol Bull 25:364–371, 1989

Gutierrez-Esteinou R, Grebb JA: Risperidone: an analysis of the first three years in general use. International Clinical Psychopharmacology 12(suppl 4):3–10, 1997

Hagerman RJ, Sobesky WE: Psychopathology in Fragile-X syndrome. Am J Orthopsychiatry 59:142–152, 1989

Hasan S, Buckley P: Novel antipsychotics and the neuroleptic malignant syndrome: a review and critique. Am J Psychiatry 155:1113–1116, 1998

Hemming H: Psychotropic medication needs of mentally retarded adults before and after transfer from institutions to new small units, in Perspectives and Progress in Mental Retardation, Vol 2. Edited by Berg JM. Baltimore, MD, Park Press, 1984, pp 349–356

Intagliata J, Rinck C: Psychoactive drug use in public and community residential facilities for mentally retarded persons. Psychopharmacol Bull 21:268–278, 1985

Keks NA, Copolov DL, Burrows GD: Discontinuing antipsychotic therapy: a practical guide. Central Nervous System Drugs 4:351–356, 1995

Kolmen BK, Feldman HM, Handen BL, et al: Naltrexone in young autistic children: Replication study and learning measures. J Am Acad Child Adolesc Psychiatry 36:1570–1578, 1997

Langee HR: A retrospective study of mentally retarded patients with behavioral disorders who were treated with carbamazepine. Am J Ment Retard 93:640–643, 1989

Langee HR, Conlon M: Predictors of response to antidepressant medications. Am J Ment Retard 97:65–70, 1992

Lewis L: Warning on cyproterone. Lancet 345:247, 1995

Linnoila M, Higley D, Nielsen D, et al: Serotonin and impulse control: from clinic to clone. Eur Neuropsychopharmacol 3:161, 1993

Linter CM, Linter SPK: Severe lactic acidosis following paraldehyde administration. Br J Psychiatry 149:650–651, 1986

Lund J: The prevalence of psychiatric morbidity in mentally retarded adults. Acta Psychiatr Scand 72:563–570, 1985

Lund J: Psychopharmacological approaches to the treatment of depression in the mentally retarded, in Depression in Mentally Retarded Children and Adults. Edited by Dosen A, Menolascino FJ. Leiden, Netherlands, Logan Publications, 1990, pp 331–339

Lynch DM, Eliatamby CLS, Anderson AA: Pipothiazine palmitate in the management of aggressive mentally handicapped patients. Br J Psychiatry 146:525–529, 1985

Malt UF, Nystad R, Bache T: The effectiveness of zuclopenthixol compared with that of haloperidol in the treatment of behavioral disturbances in mentally retarded patients: a double blind crossover study. Br J Psychiatry 166:374–377, 1995

Manchester D: Neuroleptics, learning disability and the community: some history and mystery. BMJ 307:184–187, 1993

Mauk JE: Autism and pervasive developmental disorders. Pediatr Clin North Am 40(3):567–578, 1993

Neppe VM: The serotonin 1A neuromodulation of aggression: bomodal buspirone dosage as a prototype anti-irritability agent in adults. Australian Journal of Psychopharmacology 9:8–25, 1999

O'Neil M, Page N, Adkins WN, et al: Tryptophan-trazodone treatment of aggressive behavior. Lancet 2:859–860, 1986

Panksepp J, Lensing P: Brief report: a synopsis of an open trial of naltrexone treatment of autism with four children. J Autism Dev Disord 21:243–249, 1991

Price LH, Charney DS, Henninger GR: Variability of response to lithium augmentation in refractory depression. Am J Psychiatry 143:1387–1392, 1986

Ratey JJ, Sovner R, Parks A, et al: Buspirone treatment of aggression and anxiety in mentally retarded patients: a multiple baseline, placebo lead-in study. J Clin Psychiatry 52:159–162, 1991

Reid AH: Psychiatry and mental handicap, in Mental Handicap. Edited by Craft M, Bicknell J, Hollins S. London, Bailliere Tindall, 1985, pp 317–332

Reid AH, Naylor GJ, Kay DSG: A double-blind placebo-controlled crossover trial of carbamazepine in overactive, severely mentally handicapped patients. Psychol Med 11:109–113, 1981

Rinck C, Guidry J, Calkins CF: Review of states' practices on the use of psychotropic medication. Am J Ment Retard 93:657–668, 1989

Ritvo ER, Freeman BJ, Yuwillier A, et al: Fenfluramine treatment of autism: UCLA collaborative study of 81 patients at nine medical centers. Psychopharmacol Bull 22:1333–1340, 1987

Sachdev P: Drug-induced movement disorders in institutionalized adults with mental retardation: clinical characteristics and risk factors. Aust N Z J Psychiatry 26:242–248, 1992

Sandler AD, Sutton KA, DeWeese J, et al: Lack of benefit of a single dose of synthetic human secretin in the treatment of autism and pervasive developmental disorder. N Engl J Med 341:1801–1806, 1999

Sandman CA, Barron JL, Colman H: An orally administered opiate blocker, naltrexone, attenuates self-injurious behavior. Am J Ment Retard 95:93–102, 1990

Santosh PJ, Baird G: Psychopharmacotherapy in children and adults with intellectual disability. Lancet 354(1): 233–242, 1999

Shriqui CL, Bradwejn J, Jones B: Tardive dyskinesia: legal and preventive aspects. Can J Psychiatry 35:576–580, 1990

Singh NN, Ellis CR, Donatelli LS et al: Professionals' perceptions of psychotropic medication in residential facilities for individuals with mental retardation. J Intellect Disabil Res 40:1–7, 1996

Sloman L: Use of medication in pervasive developmental disorders. Psychiatr Clin North Am 14:165–182, 1991

Sovner R, Hurley AD, Labrie R: Is mania incompatible with Down's syndrome? Br J Psychiatry 146:319–320, 1985

Stein G: Drug treatment of the personality disorders. Br J Psychiatry 161:167–184, 1992

Thomas H: Droperidol vs haloperidol for chemical restraint of agitated and combative patients. Ann Emerg Med 21:407–413, 1992

Thuresson K, Farnstrand M: A follow-up of medical treatment of persons with psychiatric health oproblems and mental; retardation. Nordic Journal of Psychiatry 53:127–130, 1999

Tschen AC, Rieder MJ, Oyewumi LK, Freeman DJ: The cytotoxity of clozapine metabolites: implications for predicting clozapine-induced agranulocytosis. Clin Pharmacol Ther 65:526–532, 1999

Tu J-B, Partington MW: 5-Hydroxyindole levels in the blood and CSF in Down's syndrome, phenylketonuria, and severe mental retardation. Dev Med Child Neurol 14:457–466, 1972

Tu J-B, Hartridge C, Izqwa J: Psychopharmacogenetic aspects of Prader-Willi syndrome. J Am Acad Child Adolesc Psychiatry 31:1137–1140, 1992

Tyrer SP: The assessment and physical treatment of affective disorder. British Journal of Hospital Medicine 42:184–194, 1989

Tyrer SP: Lithium intoxication: appropriate treatment. Central Nervous System Drugs 6:426–439, 1996

Tyrer SP: The management of aggression. Primary Care Psychiatry 4:109–119, 1998

Tyrer SP, Dunstan J: Schizophrenia, in The Psychiatry of Learning Disability. Edited by Read SG. London, WB Saunders 1997, pp 185–215

Tyrer SP, Moore PB: Eltoprazine improves autistic symptoms in self-injurious mentally handicapped patients (abstract). Eur Neuropsychopharmacol 3:384, 1993

Tyrer SP, Walsh A, Edwards DE, et al: Factors associated with a good response to lithium in aggressive mentally handicapped subjects. Progress in Neuro-psychopharmacology and Biological Psychiatry 8:751–755, 1984

Tyrer SP, Aronson ME, Lauder J: Effect of lithium on behavioral factors in aggressive mentally handicapped subjects, in Lithium in Medicine and Biology. Edited by Birch NJ, Padgham C, Hughes MS. Carnforth, UK, Marius Press, 1993, pp 119–125

Van den Borre R, Vermote R, Butiens M: Risperidone as add-on therapy in behavioral disturbances in mental retardation: a double-blind placebo-controlled cross-over study. Acta Psychiatr Scand 87:167–171, 1993

Vanstraelen M, Tyrer SP: Rapid cycling bipolar affective disorder in people with intellectual disability: a systematic review. J Intellect Disabil Res 43:349–359, 1999

Verhoeven WMA, Tuinier S: The effect of buspirone on challenging behaviour in mentally retarded patients: an open prospective multiple case study. J Intellect Disabil Res 40:502–508, 1996

Willemsen-Swinkels SHN, Buitelaar JK, Nijhof GJ, et al: Failure of naltrexone hydrochloride to reduce self-injurious and autistic behaviuor in mentally retarded adults: double-blind placebo controlled studies. Arch Gen Psychiatry 52:766–773, 1995

Wirshing DA, Marshall BD Jr, Green MF, et al: Risperidone in treatment: refractory schizophrenia. Am J Psychiatry 156:1374–1379, 1999

Wressell SE, Tyrer SP, Berney TP: Reduction in antipsychotic drug dosage in mentally handicapped patients: a hospital study. Br J Psychiatry 157:101–106, 1990

4 Behavioral Therapies

Individualizing Interventions Through Treatment Formulations

William I. Gardner, Ph.D.
Janice L. Graeber-Whalen, Ph.D.
Debby R. Ford, Ph.D.

Reports of the successful application of the behavioral therapies to the treatment of emotional and behavioral disorders presented by persons with mental retardation began to appear with some regularity during the 1950s and 1960s. Gardner (1970) offered the following impressions of the impact of this early work:

> Recent results of the application of behavior modification techniques described in the clinical and research literature provide illustration of behavior change of a range, degree, and rate that most psychiatric, psychological, and rehabilitation professionals had not thought possible due to the presumed inherent limitations of those with mental retardation. These reports suggest that at least a significant degree of the behavioral limitations of persons with mental retardation reflects the effects of an inappropriate or limited learning environment, rather than being an unalterable manifestation of the person's retardation. As a result of treatment programs involving the systematic application of behavior modification procedures, persons with severe and profound levels of mental retardation, previously viewed as being beyond help or hope, developed language, motor, perceptual, cognitive, affective, and social skills that rendered them increasingly independent and able to experience a more meaningful personal and social existence. Additionally, other less disabled persons exhibiting an array of maladaptive behavior patterns have responded favorably to behavior modification programs. (pp. 250–251)

Ms. Graeber-Whalen died in early 2000, shortly after beginning her professional career. This chapter is dedicated to her.

In the ensuing years, the behavior therapies and their applications to psychological problems presented by persons with mental retardation have undergone notable advances (Gardner 1988, 2000; Gardner and Graeber 1994). These advances involve 1) an increased emphasis on interventions based on hypothesized instigating and maintaining factors (Carr 1977; Carr and Durand 1985); 2) the expansion of the unimodal (operant) behavioral model to include other psychological, biological, and socioenvironmental contributions to aberrant behavior (Bailey and Pyles 1989; Carr et al. 1996; Gardner et al. 1996; Griffiths et al. 1998); 3) development of multimodal models that systematically guide the diagnostic intervention formulation process to ensure appropriate staging and integration of behavioral interventions with those addressing biomedical and socioenvironmental influences (Gardner and Sovner 1994; Gardner and Whalen 1996); and 4) adoption of a skill deficit perspective with a concurrent habilitative intervention focus of teaching social and coping competency skills to replace aberrant responding (Gardner 2000; Gardner et al. 1996). A collateral of the latter trend has been an increased emphasis on teaching self-management skills and providing choices as self-controlled alternatives to external management procedures (Gardner and Cole 1989; Harchik et al. 1993; Kogel et al. 1996).

Contemporary behavior therapies represent a constellation of clinical procedures derived from operant, classical, social, and cognitive learning and related theoretical models of human functioning. Such terms as *applied behavior analysis, behavior management, behavior modification, behavior therapy, behavioral treatment, cognitive-behavioral therapy, contingency management, emotional retraining, reinforcement therapy,* and *social skills training* are used by various writers either to refer to specific groups of procedures or as generic labels to encompass the entire range of behavior analysis and change procedures and their major conceptual foundations.

The major assumption underlying behavior therapy procedures is that behavioral and emotional difficulties reflect the effects of faulty or deficient learning experiences. The behavior therapies are used to offset the effects of these (Gardner 1988; Gardner and Cole 1984; O'Donohue and Krasner 1995; Repp and Horner 1999). To accomplish this objective, the behavior therapist selects specific therapeutic procedures from an array of the ones available. This selection is guided by the results of a diagnostic study of the specific personal and environmental contexts of a person's symptoms. As illustrations, on the basis of client-specific diagnostic formulations of instigating, vulnerability, and maintaining conditions, a therapist may choose: 1) systematic desensitization and related stimulus exposure procedures (respondent-based learning paradigm) to eliminate clinically significant fears and obsessive-compulsive behaviors for some clients (Erfanian and Miltenberger 1990; Hiss and Kozak

1991), 2) a skills training program (operant-based learning paradigm) to teach alternative functional communication skills to replace self-injurious and aggressive symptoms for a second client (Bird et al. 1989; Carr et al. 1994), 3) a social skills program (social learning paradigm) to teach prosocial interpersonal skills as alternatives to aggressive and other disruptive responding of adults with a dual diagnosis of psychosis and mental retardation (Matson and Stephens 1978), 4) a self-management program (cognitive-behavioral learning paradigm) to teach coping alternatives to multiple behavioral and emotional symptoms for clients with chronic and severe behavior disorders (Benson 1992; Cole et al. 1985; Jackson and Altman 1996; Koegel and Koegel 1990; Reese et al. 1984; Woods et al. 1996). Primary sources providing more comprehensive descriptions of these and related applications to persons with mental retardation include Cipani (1989), Gardner and Cole (1993), Gardner and Sovner (1994), Jacobson and Mulick (1996), Luiselli et al. (1992), Matson and Barrett (1993), Nezu et al. (1992), and Thompson and Gray (1994).

■ MULTIMODAL CONTEXTUAL APPROACH

Historically, behavioral and emotional symptoms presented by those with mental retardation have been viewed from either a biomedical *or* a behavioral perspective, with the frequent result that behaviorally responsive symptoms/disorders were "medicalized" and biomedically responsive symptoms/disorders were "behavioralized." The overuse of psychotropic medications and the misuse of behavioral procedures to suppress symptoms in the absence of a diagnostic understanding of the specific and frequently multiple factors influencing symptom presentation resulted. Dissatisfaction with these isolated approaches has resulted in an integrative *multimodal* alternative to diagnosis and treatment selection. This multimodal alternative reflects a *bio-psycho-social* view of human behavior in emphasizing that behavioral and emotional difficulties represent the influences of a person with psychological and biomedical, including psychiatric and neuropsychiatric, characteristics as he or she interacts with physical and psychosocial environments (Gardner and Sovner 1994; Gardner and Whalen 1996; Gardner et al. 1996).

To illustrate the interaction of these multiple influences, biologically based psychiatric conditions such as schizophrenia or a bipolar disorder may result in changes in cognitive functions, mood and affective states, emotional regulation, and psychomotor behaviors. These changing psychological and physical characteristics may result in new behavioral or emotional difficulties or may influence the occurrence or increased severity of problems that predated the current psychiatric episode (Lowery and Sovner 1991a). These symptoms in turn create more than usual changes in the manner in which the social environment responds to and interacts with the person and his or her problem behaviors. These experiences with the social environment may in a reciprocal manner strengthen the problem behaviors or intensify the emotional arousal and the person's perceptions of the social feedback. An effective treatment program must be sensitive to these reciprocal interrelationships and provide attention to each set of influences (Gardner and Sovner 1994).

A closely related concept of the multimodal approach to treatment selection is the interactive nature of the psychological components of this bio-psycho-social triad. Although a person's behavioral symptoms such as aggression or self-injury frequently are those that create most concern to the clinician, the functional approach recognizes the interactive effects of *behaviors, emotions,* and *cognitions.* A person's behavior (e.g., physical aggression) influences his or her feelings (e.g., anger, anxiety) and cognitions (e.g., "He deserved that") just as the person's feelings and/or cognitions may influence his or her behaviors.

Therapeutic intervention may be directed toward changing any one or each of these interacting psychological components as a means of reducing the clinical problem. As described by Benson and Valenti-Hein in Chapter 5 of this book, if a person's aggression is influenced by anger arousal, the focus of behavior therapy becomes one of teaching the person to control or reduce his or her anger and, as a result, reduce the likelihood of aggressive behavior. In other instances, a person may engage, for example, in the repetitive thoughts that a co-worker is dangerous and attempting to harm him or her. As a result of this perceptual set, the person may act aggressively if provoked by the co-worker. Modification of the ruminative thinking through the use of either behavior therapy or psychoactive medication may remove critical instigating conditions for the aggressive acts. A decrease in aggression would be expected (Gardner et al. 1983b). Finally, a person's aggressive behaviors may be followed immediately by the self-delivery of negative consequences. These experiences may result in the inhibition of future impulses for aggressive acts, changes in the person's cognitions (e.g., "I'll not hit him because I'll lose my bonus"), and a reduction in the level of anger, which, in turn, may result in a decrease in aggressive responding (Cole et al. 1985).

In sum, regardless of the specific type or focus of behavioral intervention, it is recognized that each component of a person's psychological triad (behaviors, emotions, cognitions) may be influenced. Thus, psychological, or medical when addressing biomedically related influences, intervention efforts address one or a combination of these interactive conditions viewed as critical in influencing symptom occurrence (Gardner and Whalen 1996; Sovner and Hurley 1992).

■ EXPLANATION OF MALADAPTIVE PSYCHOLOGICAL FEATURES

In seeking to understand a person's presenting symptoms, the major preintervention diagnostic focus of the behavior therapist is that of developing a contemporary explanation derived from a comprehensive *contextual analysis*. This analysis involves identifying the current external and internal conditions that influence the occurrence and persistence of these problem behaviors. In this diagnostic process, care is taken to distinguish *description* from *explanation*. It may be observed that an adolescent's episodes of verbal and physical aggression are accompanied by an agitated state of anger. It might be tempting to suggest, "He fights because he is angry," thus using a description of one characteristic as an explanation for another. Being angry may be *one* of the conditions that increases the likelihood of fighting, but anger would not be viewed as an adequate explanation of the behavior. The behavior therapist would identify other *preceding* events or conditions (e.g., teased by a physically smaller peer; reprimanded by staff when in an irritable emotional state), *consequences* (e.g., the aggressive acts are functional in terminating the teasing), and *personal vulnerability features* (e.g., the adolescent has limited alternative skills of coping with his anger or of eliminating the teasing) as a basis for developing a more useful complex of interrelated explanations and therapeutic interventions.

■ FOCUS OF BEHAVIOR THERAPY

A major objective of the behavior therapies is one of teaching coping skills that serve as functional alternatives for excessively occurring behavioral and emotional symptoms. This is accomplished through addressing the factors presumed to produce the symptoms. In illustration, an adult who is displaying temper tantrums in his home is taught both to "control his temper" and to express his emotions in a more acceptable manner. If a child is physically aggressive when she becomes jealous of the social attention provided to her peers, and as a result is isolated by them, the behavior therapy goals would consist of teaching the child alternative socially appropriate and personally enhancing skills of relating both to her feelings and to her peers (Gardner and Moffatt 1990).

Support for an intervention focus on teaching prosocial replacement behaviors rather than one that merely attempts to suppress or eliminate the occurrence of inappropriate behaviors is found in the observation that the elimination or suppression of symptomatic behaviors offers no assurance that appropriate behaviors will begin to occur. The person with developmental disabilities simply may have no prosocial functionally equivalent alternatives in his or her coping skills repertoire. Thus behavior suppression through either medication or aversive environmental contingencies may leave the person without effective coping behaviors and even more vulnerable to demonstrating maladaptive responding (Carr et al. 1994; Gardner and Cole 1989).

■ CONTEXTUAL DIAGNOSTICS: OVERVIEW

As there is no single or simple psychological or biomedical mechanism that underlies emotional and behavioral symptoms, a diagnostic assessment includes evaluation of the various personal and environmental contexts in which these occur, namely, 1) the complete stimulus complex that precedes and serves to instigate these symptoms, 2) the person's biopsychosocial vulnerabilities or risk factors for engaging in these symptoms when confronted with the instigating stimulus complex, and 3) those proximate consequences that follow behavioral occurrences and contribute to their functionality and strength. In developing an understanding of a person's aberrant symptoms as a basis for selecting person-specific interventions, a set of diagnostic intervention formulations evolves from the following four-step process.

Contextual Analysis 1: Instigating Conditions

The initial diagnostic task is that of placing the behavior in the context of current external (e.g., specific task demands, reduced social attention) and internal (e.g., anxiety, premenstrual pain, dysphoric mood, anger, paranoid ideation, organically based overarousal) stimulus conditions of a biomedical, psychological, and socioenvironmental nature that contribute to the instigation of the behavioral and emotional symptoms. These conditions, as defined later, may serve either a primary or a contributing instigating function.

Contextual Analysis 2: Vulnerability Influences

Observations relating to instigating conditions are combined with those describing relevant personal characteristics (e.g., sensory impairments, anger management skills, borderline personality disorder, communication, coping skills) and socioenvironmental or ecological features (e.g., opportunity for social interaction, type and frequency of structured program activities) that by their absence, low strength, infrequency of occurrence, or pathological nature may contribute to a person's behavioral symptoms. These are viewed as vulnerability influences that place the person at risk for demonstrating the behavioral symptoms under the previously identified conditions of instigation. To elaborate, these vulnerabilities increase the risk of aberrant responding in those persons inclined to use such inappropriate responses to cope with external or internal instigating conditions. No functionally equivalent prosocial alternative behaviors may be present in the person's repertoire or, if present, may not be as effective or efficient as the behavioral symptoms in meeting the person's current needs (Horner and Day 1991). Thus, when attempting to understand and program for a person's symptoms, knowledge of these vulnerability conditions (deficit and pathology areas) guides the clinician in simultaneously pinpointing specific functionally equivalent coping skills and related cognitive, emotional, and motivational supports that will be required for continued successful social and interpersonal functioning following termination of an intervention program (Carr et al. 1994).

Contextual Analysis 3: Maintaining Conditions

Given the instigating stimulus conditions and vulnerability influences, the final focus of the contextual analysis is the identification of the purposes or functions being served by the behavioral symptoms (e.g., terminate aversive demands, modulate pain, decrease unpleasant internal arousal, ensure physical contact and other social feedback). These contingent consequences strengthen the behavioral inclination and account for the repeated occurrence of the symptoms under future similar instigating and vulnerability influences.

Diagnostically Based Treatment Formulations

These diagnostic hunches about primary and contributing instigating conditions, relevant vulnerabilities, and the functionality of the symptoms form the basis for the formulation of diagnostically based interventions addressing each of the presumed contributing influences. Major program efforts are designed to 1) remove or minimize biomedical and psychosocial instigating and maintaining conditions, 2) teach prosocial coping alternatives and increase the personal motivation to use these newly acquired skills as adaptive functional replacements for the maladaptive symptoms, and 3) reduce or eliminate pathological biomedical conditions and impoverished and abusive features of the social and physical environments that place the person at continued risk. A skill enhancement program focus to offset psychological vulnerabilities is especially pertinent for persons with highly restricted repertoires of coping behaviors. In this personal context, aberrant behavioral symptoms may represent highly effective and efficient functional behaviors and must be replaced by equally effective and efficient functionally equivalent coping skills if the symptoms are to be minimized or eliminated (Gardner 2000; Gardner and Sovner 1994; Lowery and Sovner 1991b; Repp and Horner 1999).

To summarize, the diagnostic intervention formulation process is *person focused* rather than *symptom focused*. In illustration, one person may impulsively engage in aggressive outbursts when angry or overly anxious, whereas another person's aggression may be more deliberate and goal directed. The diagnostic formulations and related interventions obviously would differ for these two persons as different influences contribute to the occurrence of the common symptom of aggression (Gardner et al. 1996).

■ TRANSLATING DIAGNOSTIC FORMULATIONS INTO INTERVENTIONS

In the remaining sections, the components of the multimodal contextual analyses required for selecting behavior therapy interventions are described and illustrated with applications from the empirical literature. As described, behavioral treatments, when diagnostically indicated, are closely interfaced with interventions of a biomedical nature (Gardner and Sovner 1994; Gardner and Whalen 1996; Gardner et al. 1996).

■ CONTEXTUAL ANALYSIS 1: INSTIGATING CONDITIONS

As noted, the initial contextual analysis seeks to identify those antecedent conditions that, individually or in combination, instigate problem behaviors. These include external physical and social environmental conditions as well as covert psychological and biomedical features of the person. These antecedent conditions may serve a primary instigating or a contributing instigating role. *Primary discriminative instigating events* refer to antecedent stimulus states that are necessary conditions for the occurrence of specific behaviors, that is, the behavior does not occur in the absence of these. *Contributing instigating conditions* refer to those antecedent stimulus conditions that while in isolation are not sufficient to instigate a behavioral occurrence but do, when present, increase the likelihood that a symptom will occur under primary instigating conditions.

Primary Instigating Conditions: Discriminative Events

Aberrant emotional and behavioral features that are currently a part of a person's repertoire do not occur randomly or haphazardly. Rather, these, as only one component of the person's total array of appropriate and inappropriate behaviors, occur in a discriminating manner at certain times, in specific places, and under certain stimulus conditions. External instigating conditions may include such physical and social events as a work supervisor's reprimands for substandard work performance, termination or reduction in frequency of staff attention, directives from a specific staff, someone staring, or taunts of a peer as well as other sources of environmental stimulation such as high noise level, overcrowding, or agitated peer models.

Covert stimulus conditions may include both transitory and more enduring affective states such as anger, depression, anxiety, chronic sadness; cognitive influences such as provocative covert ruminations and paranoid ideation; perceptual features such as auditory and visual hallucinations; and psychological distress features resulting from biomedical states such as fatigue, seizure activity, drug effects, chronic pain, overarousal and irritability associated with neurological impairment, and premenstrual discomfort. To illustrate these instigating influences, a person with severe distress associated with a high level of anxiety arousal and no functional communication skills for use in soliciting assistance from others may repeatedly engage in face and head slapping in an attempt to reduce the level of distress (Gardner and Sovner 1994; Sovner and Pary 1993).

Such specific discriminative events begin to gain influence over the occurrence of problem behaviors by being associated repeatedly with reinforcing consequences produced by these acts. As a result of this behavior-consequence relationship, specific maladaptive behaviors, instead of other responses in a person's repertoire, become increasingly likely to occur in the presence of specific physical stimuli, specific people, specific types and intensity levels of psychological distress; at certain times and places; or following other specific types of stimulus conditions such as tone of voice with which a directive is presented or the difficulty level of a task. Also, these behaviors are unlikely to appear in situations in which reinforcement has not occurred or in which contingent negative consequences have been present (Touchette et al. 1985).

In summary, primary instigating stimulus conditions (e.g., peer taunts) signal the time, place, and conditions under which specific responses (e.g., verbal aggression) are likely to result in specific consequences (e.g., removal of peer taunts). Typically, specific behavioral symptoms are instigated by multiple antecedent stimulus events. Associated with each event is a conditional probability that, when present, the behavior will occur (Gardner 1996).

Intervention Procedures Addressing Discriminative Events

Mace and Knight (1986) performed a contextual analysis of pica in "Jim," a 19-year-old profoundly retarded male. It was noted that Jim was most likely to engage in pica during times of minimal staff supervision and, paradoxically, when wearing a helmet with a face shield (the shield did not completely prevent pica; rather it served as a deterrent). Intervention consisted of providing a combination of stimulus conditions under which it had been determined that Jim was less apt to engage in pica, namely, noncontingent staff interaction consisting of talking to and/or touching (15–30 seconds once every 3 minutes) and no helmet. Pica decreased from an average of 89.0% to 14.8% of intervals under the new stimulus conditions. Contrary to suggestions offered by other writers that altering stimulus conditions by enriching environments may lead to increased alternative behaviors, Mace and Knight posit that the decrease in pica behavior in this instance was due to a change in stimulus control.

Other studies have demonstrated the value of providing alternative means of obtaining valued sensory stimulation in managing the frequency of such aberrant behaviors as self-injury and stereotypy observed under restricted or deprived stimulus conditions. In these studies, behavioral occurrence was assumed to be maintained by the sensory stimulation produced by the self-injury and stereotypy. Providing opportunity for alternative behaviors producing similar sensory stimulation resulted in a decline in the aberrant responding.

Madden et al. (1980) provided three different settings to children who had been hospitalized for lead poisoning due to pica: an enriched individual play environment, a group play environment, and an impoverished individual play environment. Rates of pica were three to five times greater in the impoverished environment than in the enriched settings. In a second illustration of this strategy of modifying antecedent stimulus conditions, Favell et al. (1982) noted that the eye-poking, hand-mouthing, and pica self-injurious behaviors (SIBs) of a group of young adults with profound mental retardation occurred primarily when alone and unoccupied. A proactive behavior management program, based on the diagnostic hypothesis that the SIBs were maintained by the resulting visual or gustatory reinforcement, altered the antecedent stimulus conditions by providing toys, which set the occasion for an appropriate alternative to SIBs. Under these enriched conditions, the adults had an opportunity to engage in toy play that provided sensory reinforcement similar to that associated with SIBs. Following demonstration of the value of this environmental alteration in producing substantial reduction of SIBs, an added treatment component of external reinforcement of more appropriate conventional toy play resulted in further reduction. In each case, the self-stimulation produced by the toys involved the same sensory modality as that associated with SIBs (e.g., clients who eye-poked used the toys to produce visual self-stimulation; those who engaged in hand-mouthing and pica began chewing the toys). These results emphasized the value of matching the sensory activities provided by the intervention program with the sensory stimulation involved in the self-injury. Lancioni et al. (1984) used a similar program approach of providing valued sensory stimulation. Under the assumption that antecedent activating stimulus conditions for severe tantrums of adults with multiple handicaps consisted of sensory deprivation, these therapists provided daily periods of gross motor activities designed to ensure varied sensory input. Tantrums reduced in frequency and duration.

Based on the hypothesis that ruminative vomiting in two men with profound mental retardation was instigated by a state of food deprivation, Jackson et al. (1975) provided double meal portions, including milk shakes, cereal, and ice cream as well as a milk shake between meals, to maintain the effect of satiation throughout the day. A 94% reduction in the frequency of rumination was obtained with one adult and a 50% improvement in the other. Success with this procedure of food satiation was also reported by Clauser and Scibak (1990) in treatment of three males with profound mental retardation, by Libby and Phillips (1979) in treatment of a 17-year-old adolescent, and by Rast et al. (1981) with adults with severe and profound mental retardation. Each ensured satiation by providing unlimited quantities of such high-caloric carbohydrates as cream of wheat, bread, and potatoes. Clauser and Scibak (1990) and Yang (1988) described successful fading procedures to return the clients to normal food intake.

Primary Instigating Conditions: Conditioned Stimulus Events

A respondent conditioning paradigm has been used to account for various escape and avoidance behaviors when a person is confronted with specific stimulus events. These antecedents serve as the instigating conditions for a number of fear and anxiety responses that accompany and provide the motivation for escape or avoidance behaviors. These stimulus conditions represent a second class of primary instigating conditions, called *conditioned stimuli*, and serve to produce a range of emotional responses such as fear, anger, anxiety, or dysphoria (Ollendick et al. 1993). Once identified, variations of a systematic desensitization procedure combined with participant modeling have been used to reduce the fear-provoking qualities of specific stimulus conditions (Benson 1990; McNally 1991; Ollendick et al. 1993). As the fear-arousing features of the stimulus conditions are reduced during behavioral treatment, the motivation for the aberrant escape/avoidance behavior decreases.

Intervention Procedures Addressing Instigating-Conditioned Stimuli

Rivenq (1974) used a modified systematic desensitization procedure to eliminate trichophobia in a 13-year-old male with a dual diagnosis of mild mental retardation and schizophrenia. The boy's fear of hair was reported to be of such intensity that he expressed a desire to have a feminine body. He turned his head away whenever exposed to the therapist's hairy arms and hands. Graduated exposure to the fear-provoking stimulus through a series of pictures depicting increasingly hairy men, combined with a counterconditioning procedure of providing candies and French pastries as each picture was exposed, resulted in the elimination of the phobia.

Freeman et al. (1976) described the elimination of a fear of physical examination in a 7-year-old male with mild retardation through the use of a systematic desensitization procedure. The child had a retinal disorder that required frequent examinations by physicians. His fear became so intense that it had become necessary to perform the biannual ophthalmologic examination under general anesthesia. An 11-step hierarchy of the ophthalmologic examination experience was developed, beginning with the boy entering the examination room and ending with having his eyes examined with an ophthalmoscope.

A nurse, with whom the boy had a positive relationship, guided him through each step in the hierarchy. If at any time the boy demonstrated signs of anxiety (e.g., lack of cooperation, running about the room), that step was completed and the session was terminated. The entire procedure was reinitiated the following day. This continued for seven sessions. Subsequently, a familiar physician performed the initial steps in the hierarchy and remained in the room while the nurse completed the examination. The nurse gradually was faded from the room as the physician assumed more and more responsibility for the examination. During the 11th session, the boy remained cooperative as the physician completed the entire examination. In addition, the positive behavioral effects generalized to unfamiliar physicians and to another type of physical examination.

Mansdorf (1976) used a modified systematic desensitization procedure to successfully reduce an extreme fear of riding in cars in a 35-year-old woman with moderate retardation. Prior to treatment, the woman spent most of her time "confined to her room." Her extreme fear became apparent following a vocational counselor's suggestion that she become involved in a workshop program that required daily travel in an automobile. The woman appeared apprehensive when approaching a car and expressed negative statements about riding in a car. A 19-item graduated exposure hierarchy depicting the client's car-riding phobia was constructed. The usual procedure of pairing a state of relaxation with successive steps in the hierarchy was replaced by token reinforcement following completion of each step. Only 9 of 19 items, ranging from "Talking to therapist in office about cars" through "Talking to therapist with car door open and both inside," were completed before the behavioral objective of "Taking ride to workshop" was attained. A 10-month follow-up revealed that the client continued to use automobile transportation to attend community programs.

Erfanian and Miltenberger (1990) used contact desensitization for the treatment of an intense fear of dogs in two individuals with mental retardation. Both clients' extreme fear of dogs interfered with their adjustment to the community. Upon seeing a dog, the clients would become agitated until the dog was out of sight. If forced to approach the dog, or if the dog approached them, both clients would run away. On several occasions, upon unexpectedly seeing a dog, both clients had risked their lives by running across the street without looking out for traffic.

Both clients dramatically decreased avoidance of the dog after treatment, approaching within 1 foot of the dog while showing no signs of distress. Furthermore, during the treatment and later testing sessions, clients were able to pet the dog on its back upon request. Generalization and follow-up recordings were taken in a natural setting at 2 weeks and again 2 months after treatment. In each case, a dog was present outside the clients' work site or school, and their avoidance was measured as they took a walk with a teacher or staff person and passed by a 55-pound dog held on a leash by its owner. Both clients looked at the dog and both seemed vigilant during each assessment, but neither client engaged in any avoidance behavior or showed signs of fear or distress. Each was able to pass within 2 feet of the dog. Anecdotal reports from staff indicated that following treatment neither client showed any further avoidance behavior upon seeing a dog in public.

Matson (1981a) used a participant modeling technique of teaching relevant social skills to 24 adults with mental retardation and successfully eliminated the excessive fear of participating in community-based activities. Prior to treatment, all persons were identified as experiencing fear of approaching stores and as being unable to perform overall shopping skills. Such fears resulted in reduced community adaptation and interfered with independent living. Matson (1981b) also used participant modeling for the treatment of social phobias presented by children with moderate mental retardation who were living at home with their parents. The children had been referred to a mental health center for debilitating fears, which limited their ability to function normally at home and at school. Considerable "general fear" was also evident based on parental reports using a fear survey schedule.

Contributing (Setting) Instigating Conditions

As noted earlier, antecedent conditions in addition to primary stimulus states may contribute to a person's aberrant responding. These additional antecedent stimulus conditions are defined as *contributing* or *setting* events. While, in isolation, they may be insufficient conditions for producing behavioral symptoms, the presence or absence of these antecedents provide a set, activation, or inclination for the person to behave in a particular manner when exposed to primary discriminative stimuli. These contributing or setting events may represent historical, durational, and covert (physical, affective, cognitive, perceptual) conditions (Carr et al. 1996; Gardner et al. 1986; Kennedy and It-konen 1993; O'Reilly 1995; Sprague and Horner 1999).

A person's behavioral history may set the person up to behave in either a positive or negative manner when exposed to current stimulus events. The effects of these historical setting events thus may either facilitate or inhibit the occurrence of existing stimulus-response functions that follow the setting events. Use of behavioral histories in minimizing aversive qualities of primary stimulus events for aberrant responding has been reported with children and adults in a range of settings. Dunlap and Koegel (1980), Dunlap et al. (1991), and Winterling et al. (1987) demonstrated one variation consisting of initially presenting 24 trials of tasks that children with autism have already mastered and following these with a new, more difficult task. This procedure resulted in an improvement in the acquisition of new tasks and facilitated reduction in aggressive behavior during instruction.

Engelmann and Colvin (1983) described a similar strategy that involved the delivery of three to five requests immediately prior to presenting a difficult task or situation. Singer et al. (1987) used this procedure with elementary school–age students with moderate and severe disabilities to increase compliance to return to work from recess and decrease aggression. Three to five easy requests preceded instruction to return to work. Storey and Horner (1988) further suggested that these requests should "(a) require responses that take no more than a few seconds to complete, (b) be responses that the learner has a history of performing with a high probability of accuracy and speed, (c) be followed by praise, (d) be delivered in rapid succession, and (e) be delivered immediately prior to the presentation of the difficult task or situation" (p. 266). With this approach, success and praise are experienced immediately prior to the presentation of the task with aversive qualities.

In an earlier illustration of this approach, Carr et al. (1976) demonstrated that an 8-year-old boy with a dual diagnosis of schizophrenia and mild mental retardation consistently engaged in a high rate of self-injurious head and face slapping and hitting when presented with various verbal directives requiring motor responses. During free time and when presented with verbal statements that did not require a response, near zero rates of SIBs were evident. Under the hypothesis that the SIBs were escape motivated, these therapists embedded the demands in the context of positive ongoing interactions. Under this condition, the therapist would relate a simple story in an animated cheerful and entertaining manner and then present a directive within this positive context. The SIBs immediately dropped to a low level.

When alternating the verbal directives alone with a condition in which these demands were presented within the positive context, there was always an abrupt decrease in the rate of hitting in the positive context and an equally abrupt increase in the alone condition. The therapists thus demonstrated that the SIBs could be managed by altering the aversiveness of the directives. Apparently the positive context produced emotional responses that served as setting conditions for compliance behaviors. In support of this thesis, the therapists described the child as smiling and laughing and appearing to be quite happy. On removal of this setting event, however, the presentation of a directive resulted in SIBs. There had been no lasting reduction in the aversive qualities of the verbal directives.

The influence of temporally distant setting conditions is illustrated by Kennedy and Itkonen (1993). These clinicians demonstrated that various severe and chronic problem behaviors of two young adults with severe disabilities were related to specific experiences occurring earlier in the day prior to arriving at a day program. Removal of these earlier occurring setting conditions resulted in a significant reduction of problem behaviors in the school program. Similar results were reported by Gardner et al. (1986) and Sprague and Horner (1999).

In addition to the earlier occurring events that "set" the person to behave in a specific manner, durational events such as the mere presence of certain people or conditions (e.g., female staff member, reinforcement contingency, specific production requirement in the work setting, noisy or crowded environment, infrequent social attention) may influence how a person will react to various other current stimulus conditions. Other potential durational events include general environmental conditions such as amount of space, availability of competing activities, staff/client ratio, time of day, presence or absence of leisure materials, level of difficulty of classroom or workshop tasks, and behaviors of staff or peers (Gardner et al. 1986).

Touchette et al. (1985) provide illustration of the influence of a durational setting condition on aberrant responding. Conducting an initial analysis of the times and situations in which the SIBs and other agitated disruptive responding of a young adult occurred, it was discovered that the self-abuse was evident principally during the late afternoon and evening hours. Increased self-hitting correlated with the staff person assigned, the afternoon activities, and the number of peers present. In an attempt to alter the controlling antecedents, the morning staff was assigned to the late afternoon and the afternoon staff worked during the morning. All other correlated events remained the same. With this change in staff, the SIBs now occurred predominately in the morning. A second reversal of staff assignments correlated again with a total reversal of the times during which the self-abuse occurred. In this instance, the therapists were able to manage the SIBs by identifying and removing the specific staff that were highly correlated with the occurrence of the SIBs. This management of this secondary setting influence is incomplete as an intervention approach because it leaves the person vulnerable to future exposure to the controlling effects of the stimulus conditions. Additional approaches designed to reduce or remove the aversive components of these antecedent conditions or to teach the person functional alternatives when confronted with these events would be necessary.

The covert stimulus states described earlier as representing primary psychological, psychiatric, and medical instigating conditions for aberrant behaviors may also serve as contributing instigating events. Increased irritability related to menses, to a seizure medication, or to central nervous system damage may render a person generally more likely to engage in maladaptive behaviors when confronted with other specific primary environmental or interpersonal stressors. Reduction of this organically based overarousal by medication or medication change may decrease the frequency, duration, and intensity of these episodes on exposure to primary instigating conditions (Carr et al. 1996; Gardner and Whalen 1996; Peine et al. 1995; Sovner 1988; Sovner and Fogelman 1996).

Instigating Conditions: Summary

When assessing external and internal events that may serve to instigate aberrant behaviors, it is highly unusual to identify any specific primary discriminative event reflecting either a physical or psychological condition in the presence of which these behaviors always occur. In most instances, a stimulus complex occasions maladaptive reactions. This complex frequently involves both primary and contributing influences representing both internal and external stimulus conditions. As noted, instigating conditions vary in the probability of producing the behaviors. In illustration, an adolescent with severe mental retardation who is highly prone to engage in SIBs under conditions of negative social provocation may behave appropriately on some occasions when in a state of positive emotional arousal even when taunted by a peer. When aroused negatively (e.g., being angry or irritable over prolonged verbal rumination concerning a previous reprimand by a teacher), the same adolescent under the same external provocation is more likely to engage in self-injury. This diagnostic information would suggest that the critical variable requiring treatment is the person's lack of coping skills under the dual conditions of negative emotional arousal and peer teasing.

Of importance is the observation that instigating events are not constant across persons, or even for the same person across time and situations. In illustration, the mere presence of a physically large male staff member (as a durational setting event) may serve to inhibit violent outbursts in a client who is likely to become physically aggressive when reprimanded by other staff. However, this same large male staff member may have no such "setting" effect on another person under the same reprimand stimulus conditions. These instigating events thus must be empirically and individually defined and identified (Gardner et al. 1986).

■ CONTEXTUAL ANALYSIS 2: VULNERABILITY INFLUENCES

Also of interest are those deficit skill areas, such as communication, social, and related problem-solving and coping skills, that, due to their low strength or absence, contribute to the vulnerability of the person to engage in inappropriate responding under various conditions of provocation. As suggested earlier, in the context of an impoverished repertoire of alternative functional skills, aberrant behaviors may be the most effective and efficient means of coping with various sources of provocation. This correlation between skill deficits and maladaptive responding suggests a program focus on teaching alternative functional coping skills as a means of reducing the person's vulnerability (Cole et al. 1985).

Intervention Procedures for Addressing Vulnerabilities

In persons with severely and profoundly impaired cognitive features, limited communication skills, and few alternative social behaviors, aberrant responding may represent effective and efficient means of ensuring social feedback or of communicating about one's needs. In fact, a number of writers (e.g., Carr et al. 1994) suggest that such severe behavior problems as aggression, self-injury, and agitated/disruptive episodes may serve the same functions as other socially acceptable forms of verbal and nonverbal communication. The socially appropriate forms of communication either are not in the person's repertoire or are relatively ineffective or inefficient means of communication. The aberrant behaviors in these instances may represent means of communicating wishes, concerns, or physical/psychological states such as pain or dysphoria. This *communication hypothesis*, using communication as a metaphor, suggests the program strategy of replacing the aberrant behaviors with alternative functionally equivalent forms of communicative skills of obtaining individually relevant positive consequences or of reducing, terminating, or avoiding conditions that are aversive to specific persons. For the individual with minimal functional social or expressive language skills, this would involve teaching the person specific other means of expressing his or her needs or wishes through the use of verbal or nonverbal communication skills. To emphasize, this communication hypothesis of aberrant behaviors results in an educative skill development focus of intervention. Once acquired, these new communicative skills may serve to produce the same or similar results for the person as previously produced by the aberrant behaviors. Merely teaching new communicative skills, however, does not ensure that a person will begin to use these as functional alternatives to chronically occurring aberrant behaviors. This was illustrated by Duker et al. (1991) in a training effort to decrease self-injurious and other disruptive behaviors in a group of children and adults (14 subjects ranging in age from 11 to 35 years) with severe and profound mental retardation. The authors assumed that the aberrant behaviors were serving a communicative function and therefore taught the clients a number of gestures (signs) that would enhance their ability to communicate wants and needs to caretakers. Whereas self-injury and destructive behaviors showed decreases following training, other inappropriate behaviors (e.g., aggression, screaming, stereotypic behaviors, throwing objects, tearing clothes, and pica) were not significantly affected. These results would support the need to determine the specific function served by each aberrant behavior as a basis for selecting behavior-specific interventions to address the specific instigating and maintaining conditions. Simply teaching communicative behaviors in an attempt to reduce aberrant behaviors in the absence of a thorough functional analysis is unlikely to yield consistent results among persons who present chronic behavior difficulties.

Other studies emphasize the need to teach functionally equivalent communicative behaviors under the stimulus conditions in which aberrant behaviors occur. This was illustrated by Horner and Budd (1985) who taught an 11-year-old nonverbal boy diagnosed as "autistic" to communicate wants and needs with manual signs. Systematic observation of antecedents and consequent events associated with the aberrant behaviors of grabbing and yelling indicated that these occurred under five different stimulus conditions such as the presentation of food at lunch or the beginning of language session.

Initially the boy, under conditions designed to simulate those under which grabbing and yelling occurred, was taught an American Sign Language manual sign appropriate to each of the five sets of stimulus conditions. Although sign learning occurred in this simulated setting, there was no generalization to natural settings in which the aberrant behaviors continued to occur. Following training of these communicative behaviors in the natural settings, however, grabbing and yelling dropped to a near zero level. The authors concluded that the communicative behavior "was brought under control of the same stimuli (in Natural Setting Training) as the inappropriate behavior, and resulted in the same consequences (i.e., teacher attention, access to target object) as the inappropriate behavior" (p. 44). These data support the previously stated conclusions that training programs must lodge communicative behaviors in the specific context (instigating and maintaining) under which the aberrant behaviors have gained functionality. This practice is further illustrated in the final section addressing the functionality of aberrant behaviors.

A number of studies have demonstrated the therapeutic value of combining various self-management procedures with more traditional approaches in the treatment of severe conduct and related agitated-disruptive behaviors. A skill-deficit rationale underlies these studies, with the assumption made that skills of self-management would serve as functional alternatives to the impulsive aggressive reactions to sources of provocation.

Harvey et al. (1978) used various external and self-managed procedures to eliminate violent outbursts in a 38-year-old woman with moderate mental retardation. Gardner et al. (1983a, 1983b) used a multi-component self-management package to reduce high-rate conduct problems in adults with moderate mental retardation. Cole et al. (1985) demonstrated the therapeutic value of a self-management intervention program with mildly and moderately impaired adults whose chronic and severe conduct difficulties prevented their participation in community vocational rehabilitation programs. The skills training package included the self-management skills of self-monitoring, self-evaluation, and self-consequation of the patients' own appropriate and inappropriate work-related behaviors. In addition, these adults were taught to self-instruct prosocial behaviors that served as alternatives to aggression under specific conditions of provocation. In addition to a significant reduction of verbal and physical aggression, two collateral behaviors not specifically treated (on-task behavior and work productivity) showed positive effects. In a similar demonstration of the value of a multi-component behavior therapy program involving self-management, Jackson and Altman (1996) reported a reduction in aggression that allowed a young dually diagnosed adult to maintain competitive employment and a personal residence.

Benson (1986) and Benson et al. (1986) provide a final example of a self-control intervention program designed to teach alternative prosocial behaviors. The program, termed *anger management training*, teaches clients self-control skills that will enable them to handle anger-arousing situations in socially acceptable ways. Clients are taught not only to modify their outward behaviors (e.g., hitting someone) but also to modify the cognitions (thoughts) that accompany those behaviors.

■ CONTEXTUAL ANALYSIS 3: MAINTAINING CONDITIONS

The final set of variables evaluated are those psychosocial and biomedical factors that may contribute to the functionality of the problem behaviors. Aberrant behaviors may become functional in producing positive consequences. Additionally, empirical demonstrations support clinical observations that in other instances recurring patterns of maladaptive behaviors may be strengthened by their effectiveness in removing or reducing aversive events. These reinforcing events may be located in the external environment or may represent internal conditions. In illustration, agitated outbursts may be strengthened if followed by immediate staff attention or in other instances by the immediate removal of an aversive teacher directive. These same reactions may gain functionality if they produce a contingent reduction in physical pain or emotional distress (Carr and Carlson 1993; Carr et al. 1999; Sovner and Hurley 1992).

Analysis of various aberrant behaviors implicates a range of maintaining stimulus conditions that contribute to the functionality of behaviors as these serve to

- Produce such reinforcing conditions as social attention, access to activities, and tangibles (Durand and Carr 1992)
- Produce sensory stimulation (Steege et al. 1989)
- Decrease aversive levels of internal arousal or agitation such as fear, anxiety, and dysphoria (Benson 1990; Lowery and Sovner 1991a; Ollendick et al. 1993)
- Decrease aversive environmental conditions such as noise level, staff or task demands, excessive activity, or taunting from peers (Bird et al. 1989; Carr and Durand 1985; Horner and Day 1991)

Unless these individually relevant positive and/or negative reinforcement maintaining conditions are removed or modified in influence or unless effective or efficient alternative ways of producing these reinforcing conditions are forthcoming, the aberrant behaviors are likely to continue. Identification of the specific maintaining positive or negative reinforcers of the aberrant behavior (e.g., receives attention, nonpreferred task is removed, sensory stimulation is provided) offers direction in the selection of condition-specific procedures for decreasing the aberrant behaviors through teaching prosocial alternatives.

Intervention Procedures for Changing Functionality

As illustrated briefly in the previous section on programming for vulnerabilities, functionally equivalent alternatives to the aberrant behaviors may be taught as means of gaining access to either the maintaining events or their equivalents. In functional equivalence training, an initial assessment is completed to identify the consequences that maintain a specific problem behavior. Assessment information is used to devise a training program to teach a functionally equivalent and socially appropriate replacement for the aberrant behavior that produces similar consequences. Once acquired, this new skill will be controlled by the same instigating stimuli and consequences that previously controlled the problem behavior. These functional alternatives may consist of motor responses that result in equivalent reinforcing events or may involve functionally equivalent communicative behaviors of either a nonverbal or verbal nature (Carr et al. 1990).

Steege et al. (1989) reported a significant reduction in the chronic self-injurious mouthing and biting of a severely multiply handicapped 8-year-old boy (Ron) who attended a public school program. Functional diagnostics indicated that Ron engaged in a high rate of self-injury when in solitary conditions (toileting and positioning), resulting in the hypothesis that the SIBs served a self-stimulatory function. The SIBs were replaced by an alternate response of pushing a microswitch that activated either a fan or a radio, both stimulus conditions that previously had been demonstrated to be reinforcing to Ron. This alternative functional motor response of producing sensory stimulation was still dominant over the SIBs at the 6-month follow-up.

Functional communication training, as suggested earlier, involves the teaching of alternative and functionally equivalent communicative responses as replacements for problem behavior (Bird et al. 1989; Durand and Kishi 1987). Functional communication training differs from other differential reinforcement procedures. Of significance is that the schedule of reinforcement is controlled by the participant. Carr and Durand (1985) and Wacker et al. (1990) suggest that this control feature of functional communication training reflecting the active participation of the client represents a primary variable in its success. Although these procedures involve reinforcement of behaviors other than the aberrant behavior, the nature of the behavior selected as the target for reinforcement has specific qualities. In identifying the alternative responses to be reinforced in functional communication training, behaviors are selected that are functionally equivalent to the aberrant behaviors, that is, ones that will produce the same results for the person. This selection requires functional diagnostics to identify the specific function or functions served by the target aberrant behavior(s). Once this function is identified (or presumed), any behavior, verbal or nonverbal, that produces the same effect may be selected as the teaching target.

Critical in this analysis is the identification of the specific positive or negative reinforcers that are produced by the aberrant behaviors, that is, those that represent the maintaining conditions (e.g., preferred activities, attention, assistance, time away from an activity, and tangibles). Initially, for an alternative functionally equivalent behavior to be learned, the type of reinforcers provided must be specific to the person's communicative request. In addition, the reinforcers must be delivered on a schedule determined by the person's newly acquired communication requests. Reinforcement occurs on a continuous reinforcement schedule with a minimum of delay between the communicative behavior and reinforcement. As noted by Bird et al. (1989) "as a result, at the *specific* time when a *specific* environmental change is desired by the subject, a *specific* communicative response is available that can change the environment as consistently as his maladaptive behavior had in the past" (p. 46). Under these conditions, the alternative communicative response gradually becomes as effective and efficient, and as habitual or automatic, as the previously exhibited aberrant behaviors.

Experience with functional communication training has demonstrated convincingly that functional equivalents for aberrant behaviors become the most dominant behavior only after the person begins to demonstrate spontaneous use of these replacement behaviors rather than relying on prompts from others. This observation emphasizes that even though alternative means of communicating concerns are in the person's repertoire, these are unlikely to become predominant over the aberrant responses until the person has experienced consistent success in the spontaneous use of these behaviors. Shifting the control of the reinforcing events to the person's alternative behavior and ensuring, at least initially, that it is as effective and efficient in gaining access to these appear to be critical components in the success of functional communication training (Bird et al. 1989; Carr 1988; Horner and Day 1991).

Durand and Kishi (1987) taught young adults with severe/profound mental retardation and dual sensory impairments either to sign or to present a token as a means of communicating their requests for staff attention or access to favorite objects. Alternative forms of communication were selected as each had previously been unsuccessful in verbal language training. Functional diagnostics had produced the hypothesis that SIBs were serving these communicative functions prior to training. Following training, significant reductions in SIBs were observed in those instances in which the staff consistently responded to the communicative requests.

Bird et al. (1989) used functional communication training to treat high levels of several SIBs exhibited by Greg, a 27-year-old male with diagnoses of autistic disorder and profound mental retardation. Greg's expressive language skills were limited to approximately 15 one-word utterances that were seldom spontaneous and often difficult to interpret. He required physical prompting to complete most of his activities of daily living routines while attending a day program. Greg's SIBs had resulted in detachment of both retinas, leaving him blind. At the initiation of functional communication training, he was provided one-on-one staffing due to the severity of his SIBs. A range of medical and behavioral interventions had been attempted with only minimal success. The most recent behavioral interventions in effect prior to initiating the functional communication skills training program consisted of differential reinforcement procedures combined with response interruption, reprimand, and overcorrection.

Assessment of the possible functions served by Greg's SIBs suggested an escape from task demands hypothesis. The functional communication training program taught Greg an alternative nonverbal (exchanging a plastic token) but functionally equivalent means of obtaining a break from task demands presented in his classroom program. An immediate and substantial reduction in self-injurious episodes was obtained. These results were maintained with introduction of successive task demands of increasing difficulty and duration and also generalized across the three teachers who worked with Greg. Additionally, there was a concurrent increase in 1) Greg's spontaneous verbal request to initiate work even during periods of time when he had an opportunity to avoid work demands completely, and 2) spontaneous verbal requests for food, a behavior that seldom occurred prior to the training program.

Carr and Durand (1985) demonstrated through functional diagnostics that, when provided with task demands in an educational setting, a group of four children with developmental disabilities frequently engaged in various disruptive behaviors. It was hypothesized that the disruptive behaviors of two of the children were serving as nonverbal means of communication that had become functional in obtaining teacher attention. These children were taught a verbal communication response, "Am I doing good work?" to solicit the teacher attention that previously had followed the disruptive behaviors. This communicative inquiry resulted in prompt teacher response consisting of variations of the sentence, "I like the way you're working today. You're putting all the pictures where they belong!" Verbal praise was accompanied by smiles and nods as well as physical approval such as tickling and pats on the back. The self-injury and other disruptive behaviors reduced to infrequent occurrence as the newly acquired verbal communication skills replaced the function served previously by the problem behaviors.

In a later evaluation focusing on maintenance of the newly acquired functional communication response, these researchers (Durand and Carr 1992) taught six preschool children attending an educational program a functional communicative alternative to various problem behaviors. Each child's motivational analysis had implicated the problem behaviors as being maintained by teacher attention. After training each child to solicit teacher attention ("Am I doing good work?"), problem behaviors reduced to infrequent occurrence as this functionally equivalent behavior served to gain teacher attention. It is of significance to note that the communicative response of soliciting attention was maintained across new teachers who were unaware that these alternative functional behaviors had been taught. Even without any training, the new teachers responded with attention when recruited by the students. As a result, inappropriate behaviors remained at low levels. The writers suggested "Teaching students to recruit the stimuli maintaining their challenging behaviors in a more appropriate manner may not only reduce these problem behaviors initially but may also facilitate maintenance" (p. 790). In contrast, the problem behaviors of a group of control children that had been reduced through the use of a reactive treatment (timeout) procedure quickly returned to previous levels following exposure to educational tasks provided by naive trainers who did not implement the punishment contingency. The suppressive effects of this reactive treatment procedure were short-lived following termination of the contingency.

In an additional demonstration of teaching a functionally equivalent communicative behavior to replace aberrant behaviors maintained by positive reinforcement, Day et al. (1988) utilized functional communication training to decrease self-biting in a 9-year-old boy with autism and moderate mental retardation. Functional assessment revealed that the SIBs were reinforcement motivated in that high rates were observed under positive reinforcement conditions (SIBs resulted in access to edibles, objects, or activities that previously had been offered to the subject's peers in a group situation) and particularly following removal of the reinforcer. Training verbal responses to the phrase "Tell me what you want" following removal of a reinforcer (reinforcer request training) and to request alternative reinforcers when the initial request was denied (denial training) resulted in significantly lower rates of SIBs, which were sustained over the 5-month intervention. Additionally, the duration of self-injurious episodes decreased from baseline levels of up to 30 minutes to single, brief responses in most instances following training.

Carr and Durand (1985) demonstrated the value of teaching an alternative verbal communication response to reduce escape-motivated SIBs. After initially demonstrating that the children with developmental disabilities who were attending a day school program engaged in SIBs when they were presented with difficult instructional tasks, the children were taught a verbal response as a means of soliciting teacher assistance. This training consisted of three stages. The child initially was prompted by the teacher to say "I don't understand." Following consistent correct imitation of this verbal behavior, the child was presented with a difficult task. When an error was made, the teacher said "That's not correct!" and added "Do you have any questions? Say 'I don't understand.' " When correctly imitated, the teacher replied "OK. I'll show you" and, through use of gestures and verbal statements, demonstrated the correct response. In the final training stage, the teacher's verbal prompts were faded until the child responded correctly to the inquiry "Do you have any questions?" Following training, SIBs and other disruptive behaviors reduced to infrequent occurrence. Through learning an alternative verbal response that resulted in adult assistance on difficult tasks, the children experienced less failure. This reduction in aversiveness of the tasks reduced the motivation for the SIBs.

In a successful replication of these results demonstrating functionally equivalent skill development as replacements for aberrant behaviors maintained by negative reinforcement, Durand and Carr (1991) also assessed maintenance and transfer across teachers and classrooms over 18–24 months. The challenging behaviors (SIBs, tantrums, screaming, physical aggression) of three boys attending a school program for children with developmental disabilities were assessed as being maintained by escape from academic demands. Each child was taught alternative functional communication responses that resulted in teacher assistance ("I don't understand" or "Help me"). Following training of these new communicative skills, a substantial reduction in challenging behaviors of each boy was noted. Further, these results transferred across new tasks, environments, and teachers. Finally, the results were generally maintained for 18–24 months following functional communication training. In one instance, brief booster sessions were used to reduce articulation difficulties of a child to ensure that the functional communicative response was understandable to the teacher. The writers suggested that the maintenance and transfer of the intervention gains to new settings could be attributed to the introduction of natural maintaining conditions. The new communicative behaviors served to solicit the desired consequences even from teachers who were unaware of and untrained in the functional communication training procedures.

Often the functional analysis of aberrant behaviors yields not one but several instigating and/or maintaining factors. Assessment may show, for instance, that although the behaviors occur at high rates under certain conditions (decreased staff attention), they may also occur during seemingly contrary conditions (staff interactions, requests, or demands). Functional diagnostics may suggest that at times the behavior is reinforcement motivated but on other occasions escape motivated. In such cases, addressing one factor through intervention typically leads to decreases in the problematic behavior; however, these decreases may not be sustained or sufficiently clinically significant until additional contributing factors are targeted.

Day et al. (1988) used functional diagnostics to discover multiple determinants of SIBs in several children with mental retardation. Functional assessment conditions employed included positive and negative reinforcement, and sensory input both alone and with a trainer present. In one case, Mary, a 15-year-old profoundly impaired adolescent with a history of SIBs since infancy, demonstrated high rates of SIBs under the positive reinforcement condition. Initial intervention consisted of teaching Mary to clap her hands in order to obtain trainer attention and then to label or sign for desired items. Although this *request training* produced a significant decrease in SIBs, the effect was not sustained. Functional assessment of the behavior had also revealed a moderate level of responding during task demand situations. Therefore, *protest training*, in which Mary was taught to say "no" to terminate undesired tasks, was additionally implemented. The combination of the two procedures resulted in consistently low rates of SIBs.

A second case reported by Bird et al. (1989) further illustrates the need to address multiple contributing conditions. Functional communication skills were taught to a 36-year-old profoundly retarded male, Jim, who displayed severe aggression and SIBs. Assessment had determined that Jim's behavior was escape motivated (from demand situations) as well as reinforcement motivated (desire for tangible rewards). Training, consisting initially of teaching Jim to sign for a break from task demands, resulted in immediate reductions in his aberrant behaviors. Jim was also trained in using signs to request reinforcers (music, food, bathroom, and work). As these alternative communicative behaviors became a functional part of Jim's behavioral repertoire, continued decreases in problem behaviors were seen. These low levels of 5 or less incidents per week compared with 2,575 incidents per week prior to training were maintained even when task demands, difficulty, level, and length were increased. Maintenance and transfer were also observed across changes in staff, programs, classroom site, and as the staff-to-client ratio decreased. A discrimination training component was added (red/green signs) to inform Jim of when his requests would be granted and when they would not. In addition to the decreases in aggression and SIBs, positive effects of training included an increase in Jim's on-task behavior and an overall increase in his spontaneous signing.

■ CONCLUSIONS

A multimodal contextual diagnostic and intervention model is offered to guide the clinician in understanding psychological symptoms presented by persons with mental retardation. Interventions are derived from a set of diagnostic formulations about instigating, vulnerability, and maintaining conditions reflecting psychological, biomedical, and socioenvironmental influences. Applications of a variety of behavior therapy procedures are described to address psychosocial influences.

■ REFERENCES

Bailey JS, Pyles DAM: Behavioral diagnostics, in The Treatment of Severe Behavior Disorders. Edited by Cipani E. Washington, DC, American Association on Mental Retardation, 1989, pp 85–107

Benson BA: Anger management training. Psychiatric Aspects of Mental Retardation Reviews 5:51–55, 1986

Benson BA: Anxiety disorders and depression, in Handbook of Behavior Modification With the Mentally Retarded, 2nd Edition. Edited by Matson JL. New York, Plenum, 1990, pp 391–420

Benson BA: Teaching Anger Management to Persons With Mental Retardation. Worthington, OH, International Diagnostic Systems, 1992

Benson BA, Rice CJ, Miranti SV: Effects of anger management training with mentally retarded adults in group treatment. J Counseling and Clinical Psychology 54:728–729, 1986

Bird F, Dores PA, Moniz D, et al: Reducing severe aggressive and self-injurious behaviors with functional communication training. Am J Mental Retardation 94:37–48, 1989

Carr EG: The motivation of self-injurious behavior: a review of some hypotheses. Psychol Bull 84:800–816, 1977

Carr EG: Functional equivalence as a mechanism of response generalization, in Generalization and Maintenance. Edited by Horner R, Koegel R, Dunlap G. Baltimore, MD, Paul H. Brookes, 1988, pp 221–241

Carr EG, Carlson JI: Reduction of severe behavior problems in the community using a multi-component treatment approach. J Appl Behav Anal 26:157–172, 1993

Carr EG, Durand VM: Reducing behavior problems through functional communication training. J Appl Behav Anal 18:111–126, 1985

Carr EG, Newsom DD, Binkoff JA: Stimulus control of self-destructive behavior in a psychotic child. J Abnorm Child Psychol 4:139–153, 1976

Carr EG, Robinson S, Palumbo LW: The wrong issue: aversive versus nonaversive treatment. The right issue: functional versus nonfunctional treatment, in Perspectives on the Use of Nonaversive and Aversive Interventions for Persons With Developmental Disabilities. Edited by Repp AC, Sigh NN. Sycamore, IL, Sycamore Publishing, 1990, pp 361–379

Carr EG, Levin L, McConnachie G, et al: Communication-Based Intervention for Problem Behavior. Baltimore, MD, Paul H. Brookes, 1994

Carr EG, Reeve CE, Magito-McLaughlin D: Contextual influences on problem behavior in people with developmental disabilities, in Positive Behavioral Supports: Including People With Difficult Behavior in the Community. Edited by Koegel LK, Koegel RL, Dunlap G. Baltimore, MD, Paul H. Brookes, 1996, pp 403–423

Carr EG, Langdon NA, Yarbrough SC: Hypothesis-based intervention for severe problem behavior, in Functional Analysis of Problem Behavior. Edited by Repp AC, Horner RH. Belmont, CA, Wadsworth Publishing, 1999, pp 9–31

Cipani E (ed): The Treatment of Severe Behavior Disorders. Washington, DC, American Association on Mental Retardation, 1989

Clauser B, Scibak JW: Direct and generalized effect of food satiation in reducing rumination. Res Dev Disabil 11:23–36, 1990

Cole CL, Gardner WI, Karan OC: Self-management training of mentally retarded adults presenting severe conduct difficulties. Applied Research in Mental Retardation 6:337–347, 1985

Day R, Rea J, Schuster N, et al: A functionally based approach to the treatment of self-injurious behavior. Behav Modif 12:565–589, 1988

Duker P, Jol K, Palmen, A: The collateral decrease of self-injurious behavior with teaching communicative gestures to individuals who are mentally retarded. Behavioral Residential Treatment 6:183–196, 1991

Dunlap G, Koegel RL: Motivating autistic children through stimulus variation. J Appl Behav Anal 13:619–627, 1980

Dunlap G, Kern-Dunlap L, Clarke M, et al: Functional assessment, curricular revision, and severe behavior problems. J Appl Behav Anal 24:387–397, 1991

Durand VM, Carr EG: Functional communication training to reduce challenging behaviors: maintenance and application in new settings. J Appl Behav Anal 24:251–264, 1991

Durand VM, Carr EG: An analysis of maintenance following functional communication training. J Appl Behav Anal 4:777–794, 1992

Durand VM, Kishi G: Reducing severe behavior problems among persons with dual sensory impairments: an evaluation of a technical assistance model. Journal of the Association of Severely Handicapped 12:2–10, 1987

Engelmann S, Colvin D: Generalized Compliance Training: A Direct-Instruction Program for Managing Severe Behavior Problems. Baltimore, MD, Paul H. Brookes, 1983

Erfanian N, Miltenberger RG: Brief report: contact desensitization in the treatment of dog phobias in persons who have mental retardation. Behavioral Residential Treatment 5:55–60, 1990

Favell JE, McGimsey JF, Schnell RM: Treatment of self-injury by providing alternate sensory activities. Analysis and Intervention in Developmental Disabilities 2:83–104, 1982

Freeman BJ, Roy RR, Hemmick S: Extinction of a phobia of physical examination in a seven-year-old mentally retarded boy: a case study. Behav Res Ther 14:63–64, 1976

Gardner WI: Use of behavior therapy with the mentally retarded, in Psychiatric Approaches to Mental Retardation. Edited by Menolascino FJ. New York, Basic Books, 1970, pp 250–275

Gardner WI: Behavior therapies: past, present, and future, in Mental Retardation and Mental Health: Classification, Diagnosis, Treatment, Services. Edited by Stark JA, Menolascino FJ, Albarelli MH, et al. New York, Springer-Verlag, 1988, pp 161–172

Gardner WI: Nonspecific behavioral symptoms in persons with a dual diagnosis: a psychological model for integrating biomedical and psychosocial diagnoses and interventions. Psychology in Mental Retardation and Developmental Disabilities 21:6–11, 1996

Gardner WI: Behavioral therapies: using diagnostic formulation to individualize treatment for persons with developmental disabilities and mental health concerns, in Therapy Approaches for Persons With Mental Retardation. Edited by Fletcher RJ. Kingston, NY, NADD Press, 2000, pp 1–25

Gardner WI, Cole CL: Aggression and related conduct difficulties in the mentally retarded: a multicomponent behavioral model, in Advances in Mental Retardation and Developmental Disabilities: A Research Annal, Vol 2. Edited by Breuning SE, Matson JL, Barrett RP. Greenwich, CT, JAI Press, 1984, pp 41–84

Gardner WI, Cole CL: Self-management approaches, in The Treatment of Severe Behavior Disorders: Behavior Analysis Approaches. Edited by Cipani E. Washington, DC, American Association on Mental Retardation, 1989, pp 19–35

Gardner WI, Cole CL: Aggression and related conduct disorders: definition, assessment, treatment, in Psychopathology in the Mentally Retarded, 2nd Edition. Edited by Matson JL, Barrett RP. Boston, MA, Allyn & Bacon, 1993, pp 213–252

Gardner WI, Graeber JL: Use of behavioral therapies to enhance personal competencies: a multimodal diagnostic and intervention model, in Mental Health in Mental Retardation: Recent Advances and Practices. Edited by Bouras N. Cambridge, UK, Cambridge University Press, 1994, pp 205–223

Gardner WI, Moffatt CW: Aggressive behavior: definition, assessment, treatment. International Review of Psychiatry 2:91–100, 1990

Gardner WI, Sovner R: Self-Injurious Behaviors: Diagnosis and Treatment. Willow Street, PA, Vida Publishing, 1994

Gardner WI, Whalen JP: A multimodal behavior analytic model for evaluating the effects of medical problems on nonspecific behavioral symptoms in persons with developmental disabilities. Behavioral Interventions in Community Settings 11:147–161, 1996

Gardner WI, Clees T, Cole CL: Self-management of disruptive verbal ruminations by a mentally retarded adult. Applied Research in Mental Retardation 4:41–58, 1983a

Gardner WI, Cole CL, Berry DL, et al: Reduction of disruptive behaviors in mentally retarded adults: a self-management approach. Behav Modif 7:76–96, 1983b

Gardner WI, Cole CL, Davidson DP, et al: Reducing aggression in individuals with developmental disabilities: an expanded stimulus control assessment and intervention model. Education and Training of the Mentally Retarded 21:3–12, 1986

Gardner WI, Graeber JL, Cole CL: Behavior therapies: a multimodal diagnostic and intervention model, in Manual of Diagnosis and Professional Practice in Mental Retardation. Edited by Jacobson JW, Mulick JA. Washington, DC, American Psychological Association, 1996, pp 355–370

Griffiths DM, Gardner WI, Nugent JA (eds): Behavioral Supports: Individual Centered Interventions. Kingston, NY, NADD Press, 1998

Harchik AE, Sherman JA, Sheldon JB, et al: Choice and control: new opportunities for people with developmental disabilities. Ann Clin Psychiatry 5:151–162, 1993

Harvey JR, Karan OC, Bhargava D, et al: Relaxation training and cognitive behavioral procedures to reduce violent temper outbursts in a moderately retarded woman. J Behav Ther Exp Psychiatry 9:347–351, 1978

Hiss H, Kozak MJ: Exposure treatment of obsessive-compulsive disorders in the mentally retarded. The Behavior Therapist 14:163–167, 1991

Horner RH, Budd CM: Acquisition of manual sign use: collateral reduction of maladaptive behavior, and factors limiting generalization. Education and Training of the Mentally Retarded 20:39–47, 1985

Horner RH, Day HM: The effects of response efficiency on functionally equivalent competing behaviors. J Appl Behav Anal 24:719–732, 1991

Jackson GM, Johnson CR, Ackron GS, et al: Food satiation as a procedure to decelerate vomiting. American Journal of Mental Deficiency 80:223–227, 1975

Jackson TL, Altman R: Self-management of aggression in an adult male with mental retardation and severe behavior disorders. Education and Training in Mental Retardation and Developmental Disabilities 31:55–65, 1996

Jacobson JW, Mulick JA (eds): Manual of Diagnosis and Professional Practice in Mental Retardation. Washington, DC, American Psychological Association, 1996

Kennedy CH, Itkonen T: Effects of setting events on the problem behavior of students with severe disabilities. J Appl Behav Anal 26:321–328, 1993

Koegel RL, Koegel LK: Extended reduction in stereotypic behavior through self-management in multiple community settings. J Appl Behav Anal 23:119–127, 1990

Koegel JK, Koegel RL, Dunlop G: Positive Behavioral Supports. Baltimore, MD, Brooks Publishing, 1996

Lancioni GE, Smeets PM, Ceccaranin PS, et al: Effects of gross motor activities on the severe self-injurious tantrums of multihandicapped individuals. Applied Research in Mental Retardation 5:471–482, 1984

Libby DG, Phillips E: Eliminating rumination behavior in a profoundly retarded adolescent: an exploratory study. Ment Retard 17:94–95, 1979

Lowery MA, Sovner R: Severe behavior problems associated with rapid cycling bipolar disorder in two adults with profound mental retardation. J Intellect Disabil Res 36:269–281, 1991a

Lowery MA, Sovner R: The functional significance of problem behavior: a key to effective treatment. The Habilitative Mental Healthcare Newsletter 10:119–123, 1991b

Luiselli JK, Matson JL, Singh N (eds): Self-Injurious Behavior: Analysis, Assessment, and Treatment. New York, Springer-Verlag, 1992

Mace FC, Knight D: Functional analysis and treatment of severe pica. J Appl Behav Anal 19:411–416, 1986

Madden NA, Russo DC, Cataldo MF: Environmental influences on mouthing in children with lead intoxication. J Pediatr Psychol 5:207–216, 1980

Mansdorf IJ: Eliminating fear in a mentally retarded adult by behavioral hierarchies and operant techniques. J Behav Ther Exp Psychiatry 7:189–190, 1976

Matson JL: A controlled outcome study of phobias in mentally retarded adults. Behav Res Ther 19:101–107, 1981a

Matson JL: Assessment and treatment of clinical fears in mentally retarded children. J Appl Behav Anal 14:287–294, 1981b

Matson JL, Barrett RP (eds): Psychopathology in the Mentally Retarded. Boston, MA, Allyn & Bacon, 1993

McNally RJ: Anxiety and phobias, in Handbook of Mental Retardation, 2nd Edition. Edited by Matson JL, Mulick JA. New York, Pergamon, 1991, pp 413–423

Nezu CM, Nezu AM, Gill-Weiss MJ: Psychopathology in Persons With Mental Retardation. Champaign, IL, Research Press, 1992

O'Donohue W, Krasner L (eds): Theories of Behavior Therapy: Exploring Behavior Change. Washington, DC, American Psychological Association, 1995

Ollendick TH, Oswald DP, Ollendick DG: Anxiety disorders in mentally retarded persons, in Psychopathology in the Mentally Retarded, 2nd Edition. Edited by Matson JL, Barrett RP. Boston, MA, Allyn & Bacon, 1993, pp 41–86

O'Reilly MF: Functional analysis and treatment of escape-maintained aggression correlated with sleep deprivation. J Appl Behav Anal 28:225–226, 1995

Peine HA, Darvish R, Adams K, et al: Medical problems, maladaptive behavior and the developmentally disabled. Behavioral Interventions 10:149–159, 1995

Rast J, Johnston JM, Drum C, et al: The relation of food quality to rumination behavior. J Appl Behav Anal 14:121–130, 1981

Reese RM, Sherman JA, Sheldon J: Reducing agitated-disruptive behavior of mentally retarded residents of community group homes: the roles of self-recording and peer prompted self-recording. Analysis and Intervention in Developmental Disabilities 4:91–108, 1984

Repp AC, Horner RH (eds): Functional Analysis of Problem Behavior. Belmont, CA, Wadsworth Publishing, 1999

Rivenq B: Behavioral therapy of phobias: a case with gynecomastia and mental retardation. Ment Retard 12:44–45, 1974

Singer GH, Singer J, Horner RH: Using pretask requests to increase the probability of compliance for students with severe disabilities. Journal of the Association for Persons with Severe Handicaps 12:287–329, 1987

Sovner R: Anticonvulsant drug therapy for neuropsychiatric disorders in mentally retarded persons, in Use of Anticonvulsants in Psychiatry: Recent Advances. Edited by McElroy SL, Pope HG. Clinton, NJ, Oxford Health Care, 1988, pp 56–70

Sovner R, Fogelman S: Irritability and mental retardation. Seminars in Clinical Neuropsychiatry 1:105–114, 1996

Sovner R, Hurley AD: The diagnostic treatment formulation for psychotropic drug therapy. The Habilitative Mental Healthcare Newsletter 11:81–86, 1992

Sovner R, Pary RJ: Affective disorders in developmentally disabled persons, in Psychopathology in the Mentally Retarded. Edited by Matson JL, Barrett RP. Boston, MA, Allyn & Bacon, 1993, pp 87–147

Sprague JR, Horner RH: Low-frequency high-intensity problem behavior: toward an applied technology of functional assessment and intervention, in Functional Analysis of Problem Behavior. Edited by Repp AC, Horner RH. Belmont, CA, Wadsworth Publishing, 1999, pp 98–116

Steege MW, Wacker DP, Berg WK, et al: The use of behavioral assessment to prescribe and evaluate treatment for severely handicapped children. J Appl Behav Anal 22:22–23, 1989

Storey K, Horner RH: Pretask requests help manage behavior problems. Direct Instruction News 7:1–3, 1988

Thompson T, Gray D (eds): Treatment of Destructive Behavior in Developmental Disabilities, Vol 2. Thousand Oaks, CA, Sage Publishing, 1994

Touchette PE, MacDonald RF, Langer SN: A scatter plot for identifying stimulus control of problem behavior. J Appl Behav Anal 18:343–351, 1985

Wacker DP, Steege MW, Northup J, et al: A component analysis of functional communication training across three topographies of severe behavior problems. J Appl Behav Anal 23:417–429, 1990

Winterling V, Dunlap G, O'Neill R: The influence of task variation on the aberrant behavior of autistic students. Education and Treatment of Children 10:105–119, 1987

Woods DW, Miltenberger RG, Lumley VA: Sequential application of major habit-reversal components to treat motor tics in children. J Appl Behav Anal 29:483–493, 1996

Yang L: Elimination of habitual rumination through the strategies of food satiation and fading: a case study. Behavioral Residential Treatment 3:223–234, 1988

5 Cognitive and Social Learning Treatments

Betsey A. Benson, Ph.D.
Denise Valenti-Hein, Ph.D.

Behavioral analysis dominated psychological interventions and habilitation in mental retardation in the United States in the 1960s and 1970s, and tremendous advances were made in teaching self-care skills and in reducing maladaptive behaviors. However, there was some dissatisfaction with this approach for those who believed that it ignored important aspects of the individual by focusing only on observable behaviors. Concurrently, the study of information-processing models of human behavior and cognitive psychology attracted the interest and attention of researchers. The research shift was so great that Mahoney (1977) called it a "cognitive revolution." In recent years, considerable work has been done to integrate cognitive concepts into psychological interventions in nonretarded persons. To a lesser extent, this influence has been felt in the field of mental retardation.

Behavioral interventions typically focus on stimulus-response or response-consequence relationships. Observable behaviors are the targets of change. In cognitive and social learning interventions, the targets of change may be thoughts, behaviors, or a combination of the two, and behavioral principles are applied to effect changes in these as well.

Most applications of cognitive and social learning interventions in the field of mental retardation have been with adolescents or adults who are verbal and functioning in the borderline to high moderate range. There have been instances, however, in which nonverbal persons or those with severe mental retardation have profited from the techniques. Adaptations of the interventions are necessary and should be consistent with the developmental level of the individual.

■ TREATMENT TECHNIQUES

In this section, we review four techniques of cognitive-behavioral treatment that have a history of application with people with mental retardation: self-instruction, problem solving, modeling, and relaxation training.

Self-Instruction

The observation that people direct their own behavior by covert self-directed statements was introduced by Vygotsky (1962) and applied to clinical problems by Meichenbaum (1969). Much data have been gathered to support the use of self-instructions for a variety of academic (Grimm et al. 1973), psychiatric (Meichenbaum and Cameron 1973), and behavioral (Bornstein and Quevillon 1976) problems.

Typically, self-instruction involves using prompts and reinforcers to teach people to repeat statements that will help guide their behavior. For example, in learning to act less impulsively, patients are told to say something to themselves that will slow them down. A patient is first encouraged to formulate his or her own statements and repeat them overtly. The therapist then introduces a situation followed by the prompt, "What do you say to yourself?" If the patient responds with the self-instructional statement, the patient is given praise or other suitable reinforcers. As self-statements become more automatic, the prompts and reinforcers are gradually faded, and finally the patient is told to speak covertly.

Self-instructional statements can take several forms. They can involve questions regarding the demands of the situation ("What do they want me to do?"), self-affirmation ("I know I can do it"), self-control ("Take a deep breath and say 'relax' "), coping statements to handle errors and frustration ("Well, that was hard, but I'll do better next time"), or self-reinforcing statements ("I did a good job!"). Often a variety of self-instructional statements are taught. In this case, the solution steps themselves may also be rehearsed and repeated covertly. For example, in working through a math problem, students might learn a running commentary of statements such as, "The first step is to see what kind of problem it is. It's subtraction. Next, I look at the first row of numbers. . . ." Commentaries are acquired using chaining techniques, in which each phrase is learned individually and added to the phrase before it.

The use of self-instructional statements with people who are mentally retarded requires some special considerations and alterations in procedures. Primarily, the therapist must be more active and explicit in prompting and guiding responses. The therapist must also be aware of the need to work slowly. For example, Rusch and colleagues (1985) systematically faded prompts by first having cafeteria workers repeat self-instructions aloud, next repeat them in a whisper, then use only lip movements, and finally repeat them covertly. Another consideration is whether the patient has the verbal ability to self-instruct. A limited verbal repertoire will render this technique less appropriate for lower functioning patients. When that is the case, self-instruction using picture prompting cards has been a successful alternative (Robinson-Wilson 1977). Picture prompts are also useful for multistep, complex tasks, such as meal preparation (e.g., Martin et al. 1982). The therapist must assess whether the patient is developmentally ready to learn the task that the self-instruction is meant to facilitate. If he or she is not, no amount of symbolic mediation will help.

Self-instructional techniques for people with mental retardation have proven successful in limited applications (e.g., Burgio et al. 1980; Johnston et al. 1980; Rusch et al. 1985). It is likely, however, that self-instructional training could be useful for many problems experienced by persons with mental retardation.

Problem Solving

Improving one's ability to solve problems is a central goal of psychotherapy. Problem solving has been defined by D'Zurilla and Goldfried (1971, p. 180) as a cognitive and behavioral process that makes a variety of potentially effective response alternatives available and increases the probability of selecting the most effective response from these alternatives. Whereas some consider problem solving to be one aspect of social skills (Spivack et al. 1976), others view it as a process of choosing which social skills to employ (Castles and Glass 1986). In either case, most researchers agree that problem solving consists of several steps: 1) identifying the problem, 2) identifying the solutions, 3) evaluating the consequences of the solutions, and 4) choosing and enacting the best solution (Shure and Spivak 1982).

Problem situations are identified by reviewing the literature, consulting with the staff, or asking the patients to describe their concerns. Therapists then guide the patient through the problem-solving process. For example, the therapist may prompt the generation of solutions by saying, "That's one way to solve the problem. Can you think of another?" The patient is assisted in visualizing the consequences of each alternative, by either discussion or role-playing. As the focus of problem-solving training is often interpersonal, group training is generally preferred. Moreover, studies suggest that peer interaction (Foss et al. 1989) and group consensus of solution choices (Mueser et al. 1986) are both important to successful problem-solving training.

Outcome research of problem-solving training for people with mental retardation is complicated by the fact that some studies do not train all the components of problem solving. Ross and Ross (1978) note that much of the research focuses on the tasks of generating solutions or selecting the best alternative. In two separate studies, Ross and Ross (1973, 1978) found that both elements could be successfully trained in children with mild mental retardation when training focused on teaching the specific component. Tymchuk et al. (1988), however, reported that when adult subjects with mental retardation were given general problem-solving training, the skills of generating alternatives and considering consequences were still impaired despite the ability to successfully generate an appropriate solution to a problem. This finding is particularly striking when one considers the direct positive relationship between the number of solutions generated and the ability to pick a best solution (Castles and Glass 1986; Shure and Spivack 1982).

Another consideration is whether patients should practice the solution chosen as part of the problem-solving process. If so, therapists may need to role-play the best solution with patients. Whereas some studies suggest that behavioral rehearsal is not needed for successful problem solving (Foss et al. 1989), others suggest that rehearsal strongly improves the effects over that of verbally discussing the solution (Castles and Glass 1986).

A final issue involves the level of mental retardation of the persons in training. Whereas many studies focus on a combined group of persons with mild or moderate mental retardation, few have evaluated how cognitive functioning affects treatment outcome. Surprisingly, in one study in which such differences were analyzed, greater improvement was found in moderately retarded patients (Castles and Glass 1986), suggesting that a ceiling effect to the acquisition of problem-solving skills may exist. The type of problem to be solved is also a consideration. After reviewing the research findings, Beveridge and Conti-Ramsden (1987) concluded that "formal measures of IQ, language, and reasoning ability and social maturity are not clearly predictive of their ability to solve real problems, and that both absolute performance of retarded persons and the difference between them and the nonhandicapped population are related to the type of problem situation presented" (p. 104).

Modeling

Modeling, or observational learning, involves learning "through observation of other persons' behavior and its consequences for them" (Bandura 1969, p. 118). Through modeling, new behaviors are learned, fearful or avoidant behaviors can be reduced, and previously learned behaviors can be facilitated.

The fears of persons with mental retardation have been reduced through modeling interventions in which therapists, peers, or parents served as models. The subject observes the model approach the feared object or situation. It has been hypothesized that anxiety is reduced and approach responses are disinhibited because the patient observes that the model does not experience negative consequences and because the model's response has informational value (Bandura and Barab 1973).

Fears treated with modeling interventions include fear of dogs (Jackson and Hooper 1981), toilets (Wilson and Jackson 1980), escalators (Runyan et al. 1985), strangers (Matson 1981a, 1981b), and entering stores (Matson 1981a, 1981b). Typically individuals are reinforced with praise or tangible rewards for making approach responses to the feared object or situation.

Two variations of modeling include participant modeling and self-modeling. In participant modeling, the model guides the subject through the approach response. This type of modeling has been more effective for nonretarded children than simply observing the model (Ollendick 1979). It may be especially useful when skill deficits accompany the avoidance behavior. Reducing the avoidance behavior may not be sufficient to improve functioning without also providing instruction in appropriate behavior in the situation.

Self-modeling, a procedure in which the individual serves as a model for him- or herself, has proven to be as successful as peer modeling in work with persons with developmental disabilities (Dowrick 1991). The subject views videotapes of him- or herself to improve subsequent behavior. In positive self-review, the video recording is edited to show the best examples of the target skills that are currently in the individual's response repertoire but infrequently displayed. In feedforward, editing takes component behaviors in the current repertoire and creates images of behaviors that are not yet performed. The videotapes are short, only 2–5 minutes, and are viewed by the subject several times during a 1- to 2-week period. Applications of video self-modeling for persons with mental retardation have focused on skills training, such as learning to eat with a spoon and learning to make safe decisions in interactions with strangers (Dowrick 1991). It has also been used in interventions with self-injurious behavior, temper tantrums, and general disruptive behavior (Krantz et al. 1991).

Relaxation Training

Relaxation training is a general category of treatment intervention that focuses on reducing anxiety. Anxiety-related behaviors occur at a higher frequency in people with mental retardation than in those who are not disabled (Donaldson and Menolascino 1977; Peck 1977), suggesting a need for anxiety reduction therapies.

Anxiety reduction is achieved by several techniques (Benson and Havercamp 1999). Some methods, such as deep diaphragm breathing, are quickly learned and provide immediate short-term benefits (e.g., reducing stuttering). Others, such as progressive muscle relaxation (PMR), require some time to learn a series of easy-to-monitor physical exercises that trigger muscle relaxation. Still others, such as the use of guided imagery, can be very pleasurable and are engaging for patients. Finally, autogenics invoke the suggestion of relaxed feelings to reduce anxiety. Some of these methods have been enhanced with the use of biofeedback devices. Although theoretically distinct, most techniques are used in combination with one another.

Research on the use of relaxation training with mentally retarded persons has generally focused on case studies in which the techniques have been effective with many different disorders. In a review of 12 studies that employed relaxation with this population, Luiselli (1980) concluded that it seems effective in enhancing performance over that of no-treatment control subjects, but it was often no better than other "placebo" treatments such as exercise.

One problem with research in this area is that several types of relaxation training are used in combination and individual components are not compared. This is important because different methods of relaxation seem appropriate with different levels of disability. For example, Rickard and colleagues (1984) found that subjects in the lowest IQ group (40–54) had more difficulty following PMR instructions than higher IQ groups but found no difference in the acquisition of deep breathing skills. On the other hand, Calamari et al. (1987) found no difference between the levels of mental retardation using a relaxation package of biofeedback, PMR, modeling, and reinforcement. Lindsay et al. (1989) hypothesized that PMR requires an awareness of internal states that is difficult for people in the severe range of mental retardation.

Teaching relaxation techniques to the person with mental retardation requires some modifications (Cautela and Groden 1979; Harvey 1979). Simple language should be used, along with demonstration and physical prompts or guidance. Motivation can be increased via external and immediate reinforcers for participation. Finally, shaping should be used to gradually improve patient performance. For people functioning in the moderate and severe ranges of mental retardation, Lindsay et al. (1989) suggested modeling and physical guidance to help patients discriminate tense and relaxed states, a technique they called "behavioral relaxation training." The trainer shows how breathing differs when one is relaxed and not relaxed. They found that discrimination training significantly improved relaxation in patients with more limited cognitive abilities. Behavioral relaxation training was found to have a beneficial effect on short-term learning for adults with severe intellectual disability (Lindsay and Morrison 1996).

■ TREATMENT PACKAGES

Combinations of cognitive-behavioral techniques can form treatment packages focused on a particular problem area. Four of these are reviewed here: social skills training, assertiveness training, anger management training, and sociosexual skills training. All are psychoeducational skills training programs. This method has been well received by advocacy groups for persons with mental retardation because of its prosocial, nonaversive approach.

Social Skills Training

Social skills training (SST) programs can be useful for persons with mental retardation because social skill deficits are commonly observed in this population. The target behaviors in SST can be any aspect of interpersonal interaction. Training may address verbal dimensions of interactions (the content of a message and to whom and when it is given), nonverbal aspects (eye contact, gestures, body posture, interpersonal distance), and paraverbal behaviors (voice volume, voice tone). Given such a broad spectrum of behavior, it is not surprising that SST programs vary widely.

A typical SST program includes explanation of the target behavior and rationale, modeling by the trainer or others, reinforced practice with verbal (and possible video) feedback, and continued practice of the behavior with praise from the trainer or others. Tangible reinforcers may also be provided. Assignments are given to practice the behaviors between sessions. A comprehensive program would include procedures to encourage generalization of skills to other settings and would assess whether the settings would reinforce the newly acquired skills (Griffiths 1995).

The success of SST programs is determined by comparing behavior pre- and posttraining, by comparing posttreatment behavior to that of individuals judged "socially competent," or by having others rate dimensions of patient behavior after training (Kazdin and Matson 1981). Comparing the behavior of persons with mental retardation to a criterion of socially skillful behavior is difficult because there are little normative data on social skills in this population.

SST has been successfully conducted in group training programs with persons with mental retardation. Some packages have been published that are designed for specific groups or specific types of situations. These include McClennen, Hoekstra, and Bryan's program for severely retarded adults (1980) and Foxx and McMorrow's social skills game (1983). (See the section on sociosexual skills for further discussion of the Foxx and McMorrow program.)

One exemplary study of SST was conducted by Sisson et al. (1988) with a class of five multidisabled children. Thirty-minute training sessions were given three times per week that included providing a rationale, discussion, modeling, and role-playing. Trained behaviors were initiating play, sharing, asking for a toy, joining an activity, and organizing a game. Subjects improved in free play situations and maintained improvements at 6-month follow-up. Involving the entire class in the training was recommended as a way of ensuring that gains were maintained, at least among classmates.

SST has also been used to change nonverbal aspects of social interaction. Frame et al. (1982) worked with a 10-year-old depressed inpatient who was functioning in the borderline range of mental retardation. Therapist modeling, role-playing, feedback, and reinforcement of appropriate behaviors were used to change body posture, eye contact, flat affect, and poor speech quality. In each case, the specific behavior responded to the intervention once it was subject to the training contingencies.

SST is recommended for persons with mental retardation and depressed mood because research findings indicate that specific social skill deficits exist in this group (Benson et al. 1985; Laman and Reiss 1987; Schloss 1982). Further, SST is effective in the treatment of behavioral characteristics of depression (Matson et al. 1979).

It is one thing to learn a skill and quite another to perform it. Anxiety about social interaction can inhibit performance of social skills. Lindsay (1986) reported three case studies of individuals with mental retardation who seemed to be inhibited from performing social skills due to anxiety about other people's opinions of them or other negative self-statements. SST (combined with self-instruction in one case) resulted in minimal change in rated skill levels, but cognitive changes were obtained on self-report questionnaires. In addition, others reported greater frequency of social interactions following training. The author concluded that greater attention needs to be given to the cognitive factors in social interactions for people with mental retardation.

Assertiveness Training

Assertiveness is defined as the skill of "standing up for oneself and exercising one's rights in a comfortable manner without denying the rights of others" (Bregman 1985). In this conceptual framework, assertiveness is distinguished from passiveness (not standing up for one's rights) and aggressiveness (standing up for oneself in a way that violates the rights of others).

The need for persons with mental retardation to behave assertively has been addressed by several sources. Rosen et al. (1974) have pointed out the high rate of passivity and apathy that exists in this group. Similarly, Floor and Rosen (1975) suggested that such behavior patterns may be due to institutionalized living. Bregman (1984) stated that a controlled lifestyle may lead to an external locus of control.

Assertiveness training typically employs a combination of instruction, modeling, and behavioral rehearsal. It is often conducted in a group therapy setting to allow for peer feedback and social reinforcement. Training is adapted for individuals with mental retardation by simplifying the language of the didactic sections and by choosing modeling situations that reflect the real-life situations they confront. For example, a discussion of when to use assertive behavior may be explained this way:

> After you have learned HOW to be assertive, you need to learn WHEN to be assertive. It's just like riding a bicycle; once you've learned how to do it, you really enjoy it. That doesn't mean that you will always ride your bike. There are times when that would not work. You wouldn't try to ride your bike across a lake, would you? In the same way there are times when assertiveness is not the best way to handle a situation. (Miranti 1984)

The discussion is followed by a series of vignettes of daily interactions that may require an assertive response. These situations may include how to respond to criticism from the supervisor at the vocational center, how to request information when one is lost, or what to do when approached by a stranger. Sample responses are labeled as passive, aggressive, or assertive. Patients are then invited to rehearse an assertive response, with feedback solicited from other group members.

Research found that people with mental retardation benefit from assertiveness training. Unfortunately, much of this research was poorly controlled or ill conceived. For example, Granat (1978) conducted an assertiveness program for seven mentally retarded patients but did not use objective assessment tools and did not employ a control group. Later, Gentile and Jenkins (1980) included a role-play assessment in their study of assertiveness training but neglected to include a control group. In 1982, Kirkland and Caughlin-Carver both used a control group and videotaped role-plays, finding improvement on several measures of role-play ratings. Unfortunately, while attempting to assess generalization to new situations, groups were compared on different role-play vignettes. Bregman (1985) found that people with mental retardation could learn to communicate more assertively but had more difficulty in learning to discriminate assertive from nonassertive behavior when compared with nondisabled peers.

In the best controlled study to date, Nezu et al. (1991) provided five sessions of group training each in assertiveness and in problem solving of anger-arousing situations to adults with mild mental retardation and psychiatric diagnoses. Both interventions resulted in improvements on multiple self-report measures and caregiver ratings of adaptive behavior compared with a waiting list control group. The observed gains were maintained at a 3-month follow-up test.

Although it is possible to show that assertiveness training is effective with mentally retarded persons, it is another matter to show that it is the best treatment for a patient. In one study that compared relaxation therapy with assertiveness training (Miranti and Freedman 1984), relaxation therapy was superior in reducing anxiety and resulted in quicker learning. This finding suggests that the therapist should carefully assess the patient's needs before selecting a treatment.

Anger Management Training

Studies indicate that people with mental retardation are frequently referred for treatment because of aggressive behavior (Benson 1985). The Anger Management Training Program (AMT) is a cognitive-behavioral intervention to improve self-control of anger in persons with mental retardation. Based on the work of Raymond Novaco (1975, 1978) with nonretarded adults and the work of Camp and colleagues (1977) with nonretarded children, the program combines relaxation training, self-instructional training, and problem-solving training to improve interpersonal functioning. Both group interventions and individual training programs have been used with adolescents and adults who are functioning in the mild to moderate range of mental retardation (Benson 1986, 1992; Benson and Havercamp 1999; Benson et al. 1986; Rose 1996).

Early training sessions focus on identification of feelings, including happiness, sadness, and anger. Anger is viewed as one of many emotions that everyone experiences at times. Persons are asked to self-monitor feelings each day and discuss these in the weekly sessions. Through discussion, the individual is encouraged to identify connections between events and feelings and between feelings and behaviors. Patients must first recognize when they are angry, and preferably when they are starting to become angry, in order to activate the self-control skills.

The second component of the program is relaxation training. PMR with 10 muscle groups is used with the trainer modeling and guiding the individual through the exercises at first. Audiotapes of the relaxation instructions are provided for home practice once the exercises are performed correctly in the session. Individuals role-play anger-arousing situations while practicing relaxation in the sessions.

The self-instructional training component of the program begins with instruction and practice in discriminating between "coping statements" and "trouble statements." Coping statements are self-statements that help one to stay calm, whereas trouble statements serve to arouse or maintain anger. Coping statements may include, "Take it easy," "Stay calm," "I can handle it," or "Be cool." Some examples of trouble statements are, "Who does he think he is?" "I'm not going to take that from her!" and "I won't let him get away with it!" Although several examples of coping statements are provided to individuals in the training program, participants are encouraged to construct their own statements. Coping statements are practiced first aloud, then silently during role-playing of problem situations.

ing the question, "Let's pretend that you really want to go see one movie, but your boy/girlfriend would prefer to see another. How could you solve this problem?" Patients are then invited to generate as many solutions as they can to the situation, no matter how silly or farfetched. All solutions are written on a board. Next, therapists enact less appropriate solutions to the problem while patients observe. Participants judge how well the solution works by deciding whether it was helpful in solving the problem. In this way, patients are helped to think through the consequences of possible actions. Finally, more appropriate responses are role-played and the best response is agreed upon. Participants pair up to rehearse the best response while other group members are guided into giving positive feedback.

DSP is unique in many respects. Training is provided on a wide range of skills that change as intimacy levels change. Skills progress from less to more intimate, the progression seen in real-life situations. This suggests that people must first become friends before moving on to intimate relationships. Moreover, the program uses modeling and role-playing to implement both verbal and nonverbal skills, which aids in generalization to other settings. Another unique aspect is the combination of social skills with problem solving by treating social situations as problems to be solved. Using problem solving for these skills, patients learn to make their own decisions and are given a coping mechanism to deal with diverse situations that can arise in intimacy.

A final unique aspect of DSP is that it has a supportive research base. In 1986, the program was compared to a relaxation treatment for reducing social anxiety (Mueser et al. 1986). Patients were compared on several verbal and nonverbal aspects of social skills using a role-play test. Interaction patterns were also monitored during a mid-session break. Only DSP participants showed a trend toward improvement on behavior rating scales. This group also demonstrated a higher rate of interaction at mid-session breaks. Ratings of physical attractiveness, a characteristic that is presumed stable, also improved.

In a second study, Valenti-Hein et al. (1994) compared DSP to a waiting-list control condition. DSP participants again improved across all behavior rating scales, and ratings of physical attractiveness improved. Patients in DSP also reallocated their time, spending more time talking to opposite-sex peers following training. Comparing the performance of the groups across the two studies, DSP was superior to the relaxation training program and the waiting-list control group (Valenti-Hein 1989). Moreover, relaxation training appeared to be detrimental to later performance, as measured by a role-play test.

Much research remains to be done in evaluating social/sexual skills in persons with disabilities. The next few years will be critical in the development of new assessment and treatment techniques to deal with this issue.

■ CONCLUSIONS

People with mental retardation experience the full range of emotional distur-bance (Philips 1967). It is important that they have access to all effective treat-ments. As reviewed here, research shows that cognitive and social learning interventions can be effective with mentally retarded persons. For the most part, these interventions have been used with verbal persons functioning in the borderline to high moderate range, although some techniques have been adapted for less verbal individuals. Of course, the cognitive level of the indi-vidual must be taken into account in the design and implementation of the in-terventions, and some creativity is required in adapting techniques. Additional research should outline the range of application of cognitive and social learn-ing techniques with mentally retarded persons. The present state of knowl-edge indicates that cognitively based interventions must be added to the treatment armamentaria of the clinician who works with people with mental retardation.

■ REFERENCES

Bandura A: Principles of Behavior Modification. New York, Holt, Rinehart, & Win-ston, 1969

Bandura A, Barab PG: Processes governing disinhibitory effects through symbolic modeling. J Abnorm Psychol 82:1–9, 1973

Benson BA: Behavior disorders and mental retardation: associations with age, sex, and level of functioning in an outpatient clinic sample. Applied Research in Mental Retardation 6:79–85, 1985

Benson BA: Anger management training. Psychiatric Aspects of Mental Retardation Reviews 5(10):51–55, 1986

Benson BA: Teaching Anger Management to Persons With Mental Retardation. Wor-thington, OH, IDS Publishing, 1992

Benson BA, Havercamp SM: Behavioral approaches to treatment: principles and prac-tices, in Psychiatric and Behavioural Disorders in Developmental Disabilities and Mental Retardation. Edited by Bouras N. Cambridge, UK, Cambridge University Press 1999, pp 262–278

Benson BA, Reiss S, Smith DC, et al: Psychosocial correlates of depression in mentally retarded adults; II: poor social skills. American Journal of Mental Deficiency 89:657–659, 1985

Benson BA, Rice CJ, Miranti SV: Effects of anger management training with mentally retarded adults in group treatment. J Consult Clin Psychol 54:728–729, 1986

Beveridge M, Conti-Ramsden G: Social cognition and problem-solving in persons with mental retardation. Australia and New Zealand Journal of Developmental Disabilities 13:99–106, 1987

Bornstein PH, Quevillon RP: The effects of a self-instructional package on overactive preschool boys. J Appl Behav Anal 9:179–188, 1976

Bregman S: Assertiveness training for mentally retarded adults. Ment Retard 22:12–16, 1984

Bregman S: Assertiveness training for mentally retarded adults. Psychiatric Aspects of Mental Retardation Reviews 4:43–48, 1985

Burgio LD, Whitman TL, Johnson MR: A self-instructional package for increasing attending behavior in educable mentally retarded children. J Appl Behav Anal 13:443–459, 1980

Calamari JE, Geist GO, Shahbazian MJ: Evaluation of multiple component relaxation training with developmentally disabled persons. Res Dev Disabil 8:55–70, 1987

Camp BW, Blom GE, Hebert F, et al: "Think aloud": a program for developing self-control in young aggressive boys. J Abnorm Child Psychol 5:157–169, 1977

Castles EE, Glass CR: Empirical generation of measures of social competence for mentally retarded adults. Behavioral Assessment 8:319–330, 1986

Cautela JR, Groden J: Relaxation: A Comprehensive Manual for Adults, Children, and Children With Special Needs. Champaign, IL, Research Press, 1979

Champagne M, Walker-Hirsch L: Circles. Santa Barbara, CA, James Stanfield, 1988

Donaldson JY, Menolascino FJ: Emotional disorders in the retarded. International Journal of Mental Health 6:73–95, 1977

Dowrick PW: Feedforward and self-modeling, in Practical Guide to Using Video in the Behavioral Sciences. Edited by Dowrick PW. New York, Wiley, 1991, pp 109–126

D'Zurilla TJ, Goldfried MR: Problem solving and behavior modification. J Abnorm Psychol 78:107–126, 1971

Floor L, Rosen M: Investigating the phenomenon of helplessness in mentally retarded adults. American Journal of Mental Deficiency 79:565–572, 1975

Foss G, Auty WP, Irvin LK: A comparative evaluation of modeling, problem solving, and behavior rehearsal for teaching employment-rated interpersonal skills to secondary students with mental retardation. Education and Training in Mental Retardation 24:17–27, 1989

Foxx RM, McMorrow MR: Stacking the Deck: A Social Skills Game for Retarded Adults. Champaign, IL, Research Press, 1983

Frame C, Matson JL, Sonis WA, et al: Behavioral treatment of depression in a prepubertal child. J Behav Ther Exp Psychiatry 13:239–243, 1982

Gentile C, Jenkins JO: Assertive training with mildly mentally retarded persons. Ment Retard 18:315–317, 1980

Granat JP: Assertiveness training and the mentally retarded. Rehabilitation Counseling Bulletin 22:100–107, 1978

Griffiths DM: Teaching generalization of several skills with persons who have developmental disabilities. Developmental Disabilities Bulletin 23(2):43–58, 1995

Griffiths DM, Quinsey VL, Hingsburger D: Changing Inappropriate Sexual Behavior: A Community-Based Approach for Persons With Developmental Disabilities. Baltimore, MD, Paul H. Brookes, 1989

Grimm J, Bijou S, Parsons J: A problem-solving model for teaching remedial arithmetic to handicapped young children. J Abnorm Child Psychol 7:26–39, 1973

Harvey JR: The potential of relaxation training for the mentally retarded. Ment Retard 17:71–76, 1979

Jackson HJ, Hooper JP: Some issues arising from the desensitization of a dog phobia in a mildly retarded female: or should we take the bite out of the bark? Australia and New Zealand Journal of Developmental Disabilities 7:9–16, 1981

Johnston MB, Whitman TL, Johnson M: Teaching addition and subtraction to mentally retarded children: a self-instruction program. Applied Research in Mental Retardation 1:141–160, 1980

Kazdin AE, Matson JL: Social validation in mental retardation. Applied Research in Mental Retardation 2:39–53, 1981

Kempton W: Life Horizons. Santa Barbara, CA, James Stanfield, 1990

Kirkland K, Caughlin-Carver J: Maintenance and generalization of assertive skills. Education and Training of the Mentally Retarded 17:313–318, 1982

Krantz PJ, MacDuff GS, Wadstrom O, et al: Using video with developmentally disabled learners, in Practical Guide to Using Video in the Behavioral Sciences. Edited by Dowrick PW. New York, Wiley, 1991, pp 256–266

Laman DS, Reiss S: Social skills deficiencies associated with depressed mood in mentally retarded adults. American Jpurnal of Mental Deficiency 92:224–229, 1987

Lindsay WR: Cognitive changes after social skills training with young mildly mentally handicapped adults. Journal of Mental Deficiency Research 30:81–88, 1986

Lindsay WR, Morrison FM: The effect of behavioral relaxation on cognitive performance in adults with severe intellectual disabilities. J Intellect Disabil Res 40:285–290, 1996

Lindsay WR, Baty FJ, Michie AM, et al: A comparison of anxiety treatments with adults who have moderate and severe mental retardation. Res Dev Disabil 10:129–140, 1989

Luiselli JK: Relaxation training with the developmentally disabled: a reappraisal. Behavior Research of Severe Developmental Disabilities 1:191–213, 1980

Mahoney M: Reflections on the cognitive learning trend in psychotherapy. Am Psychol 32:5–13, 1977

Martin JE, Rusch FR, James VL, et al: The use of picture cues to establish self-control in the preparation of complex meals by mentally retarded adults. Applied Research in Mental Retardation 3:105–119, 1982

Matson JL: A controlled outcome study of phobias in mentally retarded adults. Behav Res Ther 19:101–107, 1981a

Matson JL: Assessment and treatment of clinical fears in mentally retarded children. J Appl Behav Anal 14:287–294, 1981b

Matson JL, Dettling J, Senatore V: Treating depression of a mentally retarded adult. British Journal of Mental Subnormality 16:86–88, 1979

McClennen SE, Hoekstra RR, Bryan JE: Social skills for severely retarded adults: an inventory and training program. Champaign, IL, Research Press, 1980

Meichenbaum D: The effects of instructions and reinforcement on thinking and language behaviors of schizophrenics. Behav Res Ther 7:101–114, 1969

Meichenbaum D, Cameron R: Training schizophrenics to talk to themselves: a means of developing attentional controls. Behav Res Ther 4:515–534, 1973

Miranti SV: Learning and anxiety reduction with highly anxious mentally retarded subjects. Unpublished master's thesis, University of Illinois at Chicago, 1984

Miranti SV, Freedman P: Effects on learning of relaxation training with mentally retarded adults (ERIC Document Reproduction Service No. ED 249 412). Paper presented at the Midwestern Psychological Association, Chicago, IL, 1984

Mueser KT, Valenti-Hein DC, Yarnold PR: Dating skills groups for the developmentally disabled: social skills and problem solving vs. relaxation training. Behav Modif 11:200–228, 1986

Nezu CM, Nezu AM, Arean P: Assertiveness and problem-solving training for mildly mentally retarded persons with dual diagnoses. Res Dev Disabil 12:371–386, 1991

Novaco RW: Anger Control. New York, Lexington Books, 1975

Novaco RW: Anger and coping with stress, in Cognitive Behavior Therapy: Research and Application. Edited by Foreyt JP, Rathjen DP. New York, Plenum, 1978, pp 135–173

Ollendick TH: Fear reduction techniques with children, in Progress in Behavior Modification, Vol 8. Edited by Hersen M, Eisler RM, Miller PM. New York, Academic, 1979, pp 127–168

Peck CL: Desensitization for the treatment of fear in the high level adult retardate. Behav Res Ther 15:137–148, 1977

Philips I: Psychopathology and mental retardation. Am J Psychiatry 124:29–35, 1967

Rickard HC, Thrasher KA, Elkins PD: Responses of persons who are mentally retarded to four components of relaxation instruction. Ment Retard 5:248–252, 1984

Robinson-Wilson MA: Picture recipe cards as an approach to teaching severely and profoundly retarded adults to cook. Education and Training of the Mentally Retarded 12:69–73, 1977

Rose J: Anger management: a group treatment program for people with mental retardation. Journal of Developmental and Physical Disabilities 8(2):133–149, 1996

Rosen M, Floor L, Zisfein L: Investigating the phenomenon of acquiescence in the mentally handicapped; I: theoretical model, test development and normative data. British Journal of Mental Subnormality 20:58–65, 1974

Ross DM, Ross SA: Cognitive training for the EMR child: situational problem solving and planning. American Journal of Mental Deficiency 78:20–26, 1973

Ross DM, Ross SA: Cognitive training for the EMR child: choosing the best alternative. Am J Ment Def 82:598–601, 1978

Runyan MC, Stevens DH, Reeves R: Reduction of avoidance behavior of institutionalized mentally retarded adults through contact desensitization. American Journal of Mental Deficiency 90:222–225, 1985

Rusch FR, Morgan TK, Martin JE, et al: Competitive employment: teaching mentally retarded employees self-instructional strategies. Applied Research in Mental Retardation 6:389–407, 1985

Schloss PJ: Verbal interaction patterns of depressed and non-depressed institutionalized mentally retarded adults. Applied Research in Mental Retardation 3:1–12, 1982

Shure MB, Spivack G: Interpersonal problem-solving in young children: a cognitive approach to prevention. Am J Community Psychol 10:341–356, 1982

Sisson LA, Babeo TJ, Van Hasselt VB: Group training to increase social behaviors in young multihandicapped children. Behav Modif 12:497–524, 1988

Spivack G, Platt JJ, Schure MB: The Problem-Solving Approach to Adjustment. San Francisco, CA, Jossey-Bass, 1976

Tymchuk AJ, Andron L, Rahbar B: Effective decision making/problem-solving training with mothers who have mental retardation. Am J Ment Retard 6:510–516, 1988

Valenti-Hein D: An evaluation of treatment approaches for romantic loneliness of mentally retarded adults. Doctoral dissertation, University of Illinois at Chicago, 1988. Dissertation Abstracts International 50–5:2170B, 1989

Valenti-Hein D, Mueser K: The Dating Skills Program: Teaching Social-Sexual Skills to Adults With Mental Retardation. Worthington, OH, IDS Publishing, 1990

Valenti-Hein D, Yarnold P, Mueser K: Evaluation of the Dating Skills Program for improving heterosocial interactions in people with mental retardation. Behav Modif 18:32–46, 1994

Vygotsky LS: Thought and Language. Boston, MA, MIT Press, 1962

Wilson B, Jackson HJ: An in vivo approach to the desensitization of a retarded child's toilet phobia. Australia and New Zealand Journal of Developmental Disabilities 6:137–141, 1980

6 Working With Families and Caregivers of People With Severe Mental Retardation

Ann Gath, M.D., F.R.C.Psych., D.P.M., D.C.H.

Children and adults with severe mental retardation are cared for at home to an increasing degree. In a study in a region of England (Farmer et al. 1991), 41.6% of those registered as eligible to use mental retardation services were living in their family homes, being looked after by their parents and occasionally siblings. The vast majority, nearly 90%, of the children under age 15 years lived with their families, but the proportion still at home dropped steadily with age in adult life.

Treatment of parents begins with the first encounter when the parents first learn of the probability that their child will have a serious disability. However, the breaking of the news is only the first step in the long-term support of the parents through the life span of that disabled child. More directed treatment will be required at specific stages or for particular problems as they arise (see also Chapter 10 of this book).

■ THE FIRST IMPACT ON THE PARENTS

Natural parents have been the subject of most research. They differ from other caregivers in that they have made no choice to take on the work, which, for most of them, comes to take over much of their lives. Initially, the realization that a child, usually the result of a planned and welcome pregnancy, has a lifelong disability likely to produce significant problems in attaining the ordinary goals of life comes as a severe shock. In understanding the psychological reactions of parents, it is necessary to be able to tease out this initial shock from the toll taken by the increased work that starts very early in the life of the child (Gath 1978).

Parents' initial reaction to revelation of a child's mental retardation has been regarded as being similar to grief. The stages often seen in grief reactions may also be observed in the reactions of parents to the news of their child's diagnosis, which brings with it the prognosis of a lasting disability. However, as in other grief reactions, people vary greatly in their speed of passage through the stages and may, without evidence of pathological reaction, omit certain stages altogether. There is, therefore, no distinct "normal" path along which parents should be guided to assist their eventual adaptation. It is also common for parents to experience grief and manifest their outward feelings in very different ways from each other.

The way that the news is broken to the parents has been shown to be crucial in determining early adaptation and later attitudes (Cunningham et al. 1984; Nursey et al. 1990; Quine and Pahl 1987). Interviews recorded 14 years after the event show much of the same flavor as those recorded shortly after the birth of a child with Down's syndrome (Gath 1990). Currently little training is offered to those likely to be faced with breaking such news.

■ THE ROLE OF MEDICAL DIAGNOSIS

The role of the doctor in supporting parents depends on his or her knowledge of the cause of the retardation and how that affects the future. An understanding of the normal process of grief and possible deviations is essential.

Much of the work on the early reactions of parents has been done on families into which a child has been born with an easily recognizable disorder, such as Down's syndrome with its characteristic facial stigmata and well-known association with moderate mental retardation. Other disorders either are recognized only gradually as development deviates more and more from the norm or are related to events taking place later in childhood following a period of apparently normal development, as in posttraumatic brain damage. Parental adjustment to the fact of the permanent nature of a disability following a traumatic event or a sudden acute illness will develop as the converse of the hope of a complete recovery slowly fades.

Most parents find it easier to accept the implications of a lasting disability if there is a medical explanation and preferably a clear diagnosis with causal etiology and prognosis carefully spelled out. Such a label can help to absolve them from blame, provide an explanation for bemused and sometimes even hostile relations, and facilitate membership of a supportive club, such as the Down's Association, the Fragile X Association, and those associated with tuberous sclerosis, Rett's syndrome, spina bifida, and many other conditions. Such groups, which are steadily increasing in number, help in ending the isolation of the distressed parents as well as in offering positive reactions by assisting with and funding research.

■ SOCIOCULTURAL DISADVANTAGES

However, much learning disability is not explainable in medical terms. Mild mental retardation less commonly carries evidence of a medical cause (Broman et al. 1987) and is more often associated with subcultural factors. Sociocultural disadvantages, however, are by no means confined to this group. Severely mentally retarded children with no known medical diagnosis matched for verbal and nonverbal abilities with children with Down's syndrome in the same school class had families with high incidence of poverty, poor housing, and parents with low educational achievement as well as high incidence of marital disharmony and parental ill health (Gath and Gumley 1986).

The problems of caring for a child with mental retardation are greatly compounded by the living conditions described by young mothers who are themselves intellectually limited (British Institute of Medical Handicap 1990). Even when rehoused by a local authority believed to be aware of their problems, these mothers have no access to a telephone even for emergencies and no external security to their home, with kitchens and bathroom that are shared, thus making the aftercare and control of even normal young children very difficult and that of a hyperactive retarded child impossible.

■ HELPING PARENTS COPE MORE EFFECTIVELY

Recent research has moved away from looking at "stress-related" signs of ill health in parents and instead seeks to identify strengths and effective coping measures (Birchwood and Cochrane 1990). Such work offers some chance of finding solutions to the problems faced by parents as caregivers of their disabled children.

Early intervention programs in which parents are taught how to assist their child's motor and intellectual development have also been shown to increase parental self-esteem, lessen the ill effects of a grief reaction, and aid them in coping better with later problems (Seifer et al. 1991). Successful programs are those that enhance the confidence and competence of parents without the emphasis being entirely on intellectual enhancement. In the United Kingdom, the Portage system is most commonly used to deliver an early intervention service (Sturmey and Crisp 1986).

■ PROBLEMS OF HEREDITY

Stepparents and foster or adoptive parents share many of the problems faced by the biological parents. They are, however, spared the distress and questioning anxiety about their role in bringing about the underlying cause of the disability. Inherited disorders have always been a source of painful family secrets and, as such, for many years provided fodder for dramatic fiction. Nowadays with the discovery of genes occurring relatively frequently and the full human genetic map expected within the decade, there is the hope and, in some cases, the practical expectation of prevention of genetic disorders. However, such possibilities can be oversimplified. If, for example, carrier status can be clearly demonstrated in a female fetus with fragile X syndrome, what is the advice to be given regarding the future life chances of such a fetus? From what is now known, such a woman may herself have only minor intellectual disability although the fate of the affected male fetus is probably more clear. The "new genetics" quite definitely add major moral and ethical dilemmas to the existing problems of natural parents.

■ SUBSTITUTE PARENTS

In clinical situations, stepparents, adoptive parents, and foster parents are often encountered as highly motivated, supportive, and hardworking caregivers. A number of studies have testified to their resourcefulness and sometimes unconventional nature (Gath 1983; Wolkind and Kozaruk 1983). However, when not fully informed or when events overtake their initial decision to take on a child that is not their own, serious problems can occur. A common example is that of adoptive parents who, after years of increasing despair at their infertility, suffer still more frustrating years before being accepted as prospective adopters; they finally take into their care a seemingly normal baby only to realize later after formalities are over that the child has severe problems. Such a history preceding the realization of disability prejudices the chances of the parents being able to meet the repeated challenges as caregivers for a child with major disabilities. Nonetheless, there is much to be learned from those adoptive parents whose commitment to a severely disabled child is robust and lifelong.

■ BURDEN OF CARE

Everyone caring for a child or adult with severe mental retardation and the commonly associated problem of behavior disturbance in their own homes encounters what has been termed the *burden of care*. This has been well described by research workers who have studied the hour-by-hour practical tasks facing the caregivers (Dupont 1986) and can be summarized as extremely hard work with virtually no carefree time off. The usual situation is for the mother to take the greater part of the burden. Physical wear and tear, particularly backache, is highly likely to be a prominent feature when the caregiver has a physically disabled adult or adolescent at home.

■ FOCUSED WORK WITH PARENTS AND CAREGIVERS ON SPECIFIC PROBLEMS

The Portage approach (Sturmey and Crisp 1986), which includes many positive features with the teaching of new skills, can assist parents in the eradication of some problem behaviors before they become difficult. Successful treatment programs have been developed to treat sleep disorders in mentally retarded children. Follow-up of the participants also revealed clear beneficial effects on the general well-being of the parents (Quine 1992). Behavioral interventions using parents as therapists are more difficult when the target behaviors are more serious and involve aggressive or self-injurious behavior. Initial gains rarely generalize and frequently do not persist. The parents' understandable distress and any coexisting family psychopathology can interfere with treatment (see Chapter 10 of this book).

■ MOTHERS ON THEIR OWN

Mothers on their own have other specific difficulties. It is common, indeed normal, for young males to assert their independence and reject maternal caring that is perceived as not being appropriate for their age. In normal childhood, the first such assertions come in the third year so often referred to as the Terrible Twos. Rebellion at this age and size is not a major problem, but the same sort of protest by a mentally retarded youngster who exceeds his mother in weight and strength can present very real difficulties (Donovan 1988). Later, the need for dependence on the mother, particularly for intimate self-care, can conflict with emerging sexuality, adding to the confusion.

■ DIVORCE

In divorce cases involving a child with special needs, it is usual for the mother to be "given care and control." But this often means unrelieved responsibility without even the relief afforded by "staying access" that fathers usually insist on for the normal sibling. A second wife rarely sees herself as having volunteered to take on the role of caregiver to a child who is often the scapegoat for the breakup of the first marriage. The United Kingdom Children Act 1989 provides that a child "with needs" has the opportunity of consideration of his or her welfare as paramount, in the same way as the "normal" siblings.

■ RELIEF CARE

All parents/caregivers must be given the opportunity to receive the relief care that they find acceptable. Link families (who in many ways should be modeled on the ideal extended family) are ordinary families in the community who are prepared to get to know a disabled child and to accept him or her into their home as a guest for weekends or holidays. Some of these arrangements have been so successful that the two sets of families have become good friends and "ordinary" normal siblings have clamored to be allowed to make the visits, too. Link families are very difficult to recruit in areas where there is either much social deprivation or conversely overemphasis on material competition. Respite care appears to work best if managed largely by parents themselves, ensuring equitable access. Unpredictable or excessive use of respite care is associated with emotional disturbance within the family (Dossetor and Nicol 1989).

■ CHANGES IN FAMILIES WITH TIME

As the children grow into adulthood, the roles of parents/caregivers and other members of the family change. Older siblings who may have taken a major role in the care of the child in the past will, in the ordinary course of events, leave home, marry, and have children of their own. Many families describe how the retarded member of the family finds new friends and companions among the new generation of nephews and nieces and enjoys the love and attention of an ever-expanding family circle. But those whose mental retardation is complicated by severe problems in social relationships or by other forms of psychiatric disturbance fit badly into a family attempting to adjust to new members, especially babies and very young children. Older mothers who have struggled for years with a difficult and dependent son or daughter have a bitter, particularly tragic disappointment when the hostility of the one still at home prevents them from enjoyment of their grandchildren.

Aging parents who have worked so hard to keep "community care" going are increasing in numbers and will eventually require relief before the situation becomes impossible or even dangerous (Farmer et al. 1991). There is little evidence of any coherent planning to meet the needs of this group.

■ PROBLEMS IN OTHER CULTURES OR ETHNIC GROUPS

It is clear that in all countries where some research has taken place, many of the same problems beset all caregivers. The ideal of the accepting village community is a myth, and the work done in India shows the usefulness of help focused on acceptable local workers. Families there appear to have problems similar to families in more developed countries (Singh et al. 1990).

Isolated groups whose culture appears to be in marked contrast to that of their neighbors are particularly disadvantaged and at risk. Women who fail to learn the language of their new country or whose role prevents them from venturing out from the home are unable to benefit from many of the programs designed to help caregivers.

■ MENTALLY RETARDED PARENTS

Only recently have the problems of parents who are intellectually impaired themselves been addressed in a positive way. Mental retardation is no absolute bar to parenting (Dowdney and Skuse 1993; Gath 1988, 1996a), but those who also have major social or economic deprivation will require a broad range of help. However, if such a group of parents are allowed to speak for themselves, it quickly becomes clear that ill-informed professionals are putting up many of the barriers to their success as parents (British Institute of Medical Handicap 1990). Positive interventions can assist in preventing the breakup of families while maintaining the best interests of children (Gath 1996a).

■ PARENTS WHO BECOME MENTALLY ILL

The strain of looking after children whose dependency lasts so much longer than expected is often manifested as chronic depression. Acute distress at the time of the news is so common as to be universal. Depression of clinical severity in the first 2 years after the birth of a child known to have the likelihood of lifelong disability is not significantly more common than in a matched group of women with normal babies (Gath 1978). As the years wear on, some drift into chronic depression, but others sometimes make surprising changes (Gath 1990). The factors influencing such change were suggested in a small prospective study (Gath 1990) and appear to be supported by the larger sample in the cross-sectional study (Gath and Gumley 1986). A supportive marriage, reasonable income, and a freedom from other causes of social disadvantage were found to be protective. Adaptable and sensitive interventions individually tailored to the family's need at that particular time have major beneficial effects, whereas more stereotyped interventions based on a generalized plan have all too often increased the difficulties and prolonged the ill health. Psychiatric disorders were found to be more common in mothers caring for older children with mental retardation. Fathers were not found to be more vulnerable.

Psychiatric ill health certainly impedes the ability of anyone to care adequately for another. Severe mental illness in a caregiver can seriously threaten the well-being or even life of a dependent. The case of Beverley Lewis, a severely multidisabled adult who died when in the care of her mentally ill mother, aroused great controversy (Wiley 1992).

■ ABUSE OF PEOPLE WITH MENTAL RETARDATION

Ill treatment of patients with severe mental retardation and other disabilities was the cause of the inquiries into institutional care that preceded the strongly motivated drive toward care in the community for people with mental retardation.

Physical abuse of children is on occasion the direct cause of the brain damage leading to their cognitive impairment and other disabilities. However, it is clear that children who are slow to develop are at an increased risk of physical abuse from their caregivers.

Although there is no direct reference to children with learning disabilities in the reports following inquiries into sexual abuse, it is now quite clear that both adults and children are as much at increased risk of sexual abuse as they are to physical and emotional ill treatment. The abuse can take place at home and in children's homes, schools, or other institutions (McCune and Walford 1991).

■ PAID CAREGIVERS

Most people who are paid to care for others with mental retardation are paid to do the job on a part-time basis. Teachers see the children only during school and then only for a comparatively short period each morning and afternoon. Nurses, however, work for longer hours, though they are on shifts and rarely work excessive hours. Some residential care workers have excessive shifts and on their time off may be expected to sleep in. Pay and prospects are least for residential care workers.

There is insufficient evidence to draw conclusions about the effect of such work on the paid caregivers, although there have been some studies comparing "stress" on nurses in a hospice for the dying with those who worked with patients who were described as "mentally handicapped" (Power and Sharp 1988). Both groups were distressed about the "purposelessness" of nursing people who would never be cured. The nurses of those with mental retardation were found to be less well off on almost all measures except for pay and prospects. The recognition that hospice work could be distressing for nurses as well as patients and families has meant that major efforts were made to support nurses and to build up mutual support as well as to introduce specific psychotherapeutic interventions from outside. Thomson (1987) looked at nurses trained in the care of those with mental retardation and confirmed Power's finding that physical environment was important to morale. She found that the nurses working in the community were most disheartened when they found poor services and had physical environments contrary to their expectations of what "community care" had to offer. Short staffing was very common, with disproportionate ratios in the number of patients and staff. Twenty percent of the staff in Thomson's study had a relative with mental retardation.

■ FELLOW PATIENTS AS CAREGIVERS

The idea of another, perhaps less retarded, individual helping to care for a resident in the same place is now considered to be largely unacceptable. It was certainly not uncommon in the old, large institutions when patients would feed and sometimes dress others in wards that were being poorly staffed. It is clear from the story of Joey Deacon, who was severely disabled with cerebral palsy but able to dictate to another who translated Joey's words to a third patient who wrote down what eventually became Joey's book, that the three of them understood each other's strengths and problems much better than the staff in their institution did.

On the Island of Leros, one patient, recognized as having Prader-Willi syndrome, was made responsible by the paid staff for locking the other patients into a restraining apparatus at night and for unlocking them in the morning (Gath 1992). He also had the keys to the refrigerator, an arrangement not conducive to his own well-being, as he was grossly obese.

Abuse of people with mental retardation as unpaid and perhaps unsafe caregivers cannot, of course, be tolerated. However, expressions of affection and chances of showing concern for others by acts of kindness must not be denied them.

■ MAINTAINING THE MORALE OF CAREGIVERS

All the caregivers, family or paid outsiders, require reasonable conditions to work in and adequate time off to function properly when looking after severely mentally retarded people. This applies just as much to young single mothers, often with mental retardation themselves, as to the trained nurses still working in institutions where only the most disabled remain. They all also require information about the job they are undertaking, including knowledge about the disabilities themselves. Finally, all need to feel respected for what they are doing. Even in the case of the higher paid professionals, this cannot be taken for granted, particularly when resources are constantly threatened by spurious comparisons with quick turnover specialties with more visible outcome measures.

■ CONCLUSIONS

There have been many changes in the care of those severely disabled by mental retardation and their associated problems. It is recognized that the management of parents is based on a long-term partnership over the life span of mentally retarded people. Caregivers themselves become frail, but only recently has it been recognized that changes in life expectancy can result in an elderly person with mental retardation being the sole caregiver of a very old parent. Nonetheless, a not insignificant group of people reach old age having spent their lives caring for a permanently dependent child and are able to look back with satisfaction at a job well done and forward with more equanimity than most (Seltzer and Krauss 1989).

Care in the community is also put at risk by the high sickness rates and rapid turnover of staff in small group homes. Rapid expansion of privately owned establishments has meant that staff can be poorly trained and without adequate support. The well-being of the residents depends on the integrity, morale, and good health of their caregivers, the maintenance of which must be far higher up on the agenda of community-placed support teams.

■ REFERENCES

Birchwood M, Cochrane R: Families coping with schizophrenia: coping styles, their origins and correlates. Psychol Med 20:857–865, 1990

British Institute of Medical Handicap: Proceedings of a Conference on Parents With Learning Disability, Kidderminster, UK, 1990

Broman S, Nichols PL, Shaughnessy P, et al: Retardation in Young Children: A Developmental Study of Cognitive Deficit. New Jersey, Lawrence Erlbaum Associates, 1987

Cunningham CC, Morgan PA, McGucken RB: Down's syndrome: is dissatisfaction with disclosure of diagnosis inevitable? Dev Med Child Neurol 26:33–39, 1984

Donovan AM: Family stress and ways of coping with adolescents who have handicaps: maternal perceptions. Am J Ment Retard 92:502–509, 1988

Dossetor DR, Nicol AR: Dilemmas of adolescents with developmental retardation: a review. J Adolesc 12:167–185, 1989

Dowdney L, Skuse D: Parenting provided by adults with mental retardation. J Child Psychol Psychiatry 34:25–48, 1993

Dupont A: Sociopsychiatric aspects of the young severely mentally retarded and the family. Br J Psychiatry 148:227–234, 1986

Farmer R, Rohde J, Sacks B: Dimensions of Mental Handicap: A Study of People With Mental Handicaps in the North West Thames Region. London, North West Thames Regional Health Authority, 1991

Gath A: Down's Syndrome and the Family: The Early Years. London, Academic, 1978

Gath A: Mentally retarded children in substitute and natural families. Adoption and Fostering 7:35–40, 1983

Gath A: Mentally handicapped people as parents: is mental retardation a bar to adequate parenting? J Child Psychol Psychiatry 29:739–744, 1988

Gath A: Down syndrome children and their families. Am J Med Genet (suppl 7):314–316, 1990

Gath A: Guest editorial. Journal of Mental Deficiency Research 36:3–5, 1992

Gath A: Enhancing the parenting skills of people with a learning disability, in Parental Psychiatric Disorder. Edited by Gopfest M, Webster J, Seeman M. Cambridge, UK, Cambridge University Press, 1996a, pp 246–258

Gath A: Parents with learning disability, in Assessment of Parenting, Psychiatric and Psychological Contributions. Edited by Reder P, Lucey C. London, Routledge,1996b, pp 203–215

Gath A, Gumley D: Family background of children with Down's syndrome and of children with a similar degree of mental retardation. Br J Psychiatry 149:161–171, 1986

McCune N, Walford G: The role of the psychiatrist in child sexual abuse. Irish Journal of Psychological Medicine 8:93–98, 1991

Nursey AD, Rhode JR, Farmer RD: A study of doctor's and parent's attitudes to people with mental handicaps. Journal of Menatl Deficiency Research 34:143–155, 1990

Power KG, Sharp GR: A comparison of sources of nursing stress and job satisfaction among mental handicap and hospice nursing staff. J Adv Nurs 13:726–732, 1988

Quine L: Helping parents to manage children's sleep disturbance: an intervention trial using health professionals, in The Children Act 1989 and Family Support: Principles into Practice. Edited by Gibbons J. London, Her Majesty's Stationary Office, 1992, pp 101–137

Quine L, Pahl J: First diagnosis of severe mental handicap: a study of parental reactions. Development Medicine and Child Neurology 29:232–242, 1987

Seifer RD, Clark GN, Sameroff AJ: Positive effects of interaction coaching on infants with developmental disabilities and their mothers. Am J Mental Retard 96:1–11, 1991

Seltzer MM, Krauss MW: Aging parents with adult mentally retarded children: family risk factors and sources of support. Am J Ment Retard 94:303–312, 1989

Singh PD, Goyal L, Peshad D, et al: Psychosocial problems in families of disabled children. Br J Med Psychol 63:173–182, 1990

Sturmey P, Crisp P: Portage guide to early intervention: a review of research. Educational Psychologist 6:139–157, 1986

Thomson S: Stress in staff working with mentally handicapped people, in Stress in Health Professionals. Edited by Payne R and Firth-Cosens J. Chichester, UK, Wiley, 1987, pp 151–156

Wiley Y: The Beverley Lewis case: an outline of some of the medico-legal aspects, in A Double Challenge: Report of a Joint CCETSW/Royal College of Psychiatrists Symposium. London, UK, CCETSW Paper 19.27, 1992a, pp 13–15

Wiley Y: The case of Beverley Lewis. Article presented at a joint meeting with the British Association of Social Work and Royal College of Psychiatrists, 1992b, pp 13–15

Wolkind S, Kozaruk A: The adoption of children with mental handicap. Adoption and Fostering 32–35, 1983

Psychotherapeutic Methods

7 Psychoanalytic Therapies

Richard Ruth, Ph.D.

Methods of psychoanalytic therapies have already been described in Chapter 2 of this book. In this chapter, I explore ways in which psychoanalytic conceptualizations and a range of psychoanalytically oriented therapies, consultation, individual therapy, and group therapy can be helpful in working with persons with mental retardation. Although these treatments have not been systematically employed or researched with this population (existing literature is confined to theoretical writings and case studies), there has been in recent years a resurgence of interest in psychoanalytically oriented work with people with mental retardation. This seems to flow from a sense that there are gaps in the results that can be achieved with other intervention methods, and from changes in psychoanalytic theory and technique that make effective therapeutic work with persons with mental retardation more possible.

■ CONCEPTUAL ISSUES

Psychoanalysis has several meanings or facets: a general framework of clinical thinking; the specific method of classical psychoanalysis; a body of knowledge accumulated through psychoanalytic clinical work and research; the body of clinicians who refer to themselves as psychoanalysts and the organizational structures in which they work. In this chapter, I deal primarily with the application of a psychoanalytic orientation to clinical work, emphasizing open-ended exploration of unconscious material through the methods of free association and interpretations of transference, dreams, resistance, and defense. To my knowledge, there is little classical analysis practiced with persons with mental retardation, though there is much application of psychoanalytic methods (Gaedt 1995, 1997). The Jungian perspective will not be included as it lies outside my area of competence, although some Jungian-oriented writers (Baum 1990) have written in this area. For similar reasons contributions by non–English-speaking analysts are not included, although there is significant interest in work with persons with mental retardation among Francophone analysts.

Although few psychoanalysts work in the area of developmental disabilities, those who do include psychoanalytic clinicians of varying theoretical leanings. In this chapter, the contributions of Kleinians, Lacanians, and clinicians associated with the British Independent, classical Freudian, self-psychology, and other schools will be mentioned.

■ INDICATIONS FOR PSYCHOANALYTICALLY ORIENTED THERAPIES

Current renewal of interest in applications of psychoanalytic work to persons with mental retardation seems to stem from two sources. One, which may be conceptualized as coming from within psychoanalysis, has to do with advances in psychoanalytic theory and techniques—in particular, understanding of deficit states, active agency in primitive mental life, the impact of external trauma on psychological functioning, and the workings of therapeutic empathy—which address some of the technical problems of working analytically with people with retardation (for a fuller discussion see Ruth 1990). In some sense, this is part of a general trend in psychoanalysis in the modern period oriented to undertaking work with more severely impaired patients.

The other source has its underpinnings in pressures that are external to analysis. Currently, in the United States, and I suspect elsewhere, there is a generation of people with retardation who graduate from behaviorally oriented special education programs and expect to spend their lives in the community, supported by appropriate services. Many have unquestionably benefited from this. They participate in the community, they work, they achieve gratifications and levels of independence almost unthinkable 20 or 30 years ago.

Yet, in ways that often are evocative of the experience of Freud's discontented Viennese bourgeoisie, their lives can seem empty and unsatisfying. Their advances in behavioral competency are often not accompanied by similar levels of competence in their emotional or inner lives. Thus, a common indication for psychoanalytic psychotherapy in a person with mental retardation would be when good behaviorally oriented programming and adequate supportive services leave unresolved problems in emotional functioning.

For an in-depth history of psychoanalytic work with people with mental retardation, the interested reader is referred to the writings of Alvarez (1992), Ruth (1990), and Sinason (1992). However, it should be noted that, among earlier generations of psychoanalytic clinicians, there were those who believed that mental retardation itself was a neurotic phenomenon, that is, a syndrome developed as a defense against potentially analyzable unconscious wishes and conflicts. Related to this was the belief that inappropriate parental behavior often caused mental retardation. This is *not* the belief of contemporary analytically oriented clinicians working with people with mental retardation.

Mannoni (1970, 1972) and Symington (1981) moved psychoanalytic thinking into a different direction by focusing on their intersubjective experiences in therapy with patients with mental retardation. Through the use of experiments, they describe intensive, protracted, and analytically oriented attempts to work with persons with retardation. Leaving aside prior opinions as to whether their patients had the capacity to demonstrate psychodynamically determined phenomena, to benefit from interpretation, or to demonstrate insight or change, their attempt was more fundamentally to engage with their patients authentically, empathically, and with the ever-hovering attention to dynamic phenomena that analysts strive to practice.

Both Mannoni and Symington felt that their patients did present analyzable material and showed a capacity to benefit from both analytic relationships and dynamic interpretations. Current workers in this area tend very much to follow this direction (Gaedt 1997; Mawson 1986; Ruth 1990; Sinason 1986, 1990, 1992; Spensley 1985). The focus is not on a theoretical debate about whether retardation is psychodynamically caused or whether analytically informed treatment can remove cognitive deficiencies so much as on understanding the meaning of a specific phenomenon in a specific person. This search for unique dynamic meanings is at the heart of all contemporary psychoanalytically informed intervention with persons with mental retardation.

More specifically, Sinason's (1986) notion of secondary mental disability has been widely found to be extremely useful clinically:

> Opening your eyes to admitting you look, sound, walk, talk, move, or think differently takes reserves of courage, honesty, and toleration of envy. It can be easier to behave like the village idiot and make everyone laugh than to expose the unbearable discrepancy between normal and not normal. In handicap there may be organic or traumatic damage that affects the person concerned. However, there is also a particular use that the person makes of any original organic or traumatic damage. (p. 132)

This latter phenomenon is at the heart of the concept of secondary disability. Sinason further describes three subtypes of secondary mental disability: 1) mild secondary disability, conceptualized as a type of neurotic character defense used by persons with mental retardation who "have compliantly exacerbated their original disability to keep the outer world happy with them" (p. 134); 2) opportunist disability, or more severe character pathology, developed to protect an inner core of the psyche against the intolerable ego awareness of the focal mental disability, the constitutional deficiencies related to it, and the painful experiences it meets from the environment; and 3) disability as a defense against trauma.

It is precisely in addressing issues such as these that psychoanalytic therapies with people with mental retardation can have their greatest utility. As is the case with other applications of psychoanalytic psychotherapy, the aim is to attempt to unblock developmental stalemates, to resolve unconscious emotional conflicts that constrict the patient's options and life space, and to foster a capacity to love as well as to work. The concern is thus not with promoting or repressing certain behaviors but with understanding the inner life of the patient.

■ PSYCHOANALYTICALLY INFORMED CONSULTATION

This modality refers to a limited contact, either with a patient or with a caretaking or educational system, for the purposes of clarifying the psychodynamics that underlie functioning. The methodologies used include observation and interview as well as theoretical concepts that are brought to bear to help the consulted understand the unconscious factors at play (Gaedt 1995, 1997). Underlying assumptions are that understanding the source and dynamics of a behavior may facilitate its positive transformation, and that tracing behaviors to their source in the inner and unconscious life of a person with mental retardation may be productive and useful, as in the following example:

> B, a 45-year-old woman with profound mental retardation had been a nursing home resident for many years. She had no speech or observable receptive language, almost no capacity for gestural communication, close to no adaptive or social competencies, and an affective life of very little range. B spent most of her time in bed; on the occasions when the nursing staff sat her up or took her to the dayroom or hallway so she could be at least exposed to a bit more of life, they had little sense of any recompense for their efforts. B was fed via a gastric tube because of her tendencies to ruminate and aspirate food. The presenting problem was that she had begun flinching and slapping at nursing staff when they attempted to care for her and poked and pulled at the gastric tube in a manner that had the potential to cause serious medical problems.
>
> The intervention began with several sessions sitting at B's bedside and watching her. It became apparent that her problematic behaviors were simultaneously expressing her own spark of life. Picking at herself or flailing at her tube seemed to serve the purpose of affirming that she had life and sensation, as opposed to a feeling of nothingness. Hitting at both her human caretakers and the caretaking tube seemed similar to the attempts of an infant, on the cusp between primary symbiosis and first autonomous acts, to define a primitive boundary between "me" and "not me"; a template experience would be an infant's biting the nipple to clarify in his or her own experience the boundary between self and breast. B's rumination of her food seemed to enact an unconscious conflict between experiencing the food as a potential toxic in-

troject, derived from the split-off part-object of "bad breast," and positively cathecting it as nourishment.

Interpreting these phenomena to the nurses provided a basis for beginning to understand B, and this in itself made for less frustration and more empathy in their care of her. Furthermore, these few insights helped the nurses begin to think creatively about how they might productively influence B's problematic behaviors. One strategy they developed was to have one nurse, the same each day, sit by her bedside during feedings, stroking her arm and speaking to her in a soothing voice. This seemed to function as an analog experience of a mother holding an infant during a feeding, the intimacy forming a containing structure against and within which the infant can begin to tolerate the confusing, disorganizing, and anxiety-provoking experiences of feeding before there is a cognitive structure in place to enable one to make sense of this rush of sensation. In analytic terms, this is referred to as the *skin* or *envelope* function of the ego (Anzieu 1989).

The strategy helped reduce B's resistance to feeding, and there was an impression that the containing presence of the nurse helped her integrate and synthesize the previously unmetabolized elements of her experience.

Another application of psychoanalytically informed consultation involves the counseling of parents of children with mental retardation (Fajardo 1987; Solnit and Stark 1962). Here, the focus is not on imparting information or instruction in behavioral management techniques but on helping the parents understand the workings of the child's inner life, their own unconscious reactions to the child, and how the two sets of issues articulate with each other, so that, from this understanding, more adaptive and satisfying patterns of interaction can emerge.

A review of the literature has not uncovered instances of analytically oriented workers attempting short-term or focal psychodynamic psychotherapy with persons with mental retardation. Theoretically, however, this type of approach may well have potential applications.

▪ INDIVIDUAL PSYCHOANALYTIC PSYCHOTHERAPY

In most aspects, individual psychoanalytic therapy with a person with mental retardation is little different from similar therapies with other patients. Careful attention should be paid to ground rule issues, such as preserving the boundaries of a predictably regular hour, allowing no outside interruptions, and eliminating (or, if this is not possible, reducing to the extent feasible) contact between patient and therapist outside the session. Patients are encouraged to say anything and everything that comes to mind; children are offered art and play materials if they are at an age when they express their thoughts and feelings more in play than verbally. The therapist provides attention from a stance of empathic abstinence and focuses on providing interpretations rather than support, reassurance, advice, or suggestion. Treatment is typically long term, and the sessions may take place more frequently than once a week. Orientation is toward process: understanding the patient's subjective reality, interpreting patterns of behavior that seem to have developed in response to early conflictual experience, freeing up areas of developmental or neurotic blockage, and unraveling ways in which current experience in the therapy replicates past experience in primary relationships. Symptom resolution and behavior change, although important and valued, are not seen as the critical nexus of therapy nor is their resolution seen as defining the stopping point.

What is different in doing this type of work with a person with mental retardation? Certainly the therapist should choose language that is accessible to the patient and avoid technical or sophisticated terminology that the patient would be unlikely to comprehend—which is actually what would happen in psychoanalytically oriented child therapy or in therapy with someone who was speaking a second language. The therapist might have more contact with parents, school, and residential or vocational facilities than might be the case in other psychoanalytic therapies—and here again this is not unlike what is typical in child therapy. To the extent that there are contacts outside the therapy hour, the emphasis should be on helping the interlocutor understand the inner world of the patient—its expressions and its exigencies—and helping caregivers and others develop ways of interacting with the patient resonant with these dynamics and needs rather than providing information or instruction in techniques. Some therapists might become attuned to watching for ways in which specific intellectual or cognitive deficits articulate with underlying dynamic patterns, and in particular for instances of secondary mental disability. This would be somewhat similar to ways in which psychoanalytic psychotherapists who work with patients with somatic involvements become attuned to a somewhat similar range of phenomena or in which analysts working with abused or traumatized patients become attuned to derivatives of these key experiences.

In many ways, however, it has been the experience of a number of psychoanalytically oriented clinicians that patients with mental retardation seem to fit well with a very classical style of work in psychoanalytic psychotherapy. They most often come to therapy, although not always defining this clearly, with the hope of freeing up some area of constriction or limitation in their lives, similar to the classically neurotic, character disordered, or posttraumatic patients commonly seen in present-day general clinical practice.

Mannoni (1970), Symington (1981), and Sinason (1986, 1990, 1992) have published rich and instructive case histories describing this kind of treatment in depth. Among the striking aspects of their reports is that a rise in the intellectual level over the course of therapy is further removed from the heart of the treatment than the working through of conflictual blockages and primitive patterns of object relations and character structure in sufficient degree to make it possible for the patient to enjoy a less constricted and emotionally richer life.

Issues of organic involvement do not necessarily determine the course of treatment or constitute a contraindication for psychoanalytic psychotherapy with persons with mental retardation. Organic deficits may or may not be present, but they often assume a background position. It has been suggested that this is because the typical material worked with in psychoanalytic psycho-therapy is more affectively than cognitively rooted. Others have suggested that the work of therapy can be usefully conceptualized as addressing the va-riety of fantasies, beliefs, defenses, experiences, and parapraxic distortions that get organized over time around a core of neuropsychological deficit and that can be structuralized into neurotic or characterologic maladaptations.

Sinason (see especially 1990) in particular, in her work focusing on persons with relatively severe intellectual deficiencies, has found that the severity of the deficit does not seem to have a major impact on the efficacy of the method. Analysts (Khan 1982–1983) working in other realms have reported work with nonverbal or minimally verbal patients and were able to decode psychody-namic meanings of body language, nonverbal behaviors, holophrasic or tele-graphic verbalizations, or for that matter silences and were often able to detect observable and dynamically comprehensible phenomena within the special in-terpersonal field of psychoanalytic therapy and not infrequently of impressive power when interpreted. A vignette can give some flavor to both the method-ology and phenomenology of this type of work:

> C, a 25-year-old woman with mild mental retardation, is currently in her fourth year of twice-weekly psychoanalytic psychotherapy. She lives in a group home, works (with somewhat uneven functioning) at semiskilled office jobs, supported by a job coach, and has little social network beyond the resi-dents of her group home. She was referred to treatment because of tenden-cies to explode with rage, appearing sad to her residential counselor, and resisting compliance with the demands of her residential facility. C has a sta-ble neurological condition with well-controlled seizures, wide and awkward gait, perseverative and concrete thinking, jerky fine-motor skills, and mild to moderate dysarthria as the primary symptoms. She is from an upper-middle-class background and graduated from a sophisticated private special educa-tion secondary school.
>
> During the first stage of therapy, C was painfully shy; she would sit as far from me in the therapy room as she could, with lowered head and close to inaudible speech. As this stance was explored over several months, what came to be understood was that the intimacy of the contact with the therapist flooded her with an almost intolerable awareness of the impact of her cogni-tive and social disabilities on the quality of her life. Her daily experience, liv-

ing in the world as a young adult woman with mental retardation, was one of discrimination, rejection, inadequacy, rage, confusion, and shame. To the extent she found it difficult to have this disclosed in the interpersonal field of the therapy, her presence in the room had the flavor of hiding. To the extent she had some emerging awareness that, in therapy, not only would she not be rejected but that the therapist's ability to tolerate these feelings and experiences empathically had the potential somehow to make them more tolerable and changeable, she remained in the room. This is what is classically described as the containment phenomenon.

As treatment progressed, C developed some capacity to describe feeling states and inner experiences verbally. Thus, for example, she was able to articulate that her tendency to perseverate (not her term) became exacerbated when she was anxious and attenuated when she was tranquil and felt respected and safe, and she was able to understand that her tantrums were worse when a current request provoked memories of an early painful experience, often one of covert rejection. In other words, these were phenomena of secondary, not primary, mental handicap. C's language in discussing this material was at the expected level given her cognitive deficits but no less effective or poignant for that.

▪ ANALYTICALLY ORIENTED GROUP THERAPIES

Hollins (1990), Pantlin (1985), and Stammler (1990) have all described applications of analytically oriented group therapies with persons with mental retardation (see also Chapter 2 of this book). Once again, these are more similar to than distinct from analytically oriented group therapies employed with other populations. Use is made of transference and countertransference, and of interpretations of group process. The primary distinctions derive from the material group members typically bring to treatment—experiences of institutional care on group living, for instance, or in confronting idealized images of nondisabled persons.

Groups of persons with mental retardation are often reported to have a "primitive" quality, frequently straying from a theme, maintaining long periods of boredom or silence (and provoking similar countertransferential responses from the group therapist), raising questions well into the treatment about what the group is for or why they are there, raising sensitive topics with an embarrassing (to the therapist, principally) directness, or raising topics seemingly not germane to the therapeutic purpose. However, such groups often have a similar flavor to what is found in in-depth group analytic experiences with very sophisticated patients, who find, perhaps uniquely in group-process material, points of contact with the primitive underpinnings of daily life (Bion 1959). The literature is fairly consistent in reporting that intellectual or adaptive levels do not seem to preclude the interpretability of such primitive phenomena or a patient's capacity to derive benefit from such interpretation. The main constraint to the wider use of group methods, reported quite consistently in the literature, has to do with the demands such work poses on the therapist, who is called on to come into contact with very elemental forces and often very painful material. Good training and supervision are essential prerequisites to undertaking such work.

As an example: in my third year of once-a-week analytically oriented group therapy with five adults with retardation ranging from moderate to mild, the group began discussing why they had difficulty allowing the members to speak in turn and why they often strayed from one topic to another without reaching closure. Each member participated actively in the conversation, and the therapist's participation was minimal. Various hypotheses were developed: that the group members were "too stupid" to wait their turn; that the topic from which they were straying was "boring"; that alternate topics, such as one member's discourse on his relationship with his girlfriend or another's about tensions at work, were introduced because the main theme was "too sensitive" or "too complicated." Midway through the session I observed that perhaps this topic had arisen because the group had reached an important turning point in its maturation. They were now able to reflect on the process of their conversation as well as its content, and thus to experience and examine more carefully their interactions as a group. Further, the emergence of strong feelings (of "being stupid" or "things being too complicated") might be related to an awareness of having reached this marking point of collective maturation. The members were able to work productively with this group-as-a-whole interpretation for the remainder of the session and in the following weeks often made reference to it as a benchmark experience, both in their collective process as a group and in their personal life experiences. One member, for example, remarked that it helped her "control (her) angaries" when she remembered, during the week, what she had achieved in group.

Whereas this example has presented a relatively high-functioning group, Stammler (1990) has described the applicability of a similar methodology to a group of severely to profoundly retarded nonverbal children, describing group treatment as uniquely capable of "opening . . . a space for each child and a movement on the road to simple humanisation."

■ CONCLUSIONS

In this chapter, I have attempted to describe methods of psychoanalytically informed consultation and individual and group psychoanalytic psychotherapy with persons with mental retardation. I have emphasized throughout that these are, in general, little different from other psychoanalytic therapies, the main differences deriving from the unique life experiences of persons with mental retardation. Sinason's (1986) notion of secondary mental disability, a concept of great heuristic value to many clinicians working analytically with this population, is an example of such a specificity. Rationales for viewing intellectual level as no obstacle to analytically informed work have been explored, and attention has been drawn to the potential of psychoanalytic therapies to improve the emotional well-being and sense of inner satisfaction of people with mental retardation—issues that are often given insufficient emphasis in special education and behaviorally informed programs. The difficult feelings such clinical work often evokes for therapists have also been touched on.

The presence of a chapter on this topic in a volume such as this bespeaks a renewal of interest in the application of analytic thinking and methods to people with mental retardation. What must be emphasized in closing, however, is that this is still a relatively new area of work, inviting new thinking, new clinicians, and much research.

■ REFERENCES

Alvarez A: Live Company. New York, Routledge/Tavistock, 1992

Anzieu D: The Skin Ego: A Psychoanalytic Approach to the Self. New Haven, CT, Yale University Press, 1989

Baum NT: Therapy for people with dual diagnosis: treating the behaviors of the whole person? in Treatment of Mental Illness and Behavioral Disorder in the Mentally Retarded. Edited by Došen A, Van Gennep A, Zwanikken GJ. Leiden, Netherlands, Logon, 1990, pp 143–156

Bion W: Experiences in Groups. New York, Basic Books, 1959

Fajardo B: Parenting a damaged child: mourning, regression and disappointment. Psychoanal Rev 74:19–43, 1987

Gaedt C: Psychotherapeutic approaches in the treatment of mental illness and behavioural disorders in mentally retarded people: the significance of a psychoanalytic perspective. J Intellect Disabil Res 39(3):233–239, 1995

Gaedt C: Psychodynamic oriented psychotherapy in people with learning disability, in Issues in Service Provision for People With Learning Disabilities: Papers on Philosophy, Social Psychology, and Psychiatry. Edited by Gaedt C. Neuerkerode, Germany, Evangelische Stiftung Neuerkerode, 1997, pp 50–79

Hollins S: Group analytic therapy with people with mental handicap, in Treatment of Mental Illness and Behavioral Disorder in the Mentally Retarded. Edited by Došen A, Van Gennep A, Zwanikken GJ. Leiden, Netherlands, Logon, 1990, pp 81–89

Khan MMR: Speech, the psychoanalytic method and madness: a "case history." International Journal of Psychoanalytic Psychotherapy 9:447–473, 1982–1983

Mannoni M: The Child, His "Illness," and the Others. New York, Pantheon, 1970

Mannoni M: The Backward Child and His Mother. New York, Pantheon, 1972

Mawson C: The use of play technique in understanding disturbed behavior in school. Psychoanalytical Psychotherapy 2:53–61, 1986

Pantlin AW: Group-analytic psychotherapy with mentally handicapped patients. Group Analysis 28:44–53, 1985

Ruth R: Some trends in psychoanalysis and their relevance for treating people with mental retardation, in Treatment of Mental Illness and Behavioral Disorder in the Mentally Retarded. Edited by Došen A, Van Gennep A, Zwanikken GJ. Leiden, Netherlands, Logon, 1990, pp 167–177

Sinason V: Secondary mental handicap and its relationship to trauma. Psychoanalytical Psychotherapy 2:131–154, 1986

Sinason V: Individual psychoanalytical psychotherapy with severely and profoundly handicapped residents, in Treatment of Mental Illness and Behavioral Disorder in the Mentally Retarded. Edited by Došen A, Van Gennep A, Zwanikken GJ. Leiden, Netherlands, Logon, 1990, pp 71–80

Sinason V: Mental Handicap and the Human Condition: New Approaches From the Tavistock. London, Free Association Books, 1992

Solnit A, Stark M: Mourning and the birth of a defective child. Psychoanal Study Child 17:523–537, 1962

Spensley S: Mentally ill or mentally handicapped: a longitudinal study of severe learning disorder. Psychoanalytical Psychotherapy 1:55–70, 1985

Stammler A: Portrait of small therapy group with violin, in Treatment of Mental Illness and Behavioral Disorder in the Mentally Retarded. Edited by Došen A, Van Gennep A, Zwanikken GJ. Leiden, Netherlands, Logon, 1990, pp 157–166

Symington N: The psychotherapy of a subnormal patient. Br J Med Psychol 54:187–199, 1981

8 A Rational Emotive Group Treatment Approach With Dually Diagnosed Adults

Nefeli Schneider, Ph.D.

There is growing evidence supporting the considerable success achieved in improving the social, emotional, and personal adjustment of mentally retarded persons by means of modified individual and group psychotherapeutic methods (Reiss 1994; Rubin 1983). One of these methods is rational emotive therapy (RET).

RET is a cognitive psychotherapeutic approach developed by Albert Ellis in 1962 and employs a humanistic and educative model of treatment. Initially, this approach was applied to parenting techniques in the 1950s and was then adapted and promoted with school-age children in the 1960s. In the 1970s, RET was incorporated in elementary school curriculums, where teachers as opposed to therapists could teach these concepts in a preventative approach within classroom settings. Rational emotive education (REE) became the educational derivation of RET that was applied extensively to various populations in school settings.

During the late 1970s and 1980s, more interest developed in applying rational emotive principles to specialized populations such as learning disabled students (Gerber 1985; Meyer 1982; Omizo et al. 1986), hearing impaired adolescents (Giezhels 1980), and the developmentally disabled (Eluto 1980; Wooten 1983).

REE and training have been employed with children as young as 5 years of age (Waters 1981). Many of these therapeutic techniques and strategies can effectively be adapted to address the special learning needs of the mentally retarded.

■ BASIC THEORY OF RET

RET is based on the theory that emotional experiences and subsequent behaviors are not created by the events themselves but are related to the way an individual views or perceives these events. In other words, the person's antecedent thoughts or private speech is the real cause of the emotional reactions. All too often the way that an individual looks at an event is fraught with irrational thoughts, erroneous assumptions, and illogical beliefs that lead to disabling emotions and maladaptive reactions.

RET strives to challenge these irrational beliefs and replace them with more logical and constructive thoughts. It sharply challenges irrational and antisocial behavior, discourages preoccupation with past antecedents and events, and teaches individuals to develop a more tolerant approach to life by accepting people in an imperfect world with nonblaming attitudes.

RET employs the A-B-C model to best illustrate its concepts: A is the activating event; B represents the individual's intervening perceptions, thoughts, and beliefs about the event, which result in an interpretation and perception of event A; and C is the emotional reaction and subsequent behavior(s).

It is a common misconception to assume that A (the event) causes C (the emotional reaction), when in fact it is B (the intervening interpretation and thoughts) that directly contributes to C.

Thus, people cause their own emotional reactions and consequences at C by what they tell themselves at B. By successfully challenging and changing irrational beliefs and thoughts, an individual can *moderate* the intensity of emotional reactions. It is not the intent of RET to strive for "unemotionalism" but to reduce the frequency, intensity, and duration of the negative affect so that problem solving can be implemented. Only in rational states of mind can good solutions to problems be found.

Walen et al. (1980) have helped to define and distinguish rational from irrational beliefs in the following manner:

1. Rational beliefs are true and consistent with reality and can be supported by evidence, facts, and logic. In contrast, irrational beliefs cannot be supported by facts or evidence and tend to be exaggerations and gross overgeneralizations of a situation.

2. Rational beliefs are not absolutist but conditional. They are usually stated as desires, wishes, hopes, or preferences. Irrational beliefs employ absolute commands, which are expressed in demanding statements such as "must have," "should do," or "need to be." When negative life events occur, the individual often tends to make "awfulizing" statements such as "This is awful, horrible" or "This is impossible," and "I can't live with it" or "I can't stand it." All too often, catastrophic reactions can follow.

3. Rational beliefs result in moderate as opposed to extreme emotions, which can then act as motivators for solving problems and achieving goals more effectively. Irrational beliefs lead to extreme and disturbed emotions that

can range from outrage to apathy. These unhealthy emotions interfere with and obstruct the problem-solving process and block goal attainment.

■ RET IN INDIVIDUALS WITH MENTAL RETARDATION

There are several reasons why RET can be applied in the treatment of persons with mental retardation. First, it employs a strong didactic format that enables the therapist to use any number of audiovisual teaching aids to enhance education and training. Its strong teaching and reeducational stance incorporates skill development and skill refinement—both essential tools in effecting behavior changes.

Secondly, RET assumes a strong behavioristic orientation, incorporating well-established social behavior techniques, such as systematic desensitization, modeling, and reinforcement. These behavioral techniques have proven to be effective in addressing behavioral problems in mentally retarded people with a dual diagnosis.

Thirdly, the therapist is encouraged to adopt a strong directive approach and take an active role in structuring therapeutic experiences, helping the individual process them, and challenging, guiding, and encouraging the individual at each stage of the process. This leadership style has proven to be most effective with the dually diagnosed because self-directive behavior and self-initiation tend to be weak in this population.

Finally, RET emphasizes the importance of generalization to the real world outside of the counseling relationship. This is promoted through homework assignments, reports on practice, and implementation of therapeutic ways of behaving in actual situations. In implementing RET with the persons with mental retardation, it is essential to be sensitive to and aware of the particular cognitive level of functioning at which an individual may be operating. Often, the intellectual limitations present in a mentally retarded person can lead to the development of beliefs about oneself and the world that are not rational and accurate. These beliefs are the result of having formed a conclusion based on limited evidence and having used the conclusion as an unquestioned rule for guiding subsequent behavior (Bernard and Joyce 1984).

Some basic irrational beliefs commonly shared by many mentally retarded persons include the following:

- Everyone must love me and approve of me, and it is terrible if they don't (fear of rejection and disapproval).
- I must be perfect. I must always be competent and successful, and I must never fail; otherwise, I am not a worthy person.
- Things must go my way, and I must be comfortable and without pain at all times.

- The world must be fair and just at all times.
- People are either all good or all bad. When they behave badly or unfairly, they must be blamed and punished severely.

These irrational beliefs and thoughts ultimately lead to maladaptive philosophies and behavioral responses, self-deprecation, intolerance of frustration, insufficient assumption of responsibility, and blaming and condemning of oneself and others.

Though full utility of RET at the moderate level of mental retardation (developmental age below 7 years) may not be possible, such individuals can nevertheless benefit from this approach and be helped to resolve specific psychological problems. Over time, with good instruction at the appropriate level, they can learn to become more objective, relativistic, and flexible.

Appropriate goals at this level should be oriented toward teaching the individual what to exactly tell oneself in certain problem situations. Instruction should be directed at developing rational self-statements for specific situations. Extensive rational analysis of irrational concepts is discouraged; instead, the therapist should rely on more concrete and simple materials presented in multiple mediums such as pictures, tapes, diagrams, and stories. Finally, it is important to work toward the acquisition and eventual spontaneous use of rational self-talk in the identified situations. Therefore, practice and repetition are essential.

Appropriate objectives and activities with the lower functioning individuals should address such needs as identifying emotions and developing a wider emotional vocabulary and range. Many patients lack the ability to understand and express their own emotions, let alone identify what others are feeling. Their emotional vocabulary is impoverished, essentially consisting of only three basic feelings such as "happy," "mad," and "sad." Once emotional awareness has increased, additional training should be directed at distinguishing between helpful and hurtful feelings as well as between thoughts and emotions. Another important area to train is the individual's ability to "tune in" to self-talk. Once this is accomplished, then a connection between self-talk and feelings can be established that can pave the way to learning rational coping statements for specific situations.

Individuals with mild levels of mental retardation (development age 7 years and above) will be able to deal with more complex concepts. They can coordinate more than one viewpoint at a time and be less egocentric and more objective in their evaluations.

Given these higher capabilities, goals should be oriented toward disputing irrational concepts and beliefs and focusing on the development of more rational analyses. The therapist should continually work toward spontaneously generating rational thoughts as well as generalizing rational thinking across situations.

Appropriate activities should employ the A-B-C model, "catastrophizing" and "awfulizing" concepts, recognition of demanding words, identification of misperceptions of reality, challenging irrational beliefs, generalization of rational thinking across situations, and self-acceptance that is not dependent on external factors.

It should be noted that mentally retarded individuals frequently do not function at their highest capacity for advanced thinking and suffer from performance deficiencies. Thus, it may be necessary to begin with simpler and more concrete goals and activities resembling those used with lower functioning individuals. Gradually, with appropriate sequential instruction and concept development, performance will improve and the persons can advance to more mature levels and realize his or her potential.

■ ASSESSMENT

Pre- and posttest measures are essential in evaluating the effectiveness of this treatment approach to the development of adaptive coping skills. Four types of assessments were found to be useful with this population and approach:

1. A clinical interview with the mentally retarded person should employ direct questioning and some use of role-play in order to evoke descriptions of feelings and irrational thoughts. In addition, interviews should be extended to knowledgeable persons working directly with the individual who can help identify problem situations and maladaptive reactions that are not always clearly recognized by the developmentally disabled person.
2. Use of the Rational Emotive Problem-Solving Test (REPS; Schneider 1986), which presents four stories depicting problem situations. The protagonist in each story generates irrational beliefs and statements in response to the problem, and the subject is asked to present as many rational arguments as he or she can to dispute each protagonist's statements. Responses are qualitatively evaluated and scored on the basis of adequacy and relevance of the rational arguments presented by the subject.
3. Behavior assessment of target behaviors occurring outside the group setting must be performed, utilizing clear and concise data collection by trained staff and/or family members. A self-monitoring component is essential in order to help the individuals become more aware and cognizant of their own reactions to problems, and feel more powerful once the tools for greater self-control are within reach.
4. Assessment of practical problem-solving skills can be performed through the use of two tests developed by Platt and Spivack (1977):

- The Means-Ends Problem-Solving (MEPS) procedure consists of a series of vignettes that are presented to the individual describing a problem situation and the desired outcome. The subject is then asked to make up a story that describes the intervening events and is scored for relevance and adequacy of means.
- The Optional Thinking Test (OTT) calls for a subject to generate as many solutions as possible to a set of four problem situations in which a protagonist is faced with some sort of temptation. The person is then asked to describe the thoughts and actions of the protagonist, and the responses are scored for reported awareness of the consequences of each alternative generated.

■ A STRUCTURED RET GROUP COUNSELING PROGRAM

Rational emotive concepts can be taught in a group setting. Within the structure of a group, peer interactions and socialization opportunities are enhanced, and social feedback and reality testing can effectively occur. As members are encouraged to share views and perceptions with each other, peer support systems can begin to develop that will increase independence from authority figures. A structured group setting can also provide a "safe" environment to practice new behaviors and encourage corrective learning.

The following summary outlines a basic 10-session program:

Session 1: Promote positive group dynamics; define the purpose, goals, and expectations of the group; and emphasize cooperation and participation of the members in helping each other with problems (e.g., ask everyone to describe a problem they have and would like to receive help with, and generate a short list of rules that begin with the word *do* as opposed to *don't*).

Session 2: Increase emotional awareness through the identification of a variety of emotions and the evaluation of their intensity (e.g., create a list of emotions and ask members to act them out in a game of charades, and have members share personal examples of problems evoking low, moderate, and strong emotions).

Session 3: Establish the connection between self-talk and emotional reactions (e.g., read a story in which an event evokes two opposite reactions from two individuals, and discuss the connection between thought, or what one says to oneself, and emotions).

Session 4: Review the connection between thoughts and feelings and introduce the A-B-C model to analyze this concept (e.g., ask members to share a real problem, and analyze the troublesome thoughts that may have led to negative and unhelpful reactions).

Session 5: Introduce and define *rational* versus *irrational* thoughts and beliefs (e.g., establish the criteria for evaluating the rationality of a statement: Is it true and can it be proven? Present logical and illogical statements and ask the group to identify which category they fall in, and why).

Session 6: Present five common irrational beliefs, and identify the demanding words that make them troublesome. Distinguish between wants and needs (e.g., present the five most common illogical beliefs, and discuss why they are irrational).

Session 7: Introduce the concepts of "catastrophizing" and "awfulizing" (e.g., have the group generate a list of real catastrophes in the world [Vernon 1980], and ask the group how they would rate events. Discuss how we sometimes overreact and blow events out of proportion).

Session 8: Integrate and apply challenging and disputing skills (e.g., practice disputing by presenting role-plays or stories of potential problems, and ask each member participating to generate all possible arguments and disputes against irrational statements, self-talk, and beliefs).

Session 9: Demonstrate that labeling people is not logical or helpful (e.g., present a basket containing a variety of fruit of which some are good and some rotten. Pass it around and ask if this basket is a "good" basket or a "bad" basket of fruit. Discuss the problem of labeling. Draw analogy between the basket of fruit and people).

Session 10: Present a step-by-step process for practical problem solving (e.g., generate as many solutions as possible, and evaluate these by defining the positive and negative consequences associated with each).

Homework assignments must be given at the end of each session and then reviewed at the beginning of the next. They are an important component in practicing and applying concepts outside the group. Each participant should select one or more person(s) outside the group, such as a counselor, friend, or family member, who can help plan and implement the assignment and process the results.

It is essential that staff who support the person at home or on a job, as well as family members, be trained in using these RET-based approaches so that meaningful practice and application to real-life situations can take place as situations occur. Generalization of skills is always the most challenging component of a treatment program, and the most crucial. RET can only be effective if it is supported and applied to as many aspects of life as possible.

■ RESULTS

Rational emotive group approach was implemented in a study of 18 mentally retarded adults functioning at the upper moderate to mild ranges of intelligence and exhibiting a variety of psychiatric disorders (Schneider 1986). The results demonstrated significant gains in rational and logical thinking as well as interpersonal problem-solving skills for 17 of the 18 subjects participating in the study. Additionally, the group approach enhanced social interactions, and all subjects became more socially responsive over the course of treatment. Perhaps the greatest therapeutic value that emerged was that of increased self-esteem as each individual accepted and was accepted by others in the group.

A study performed by Hajzler and Bernard (1991) reviewed 21 RET research studies conducted with learning disabled children and adolescents. Their purpose was to evaluate the efficacy of REE approaches on self-esteem, anxiety, impulsivity, or behavior problems. They found that in 88% of the studies there was a significant decrease in irrationality, 71% of the studies demonstrated increase in internal control, 80% of those studies measuring anxiety revealed significant reductions, and 50% showed marked improvements in self-esteem and behavior problems.

■ CONCLUSIONS

RET is a psychotherapeutic approach that employs a strong didactic format, a behavioristic orientation, and a directive leadership style, and it emphasizes generalization to real-life situations. These are all tools in building better coping skills and changing maladaptive patterns in the mentally retarded person. Successful implementation of RET with this population must incorporate a strong developmental approach by modifying therapeutic goals and objectives and language and techniques to the individual's level of functioning. Generalization to real-life situations is an important challenge if results are to have a long-lasting impact. It is recommended that other people who are significant to the individual's life—such as counselors, teachers, and family members—be trained in rational emotive principles so that application can occur in the natural setting. RET provides opportunities to build peer support systems, independence from authority figures, reality testing, practice of new behaviors, and self-esteem.

■ REFERENCES

Bernard M, Joyce M: Rational Emotive Therapy With Children and Adolescents. New York, Wiley, 1984, pp 26–27, 105–109

Ellis A: Reason and Emotion in Psychotherapy. New York, Lyle Stuart, 1962

Eluto ME: Effects of a rational emotive education and problem solving therapy on the adjustment of intermediate special education students. Doctoral dissertation. New York, Hoffstra University, 1980

Gerber GW: Modifying impulsivity in handicapped children through the development of rational thinking. Dissertation Abstracts International Vol 46(5A):1248, 1985

Giezhels JS: Effects of REE on a Hearing Impaired High School Population. Doctoral dissertation. New York, Hofstra University, 1980

Hajzler DJ, Bernard ME: A review of rational-emotive education outcome studies. School Psychology Quarterly 6:27–29, 1991

Meyer DJ: Effects of rational emotive group therapy upon anxiety and self esteem of learning disabled children. Doctoral dissertation. Berrien Springs, MI, Andrews University, 1982

Omizo MM, Lo-Fuang-Luan G, Williams RE: Rational-emotive education, self concept, and locus of control among learning disabled students. Journal of Humanistic Education and Development 25(2):58–69, 1986

Platt JJ, Spivack G: Measures of Interpersonal Problem Solving for Adults and Adolescents. Philadelphia, PA, Hahneman University, 1977

Reiss S: Handbook of Challenging Behavior: Mental Health Aspects of Mental Retardation. Worthington, OH, IDS Publishing, 1994

Rubin R: Bridging the gap through individual counseling and psychotherapy with mentally retarded people, in Mental Health and Mental Retardation. Edited by Menolascino F, McCann B. Baltimore, MD, University Park Press, 1983, pp 119–128

Schneider N: A rational emotive group treatment approach to problem solving with dually diagnosed adults. Doctoral dissertation. Boulder, CO, University of Colorado, Boulder, 1986

Vernon A: Help Yourself to a Healthier You. Washington, DC, University Press of America, 1980

Walen S, DiGuiseppe R, Wessler RL: A Practitioner's Guide to Rational Emotive Therapy. New York, Oxford University Press, 1980

Waters V: The living school. RETwork 1(1):11–35, 1981

Wooten BM: A Rational Approach to Counseling Mentally Retarded Persons. Edina, MN, REM Consulting Services, 1983

Pre-Therapy

*A Treatment Method for People With
Mental Retardation Who Are Also Psychotic*

Garry Prouty, Ph.D.

$P_{re\text{-}therapy}$ is a theoretical and clinical evolution in client-centered therapy that is specifically designed for severely regressed retarded-psychotic and schizophrenic patients (Peters 1992, 1996; Prouty 1976, 1990, 1995, 1996; Prouty and Cronwall 1990; Prouty and Kubiak 1988a, 1988b; Van Werde 1989, 1990a, 1990b). Application has also been made to the regressed aspects of multiple personality (Roy 1991). In this chapter, I will examine primarily the treatment of mentally retarded patients who are also psychotic or "schizophrenic."

■ HISTORICAL BACKGROUND

Considerable criticism has been made of client-centered therapy concerning its range of applicability. Generally, its use has been restricted to high-level, functional patients (i.e., the "worried well"). These criticisms are not without merit. Rogers (1942) argued that client-centered therapy was not applicable to those who were mentally retarded because these patients lacked the autonomy and introspective skills necessary for psychotherapy. Ruederich and Menolascino (1984) have argued that Rogers's views had a limiting effect on psychotherapy research with this population. It is only recently that several European therapists have produced articles applying classical client-centered therapy to patients with mental retardation (Badelt 1990; Peters 1981, 1986; Portner 1990).

Client-centered work with the schizophrenic population has also been quite limited. Little work has been done since the Wisconsin Project (Rogers et al. 1967). Although these researchers did discern some positive results, they discovered that patients did not accurately perceive the essential "Rogerian attitudes"; and, secondly, they did not observe increased "experiencing" (i.e., the central "outcome" measure). This research marked the end of Rogers's formal collaboration with American psychiatry and drew to a close any major work with the schizophrenic population. Again, as with retardation research, there are European exceptions, such as Teusch of Germany (Teusch 1990; Teusch et al. 1983). Although there are these notable exceptions in the practice of client-centered therapy with retarded and schizophrenic populations, they do not provide a *theoretical* adaptation or evolution.

■ CLIENT-CENTERED THEORY

Client-centered theory has evolved through three stages: *person-centered relationship*, *person-centered experiencing*, and *person-centered contact*.

Person-Centered Relationship

Rogers (1957) hypothesized that the "necessary and sufficient conditions" for therapeutic change were a relationships characterized by 1) unconditional positive regard, 2) empathy, and 3) genuineness. *Unconditional positive regard* refers to deep acceptance and care on the part of the therapist; *empathy* generally means an accurate understanding of the patient's "lived experience" (i.e., phenomenology); and *genuineness* refers to the therapist's authenticity. These therapist attitudes were described as the central facilitative elements in personality change.

Person-Centered Experiencing

Hart (1970) describes the evolution of person-centered theory into an "experiential phase." Gendlin (1964) theorized that client "experiencing" was the critical factor in therapy. *Experiencing* was defined as 1) concrete, 2) bodily felt, and 3) a process. *Concrete* refers to the patient's direct awareness of his or her immediate experience. *Bodily felt* means that experiencing is always organismic. The body "feels" experience. The term *process* refers to the fact that if we concretely attend to our bodily felt sense of an experience A, it will undergo a "felt shift" to experience B, etc. Experiencing is a concrete, bodily felt process. Therapy is the process of experiencing.

Generally, we can describe Rogers as having described the therapist and Gendlin as having described the patient. This is the rationale for the modern label of "person-centered/experiential therapy."

Person-Centered Contact

Rogers (1959) describes "psychological contact" as the first "necessary and sufficient" condition of psychotherapy. Watson (1984) states that if the other conditions are operationalized, and then shown to be present, there is no need to operationalize "psychological contact," even though Rogers had stated that if "psychological contact" was not present, the other conditions were meaningless. He did not provide any theoretical definitions. Also, he did not provide any techniques for developing contact in case of its absence or impairment.

Within this context, pre-therapy is a further evolution in client-centered theory. It is a theory of psychological contact (Prouty 1994). Psychological contact is the "pre" condition of therapeutic relationship/experiencing.

■ PRE-THERAPY: A THEORY OF PERSON-CENTERED CONTACT

As a theory of "psychological contact," pre-therapy is described in terms of therapeutic method (contact reflections), patient process (contact functions), and measurable behavior (contact behaviors).

Contact Reflections

Contact reflections are a "pointing at the concrete" (Buber 1964). They are predicated on a conception of the phenomenon that is conceived "as itself." The phenomenon is conceived as "naturalistic" (i.e., exactly as it appears in consciousness) (Farber 1959). It is also described as "absolutely self-indicative" (Sartre 1956). This means that the phenomenon has no meaning beyond its appearance. It is "nonsymbolic" (Scheler 1953). This construction of the phenomenon is particularly relevant because brain-damaged and schizophrenic patients evince "concrete attitudes" (Arieti 1955; Gurswitch 1966). Contact reflections are extraordinarily concrete and literal so as to respond to the "lived experience" of concretely oriented, retarded, and schizophrenic patients.

Situational Reflections

Situational reflections are oriented toward the patient's immediate situation, environment, or milieu. Their function is to facilitate the reality contact of the patient. An example would be, "You are playing with the red ball."

Facial Reflections

Many regressed patients—due to psychosocial isolation, institutionalization, and overmedication—have poor affective contact. Facial reflections have as their purpose the facilitation of "pre-expressive" emotion. An example could be, "You look sad."

Word-for-Word Reflections

Many retarded and schizophrenic patients suffer from communication disorders. The retarded psychotic and schizophrenic patients often manifest echolalia, "word salads," and neologisms. These are often mixed with periods of being incomprehensible. The rationale underlying word-for-word reflection is the restoration/development of communicative contact. An example would be from the patient: "Incoherent word," "tree," "incoherent word," "boy." The therapist would reflect word for word: "tree," "boy."

Body Reflections

Many schizophrenic or retarded schizophrenic persons evidence bodily symptoms such as echopraxia and catatonia. Such patients often have difficulty integrating their body as part of the self. Body reflections are verbal (sometimes nonverbal) reflections of the patient's "bodying" or expressive behavior. A verbal example would be a statement such as, "Your arm is in the air." A nonverbal example would be for the therapist to reflect by raising his or her own arm in the air.

Reiterative Reflections

Reiteration is not a specific technique; it is a principle. If any of the other four contact reflections are successful in producing a patient response, repeat the response. Reiterative contact is facilitative of the experiencing process. Contact facilitates experiencing and relationship. Contact is "pre-experiential" and "pre-relationship."

Contact Functions

Pre-therapy, broadly conceived, is the facilitation of contact functions. Contact reflections facilitate the contact functions. Perls (1969) defines contact as an "ego function" but fails to provide a fleshed-out description of these functions. Pre-therapy defines them as reality, affective, and communicative contact.

Contact functions are based on the philosophical assumption of Heidegger that a human is a being who is "open" to being (Boss 1963). Such an ontological description, however, lacks concrete specificity and application. Open to what concretely? A possible answer can be derived from Merleau-Ponty (1962), who describes the human phenomenal field in terms of "world," "self," and "other." Consciousness is open to "world," "self," and "other" and is open to human existence.

Again, Merleau-Ponty's description lacks concrete specificity. How does one describe "world," "self," and "other"? How does one describe these giant "existential structures of consciousness" (Prouty 1994)? The existential structures of consciousness are the natural and absolute categories of experience through which particular concrete existents manifest themselves. Psychological contact is our awareness of these. In terms of consciousness, how are we concretely aware of "world," "self," and "other"?

The *world* is manifested in existential phenomenological forms as concrete: 1) people, 2) places, 3) things, and 4) events. Awareness of people, places, things, and events is the definition of *reality contact.*

The *self* is manifested through existential phenomenological forms that differentiate as 1) moods, 2) feelings, and 3) emotions. Awareness of moods, feelings, and emotions is the definition of *affective contact.*

The *other* is powerfully related to us through human communication. We symbolize the "world" and "self" to the "other." This is communicative contact. Communicative contact is the symbolization of our *reality and affective contact to others.*

Reality, affective, and communicative contact are our awareness of existence. Pre-therapy is the resolution of existential autism (Prouty 1994). It is the restoration or development of contact with the "world," "self," or "other" (i.e., "existential contact") (Prouty 1994).

Clinical Vignette

The following rare clinical vignette is an example of using contact reflections to facilitate the contact functions. It illustrates the restoration of reality, affective, and communicative contact with a chronic schizophrenic woman.

> Dorothy is an old woman, one of the more regressed women on X ward. She was mumbling something [as she usually did]. This time I could hear certain words in her confusion. I reflected only the words I could clearly understand. After about 10 minutes, I could hear a complete sentence.
>
> **Patient:** Come with me.
> **Therapist (word-for-word reflection):** Come with me.
>
> The patient led me to the corner of the day room. We stood there silently for what seemed to be a very long time. Because I couldn't communicate with her, I watched her body movements and closely reflected these.
>
> **Patient [puts her hand on the wall]:** Cold.
> **Therapist (word-for-word reflection/body reflection) [I put my hand on the wall and repeat the word]:** Cold.
>
> She had been holding my hand all along, but when I reflected, she would tighten her grip. Dorothy would begin to mumble word fragments. I was

careful to reflect only the words I could understand. What she was saying began to make sense.

Patient: I don't know what this is anymore. [Touching the wall (reality contact).] The walls and chairs don't mean anything anymore (existential autism).
Therapist (word-for-word reflection/body reflection) [touching the wall]: You don't know what this is anymore. The chairs and walls don't mean anything to you anymore.

The patient began to cry (affective contact).

After a while the patient began to talk again. This time she spoke clearly (communicative contact).
Patient: I don't like it here. I'm so tired. . . so tired.
Therapist (word-for-word reflection) [As I gently touch her arm, this time it is I who tightened my grip on her hand. I reflect.]: You're tired, so tired.

The patient smiled and told me to sit in a chair directly in front of her and began to braid my hair.

This vignette illustrates the resolution of the problems inherent in Rogers's formulation of psychological contact. It provides a definition of contact and techniques to assist the "contact impaired" patient. It also illustrates the assertion that contact is "pre" relationship.

Reality, affective, and communicative contact are the theoretical goals of pre-therapy. In existential-phenomenological terms, pre-therapy is the restoration or development of existential contact between consciousness and the world, self or other (i.e., the resolution of existential autism).

Contact Behaviors

Contact reflections facilitate the contact functions resulting in the emergence of contact behaviors. Contact behaviors represent the operationalization necessary for measurement and scale development. Reality contact is operationalized as the verbalization of people, places, things, and events. Affective contact is operationalized as 1) the verbalization of "feeling words" (e.g., "sad") and 2) the expression of affect through bodily and facial signs. Communicative contact is operationalized through words and/or sentences.

Early pilot studies provide some evidence to support construct validity and reliability. Prouty (1994) presents data from a single case study of a mentally retarded schizophrenic patient, indicating a correlation coefficient of 0.9966 between independent raters, with a P value of 0.0001. The t value was 0.9864, with a P value of 0.3528.

A second case study of a mentally retarded schizophrenic patient yielded a correlation coefficient of 0.9847 between independent raters, and a *P* value of 0.0001. The *t* value was 2.3728, with a *P* value of 0.0526. No difference was indicated at 1% or 5% level of significance.

A reliability study in chronic schizophrenics was undertaken by De Vree (1992). She and her colleagues developed rating scores for three independent raters and three patients. They then correlated these with nonrater trained nurses. They obtained kappa scores of 0.7, 0.76, and 0.87.

An evolved form of measurement for pre-therapy has been devised (Dinacci 1994). It more directly focuses on patient expression as an outcome.

■ PRE-THERAPY APPLICATIONS

Pre-therapy is generally applied to mentally retarded patients who are overtly psychotic or manifest psychotic features. They are often referred because they lack the reality, affective, or communicative contact necessary for psychotherapy. Because of regression, acting-out, and bizarre behavior, treatment is usually within the context of more structured settings. In selected cases or circumstances, treatment may be conducted on an outpatient basis. Length and frequency of sessions vary with attention span, behavioral control, and willingness to participate.

In sharp contrast to classic patient-centered therapy, pre-therapy pays careful attention to spatial and temporal factors. Many schizophrenic-type patients are very sensitive to psychological contact. Contact reflections that are too rapid may provoke feelings of intrusion. Contact reflections that are too slow may be experienced as a lack of empathy. Spatial experience is also important. Nearness may be experienced as threatening. Entering a patient's hallucinatory space may provoke an intense reaction. Generally, the therapist needs to carefully sense out and test the patient's spatial and temporal boundaries.

Empathy is also applied differently. Empathy is for the patient a literal "pre-expressive" behavior because frequently the therapist does not know the patient's frame of reference, a classic phenomenological response is not possible. On a more subtle level, empathy is for the patient's efforts at expression and coherence.

Prouty and Kubiak (1988b) describe the use of contact reflections to resolve a psychotic crisis with a mentally retarded schizophrenic patient. The case is important because it illustrates the use of an empathic method without severe controls or tranquilizing medications.

> The patient, a woman, was one of seven on an outing from a halfway house.
> She was seated in the rear seat of the van. As I looked in the rear-view mirror,

I noticed the patient crouched down into the seat with one arm outstretched above her head. The patient's face was filled with terror and her voice began to escalate with screams.

I pulled the van off the road and asked the volunteer to take the others out of the van. I sat next to the patient, sharing the same seat. The patient's eyes were closed and her face was wincing with fear.

Patient [in escalated voice]: It's pulling me in!
Therapist (word-for-word reflection): It's pulling me in.

The patient continued to slip farther down into the seat, with her left arm outstretched. Her eyes were still closed.

Therapist (body reflection): Your body is slipping down into the seat. Your arm is in the air.
Therapist (situational reflection): We are in the van. You are sitting next to me.

The patient continued to scream.

Therapist (facial reflection): You are screaming, Carol.
Patient: It's pulling me in!
Therapist (word-for-word reflection): It's pulling you in.
Therapist (situational reflection): Carol, we are in the van. You are sitting next to me.
Therapist (facial reflection): Something is frightening you. You are screaming.
Patient: It's sucking me in!
Therapist (word-for-word reflection): It's sucking you in.
Therapist (situational reflection/body reflection): We are in the van, Carol. You are sitting next to me. Your arm is in the air.
Patient: [She begins to sob very hard. Her arms drop to her lap.] It was the vacuum cleaner.
Therapist (word-for-word reflection): It was the vacuum cleaner.
Patient: [Gives me direct eye contact.] She did it with the vacuum cleaner. [Now in a normal tone of voice.] I thought it was gone. She used to turn on the vacuum cleaner when I was bad and put the hose right on my arm. I thought it sucked it in. [Less sobbing.] [It should be noted that daily this patient would kiss her arm up to her elbow and stroke it continuously.]
Therapist (word-for-word reflection): Your arm is still here. It didn't get sucked into the vacuum cleaner.

The patient smiled and was held by the therapist.

Later that afternoon a therapy session was held, and the patient began to delve into her feelings regarding the punishment she received as a child. It should also be noted that the "kissing and stroking of the arm" behavior ceased.

This clinical vignette illustrates the application of pre-therapy techniques for managing an acute crisis in a psychotic mentally retarded patient. The patient was helped to deal with this acute exacerbation and understand how her symptoms were related to a negative childhood experience (i.e., her mother threatening her with a vacuum cleaner). The patient was able to utilize the newly acquired insightful experiences as a basis for further therapy. In addition, the meaning of symptomatic behavior (arm kissing) became clarified as trauma related; that behavior also ceased.

■ CONCLUSIONS

Pre-therapy is a development in person-centered theory and technique applicable to the psychotic mentally retarded population. Evolving from Rogers's view that psychological contact is the first condition of a therapeutic relationship, pre-therapy develops the functions necessary for psychotherapy. Consequently, it is construed as "pre" therapy.

As a theory, pre-therapy describes psychological contact. Contact is described on three levels: 1) contact reflections, 2) contact functions, and 3) contact behaviors. Contact reflections refer to very literal and extraordinarily concrete reflections. Contact functions refer to the psychological functions of the patient that involve contact with the "world," "self," or "other." The restoration and/or development of these functions are the theoretical goals of pre-therapy. Contact behaviors refer to the behavioral change of the patient that can be utilized for measurement. Preliminary pilot studies provide some evidence as to construct validity and reliability.

These developments in theory and practice help dislodge the criticism that person-centered therapy is mainly applicable to well-functioning patients and not suitable for the psychiatrically impaired patient. It also highlights the restoration/development of reality, affective, and communicative functions necessary for psychotherapy to be undertaken with psychotic mentally retarded patients.

■ REFERENCES

Arieti S: Interpretation of Schizophrenia. New York, Robert Brunner, 1955

Badelt I: Client-centered psychotherapy with mentally handicapped adults, in Client-Centered and Experiential Psychotherapy in the Nineties. Edited by Lietaer G, Rombauts J, Van Balen R. Leuven, Belgium, Leuven University Press, 1990, pp 671–681

Boss M: A patient who taught the author to see and think differently, in Psychoanalysis and Daseinsanalysis. New York, Basic Books, Incorporated, 1963, pp 28–48

Buber M: Elements of the interhuman, in The Worlds of Existentialism. Edited by Friedman M. New York, Random House, 1964, pp 229–547

De Vree A: Pouly's pre-therapy. Master's thesis. Department of Psychology, University of Ghent, Ghent, Belgium, 1992

Dinacci A: Colloquio pre-terapeutico: legge e psiche. Rivista di Psicologia Giuridica 2(3):24–32, 1994

Farber M: Consciousness and natural reality, in Naturalism and Subjectivism. Albany, New York, State University of New York Press, 1959, pp 87–99

Gendlin ET: A theory of personality change, in Personality Change. Edited by Worchel P, Byrne D. New York, Wiley, 1964, pp 102–148

Gurswitch A: Gelb-Goldstein's concept of concrete and categorical attitude and the phenomenology of ideation, in Studies in Phenomenology and Psychology. Evanston, IL, Northwestern University Press, 1966, pp 359–389

Hart JT: The development of client-centered therapy, in New Directions in Client-Centered Therapy. Edited by Hart JT, Tomlinson TM. Boston, MA, Houghton Mifflin Company, 1970, pp 3–22

Merleau-Ponty M: The phenomenal field, in The Phenomenology of Perception. Edited by Honderich T. London, Routledge & Kegan Paul, 1962, pp 60–78

Perls FS: The ego as a function of the organism, in Ego, Hunger, and Aggression. Edited by Peals FS. New York, Vintage Books, 1969, pp 139–161

Peters H: Luisterend Helpen: Poging Tot Beter Omagaan Met de Zwakzinnigen. Lochem, Netherlands, De Tijdstrom, 1981

Peters H: Client-centered benaderingswijzen in de zwakzinningenzorg, in Droom en Werkelijkheid. Edited by Van Balen R, Leijssen M, Lietaer G. Leuven, Belgium, Acco Press, 1986, pp 205–220

Peters H: Psychotherapie Bij Geestelijk Gehandicapten. Amsterdam, Netherlands, Swets & Zeitlinger, 1992

Peters H: Prouty's pre-therapeutische methodes bij geestelijke gehandicapten. Tijdschrift voor Orthopedagogik, Kinderpsychiatrie en Klinische Kinderpsychologie 3:23–35, 1996

Portner M: Client-centered therapy with mentally retarded persons: Catherine and Ruth, in Client-Centered and Experiential Psychotherapy in the Nineties. Edited by Lietaer G, Rombauts J, Van Balen R. Leuven, Belgium, Leuven University Press, 1990, pp 559–569

Prouty G: Pre-therapy: a method of treating pre-expressive psychotic and retarded patients. Psychotherapy: Theory, Research and Practice 13:290–294, 1976

Prouty G: Pre-therapy: a theoretical evolution in the person-centered/experiential psychotherapy of schizophrenia and retardation, in Client-Centered and Experiential Psychotherapy in the Nineties. Edited by Lietaer G, Rombauts J, Van Balen R. Leuven, Belgium, Leuven University Press, 1990, pp 645–658

Prouty G: Theoretical Evolutions in Person-Centered/Experiential Therapy: Applications to Schizophrenic and Retarded Psychoses. Westport, CT, Praeger Publishing, 1994

Prouty G: Pre-therapy: an overview. Chinese Mental Health Journal 9(5):223–225, 1995

Prouty G, Cronwall M: Psychotherapy with a depressed mentally retarded adult: an application of pre-therapy, in Depression in Mentally Retarded Children and Adults. Edited by Došen A, Menolascino F. Leiden, Netherlands, Logon Publications, 1990, pp 281–293

Prouty G, Kubiak M: The development of communicative contact with a catatonic schizophrenic. Journal of Communication Therapy 4:13–20, 1988a

Prouty G, Kubiak M: Pre-therapy with mentally retarded/psychotic clients. Psychiatric Aspects of Mental Retardation Reviews 7:62–66, 1988b

Rogers C: Counseling and Psychotherapy. Boston, MA, Houghton Mifflin, 1942, pp 115–122

Rogers C: The necessary and sufficient conditions of therapeutic personality change. Journal of Consulting Psychology 21:95–103, 1957

Rogers C: A theory of therapy, personality and interpersonal relationships as developed in the client-centered framework, in Psychology: A Study of a Science, III. Edited by Koch E. New York, McGraw-Hill, 1959, pp 245–259

Rogers C, Gendlin ET, Kiesler DJ, et al: The findings in brief, in The Therapeutic Relationship and Its Impact: A Study of Psychotherapy with Schizophrenics. Edited by Rogers C. Madison, WI, University of Wisconsin Press, 1967, pp 73–93

Roy BC: A client-centered approach to multiple personality and dissociative process, in New Directions in Client-Centered Therapy: Practice with Difficult Client Populations. Edited by Fusek L. Chicago, IL, Chicago Counseling and Psychotherapy Research Center, 1991, pp 18–40

Ruederich S, Menolascino F: Dual diagnosis of mental retardation: an overview, in Handbook of Mental Illness in the Mentally Retarded. Edited by Menolascino F, Stark J. New York, Plenum, 1984, pp 45–82

Sartre JP: Being and Nothingness. New York, Washington Square Press, 1956

Scheler M: Selected Philosophical Essays. Evanston, IL, Northwestern University Press, 1953

Teusch L: Positive effects and limitations of client-centered therapy with schizophrenics, in Client-Centered and Experiential Psychotherapy in the Nineties. Edited by Lietaer G, Rombauts J, Van Balen R. Leuven, Belgium, Leuven University Press, 1990, pp 637–644

Teusch L, Beyerle U, Lange, et al: The client-centered approach to schizophrenic patients: first empirical results, in Research in Psychotherapeutic Approaches. Edited by Minsel WR, Herff W. Frankfurt, Germany, Peter Lang, 1983, pp 140–148

Van Werde D: Restauratie van het psychologisch contact bij acute psychose. Tijdschrift Voor Psychotherapie 5:271–279, 1989

Van Werde D: De Pre-Therapie Van Prouty: psychotherapie met de pre-expressieve zwakzinnige client, in Zorg Voor Geestelijke Gezondheid By Zwakzinnigen. Edited by Došen A, Flikweert DA. Groningen, Netherlands, Stichting Kinderstudies, 1990a, pp 26–32

Van Werde D: Psychotherapy with a retarded schizoaffective woman: an application of Prouty's pre-therapy, in Treatment of Mental Illness and Behavioral Disorder in the Mentally Retarded. Edited by Dosen A, Van Gennep A, Zwanikken G. Leiden, Netherlands, Logon Publications, 1990b, pp 469–477

Watson N: The empirical status of Rogers' hypotheses of the necessary and sufficient conditions for effective psychotherapy, in Client-Centered Therapy and the Person-Centered Approach. Edited by Levan R, Shlien J. New York, Praeger, 1984, pp 17–40

10 Systemic Therapy

Wilhelm Rotthaus, M.D.

Systemic therapy is the application of psychotherapy and its procedures and techniques to systemic thinking in the social process. Psychotherapy is essentially a human encounter, and the way in which systemic thinking influences the therapists and the perception of the mentally retarded persons as partners in therapy are important. The problems encountered in the families of mentally retarded persons have been already described in Chapter 6 of this book. In this chapter, I describe some essential aspects of systemic thinking. First to be outlined is the view that the systemic-oriented therapist has of mentally retarded people. Next to be considered are systemic thinking and the effects it has on the social procedure of therapy. I then discuss some systemic therapeutic constellations and close with an evaluation of the possible uses of systemic therapeutic work with mentally retarded persons.

■ CHARACTERISTICS OF SYSTEMIC THINKING

From a systemic viewpoint, a person creates the world in which he or she lives through his or her communications and interactions. In this process, the person is both the subject as well as the object of events. In the person's actions he or she is an element of a superior system of interaction on which he or she is at once dependent and influential in determining the living conditions of others. This happens recursively, such that the behavior of one person influences all others whose behavior in turn influences the person in a never-ending cycle of repeated, recursive operations, which result in a system of eigenvalues (own values)—also known as eigenbehaviors—or eigenstructures (von Foerster 1984, 1987)—of the family as well as of the larger interaction system.

The behavior of a person can be explained by identifying the interaction field that is important for him or her and that serves to preserve his or her Eigen values. The person's behavior is therefore never to be understood as being detached from his or her current field of interaction (i.e., from the field in which the person describes his or her world by his or her behavior and which the person changes or maintains in dependency on the partners in his or her interaction) (Simon 1988).

The systemic perspective compels one to think in categories of "not only, but also." On the one hand, a person is autonomous, responsible for his or her actions, and not to be influenced directly by others. According to Maturana (1975), no instructive interaction is possible, and it is not the therapist with his or her therapeutic interaction who determines the fate of a patient; rather, it is the patient who determines independently the fate of the therapeutic intervention. Similarly, it is not the educator with his or her pedagogic measures who determines the behavior of the child, but it is the child who determines independently the fate of the pedagogic intervention. On the other hand, a person is dependent on his or her environment. The individual is, as emphasized by Duss-von Werdt (1987), "not a unity of life, but theoretical, something abstract, existentially unable to live" (p. 128).

Additionally, the viewpoint of systems theory asserts that no person possesses absolute truth and absolute reality. Whatever one holds to be true or real is a construction that is worthwhile if it facilitates orientation. This view is well known in science, in which models and theories are not "true" but are only more or less "appropriate" and useful (Kuhn 1980).

Furthermore, it holds true that every description comes from an observer and is therefore unavoidably subjective. As Maturana put it, descriptions are possible only as a result of a structural coupling between the observer and the person observed; an isolated description of the person being observed is unthinkable because the observer immediately causes disturbances that are met by the one being observed by attempts to adapt. The observer and the observed depend mutually on each other. Correspondingly, one can only ascribe characteristics to a system—or a family or an individual—by including the conditions of the observer and the observation.

Thus, when an observer describes the behavior of an individual human being, he or she is dealing with a particular environmental context and is making particular judgmental statements and evaluations. Behavior belongs to the category of the observer. From the point of view of an individual as an autopoietic system, every behavior that is carried out is suitable, good, and proper so long as it serves its self-preservation, its autopoiesis, and does not lead to disintegration; terms such as *pathological, abnormal, mad,* and *handicapped* are descriptions that are made by an observer.

■ A SYSTEMIC VIEW OF THE MENTALLY RETARDED

If one applies the aforementioned guidelines of systemic thinking to the mentally retarded, it would mean that the description "mental retardation" also belongs to the category of an observer. With no observers in the environment to describe a certain individual as being "mentally retarded," there would be no mentally retarded people. The observer uses special criteria, for example, to judge someone's ability to speak and think logically, as a basis leading him or her to characterize a certain individual as being mentally retarded. If the observer used other criteria instead, such as the above-mentioned ability to survive or the abilities to smell, to taste, to feel, to laugh, to cry, to love, to have sex, the observer would perhaps describe the individual as being "normal."

The decision upon which the observer bases his or her judgmental and evaluative criteria has concrete consequences for the interaction system and especially for the individual being described. In this context, it is worth noting that "reality" is a creation of language and that psychotherapy, pedagogy, and every other form of a discourse have their own "hate language," as Lynn Hoffman put it, notwithstanding "that these expressions can be hidden well behind a brilliant facade which is borrowed from science or medicine." Hoffman (1992) goes on to say that, "Perhaps every clinical dys-description should be termed 'politically wrong.' This not only includes 'disabled,' which is today defined as 'differently abled,' i.e., as a specific ability but also terms such as 'dysfunction,' 'disorder' and 'disease' " (p. 98).

This construction by the mentally retarded person of his or her self-image is greatly influenced by the way in which the person's most important interaction partners observe him or her and the language they use in communicating with the person. Inasmuch as the mentally retarded person is a part of a superior interaction system in which he or she is dependent on others who determine the person's living conditions, his or her activities are limited and freedom to act is imposed and restricted by the other members of his or her interaction system. This has practical implications for pedagogic and therapeutic measures. Salutary measures have the greatest chance of success, if they are applied not only to the mentally retarded individual but to the whole interaction system as well (e.g., the family, the neighborhood, the group in the home).

This can be illustrated from the research and compensation/early intervention programs. Flammer (1988) summarizes the results as follows: "The various so-called compensation programs, such as the comprehensive 'headstart-project' in the USA almost all had surprising positive immediate effects on the measured IQ; but these benefits did not last after conclusion of the programs" (p. 269). Bronfenbrenner (see Flammer 1988), who led a substantial part of his research, attributed this to the fact that the programs had too little influence on the remaining social world of the children involved; he concluded, "Whoever wishes to see a lasting positive influence on the development of children, must support the people nearest to these children, the family, and the immediate environment. Developmental support of individual children functions only as developmental support of all people involved in the environment of these children" (p. 320). Bronfenbrenner gave his publication in which he described this, a remarkable title, namely, "The context of development and the development of the context."

The mentally retarded person not only is influenced by the context but also influences it. Anyone who has contact with the family of a mentally retarded person knows very well how Eigen values and Eigen structures of such families develop as a reaction to this member of the family because this person is an integral part of the structure. Therefore, the mentally retarded person acts autonomously and is correspondingly responsible for his or her actions. This constitutes his or her human dignity and includes the "dignity of risk" (Dybwad 1985). This human dignity would be endangered if we did not allow the mentally retarded person to be responsible for his or her deeds by trying to shield the person from all situations in which he or she could be hurt or otherwise overprotect him or her from all dangers.

The mentally retarded person is a unique individual with a unique biography. The mentally retarded person's unique structure decides at any moment how he or she responds to an action carried out within his or her interaction system. This structure of the individual at any given time is the product of his or her evolutionary and individual history. Functional damage may have a place in the history of a mentally retarded person that from the first day of life—indeed even before—has influenced the recursive coupling of all actions in the mutuality of the interaction systems. Social context variables—such as stigmatization, labeling, and generalization processes, as well as other aspects of allocation and taking over of the role of the retarded person—influence the interaction and are therefore an essential part of the history of this individual. The structure of the individual is determined by this unique history, and this determines the person's way of reacting at the present time. The single factors of influence cannot be isolated from the structure, and it will not be possible to say which factors of influence have affected the existence of the retardation or to what extent. In principle, the possibility of estimating more or less exactly the impact of such factors of influence on larger groups of people does not alter this stance. In addition, a knowledge of the meaning of various factors of influence in the past is in no way a necessary requirement for pedagogic or therapeutic measures to be taken in the future.

An awareness of the fact that a person's actions are determined at any point in his or her life by his structure can protect us from denying that people are different from one another and that a retarded person is different. On the contrary, it should encourage us to perceive the uniqueness of others and to accord them respect.

■ PRINCIPLES OF SYSTEMIC THERAPY

Systemic thinking as applied to psychotherapy implies understanding the behavior of the individual within the relevant field of interaction and achieving a change in behavior by influencing all members in this field of interaction. This does not mean that the behavior of someone might proceed causally from the behavior of the other by way of a stimulus reaction pattern. The interactions of all concerned can only be classified on the abstract meta-level of rules. This in no way includes the deterministic cause-effect mode of thinking because the concrete outcome is not predictable. However, it is possible to make predictions about what may possibly happen. In this respect, attention must be drawn to one of the most common and disastrous mistakes one encounters in working with families, namely the idea—possibly never articulated—that the family "causes" or has "caused" the difficulties of the mentally retarded person. Such erroneous assertions arise from the acceptance of lineal cause-effect thinking in the larger domain of the family. Goolishian and colleagues tell us that it is not the problem system (i.e., the people who are concerned with the problematic behavior of the mentally retarded person) that creates the symptom, but it is the symptom that creates the problem system (Anderson et al. 1986; Goolishian and Anderson 1987).

From a systemic point of view, the question of "why" a certain difficulty or problematic behavior occurs is principally unanswerable. In addition, the answer to this question is not a necessary requirement for therapy. The more important and intriguing question is, What is the purpose, function, and significance of the symptom? This question includes access to the "rules of the game" of a problem system, which obviously cannot keep up with the development of the system. The aim of therapy is to open up new possibilities to the system members and to alter the rigid and inappropriate rules that have become out-of-date in the course of the development process. Such a change is possible once the therapist dispenses with certain patterns of the game in contact with the problem system, using instead alternative patterns or disrupting what seems to the therapist to be the dysfunctional family patterns (and restricted family ideas) by introducing a fresh perspective.

■ SYSTEM THERAPEUTIC CONSTELLATIONS

Systemic thinking offers the counselor or therapist[1] the possibility of focusing his or her attention on and at various levels. Thus, the therapist can focus on the family of the mentally retarded member in the context of the social system or in the context of the institutions helping the family. The therapist can look at the mentally retarded person in the context of his or her family or group home, or the therapist can consider a certain behavior of a retarded individual as an expression of the individual's biological condition. For a better understanding of family problems, see Chapter 5 of this book.

The advantage of the choice of a larger context hinges on the fact that the interactions lay open and are relatively easy to observe, and that the special rules of the system can be relatively easily understood in their context. Perhaps the most decisive advantage to the therapist in his or her work with larger systems is the ability to direct his or her interventions not only to the retarded person but to numerous other persons—thereby enhancing his or her influence in achieving the desired changes.

Some constellations and patterns at various levels that can often be observed in the behavior disorders of mentally retarded children and adults are described below.

The Family of the Mentally Retarded Person in the Context of the Social System

Just as the mentally retarded person is a member of a family system, the family, too, is a member of a larger system—the social environment, with its attitudes and behaviors toward the mentally retarded and its political, social, and economic influences. The latter can sometimes be in the foreground, so that the help for finding a larger flat or obtaining regular financial support can be the most important measures for reducing the behavioral problems of the mentally retarded member.

The same applies to the family of the mentally retarded individual. The family is, indeed, on the one hand, a part of society and influences it and, on the other hand, has its own scope restricted by society. A recursive process of interaction also occurs here, often with the result that the family tries to hide the retarded person only to prevent him or her from having any "normal interaction" with the community. The family may be ashamed and restricted in its own social contacts. It is isolated or becomes isolated from stimuli and impulses from the social environment, which would normally facilitate the further development of the family and its members (see Chapter 6 of this book). As a result, behavior and family rules can develop in a bizarre way, and their "true origin" can rarely or in only some cases be uncovered. The counselor/

---

[1] When talking with retarded people and their relatives, we avoid the word *therapist* because all too often this suggests the idea that the person or his or her family is not all right, has deficiency, is ill, etc. Instead of this, we prefer such terms as *counselor, adviser, discussion leader,* and *family conversations* or *consultations.*

therapist has the opportunity to reintroduce outside perspectives through his or her own person but, importantly too, through the activation of outside contacts that may have long been neglected.

The Family of the Mentally Retarded Person in the Context of Helping Institutions

The most important contact source—and in some cases the only one—for the family of a mentally retarded member is the helpers from various professional institutions such as the youth service, the health service, the school, the clinic, or the group home. Such helpers often have the tendency to take over the responsibility of the family, which now feels that matters have been taken out of their hands. Others attempt to make the parents of the mentally retarded children assume the role of therapists.

There is often a helper system around families whose caregivers do not discuss their actions reciprocally—often giving the families contradictory instructions and advice, thereby causing a lack of confidence, creating confusion, and undermining the competence of members of the family to manage their own lives. There is often a striking contradiction—which is self-defeating—between the complaints of the family about insufficient help, on the one hand, and, on the other, the large number of caregivers who get involved with these families. What is often lacking here—as in the relationship to the mentally retarded person—is the respect for the autonomy and the responsibility of the respective partner.

Imber-Black (1987) has drawn attention to numerous further constellations. She has clearly described how helpers in the process of escalating complementarity increase more and more the initial feeling of helplessness in families. They not only fail to perceive the resources of the family and strengthen them but also offer help without considering the actual wishes of the family members until they become dependent on a series of helpers and helper systems. "Such escalating complementarity often leads to an expansion of the macro-system, as more and more helpers and specialists are enlisted" (Imber-Black 1987, p. 432).

Conversely, she describes how helpers—when giving advice and directives without considering and evaluating the individual and the special attempts of the family to solve the problem—can also enter a process of escalating symmetry, in which each person tries to pursue his or her own ideas and put them into practice. Fierce struggles, with traded blame, then ensue over who knows best. "The larger system and family may intermittently withdraw from one another, cutting off sources of information, only to reengage in the symmetrical struggle at a later time about another issue" (p. 432).

Finally, Imber-Black (1987) points out that the contradictory instructions and advice from helper systems or a symmetrical battle within a helper system are sometimes reflected in similar behavior patterns between the mother and father, who are unable to cooperate and develop suitable plans for the further development and care of their mentally retarded child. If the counselor/therapist is able to get insight into such processes, he or she may withhold apportioning blame while also using interventions that introduce more efficacious and flexible patterns.

If a mentally retarded child or young person is being cared for in a home, he or she may become enmeshed in loyalty conflicts between the group caregivers and the parents, which can manifest themselves in violent and aggressive behavior. This happens when the group caregivers of the home try to be "better parents" than the parents themselves rather than assume the role of the modest delegates of the parents (Rotthaus 1990a, 1995).

Of course, families with mentally retarded members often need help and support. However, they should be able to expect that the activities and ideas of helpers are well coordinated and that the helping relationship is, in principle, characterized by equality, partnership, and reciprocal relatedness, so that a coevolution from which both sides benefit can take place. Essentially, there should be a fixed time limit to helping families, which should be as short as possible so as not to endanger the confidence and trust that the families have in their own resources and ability to cope. Helpers should see themselves as rendering a service to their "customers"—the parents of a retarded person, the caregivers, and the retarded person him- or herself. They should provide the best possible service based on up-to-date scientific knowledge that the "customers" can accept or reject.

Unfortunately, all helpers have been trained in a long tradition of recognizing the deficits and shortcomings of others. They usually have no training in sensing the achievements and the strengths of the people they care for or discovering possibly hidden resources. However, as systemic thinking teaches us, the mentally retarded person behaves properly and adequately in a given situation (even if this behavior is condemned by all others as disturbing and in fact negatively influences his or her development in the long run) and is in a position to confront the family with the assumption that there are good reasons for his or her behavior (even if this cannot be identified at the time). It is important to recognize that parents have the primary authority for the welfare of their family, and it is useful to assume that they have at their disposal the necessary resources for the further development of the whole family even if these resources have not been used up yet. By means of an accepting, stimulating, and supportive contact with the counselor or therapist, it is often possible for family members to discover their own resources again.

Mentally Retarded Persons in the Context of Their Families

Families with a mentally retarded member experience the same developmental steps and normative crises that "normal" families do. Such normative crises include the possibility of further development and growth but also of standstill and inappropriate development. Imber-Black (1987) states that "For the mentally handicapped and their families, this perspective assumes an added dimension, because each normative transition (e.g., birth, going to school, adolescence, leaving home) also involves the family initially and in enduring ways with larger systems. Not only must the family system reorganize at each stage, but it must do so in relationship to a host of outside professionals" (p. 442). Families with a retarded member have to overcome all crises in the family cycle twofold, for example, the separation of the young family member at the end of puberty and, at the same time, the separation from the helpers. It is perhaps understandable that some helpers often have the impression that in the background of every individual disable child there is always a disabled family (Sheridan 1965). However, such attitudes easily lead to overlooking the great achievements of the family members and usually render access to them difficult if not impossible.

For many families these transitions in the family cycle are points in time when renewed mourning occurs over the loss of the "normal" child they have expected (Black 1982; Dornette 1985; Seligman and Darling 1989; Sloman and Konstantareas 1990) (see also Chapter 6 of this book). The attentive counselor or therapist is able to perceive the necessity of this mourning and helps the family release the pain and not be ashamed of doing so, but, indeed, recognize its justification. It is important to recognize that the mentally retarded child usually reaches the various stages of his or her development later than his or her nondisabled contemporaries. Sloman and Konstantareas (1990) formulate the following as one of their guidelines for family work: "At key developmental periods, for example, entry into elementary school, onset of puberty, and reaching the age 'normal' children leave home, be prepared to support the renewed anxieties, concerns, and adjustments the families may have to make" (p. 426).

The disappointment and loss of their own self-esteem as a result of having produced a dysfunctional child, the confrontation with social isolation and numerous prejudices, and, last but not least, the high financial and physical costs present serious existential burdens for the family. Nevertheless, most families seem to be able to cope with this and lead a fairly "normal" life with their children (Schubert and Tatzer 1987). This strain, however, is not without its consequences. In an empirical study, Schubert and Tatzer (1987) furnished proof of clearly weaker cohesion and adaptability in families with a disabled child compared with a control group. Families with a disabled child manifest more often "weaknesses in a family" than family members in the control group. According to the researchers, "The problems (weaknesses) apply above all to emotional areas. Difficulties reveal themselves in the exchange and expression of feelings as well as in the affective relationships between the family members" (p. 88).

The same authors (1987) also observed a significantly worse pair-relationship in families with a disabled child, particularly a pattern of "peripheral father–enmeshed mother":

> The "peripheral" father occupies an outside position as regards events in family life; he possesses less pedagogic competence; makes fewer decisions as regards the family and his interests are directed to outside the home. The "enmeshed" mother on the other hand occupies and orients herself particularly intensively towards the (retarded) child and she leads her life according to his needs. . . . Disagreement on educational questions, conflicts and alienation at pair level are thus fostered. (p. 94)

A second common variant is "dichotomy of the family":

> The father directs his attention particularly intensively towards a certain child, mostly to the non-handicapped one, while the mother directs hers usually towards the handicapped child. Rigid subsystems develop. . . . This adversely affects the marital and the sibling subsystem and favors in some circumstances a worsening of the relationship between husband and wife. (p. 94)

It is worthwhile to call attention to the results of the study as they pertain to the nondisabled siblings. Whereas the brothers and sisters judged the parent-child relationship as being significantly worse, the relationship was estimated by the parents as being better. This may be an indication that the parents of disabled children pay less attention to their nondisabled children. Nondisabled children—especially the eldest daughter—must often take on some of the physical tasks and burdens of caring for the retarded child (Black 1982). In some cases, they must even bear all the hopes and aspirations that the parents originally had for their disabled child. It is not, therefore, surprising that brothers and sisters of disabled children often develop into very independent persons with strong social and humanitarian engagement. On the other hand, they are more likely to be conspicuous from a psychiatrist's point of view.

The Disturbing Behavior of Mentally Retarded Persons in the Context of the Individual

The systemic counselor/therapist will not fail to see disturbing behavior as a consequence of the strengths and weaknesses of an individual's biologically based restrictions. For example, he or she will notice disturbances in optical and acoustic perception and will under certain circumstances consider it sensible to encourage developmental processes in this area, by means of special measures such as body gestalt therapy (Besems and van Vugt 1985) or attention interaction therapy (AIT) (Hartmann et al. 1988). It should be noted that these well-tried methods, which are primarily aimed at the disabled individual, achieve their effect from the lively interaction between the disabled person and the therapist. Careful observation always shows that behavior only takes place within relationships, regardless of how many or how few biological disadvantages an individual has (Hartmann and Jakobs 1993).

To summarize, system therapeutic work with the mentally retarded is basically no different from its use with the nondisabled. However, it is an advantage for the counselor/therapist to be aware of typical constellations that often develop in an interplay among the retarded individual, the relatives, and the broader context. Usually the systemic counselor/therapist departs from the concept of physical conspicuousness as an individual phenomenon—a concept with a very long tradition in our Western culture, going back to the end of the Middle Ages (Rotthaus 1990b). Instead, the counselor leads the behavior back to its contextual relationship in which it is easier to influence. In his work, the therapist adopts an attitude of partiality to all. The therapist avoids the one-sided coalition with the mentally retarded person that typically occurs, especially in an institution. The mentally retarded persons would in no way benefit if the therapist joined sides with them against their parents or other relatives.

The systemic therapist respects the needs of families with retarded members and carefully differentiates between his or her own needs and wishes and those of the families. In his or her work, the therapist orients him- or herself toward the resources of the families, to what they are able to do and achieve, and appreciates the solutions they offer. Instead of looking at the deficits and making the so-called pathological behaviors the therapist's main conversational topics, he or she concentrates on the situations in which disturbing behavior does not occur and tries to let these "exceptions" become the norm. Based on an attitude of partnership, which corresponds with the relationship between a customer (the mentally retarded person and his or her family) and the provider of a service (counselor/therapist), the therapist reinforces the sense of responsibility of both the retarded person and the parents and may, indeed, benefit from some favorable encounters. As Black (1982) has stated, families with a disabled member "have much to teach us about courage and endurance, and about how to find pleasure in the almost unperceptible development of the most handicapped children" (p. 437).

■ CONCLUSIONS

Mentally retarded children and adults are especially dependent on their close relatives for help and for a long period of time or indeed their entire lives. The possibility of manifold entanglements and enmeshments is especially high. Thus, I believe that the systemic approach may be very effective in revealing and unfolding the conspicuous or disturbing behavior of mentally retarded persons in the context of their individual environment. In my work with mentally retarded children, young people, and adults, as well as with their families and other relatives, I believe that this fact has been substantiated and see an increasing number of colleagues following this approach (Black 1982; Griffioen et al. 1990; Hennicke 1993, 1994, 1996; Imber-Black 1987; Rotthaus 1996; Schubert and Tatzer 1987). Since the beginning of the 1980s, at least in Germany, the systemic approach has given precedence to encouraging the early intervention in the development of retarded children and has led to a new orientation that advocates early support and includes the whole family (Gusky 1989; Krause 1986; Mangold and Obendorf 1981; Oberbeck 1981; Rotthaus 1991, 1993; Wolf 1984).

However, it must be admitted that the efficacy of systemic therapy with mentally retarded persons has not received adequate scientific scrutiny. More research is required that focuses on the effectiveness as well as on the problem-solving strategies of system therapeutic work, that embodies the integration of the retarded person in the total environment (i.e., living, working, and leisure time activities), that strives for the contentment of the retarded person and his or her relatives, that accentuates the efforts made to strengthen parental competence in solving problems, and that carries out follow-ups studies for evaluating long-term benefits.

■ REFERENCES

Anderson H, Goolishian H, Windermand L: Problem determined systems: towards transformation in family therapy. Journal of Strategic and Systemic Therapies 5:1–13, 1986

Besems T, van Vugt G: Gestaltherapie mit geistig Behinderten, in Psychotherapie mit Jugendlichen. Edited by Rotthaus W. Dortmund, Germany, Verlag Modernes Lernen, 1985, pp 251–275

Black D: Handicap and family therapy, in Family Therapy, Vol 2. Edited by Bentovim A, Barnes GG, Cooklin A. London, Academic Press, 1982, pp 417–439

Dornette W: Behinderte Jugendliche und ihre Familien im Spannugsfeld zwischen Überbe hüten und Ausklammern, in Psychotherapie mit Jugendlichen. Edited by Rotthaus W. Dortmund, Germany, Verlag Modernes Lernen, 1985, pp 101–114

Duss-von Werdt D: Von der systemischen Sicht zum therapeutischen Handeln. Psychotherapie Medizinische Psychologie 34:126–132, 1987

Dybwad G: Realitäten und Tendenzen der Betreuung geistig behinderter Menschen aus internationaler Sicht, in Geistige Behinderung und soziales Leben. Edited by Wacker E, Neumann J. Frankfurt, Germany, Campus, 1985, pp 21–42

Flammer A: Entwicklungstheorien. Stuttgart, Germany, Huber, 1988

Goolishian H, Anderson H: Language systems and therapy: an evolving idea. Psychotherapy 24:529–538, 1987

Griffioen J, de Graaf S, Gehrels JF: Treatment of severe behaviour disorder in the mentally retarded from a systems approach, in Treatment of Mental Illness and Behavioral Disorder in the Mentally Retarded. Edited by Došen A, van Gennep A, Zwanniken G. Leiden, Netherlands, Logon Publications, 1990, pp 233–239

Gusky E: Systemsicht und familienorientierung am beispiel der frühf örd erung. Geistige Behinderung 29:78–87, 1989

Hartmann H, Jakobs G: 'Dialogische Prinzip' bei der behandlung von aggression, auto aggression und autismus, in Psychotherapie und Geistige Behinderung. Edited by Hennicke K, Rotthaus W. Dortmund, Germany, Verlag Modernes Lernen, 1993, pp 36–50

Hartmann H, Kalde M, Jakobs G, et al: Die Aufmerksamkeits-interaktions-therapie (AIT), in Autismus Heute, Bd 1. Edited by Arens CH, Dzikowsi S. Dortmund, Germany, Verlag Modernes Lernen, 1988, pp 129–137

Hennicke K: System therapy for persons with mental retardation, in Mental Health Aspects of Mental Retardation. Edited by Fletcher RJ, Došen A. New York, Lexington Books, 1993, pp 402–417

Hennicke K: Therapeutische zugänge zu geistig behinderten menschen mit psychischen störungen: traditionelles und systemisches konzept. Geistige Behinderung 33:95–110, 1994

Hennicke K: Kontexte von gewalt und gegengewalt in familien mit geistig behinderten. Geistige Behinderung 35:290–306, 1996

Hoffman L: Relationale arbeit mit systemen: familientherapie mit anderer. Stimme Zeitschrift Systemische Therapie 10:97–100, 1992

Imber-Black E: The mentally handicapped in context. Family Systems Medicine 5:428–445, 1987

Krause P: Entwicklungsförderung behinderter kinder: ein familienzen triertes. Konzept Sozialpädiatrie 8:39–42, 1986

Kuhn W: Lehrbuch der Physik, III. Braunschweig, Germany, Westermann Verlag, 1980

Mangold B, Obendorf W: Bedeutung der familiären beziehungsdynamik in der früfötfrtung und therapie mit behinderten kindern. Praxis der Kinder Psychologie und Kinderpsychiatrie 30:12–18, 1981

Maturana H: The organisation of the living: a theory of a living organisation. International Journal of Man-Machine Studies 7:313–332, 1975

Oberbeck A: Familientherapeutische ansätze in der behindertenarbeit. Geistige Behinderung 21:202–213, 1981

Rotthaus W: Stationäre Systemische Kinder-und Jugendpsychiatrie. Dortmund, Germany, Verlag Modernes Lernen, 1990a

Rotthaus W: Diagnostische und therapeutische sichtweisen im wandel: die systemische perspektive. Praxis Kinderpsychologie, Kinderpsychiatrie 39:361–364, 1990b

Rotthaus W: Systemisches arbeiten bei der rehabilitation von kindern und jugendlichen. Praxis Psychomotorik 16:75–80, 1991

Rotthaus W: Menschenbild und psychische krankheit des geistigbehinderten aus systemischer sicht, in Psychotherapie und Geistige Behinderung. Edited by Hennicke K, Rotthaus W. Dortmund, Germany, Verlag Modernes Lernen, 1993, pp 195–203

Rotthaus W: Das rollenverständnis der mitarbeiterinnen in der stationärne systemischen kinder-und jugendpsychiatrie. Zeitung für Systemische Therapie 13:105–110, 1995

Rotthaus W: Systemische therapie mit geistig behinderten menschen. Behinderte 19:45–52, 1996

Schubert MT, Tatzer E: Familien mit behinderten kindern und ihre helferzwischen kompetenz und resignation, in Erziehung und Therapie in Systemischer Sicht. Edited by Rotthaus W. Dortmund, Germany, Verlag Modernes Lernen, 1987, pp 139–146

Seligman M, Darling RB: Ordinary Families, Special Children: A System Approach to Childhood Disability. New York, Guilford, 1989

Sheridan M: The Handicapped Child and His Home. London, National Childrens Home, 1965

Simon FB: Unterschiede, die Unterschiede Machen. Heidelberg, Germany, Springer, 1988

Sloman L, Konstantareas MM: Why families of children with biological defects require a system approach. Family Process 29:417–429, 1990

von Foerster H: Observing Systems. Seaside, CA, Intersystems Publications, 1984

von Foerster H: Entdecken oder Erfinden: wie läßt sich Verstehen verste hen? in Erzie Hung und Therapie in Systemischer Sicht. Edited by Rotthaus W. Dortmund, Germany, Verlag Modernes Lernen, 1987, pp 22–60

Wolf FE: Über die rolle der eltern. Frühförderung Interdisziplinär 3:70–75, 1984

Treatment of Mental Illness

11 Treatment of Schizophrenia

David J. Clarke, M.B., Ch.B., M.R.C.Psych.

Schizophrenia is more common among people with mental retardation than among the general population and often has the effect of markedly reducing adaptive functioning. Compared with the extensive literature concerning the treatment of schizophrenia among people of normal intelligence, relatively little has been written specifically about the treatment of schizophrenia in association with mental retardation. People with mental retardation often have additional disabilities or disorders (such as epilepsy, motor impairments, or autistic spectrum disorders), which make diagnosis more difficult, predispose to adverse effects when medication is employed, or place constraints on the use of other treatment strategies. The concept of schizophrenia is useful as a working model for the subclassification of psychotic disorders associated with mental retardation, but attention to diagnostic issues should not hinder the provision of effective treatment. Brockington (1992) observed that "when dealing with patients with intractable polysymptomatic illnesses—with perceptual and thinking disorders, defects, and handicaps (both primary and secondary), often associated with affective and neurotic symptoms—the psychiatrist's role is to analyze the clinical record, identify and evaluate each component of the patient's mental life, and devise a range of interventions, dealing with each on its merits." A symptom-based approach to treatment is often necessary when managing schizophrenic disorders associated with mental retardation because of the difficulty in establishing the diagnosis in accordance with current criteria such as ICD-10 (World Health Organization 1992), if the patient has difficulty communicating complex subjective experiences to the clinician. Such an approach avoids definitional debates about whether the symptoms reflect an "organic" delusional (schizophrenia-like) disorder rather than "true" schizophrenia. It is necessary when adopting such a symptom-based approach to have a broadly based assessment that identifies factors (such as epilepsy) that are relevant to treatment selection and to have a system of quantifying psychopathology or resulting behavior that allows measurement of response to treatment.

183

■ ANTIPSYCHOTIC DRUGS

Efficacy

The use of chlorpromazine and other antipsychotic or "neuroleptic" drugs from the early 1950s onward improved the quality of life of people with schizophrenic illnesses enormously. By eliminating or reducing the impact of the symptoms, these medications promoted the exodus from psychiatric hospitals to the community (and reduced the length of hospital stay for patients who were admitted). They do, however, have limitations. They act predominantly by reducing positive symptoms such as delusions and hallucinations. Most have relatively little effect on negative symptoms, such as lack of drive and emotional blunting, which can be important in determining the outcome of rehabilitation.

There is no doubt that antipsychotic drugs effectively reduce or abolish symptoms such as delusions and hallucinations. Davis (1976) summarized the results of over 200 double-blind studies comparing the antipsychotic activity of antipsychotic drugs versus placebo: antipsychotic medication was more effective in over 85% of the trials. Cole et al. (1964), in a large trial of antipsychotic medication in acute schizophrenia, found that 75% of the patients receiving antipsychotic drugs improved considerably compared with 25% of those receiving placebo. A substantial proportion of those receiving placebo became more unwell during the course of the trial. Most studies of mental illness occurring in people with mental retardation have found that antipsychotic drugs are as efficacious in the treatment of schizophrenia as they are for nonretarded people (e.g., Reid 1972), but the weight of evidence is less because there have been fewer studies. Appropriate doses for different clinical situations and the use of high doses of antipsychotic medication have been reviewed by Thompson (1994), who presented the United Kingdom Royal College of Psychiatrists' Consensus Statement.

Adverse Effects

As with all effective medications, antipsychotic compounds have unwanted effects, some of the most troublesome being movement disorders such as acute dystonia, pseudoparkinsonism, akathisia (restlessness), and tardive dyskinesia. These, and other adverse effects, are such that the prescription of antipsychotic drugs to people with mental retardation should be carefully considered and monitored. The communication problems some patients have predispose them to the development of unwanted effects because they are unable to draw attention to early manifestations of side effects and may suffer more severely. One adverse effect, tardive dyskinesia (a movement disorder), is sometimes irreversible, and another, neuroleptic malignant syndrome, may be fatal if not recognized at an early stage. There is some evidence that patients with organic brain disorder are more likely to develop tardive dyskinesia, and that people with mental retardation are susceptible to dyskinesia and other adverse effects of antipsychotic medication (Gualtieri and Hawk 1980; Gualtieri et al. 1986). Antipsychotic medications lower the convulsive threshold, and about a third of the people with severe retardation have epilepsy. Photosensitivity induced by chlorpromazine can lead to severe sunburn if a patient is immobile and exposed to the sun without adequate skin protection. Prescribers are advised to refer to data sheets and other relevant material when considering the appropriateness of a class of antipsychotic or an individual compound.

Patient Characteristics and Choice of Antipsychotic Medication

Antipsychotic medications vary in their potency (related to blockade of dopaminergic receptors) and in other effects that reflect binding to other receptors (such as anticholinergic activity). It is important to choose an antipsychotic medication that will be well tolerated because adverse effects are likely to lead to noncompliance and inadequate symptom control, in addition to the problems created directly by the medication. Individual patient characteristics must be borne in mind when a choice of antipsychotic drug is made so that the maximum benefit is gained with the lowest risk of adverse effects. Commonly encountered additional problems or disabilities include epilepsy (antipsychotics vary in the magnitude of their effect on the convulsive threshold), constipation (drugs such as thioridazine with marked anticholinergic effects should be avoided if possible and the use of antiparkinsonian agents minimized), and motor disorders such as cerebral palsy (such disorders may increase vulnerability to extrapyramidal adverse effects, especially if potent antipsychotics are prescribed). More caution than is usual in the general population is appropriate when initiating treatment or increasing doses of antipsychotic drugs. The possible increased risk of dyskinesia, including tardive dyskinesia, implies that an ongoing review of the antipsychotic dosage is wise, the aim being to use the lowest possible dose of medication that will adequately control the symptoms.

Effects on Learning

Some drugs (such as chlorpromazine) have a sedating effect when given to most people, but the degree of sedation varies markedly between individuals. If high doses are used, some impairment of cognitive functioning can be expected. This is obviously of concern when the person prescribed for has a preexisting learning disability. However, much of the published work concerning the adverse effects of antipsychotic drugs on learning and adaptive behavior in this population derives from studies of other populations or from work that has now been discredited (see Aman 1987 for a discussion). Some methodologically sound work remains that implies that antipsychotic drugs may impair cognition (e.g., Sprague 1977).

Few studies have considered the benefits and adverse effects of antipsychotic medication when used to treat schizophrenia occurring in association with mental retardation; most concern the adverse effects noted when the drugs are given to manage nonschizophrenic behavioral symptomatology. When antipsychotic drugs are used in a nonspecific way (i.e., other than to treat psychotic symptoms), greater weight needs to be given to potential risks of treatment (because the benefits have not been clearly established). It is good practice to use antipsychotic medication in the lowest dose and for the shortest time that is effective. This practice will minimize adverse effects, including the effects on learning. Potentially adverse effects are important constraints on the use of antipsychotics, but in cases in which these drugs are specifically indicated for the treatment of schizophrenia, the risks must be balanced against the undoubted benefits from treatment for the vast majority of people.

Route of Administration

Oral administration has the advantage that dose adjustments can be made swiftly, and properties such as sedation can be used to promote sleep while minimizing daytime drowsiness. However, antipsychotic drugs are stored in body fat, and after some weeks of administration dose reductions do not have immediate effect. The oral route is preferred by some patients because they regard depot injections as undignified, or because they fear intramuscular injections or choose to take day-to-day responsibility for their own treatment. Many people with mental retardation do not administer their own medication, and compliance is less of an issue than for people who have to remember (and remain motivated) to take oral medication. Depot injections circumvent the need to remember to take medication and may be more efficacious in preventing relapse among patients who stop taking medication when their insight becomes impaired or other psychotic symptoms appear, thus making rapid relapse probable. Depot administration also results in a lower total drug dose being administered (because the metabolism that occurs in the gut and liver after oral administration is avoided). Toxicity, however, may be greater with depot preparations (Falloon et al. 1978; Rifkin et al. 1977). The choice of route of administration should ideally be the patient's, informed by relevant advice from the psychiatrist. Some people may be unable to make an informed choice either about treatment or about the route of administration. If they are not subject to mental health legislation, it is good practice to consult with caregivers and with the multidisciplinary team to arrive at a consensus regarding the treatment that is in the individual's best interest.

Maintenance Treatment

Following the treatment of acute symptoms, a decision must be made about the need for maintenance treatment (to prevent further relapse) and its duration. One study found that the 2-year outcome was better if maintenance antipsychotic treatment was given for 12 months (Johnson 1979). About one-third of the patients with schizophrenia relapse over a 2-year period, despite receiving maintenance treatment. About 20% of the people with schizophrenia remain relapse free and maintain their level of functioning without medication. Unfortunately, there are no indicators that allow the patients who remain well without antipsychotics to be identified. Psychiatrists are no better at making this judgment than patients, and the decision must be weighed against the risk of, and consequences of, relapse. After 5 years, about 80% of the patients relapse when antipsychotic drugs are stopped (Johnson et al. 1983). Leff and Wing (1971) suggested that patients likely to have a poor prognosis were likely to relapse even if treated with antipsychotic medication, and Goldberg et al. (1977) produced evidence to suggest that patients with good prognosis schizophrenia benefited most from maintenance antipsychotic medication.

Polypharmacy and Prescription Review

It is considered good practice to use the fewest number of drugs and in the lowest doses possible to prevent relapse. In practice, polypharmacy appears to be relatively common. Edwards and Kumar (1984) found that 10% of day or inpatients at two mental illness hospitals were receiving two antipsychotics, and depot and oral antipsychotics were combined in 20% of the patients. Half those studied also received anticholinergics.

The need to review antipsychotic drug use to ensure treatment is rational, and uses the lowest effective dose, has led to studies to assess the impact of reviews by pharmacists and others. In most cases, such interventions promote rational treatment and reduce overall use of psychoactive medication. Inoue (1982) found that the involvement of a hospital pharmacist to review psychotropic drug use in a mental retardation facility over a 5-year period resulted in significant reductions in both the proportion of patients receiving psychoactive medication and in the numbers of drugs and dosages used. Inoue felt that a lack of feedback to prescribers about responses to drugs was something that could be overcome by the pharmacist coordinating the gathering of information about residents' behavior and the relationship of changes in behavior to changes in prescriptions. Briggs (1989) found that the use of psychotropics in an institution in the United States was reduced and maintained at about 20% over an 8-year period when a monitoring system (with interdisciplinary review, identification of target behaviors, and use of alternatives) was operating.

Withdrawal of Antipsychotic Medication

It has been argued that among the general population in which a firm diagnosis of schizophrenia can be established, the risks of discontinuing antipsychotic treatment outweigh those of continuing with treatment at a *population* level. Discontinuation of treatment may be associated with relapse and subsequent use of higher doses of medication than would have been employed had maintenance treatment been continued (Johnson et al. 1983). For people with mental retardation, however, the individual profile of problems, symptoms, response, and additional disabilities will be much more important in arriving at a decision about whether treatment should be continued. Another important consideration is the degree to which the clinician is satisfied that a diagnosis of schizophrenia is justified, compared with the possibility that auditory hallucinations, for example, were symptomatic of, for example, an acute and transient psychotic disorder (which has a much better prognosis). It is therefore important that people with mental retardation who receive antipsychotic drugs are reviewed by clinicians who have special expertise in the area.

Prescription of Anticholinergics

The use of anticholinergic drugs to counter pseudoparkinsonism and dystonic reactions to antipsychotic drugs should be confined to the following: patients at high risk because of a previous history of extrapyramidal reactions or the presence of concurrent illness predisposing to such reactions; patients prescribed high doses of antipsychotic drugs; young male patients receiving high-potency antipsychotics; and when adverse effects are still not adequately controlled despite reductions in the dosage of antipsychotic medication. The research evidence leading to these recommendations and further information on this topic can be found in Johnson (1986) and Arana et al. (1988). The incidence of extrapyramidal symptoms on stopping concurrent anticholinergic medication varies widely between studies, from 4% to 62%. Most studies indicate that whereas about 60% of patients receive anticholinergics, only about 30% derive benefit from them (Johnson 1986).

Anticholinergics are effective treatments for tremor, rigidity, and dystonia. They have no effect on akathisia (which may be made worse), have adverse effects related to anticholinergic activity, and may have a euphoriant effect. They may also reduce the effectiveness of antipsychotic drugs, worsen positive symptoms of schizophrenia, and disrupt sleep (Johnstone et al. 1983). They should therefore only be prescribed when necessary and for the shortest possible time in the lowest effective dose. It may be preferable to lower the dose of the antipsychotic drug, or change the antipsychotic medication to one less likely to produce extrapyramidal adverse effects (such as thioridazine), rather than introduce an antiparkinsonian agent. Antiparkinsonian medications have anticholinergic effects that may produce a dry mouth, blurred vision, retention of urine, constipation, euphoria (with a risk of abuse), drowsiness, or a confusional state in vulnerable individuals. Some people with mental retardation who are prone to severe constipation may have an episode of intestinal obstruction precipitated by the prescription of an anticholinergic compound. The confusional state that can be produced by anticholinergics (usually at high dose) is characterized by a rapid pulse, a dry skin, and the presence of illusions or visual hallucinations in addition to disorientation. Such symptoms should not be confused with schizophrenic symptomatology.

Newer Antipsychotic Medications and Their Role in the Treatment of Refractory Schizophrenia

Clozapine is an antipsychotic drug licensed in the United Kingdom for the treatment of patients with schizophrenia whose illness is resistant to treatment with other drugs. It is claimed to improve both positive and negative symptoms and is at least as effective as other antipsychotic drugs in the treatment of schizophrenia (Ereshefsky et al. 1989). Because of an association with neutropenia (in up to 3% of the patients) and agranulocytosis, clozapine's use is confined to patients with schizophrenia unresponsive to other treatments, and stringent hematological monitoring is required.

A large, double-blind, multicenter trial compared the effectiveness of clozapine and chlorpromazine in 268 patients with schizophrenia who had failed to respond to at least three courses of treatment with at least two antipsychotic drugs, and who also failed to respond to a single-blind trial of treatment with haloperidol. Using relevant clinical response criteria, researchers found that 30% of the patients treated with clozapine improved substantially over a 6-week period compared with 4% of the patients receiving chlorpromazine (Kane et al. 1988; Marder and Van Putten 1988). Other studies have confirmed clozapine's effectiveness in up to 60% of the people with schizophrenia who were unresponsive to other medication (Ereshefsky et al. 1989). The need for weekly hematological monitoring (and hence venepuncture) and clozapine's effect on the convulsive threshold—about 4% of the patients receiving 300–600 mg/day develop seizures, and the incidence rises with increasing dose (Haller and Binder 1990)—place some limit on its use for people with mental retardation and treatment-resistant schizophrenia. However, the enormous improvement in the quality of life that can follow remission of psychotic symptoms justifies clozapine's place in the therapeutic armamentarium, in spite of its high cost.

Risperidone is a relatively new antipsychotic drug that has combined $5\text{-}HT_2$ and D_2 antagonist properties, and that may reduce negative, as well as positive, symptoms and has less prominent extrapyramidal adverse effects than standard antipsychotics (Lieberman 1993). Kane and Freeman (1994) reviewed the newer antipsychotic drugs and the issue of treatment resistance.

■ LITHIUM

Delva and Letemendia (1982) reviewed over 20 studies that had investigated the use of lithium in the treatment of schizophrenia and about 30 studies that had considered its role in the treatment of schizoaffective, cycloid, and other "atypical" psychoses. They concluded that about half of the patients with schizophrenia in these studies benefited from lithium. Results in the treatment of schizoaffective and other atypical psychoses were even more encouraging: 73% benefited, and 14% made a full recovery. Delva and Letemendia concluded that the benefit of lithium was not confined to a reduction in affective symptoms alone. They also noted that all studies comparing lithium with placebo in the treatment of both schizophrenia and schizoaffective psychosis found lithium to be superior.

Johnstone et al. (1988), however, compared the efficacy of lithium, pimozide, both drugs together, and placebo in a trial involving 120 patients with functional psychosis. Patients were assessed for psychotic symptoms, manic symptoms, and depressive symptoms. Pimozide reduced psychotic symptoms, whereas the only significant effect of lithium was to reduce elevated mood.

There is evidently a need for further studies in this area, but in view of the impact of schizophrenic symptoms on emotional life and everyday functioning, the use of lithium appears to be fully justified as part of the management of schizophrenic symptoms that have proved unresponsive to conventional antipsychotic treatment, or when there is a marked affective component to the illness. The decision to prescribe lithium will be influenced by additional factors, such as the need for supervision of medication and the patient or caregiver's understanding of information about toxicity and drug interactions (Clarke and Pickles 1994).

■ SOCIAL AND PSYCHOLOGICAL APPROACHES

The treatment of schizophrenia involves much more than the prescription of antipsychotic medication, even when the specific treatments referred to below are not employed. Support from the psychiatrist or another professional who knows the patient and his or her problems is often valued very highly and may provide the opportunity to identify early signs of relapse. The family or caregivers will benefit from education about the illness and its treatment. Some studies show that families and caregivers can themselves be helped to identify early signs or symptoms suggesting imminent relapse, that relatives groups and family education are cost-effective interventions, and that such interventions reduce relatives' perceptions of the family burden (e.g., Leff et al. 1989; Smith and Birchwood 1987). The psychiatrist may offer support through outpatient or domiciliary contact. This support will allow the detection and treatment of schizophrenic symptoms, symptoms such as anxiety or depression that may precede relapse (Johnson 1988), and facilitate the review of medication. Norman and Malla (1993) have reviewed research concerning the relationship between stressful life events and schizophrenia, concluding that the severity of the symptoms is influenced by life events. Life events can rarely be avoided, but their impact on someone with mental retardation and a history of schizophrenia may be lessened by appropriate interventions and the sensitive handling of events such as bereavement.

The concept of expressed emotion was developed as a way to describe and measure how relatives interact with patients with schizophrenia. Critical comments, hostility, and emotional overinvolvement are assessed, and a composite score of expressed emotion is derived. An estimate of time in face-to-face contact with the relative is also made (Kuipers 1979). Studies of expressed emotion (EE) have indicated that high EE is associated with a greater risk of relapse, that relapse rates are lower for patients with high EE who spend less time in face-to-face contact with their relative, and that antipsychotic drugs exert a protective effect on patients returning to live with a high-EE relative. Studies examining the impact of interventions to reduce EE within families demonstrate that such measures can be effective (e.g., Tarrier et al. 1988). This study included a comparison between two forms of intervention to reduce EE: an *inactive* strategy (such as active teaching of relaxation techniques, with instruction in monitoring and recording) and a *symbolic* strategy (such as verbal instruction about how to relax when under stress). Both interventions were superior to routine treatment or the use of an educational package about schizophrenia. Although the impact of the two interventions (as measured by reduction in relapse) was similar, the authors concluded that there was some evidence that the inactive strategy was more effective for relatives with very high ratings of emotional overinvolvement. Expressed emotion may be a factor in relapse in living situations other than with families (e.g., in hostels and homes for people with mental retardation), and management strategies similar to those outlined above may be of benefit.

■ NONPHARMACOLOGICAL TREATMENT OF AUDITORY HALLUCINATIONS

Auditory hallucinations occurring in association with schizophrenia are often distressing and may persist in spite of treatment with antipsychotic drugs.

They may occur in isolation, without other symptoms of mental illness. The neuropsychology of auditory hallucinations has been reviewed by Slade and Bentall (1988). Several strategies have been developed to reduce or mask the impact of auditory hallucinations. Most techniques involve anxiety reduction and a shift in attention. Strategies for which there is evidence of effectiveness in some circumstances include the use of ear plugs (Birchwood 1986; Done et al. 1986), auditory stimuli such as music played from a personal cassette player via bilateral headphones (Collins et al. 1989; McInnis and Marks 1990), and vocalization tasks such as subvocal counting or singing (Margo et al. 1981). Nelson et al. (1991) compared these methods in the management of 20 people (without mental retardation) who had chronic schizophrenia with auditory hallucinations, all of whom were receiving maintenance antipsychotic drugs. The use of a portable cassette player was the most popular and effective method, but the authors pointed out that the wearing of headphones may not always be socially acceptable. Subvocal counting was the least popular method (singing may prove more acceptable).

The use of such techniques is not widespread in the treatment of schizophrenia associated with mental retardation. They could be valuable components of a management plan for some people, in view of their noninvasive nature and lack of major adverse effects. Other nonpharmacological techniques that have been proposed include operant procedures (Nydegger 1972), desensitization (Slade 1973), thought stopping (Lamontagne et al. 1983), aversive techniques (Bucher and Fabricatore 1970), and a technique centered on accepting responsibility, termed *first person singular therapy* (Greene 1978).

■ BEHAVIORAL AND COGNITIVE TREATMENTS FOR DELUSIONS

Ayllon and Haughton (1964) reported an increase in the frequency of verbal expressions of delusions in response to attention, approval, and reinforcement. When social and other reinforcers were made contingent on the nonexpression of delusions, such expression decreased in frequency. Various cognitive-behavioral methods have been suggested to modify behavior such as the expression of delusions, for example, the "belief modification" procedure described by Watts et al. (1973). Johnson et al. (1977) used a cognitive approach based on "retribution." Such approaches may be of value to some people with mental retardation and schizophrenia, but the effectiveness of strategies based on modifying attitudes or the "ownership" of experiences may need modification (in view of their reliance on the communication of abstract concepts).

■ ENVIRONMENTAL MANIPULATION AND OTHER COMPONENTS OF REHABILITATION

Wing and Brown (1970) described the handicaps that should be considered when planning a strategy of rehabilitation for someone with (or who has had) a schizophrenic illness. Premorbid handicaps include factors such as poverty or lack of education, which precede the onset of schizophrenia but which may impede rehabilitation. Primary handicaps are those that arise as a direct consequence of the illness and may be positive (such as delusions and hallucinations) or negative (such as social withdrawal and lack of motivation). Secondary handicaps occur as a result of illness but are not a direct consequence of schizophrenia (e.g., changes in behavior resulting from institutional demands, constraints, and incursions into privacy or other basic rights). It is important to be aware of premorbid and secondary handicaps as well as of the more obvious primary handicaps because they may be more amenable to intervention than the schizophrenic symptomatology itself. Relatives, caregivers, and sometimes staff may need to be educated about the affect of schizophrenia and its effect on everyday life—lack of motivation may be dismissed as "laziness" or the person may be regarded as "sick" and protected from necessary stimulation, exacerbating negative symptoms and secondary handicaps. In addition to the evidence concerning expressed emotion, there is also research to support the provision of an adequately stimulating environment, which is not so challenging or stressful as to precipitate relapse or worsen symptoms but which does not exacerbate the negative symptoms of schizophrenia through monotony and understimulation (Barton 1976; Wing and Brown 1961, 1970).

Linn et al. (1979) examined the role of day hospitals and their effectiveness in preventing relapse. Centers with an emphasis on occupational therapy and the provision of a predictable, nonthreatening environment were more effective than those with an emphasis on short-term intensive treatments such as group psychotherapy. The term *milieu therapy* is sometimes used to describe a mix of interventions, including occupational therapy, recreational activity, industrial or vocational rehabilitation, or therapy and group work. There are some grounds for believing that such an approach (if carefully tailored) has some benefit, but there have been few controlled studies of effectiveness.

■ PSYCHODYNAMIC TREATMENT

Psychoanalytic psychotherapy was felt by Freud to be unsuitable for people suffering from schizophrenia, a view shared by many psychiatrists (especially in the United Kingdom); Kendell (1988) noted that "psychotherapeutic relationships and other emotional pressures may be positively harmful to those who have recently had a schizophrenic illness and so should only be offered if it is quite clear that they are capable of responding. Emotional withdrawal is not merely a symptom; it is also a valuable protective device." Others advocated the use of psychodynamic treatment (e.g., Fromm-Reichmann 1948). Following the introduction of antipsychotic drugs, combination treatments have been used for patients with schizophrenia who possess the requisite verbal skills (e.g., Normand and Bluestone 1986). Although psychotherapy is a useful treatment resource for some emotional problems occurring in people with mental retardation, three considerations argue against its use for those with schizophrenic or similar disorders. Firstly, psychodynamically based psychotherapy is usually more effective when used to treat people who are verbally fluent (although this does not exclude people with mental retardation per se, those with additional cognitive disruption due to concurrent psychotic illness would be at a particular disadvantage). Secondly, psychodynamically oriented psychotherapy is of no proven value in the treatment of schizophrenia when used with people of normal intelligence (Mueser and Berenbaum 1990). Thirdly, there is some evidence that psychodynamic treatments may be associated with adverse effects when used in the management of schizophrenia; one study reported a high suicide rate among those so treated (Stone 1986) and another found that patients who received psychodynamic therapy spent longer in hospital than those receiving a different ("reality adaptive") therapy (Gunderson et al. 1984).

After reviewing the literature on the subject, Mueser and Berenbaum (1990) proposed a moratorium on the use of psychodynamic treatments for schizophrenia.

■ EVALUATION OF TREATMENTS

Although there are few specific rating or diagnostic instruments for schizophrenic symptomatology associated with mental retardation, it is helpful to quantify symptoms or behavior whenever possible to provide as objective an assessment of the effect of interventions as possible. One technique is to devise a rating schedule tailored to the individual patient's behavior or symptoms, with a set of possible responses to be ringed on a 10-cm line with a statement at each end (e.g., "repeatedly shouting back at 'voices'" at one end and "calm with no evidence of hallucinations" at the other). It is best if specific instructions are given regarding who rates the behavior, how frequently, at what time(s), etc. More than one rater may sometimes be advantageous, allowing ratings to be compared. Some behaviors can be rated by simply counting the frequency with which they occur. Other behaviors may require separate ratings of frequency, severity, and duration. Such rough-and-ready instruments can be criticized on many grounds, but it is often better to have some form of quantitative assessment of symptoms (or resulting behavior), however crude, rather than none. Direct observation techniques are usually of limited value and difficult to carry out reliably without considerable resources; they are usually more suited to research designs than clinical practice. Occasionally they may be of value and may be combined with interview or other indirect rating techniques.

■ HOME TREATMENT

There are advantages in treating someone with mental retardation and schizophrenia in the community rather than admitting him or her to the hospital. There is no risk of institutionalization (Barton 1976). Behavioral change due to an alteration in environment (e.g., as a result of anxiety) is avoided, aiding assessment. The family or caregivers are helped to cope with or modify behavior, rather than hand over care completely to professionals (Birchwood and Cochrane 1990). This helps to minimize caregivers' feelings of guilt. There are also disadvantages, which include a lack of acceptability to some patients or caregivers (who may feel their privacy is eroded by the presence of professionals). Home treatment works best when the patient and caregivers have confidence in the service and when it is adequately staffed and resourced. Domiciliary treatment is unwise in some circumstances and for some patients. These include patients who are extremely violent; patients who have potentially dangerous delusions concerning family members or other caregivers; when there are pathological family relationships or abuse is suspected; when there is concurrent severe physical illness requiring specialist management; and when the patient refuses to take medication or to comply with other interventions and is a danger to him- or herself or others (when detention using mental health legislation may be necessary).

Studies have found fewer symptoms and better social functioning (Stein and Test 1980) and more patient satisfaction (Reynolds and Hoult 1984) when home treatment rather than hospital admission is used. It is an appropriate response to many people with schizophrenic illnesses (Dean and Gadd 1990) and has been associated in some studies with a reduction in the family "burden" (Pai and Kapur 1982). Knapp et al. (1994) found a program of problem-oriented, home-based care for adults with severe mental illness to be cost-effective, with "mildly encouraging" outcome results over a 20-month period, but Audini et al. (1994) reported low morale and conflict between team members during the second phase of this randomized controlled trial of home-based care, although patients and relatives were more satisfied with home-based treatment. Marks et al. (1994) commenting on the same trial concluded that "home based care is hard to organize and vulnerable to many factors, and needs careful training and clinical audit if gains are to be sustained." Muijen et al. (1994) compared two patterns of working by community psychiatric nurses and found no benefit from "intensive support" for people with severe and persistent mental health problems compared with generic care, despite a higher number of contacts by the intensive support team and the use of a wider range of interventions.

Decisions about where treatment should be provided and the most effective pattern of support will depend on a careful weighing of the various factors pertinent to the particular case, with particular emphasis given to the wishes of the person in need of treatment and his or her caregiver(s), and the need to minimize potential for harm resulting from psychotic symptoms.

■ SERVICE COMPONENTS

The most appropriate components of a service for people with mental illnesses and mental retardation will vary according to local practice and resourcing but may include some or all of the following:

- A home treatment or intensive support service
- A hospital admission facility
- Access to respite care and day care with staff who have some knowledge of mental illness
- Outpatient facilities
- Liaison with the community team for people with mental retardation and other statutory and voluntary agencies

The multidisciplinary team working with such patients will need expertise in areas such as nursing, social work, psychiatry, psychology, occupational therapy, and speech therapy. There will also be a need for access to high-quality primary and secondary physical health care facilities.

Some people with mental retardation and schizophrenia will continue to have behavior that is dangerous to themselves or others, and special residential care may need to be arranged if their needs cannot be met in any other way (e.g., by intensive support in "ordinary" residential facilities). Staff perceptions and responses to behavior may need to be altered. Training in appropriate responses to aggressive or other unacceptable behavior may reduce the frequency of expression of such behavior and lessen its impact.

The proportion of resources allocated to each component of the service will depend on the availability and quality of other components. An effective day, respite, and home treatment service will probably reduce the number of people needing hospital admission, and effective staff training may reduce the frequency of exclusion of people with schizophrenia from generic mental retardation services such as day centers.

■ REFERENCES

Aman MG: Overview of pharmacotherapy: current status and future directions. Journal of Mental Deficiency Research 31:121–130, 1987

Arana GW, Goff DC, Baldessarini RJ, et al: Efficacy of anticholinergic prophylaxis for neuroleptic-induced acute dystonia. Am J Psychiatry 145:993–996, 1988

Audini B, Marks IM, Lawrence RE, et al: Home-based versus out-patient/in-patient care for people with serious mental illness: phase II of a controlled study. Br J Psychiatry 165:204–210, 1994

Ayllon T, Haughton E: Modification of symptomatic behavior of mental patients. Behav Res Ther 2:87–89, 1964

Barton R: Institutional Neurosis. Bristol, UK, Wright, 1976

Birchwood M: Control of auditory hallucinations through occlusion of monaural auditory input. Br J Psychiatry 149:104–107, 1986

Birchwood M, Cochrane R: Families living with schizophrenia: coping styles, their origins and correlates. Psychol Med 20:857–865, 1990

Briggs R: Monitoring and evaluating psychotropic drug use for persons with mental retardation: a follow-up report. Am J Ment Retard 93:633–639, 1989

Brockington I: Schizophrenia: yesterday's concept. European Psychiatry 7:203–207, 1992

Bucher B, Fabricatore J: Use of patient-administered shock to suppress hallucinations. Behav Ther 1:382–385, 1970

Clarke DJ, Pickles KJ: Lithium treatment for people with learning disability: patients' and carers' knowledge of hazards and attitudes to treatment. J Intellect Disabil Res 38:187–194, 1994

Cole J, Klerman CL, Goldberg SC: Phenothiazine treatment of acute schizophrenia. Arch Gen Psychiatry 10:246–261, 1964

Collins MN, Cull CA, Sireling L: Pilot study of treatment of persistent auditory hallucinations by modified auditory input. BMJ 229:431–432, 1989

Davis JM: Recent developments in the drug treatment of schizophrenia. Am J Psychiatry 133:208–214, 1976

Dean C, Gadd EM: Home treatment for acute psychiatric illness. BMJ 301:1021–1023, 1990

Delva NJ, Letemendia FJJ: Lithium treatment in schizophrenia and schizoaffective disorders. Br J Psychiatry 141:387–400, 1982

Done DJ, Frith CD, Owens DC: Reducing persistent auditory hallucinations by wearing an ear plug. Br J Clin Psychol 25:151–152, 1986

Edwards S, Kumar V: A survey of prescribing psychotropic drugs in a Birmingham general hospital. Br J Psychiatry 145:502–507, 1984

Ereshefsky L, Watanabe MD, Tran-Johnson TK: Clozapine: an atypical antipsychotic agent. Clinical Pharmacology 8:691–709, 1989

Falloon I, Watt DC, Shepherd M: A comparative controlled trial of pimozide and fluphenazine decanoate in schizophrenia. Psychol Med 8:59–70, 1978

Fromm-Reichmann F: Notes on the development of treatment of schizophrenics by psychoanalytic psychotherapy. Psychiatry 2:263–273, 1948

Goldberg SC, Schooler NR, Hogarty GE, et al: Prediction of relapse in schizophrenic outpatients treated by drug and sociotherapy. Arch Gen Psychiatry 34:171–184, 1977

Greene R: Auditory hallucination reduction: first-person singular therapy. Journal of Contemporary Psychotherapy 9:167–170, 1978

Gualtieri CT, Hawk B: Tardive dyskinesia and other drug-induced movement disorders among handicapped children and youth. Applied Research in Mental Retardation 1:55–69, 1980

Gualtieri CT, Schroeder SR, Hicks RE, et al: Tardive dyskinesia in young mentally retarded individuals. Arch Gen Psychiatry 43:335–340, 1986

Gunderson JG, Frank A, Katz HM, et al: Effects of psychotherapy in schizophrenia; II: comparative outcome of two forms of treatment. Schizophr Bull 10:564–598, 1984

Haller E, Binder RL: Clozapine and seizures. Am J Psychiatry 147:1069–1071, 1990

Inoue F: A clinical pharmacy service to reduce psychotropic medication use in an institution for mentally retarded persons. Ment Retard 20:70–74, 1982

Johnson DAW: Further observations on the duration of depot neuroleptic maintenance therapy in schizophrenia. Br J Psychiatry 135:524–530, 1979

Johnson DAW: Drug treatment of schizophrenia, in Contemporary Issues in Schizophrenia. Edited by Kerr A, Snaith P. London, Gaskell, 1986, pp 374–380

Johnson DAW: The significance of depression in the prediction of relapse in chronic schizophrenia. Br J Psychiatry 152:320–323, 1988

Johnson DAW, Pasterski G, Ludlow JM, et al: The discontinuation of maintenance neuroleptic therapy in chronic schizophrenic patients: drug and social consequences. Acta Psychiatr Scand 67:339–352, 1983

Johnson WG, Ross JM, Mastria MA: Delusional behavior: an attributional analysis of development and modification. J Abnorm Psychol 86:421–426, 1977

Johnstone EC, Crow TJ, Ferrier IN, et al: Adverse effects of anticholinergic medication on positive schizophrenic symptoms. Psychol Med 13:513–527, 1983

Johnstone EC, Frith CD, Crow TJ, et al: The Northwick Park "functional" psychosis study: diagnosis and treatment response. Lancet 2:119–125, 1988

Kane JM, Freeman HL: Towards more effective antipsychotic treatment. Br J Psychiatry 165(suppl 25):22–31, 1994

Kane J, Honigfeld G, Singer J, et al: Clozapine for the treatment-resistant schizophrenic: a double-blind comparison with chlorpromazine. Arch Gen Psychiatry 45:789–796, 1988

Kendell RE: Schizophrenia, in Companion to Psychiatric Studies, 4th Edition. Edited by Kendall RE, Zeally AK. Edinburgh, UK, Churchill Livingstone, 1988, pp 310–334

Knapp M, Beecham J, Koutsogeorgopoulou V, et al: Service use and costs of home-based versus hospital-based care for people with serious mental illness. Br J Psychiatry 165:195–203, 1994

Kuipers L: Expressed emotion: a review. British Journal of Social and Clinical Psychology 18:237–243, 1979

Lamontagne Y, Audet N, Elie R: Thought stopping for delusions and hallucinations: a pilot study. Behav Psychother 11:177–184, 1983

Leff JP, Wing JK: Trial of maintenance therapy in schizophrenia. BMJ 3:599–604, 1971

Leff J, Berkowitz R, Shavit N, et al: A trial of family therapy v. a relative's group for schizophrenia. Br J Psychiatry 154:58–66, 1989

Lieberman JA: Understanding the mechanism of action of atypical antipsychotic drugs: a review of compounds in use and development. Br J Psychiatry 163(suppl 22):7–18, 1993

Linn MW, Caffey EM, Klett J, et al: Day treatment and psychotropic drugs in the aftercare of schizophrenic patients. Arch Gen Psychiatry 36:1055–1066, 1979

Marder SR, Van Putten T: Who should receive clozapine? Arch Gen Psychiatry 45:865–867, 1988

Margo A, Hemsey DR, Slade PD: The effects of varying auditory input on schizophrenic hallucinations. Br J Psychiatry 139:122–127, 1981

Marks IM, Connolly J, Muijen M, et al: Home-based versus hospital-based care for people with serious mental illness. Br J Psychiatry 165:179–194, 1994

McInnis M, Marks I: Audiotape therapy for persistent auditory hallucinations. Br J Psychiatry 157:913–914, 1990

Mueser KT, Berenbaum H: Psychodynamic treatment of schizophrenia: is there a future? Psychol Med 20:253–262, 1990

Muijen M, Cooney M, Strathdee G, et al: Community psychiatric nurse teams: intensive support versus generic care. Br J Psychiatry 165:211–217, 1994

Nelson HE, Thrasher S, Barnes TRE: Practical ways of alleviating auditory hallucinations. BMJ 302:327, 1991

Norman RMG, Malla AK: Stressful life events and schizophrenia; I: a review of the research. Br J Psychiatry 162:161–166, 1993

Normand WC, Bluestone H: The use of pharmacotherapy in psychoanalytic treatment. Contemporary Psychoanalysis 22:218–234, 1986

Nydegger RV: The elimination of hallucinatory and delusional behavior by verbal conditioning and assertive training: a case study. J Behav Ther Exp Psychiatry 3:225–227, 1972

Pai S, Kapur RL: Impact of treatment intervention on the relationship between dimensions of clinical psychopathology, social dysfunction and burden on the family of psychiatric patients. Psychol Med 12:651–658, 1982

Reid AH: Psychoses in adult mental defectives; II: schizophrenic and paranoid psychoses. Br J Psychiatry 120:213–218, 1972

Reynolds I, Hoult JE: The relatives of the mentally ill; a comparative trial of community-orientated and hospital orientated psychiatric care. J Nerv Ment Dis 172:480–489, 1984

Rifkin A, Quitkin F, Rabiner C, et al: Fluphenazine decanoate, fluphenazine hydrochloride and placebo in remitted schizophrenics. Arch Gen Psychiatry 34:43–47, 1977

Slade PD: The psychological investigation and treatment of auditory hallucinations: a second case report. British Journal of Social and Clinical Psychology 13:73–79, 1973

Slade PD, Bentall RP: Sensory Deception: A Scientific Analysis of Hallucinations. London, Croon Helm, 1988

Smith JV, Birchwood MJ: Specific and non-specific effects of educational intervention with families living with a schizophrenic relative. Br J Psychiatry 150:645–652, 1987

Sprague RL: Overview of psychopharmacology for the retarded in the United States, in Research to Practice in Mental Retardation, Vol 3. Edited by Mittler P. Baltimore, MD, University Park Press, 1977, pp 199–202

Stein LI, Test MA: Alternative to mental hospital treatment; I: conceptual model, treatment programme and clinical evaluation. Arch Gen Psychiatry 37:392–397, 1980

Stone MH: Exploratory psychotherapy in schizophrenia-spectrum patients. Bull Menninger Clin 50:287–306, 1986

Tarrier N, Barrowclough C, Vaughn C, et al: The community management of schizophrenia: a controlled trial of a behavioral intervention with families to reduce relapse. Br J Psychiatry 153:532–542, 1988

Thompson C: The use of high-dose antipsychotic medication. Br J Psychiatry 164:448–458, 1994

Watts FN, Powell EG, Austin SV: The modification of abnormal beliefs. Br J Med Psychol 46:359–363, 1973

Wing JK, Brown GW: Social treatment of chronic schizophrenia: a comparative survey of three mental hospitals. Journal of Mental Science 107:847–861, 1961

Wing JK, Brown GW: Institutionalism and Schizophrenia. Cambridge, UK, Cambridge University Press, 1970

World Health Organization: Classification of Mental and Behavioral Disorders: Clinical Descriptions and Diagnostic Guidelines, 10th Edition. Geneva, Switzerland, World Health Organization, 1992

12 Treatment of Mood Disorders in Mentally Retarded Persons

Stephen Ruedrich, M.D.
Anne Des Noyers-Hurley, Ph.D.
Robert Sovner, M.D.

Since the first literature reports of mood disorders in mentally retarded patients, there has been increasing interest in treating these individuals (Carlson 1979; Došen and Menolascino 1990; Reid 1972; Sovner and Hurley 1983). Finding methods to establish a diagnosis of mood disorder has been a major thrust of research and clinical investigation because, in many cases, the diagnosis is difficult to determine. One major reason is *diagnostic overshadowing*, a term Reiss and colleagues coined to describe when clinicians are so taken with an individual's developmental disability that they neglect to see psychopathological symptoms and signs (Reiss et al. 1982). Another major diagnostic problem involves the difficulty of translating the common signs and symptoms of psychiatric illness in persons of normal intelligence into meaningful terms for mentally retarded persons. Sovner and colleagues (Lowry 1997, 1998; Pary et al. 1999b; Sovner and Hurley 1982, 1983; Sovner and Lowry 1990) have described a diagnostic schema useful for organizing diagnostic criteria into diagnostic equivalents (see Tables 12–1 and 12–2), based on DSM criteria (American Psychiatric Association 1994).

Clearly, in order to treat mood disorders, clinicians must first recognize them in the patient (Menolascino et al. 1991). Toward this end, clinicians and researchers have provided a growing body of knowledge on the treatment of mood disorders in mentally retarded persons, using both traditional and newer therapies for both unipolar and bipolar illness. In this chapter, we review these treatment types and strategies. For purposes of clarity, the terms *mood disorder* and *affective disorder* will be used interchangeably in the text, based on the current utilization of both in the literature.

Table 12–1. DSM-IV diagnostic criteria for mania and behavioral equivalents in mentally retarded persons

DSM-IV criteria	Observed equivalents in mentally retarded persons	Objective behaviors that might be monitored
Mood state:		
Euphoric/elevated/irritable mood (no minimum duration necessary).	Boisterousness or excitement may be the predominant mood state. Self-injury may be associated with irritability.	Measure rates of smiling and/or laughing.
Symptom criteria:		
At least three symptoms must be present if patient has euphoric mood. Four symptoms must be present if patient has only irritable mood.		
1. Inflated self-esteem/grandiosity	Thoughts content may be centered around mastery of daily living skills.	Measure inappropriate remarks.
2. Decreased need for sleep	Increased maladaptive behavior at usual bedtime or in early morning. Patient is dressed for work at 5:00 A.M.	Monitor sleep pattern using 30-minute intervals.
3. More talkative/pressured speech	Increased frequency of vocalization irrespective of whether patient has usable speech.	Measure rates of swearing, singing, screaming.
4. Flight of ideas/racing thoughts	Disorganized speech.	
5. Distractibility	Decrease in workshop performance.	Use workshop performance data.

Table 12–1. DSM-IV diagnostic criteria for mania and behavioral equivalents in mentally retarded persons *(continued)*

DSM-IV criteria	Observed equivalents in mentally retarded persons	Objective behaviors that might be monitored
6. Increased goal-directed activity/psychomotor agitation	Aggressive behavior and negativism may be present.	Measure aggressions, request refusals per week, pacing, etc.
7. Excessive involvement in pleasurable activities	Teasing behavior, fondling others, publicly masturbating.	Measure intervals in which the behavior occurs.

Table 12–2. DSM-IV diagnostic criteria for major depression and behavioral equivalents in mentally retarded persons

DSM-IV criteria	Observed equivalents in mentally retarded persons	Objective behaviors that might be monitored
Five or more of the following symptoms must be present for a minimum of 2 weeks. Symptom (1) or (2) must be one of the five.		
Mood state:		
1. Depressed mood, irritable mood in children or adolescents	Apathetic facial expression with lack of emotional reactivity.	Measure rates of smiling responses to preferred activities, crying episodes.
Symptom criteria:		
2. Generalized decrease in interest or pleasure by self-report or observed	Withdrawal, lack of reinforcers.	Measure time spent in room, etc.
3. Significant decrease in appetite or weight loss (5% body weight in 1 month) or significant increase in appetite or weight gain (5% of body weight in 1 month)		Measure meal refusals, change in weight.
4. Insomnia or hypersomnia	Change in total sleep time.	Use sleep chart to record sleep and time spent in bed.
5. Psychomotor activity or retardation	Agitation may present as self-injurious behavior or aggression.	Measure spontaneous verbalizations, pacing.

Table 12–2. DSM-IV diagnostic criteria for major depression and behavioral equivalents in mentally retarded persons (*continued*)

DSM-IV criteria	Observed equivalents in mentally retarded persons	Objective behaviors that might be monitored
6. Fatigue or loss of energy	Retardation may present as decreased energy, passivity.	
7. Feelings of worthlessness/ inappropriate guilt	Statements such as, "I'm retarded."	Requires expressive language to determine if symptom is present.
8. Decreased concentration/ indecisiveness/diminished ability to think	Change in workshop performance.	Use workshop performance data.
9. Recurrent thoughts of death/suicidal ideation	Perseveration on the deaths of family members and friends, preoccupation with funerals.	Requires expressive language to determine if symptom is present.

■ PSYCHOTHERAPIES FOR DEPRESSION

A number of nonsomatic (psychotherapeutic) treatments have become widely used for patients of normal intelligence suffering from mood disorders. In fact, several treatment outcome studies have shown that cognitive-behavioral therapies often fare as well as pharmacotherapy for subtypes of depression (Dobson 1989; Kovacs 1980; Kovacs et al. 1981; Murphy et al. 1984).

Treating patients with mental retardation does, however, present some challenges. In contrast to most drug therapies, all psychotherapeutic treatments must be modified to account for the patient's developmental level (Hurley 1989b). The clinician generally must speak and act concretely, use aids such as role-play and reinforcement, and involve family and treatment teams much more than would be the case in treating patients of normal intelligence. Many psychotherapeutic adaptations useful with children may be also useful with patients with mental retardation. Like children, mentally retarded adults do not ordinarily seek treatment on their own and instead are brought by staff or family members who have noticed behavioral changes, such as noncompliance or irritability. Behavioral or psychotherapeutic treatment of these persons requires adaptation to the cognitive level of the individual, in a manner similar to that used for children (DiGiuseppe 1989; Kendall 1985; Kendall and Braswell 1982).

Behavioral Treatment of Depression

Initial behavioral models of depression stressed the existence of a cluster of observable behaviors associated with the disorder (e.g., poor eye contact, self-deprecating statements). Behavioral therapists posited that punishing or ignoring behaviors characteristic of depression would decrease their frequency, and reinforcing behaviors incompatible with depression would increase such behavior. Token economy programs were devised to reinforce depressed inpatients when they exhibited behaviors incompatible with depression, such as participating in a work program (Hanaway and Barlow 1975; Hersen et al. 1973). In depressed patients of normal intelligence, reports have attested to the effectiveness of such procedures (Boyd and Levis 1980; Reisinger 1972).

Applying this approach to patients with mental retardation, Matson (1982) treated four mildly retarded adults with depression who had not responded to antidepressant medication. In this systematic but uncontrolled study, observable target behaviors were quantified: few spoken words, irritability, flat affect, poor eye contact, long speech latency, somatic complaints, negative self-statements, and poor grooming. Individual therapy sessions were undertaken in which patients would be given tokens exchangeable for rewards for nondepressed responses and for good eye contact and grooming. Following a depressed response, the patient was told the correct response and rehearsed it three times. The treatment was successful, generalized to the natural environment, and was maintained at 60-month follow-up.

In another area, work with mentally retarded patients has investigated the relationship between deficits in social skills and depression. Reiss and Benson (1985) compared 28 mildly mentally retarded adults who were depressed with 17 peers without mood abnormalities, regarding how often subjects saw or talked with friends or family, talked about feelings, and socialized. Depressed patients demonstrated significantly lower levels of social support than did control subjects. In a related study, Benson et al. (1986) showed that depressed mentally retarded adults also had poor interpersonal skills. Subsequent investigation by the same group (Laman and Reiss 1987) confirmed these earlier findings. The social interactions of depressed mentally retarded individuals were found to be inappropriate and ineffective, with social withdrawal and poor ability to initiate conversation or give positive responses to others' good fortune.

As a result of these findings, research and clinical work have focused on improving the social skills of developmentally handicapped persons, noting that such skills are often deficient due to cognitive limitations and restricted life experiences. Treatment packages to improve the social skills of clients with developmental disabilities are available (Bregman 1984; Foxx and McMorrow 1980; Foxx et al. 1983; McClennen et al. 1980; Nezu et al. 1991). These approaches typically rely on staff and clinicians to assess the patient's social strengths and weaknesses and involve role-playing, homework, and feedback in work groups as therapeutic measures. More recent work has expanded typical training approaches in order to help retarded individuals to alter their use of social skills depending on the context of the situation (Griffiths 1990a; Quinsey and Varney 1977). Unfortunately, to date there is little systematic research linking social skills treatment of mood disorders in mentally retarded adults with improvement in symptomatology.

Cognitive Therapy for Depression

Cognitive theories of depression hold that attention to life events, social cues, and the interpretation of these events are influenced by thought patterns (Ellis and Harper 1973). There are many cognitive therapies; among the most popular is that developed by Beck and colleagues (1979). This approach addresses an individual's negative thoughts and attitudes, and the way in which the patient processes information. Treatment focuses on negative thought patterns; for example, depressed patients may pay more attention to negative comments by others and minimize the importance of positive events in their lives. Mood disorders, particularly depression, may be the result of, or exacerbated by, a pervasively distorted cognitive pattern. Systematic treatment research in this area has been done primarily with patients of normal intelligence. In these depressed patients, cognitive therapy has been shown to be as effective as antidepressant medication, with possible better long-term outcome for some patients (Murphy et al. 1984). Such cognitive/behavioral techniques rely on basic intellectual and academic skills and may require extensive modification for use in mentally retarded patients. In the past, clinicians have been reluctant to use these treatments for patients with developmental disabilities, due in part to the misguided belief that patients with less than normal intelligence cannot benefit from such modalities (Hollon 1984). There is, however, evidence that patients with mental retardation can profit from treatment with cognitive therapy (Dagnan and Chadwick 1997; Kroese et al. 1997) in the areas of anger management (Benson et al. 1986), self-control (Gardner et al. 1983), and the acquisition of social skills (Foxx et al. 1983; Griffiths 1990a, 1990b) (see also Chapters 4, 5, and 17 of this book).

There are also now several reports of cognitive treatments of depressed adults with mild mental retardation. Hurley (1989a) reported the successful cognitive treatment of a depressed man with Down's syndrome who was able to use written materials and to self-monitor and record data. Matson et al. (1979) treated a 32-year-old man with a 10-year history of depression who was also concurrently treated with pharmacotherapy. During highly structured individual treatment sessions, statements indicative of depression were targeted for reduction. When the patient made positive self-statements, he was praised and was instructed to self-reinforce. When statements reflecting depressive content were made, the therapist asked him to evaluate the statements, and the therapist modeled better statements. Homework assignments were given and carried out. The authors reported a reduction in the frequency of depressive statements and an increase in positive statements, both within and outside the therapy sessions, and an increase of social activities.

Lindsay et al. (1993) reported on their treatment of two adults with mild mental retardation (male age 28, female age 20) with modified cognitive therapy. Neither patient received pharmacotherapy. Both subjects demonstrated improvement in depression ratings on the Zung Self-Rating Depression Scale immediately after treatment and at the 4-month follow-up.

Other aspects of cognitive therapy approach can be augmented through work with staff and family as supporters. Benson (1996) reported use of a daily mood check form to assist in the treatment. Although the patient him- or herself can be taught to use the form, it will be used most frequently with the help of support staff and a psychotherapist. Increases in scheduled pleasurable activities can be organized by caregivers, and feedback regarding mastery and arrangement of mastery can be scheduled as well. These augmentations can be directed by the psychotherapist and monitored at individual psychotherapy sessions.

These authors emphasized that although some modification of cognitive therapy techniques was necessary, the basic elements of the treatment remained the same. However, the lack of systematic controlled studies limits the evaluation of cognitive treatments in retarded patients. In the cases reported above, success was achieved, but none reported long-term follow-up. Also, the individuals treated above demonstrated cognitive ability in the mild range of developmental disability. It remains to be seen whether such strategies produce lasting symptom reduction/remission and whether they are of benefit in more severely mentally retarded depressed persons.

Other Psychotherapies

Gardner and Willmering (1999) summarized an integrative psychosocial model for the development of unipolar depression. In addition to incorporating previous aspects of cognitive and social models of depression, they emphasized the role of "instigating" stressors or life events in the depressogenic process. These events may include typical losses, such as loss of parents or living milieu or development of serious illness. Within the integrative treatment approach the authors recommend giving of emotional support, validation, and targeted social and behavioral support programs to promote relationships and attachment.

Dosen (1990) described the application of so-called developmental-dynamic relationship therapy (Dosen and Petry 1993), in which attachment to figures within the environment and the building of social relationships is used to address depression (see Chapter 23 of this book).

Finally, individual psychodynamically oriented, client-centered, and supportive therapies, as well as group psychotherapy, have been described as beneficial in the treatment of mentally retarded persons (Benson 1990; Buetz et al. 2000; Fletcher 1993, 1999; Hollins 1990; Hurley et al. 1998; Monfils and Menolascino 1984; Szymanski and Rosefsky 1980). At this time, there are only a few descriptions of the application of these approaches to mentally retarded persons with mood disorders (Bojanin and Ispanovic-Radojkovic 1990; Došen and Menolascino 1990; Došen and Petry 1993). For a more comprehensive description and review of all forms of psychotherapeutic treatment of mentally retarded persons, please see Chapter 2 (Hollins), Chapter 5 (Benson), and all of Part III of this book.

■ PHARMACOTHERAPY OF DEPRESSION

Among the first to discuss treatment strategies in mentally retarded persons with mood disorders was Reid (1972), who in a benchmark article identified 21 patients suffering from manic-depressive psychosis with varying degrees of mental retardation. Of these, 15 were thought to have primarily depressive episodes and were reported to benefit from tricyclic antidepressants (TCAs) and electroconvulsive therapy (ECT). Reid concluded that persons with less severe mental retardation seemed to respond more reliably. Hurley and Sovner (1979) described a 15-year-old female with mild mental retardation, anorexia nervosa, and probable major depressive disorder who responded to a combination of behavioral modification and thioridazine. A 13-year-old autistic female with moderate mental retardation and recurrent depressive episodes was successfully treated with carbamazepine, 300 mg/day, by Komoto and Usui (1984). Szymanski and Biederman (1984) described 3 patients with Down's syndrome and unipolar depression who were treated successfully with TCAs (amitriptyline, imipramine, and doxepin); two required concurrent treatment with low doses of neuroleptic medications. All three relapsed when attempts were made to reduce or discontinue TCAs but responded to reinitiation of the same medications. Field and colleagues (1986) noted the lack of empirical data regarding the treatment of depression in retarded persons and presented a single subject study of a 22-year-old moderately mentally retarded woman who responded to imipramine, 100 mg/day, as compared with placebo, with improvement in weight loss, sleep disturbance, and screaming.

In a study of 50 institutionalized elderly patients with severe and profound mental retardation, James (1986) described 11 patients with mood disorders. Six were receiving antidepressants for unipolar depression, and only 1 was also receiving a neuroleptic. All 6 had not been treated pharmacologically until they were older than 50, and 4 were not treated until they were in their 70s. The author ascribed the high incidence of mood disorder in this older sample to the persistence of bipolar disorders, which had begun in mid-life, as well as the new onset of episodes of depression in older persons.

Došen (1988), in a large study of 700 mentally retarded children, noted that 11 (1.6%) had major mood disorder characterized by depression, including both unipolar and bipolar types. Of these, 9 were treated pharmacologically, with either TCA (2), lithium carbonate (3), carbamazepine (3), or tryptophan and nicotinamide (3), and seven trials were considered successful. Thirty-one other children at the clinic were thought to have neurotic or reactive depressions, akin to DSM-III dysthymic disorder. Their treatment was primarily psychotherapeutic, with "occasional treatment supported by antidepressant drugs." Results were described as good, but no particular number or response rates were reported.

Sovner (1988) presented a 25-year-old mildly mentally retarded woman who was treated with carbamazepine for major depressive disorder. Initial treatment with nortriptyline had resulted in a major motor seizure. Subsequent carbamazepine at therapeutic levels resulted in the normalization of mood and sleep, and a decrease in self-injurious behavior. Warren et al. (1989) described five patients with trisomy 21 syndrome referred for dementia who were found to have major depression on closer examination. Three of the five were successfully treated with ECT, two of these after adequate but unsuccessful antidepressant drug trials (nortriptyline, amitriptyline). The other two patients made complete recoveries with TCA; both received amitriptyline at doses of 50 mg/day.

In an interesting review, Langee and Conlon (1992) described their experience with antidepressant treatment of severely and profoundly mentally retarded persons in an institutional setting. The authors found that 40 of 54 patients with "depressive symptoms" (sad affect, periods of withdrawal, crying, coupled with sleep and appetite change) responded on two separate occasions to trials of antidepressant therapy. Ruedrich and Wilkinson (1992) added 2 adults (28-year-old female, mild; 35-year-old female, severe) who responded to amoxapine after failed systematic trials of previous TCAs, and TCA-neuroleptic combined treatment. Howland (1992) used fluoxetine in an open trial for 6 depressed mentally retarded adults; 5 showed significant improvement and 1 partial remission. In an attempt to predict and follow treatment response, Soni et al. (1992) described 19 depressed mentally retarded adults (9 females, 10 males; 16 with mild or moderate retardation), all of whom were treated with the TCA dothiepin up to 150 mg/day. Fifteen of the 19 demonstrated significant improvement at 3 months, as measured by decreased Hamilton Rating Scale for Depression scores. Four of the 7 who were originally dexamethasone nonsuppressors (DST+) demonstrated reversal of the DST with successful somatic therapy.

Jancar and Gunaratne (1994) presented two individuals with mental retardation (moderately retarded male, mildly retarded female) who suffered chronic moderate levels of depression consistent with dysthymic disorder. Both patients had brief responses to somatic treatments (antidepressants and ECT) for superimposed major depressive episodes, but the underlying dysthymic symptoms were resistant to these somatic therapies. Finally, Puri and colleagues (1992) described their successful use of combined dothiepin and maintenance ECT for a 32-year-old mildly mentally retarded man with severe recurrent unipolar depression.

With the introduction of the selective serotonin reuptake inhibitors (SSRIs) in the 1990s, reports began appearing describing their use in individuals with mental retardation. Hamdan-Allen (1991), Ghaziuddin and Tsai (1991), and Cook et al. (1992) presented single patients with mental retardation, autism, and depression, all of whom responded to fluoxetine. Sovner et al. (1993) described two individuals with severe/profound mental retardation, depression, and self-injurious behavior who responded to fluoxetine with improvement in both areas. Howland (1992) used fluoxetine in an open trial for 6 depressed adults with mental retardation; 5 showed significant improvement and 1 showed partial remission. Ghaziuddin and colleagues (1991) reported 3 young autistic adults with depression treated with fluoxetine, 2 of whom responded but one became worse.

Meyers (1998) presented case illustrations of 28 adults with moderate to profound mental retardation, 27 of whom responded to fluoxetine treatment, and Clarke and Gomez (1999) reported 11 more inpatients who responded to antidepressants.

Masi et al (1997) described an open-label treatment of 7 adolescents with mild mental retardation with paroxetine 20–40 mg/day. All 7 responded with significant decrease in depressive symptoms.

To date there are no refereed reports of the use of other newer antidepressants (venlafaxine, bupropion, mitrazepine) to treat depression in persons with mental retardation.

The psychiatric literature now includes at least 15 reports describing the electroconvulsive therapy (ECT) treatment of 32 patients with mental retardation and depression (Cutajar and Wilson 1999). As is common with case reports, most describe successful treatment, including both single and multiple courses of ECT, as well as 8 persons who received maintenance ECT (Ruedrich and Alamir 1999). Most authors described ECT use as safe, effective, and, in severe cases, life saving (Thuppal and Fink 1999).

In a symposium describing the phenomenology and diagnosis of depression in mentally retarded persons, Day (1988) recommended that pharmacologic treatment follow a systematic approach, involving only a single treatment method at a time (e.g., ECT versus antidepressant medication, only one antidepressant at one time) and that treatment should involve adequate doses of medication, given up to the therapeutic maximum if allowed within the patient's tolerance of side effects, and an adequate response time allowed for improvement.

Since then, several other reviews have provided guidelines for the treatment of depression in persons with mental retardation (Benefield and Tramonte 1997; Mikkelsen et al. 1997; Silka and Hurley 1997). Sovner et al. (1998), noting that most antidepressants appeared to be equally effective, recommended choosing an antidepressant based on a number of factors: a biological relative with prior good response to a particular drug, the need to determine adequacy of response via blood levels side effect profiles, drug-drug interactions, and a history of previous response to a specific medication. Sung et al. (1997) reminded clinicians of the benefit of treating depression that can occur comorbidly with dementia in aging patiens with Down's syndrome. Finally, depressive episodes that are a part of bipolar illness should be treated with a combination of a mood stabilizer and an antidepressant (Rush and Frances 2000).

■ PHARMACOTHERAPY OF BIPOLAR ILLNESS

The literature addressing the pharmacologic treatment of mentally retarded persons with bipolar disorders is fairly extensive (Mayer 1985). Reid (1972), in his original report of 21 patients with various affective psychoses, referred to their successful treatment with lithium, and Reid and Naylor (1976) further described 4 bipolar patients who received lithium; 2 responded, 1 did not, and 1 developed neurotoxicity. In an oft-quoted study, Naylor et al. (1974) systematically studied 12 patients with clear or probable bipolar disorder in which each patient received 1 year of lithium and 1 year of placebo in a double-blind fashion (some other psychotropics were allowed). Lithium decreased the number of weeks of illness as well as number of affective episodes (the latter not significantly). Reid and Leonard later (1977) described successful treatment of a 29-year-old mildly mentally retarded woman with bipolar illness and cyclic vomiting. Lithium added to neuroleptic treatment provided remission not seen with the neuroleptic alone.

Rivinus and Harmatz (1979) reported on five patients with bipolar disorders who were treated with lithium in a single-blind, placebo-controlled manner over 3 years. All patients received lithium for the first year, which was then replaced by placebo for at least 90 days or until manic symptoms reappeared; lithium was then restarted. All five patients demonstrated a significant lithium response, the return of symptoms on placebo, and reimprovement when lithium was restarted. In the same year, Hasan and Mooney (1979) presented three additional mentally retarded adults with bipolar illness who responded to lithium (all patients also received fluphenazine decanoate). Carlson (1979), in a comprehensive review of the case report literature to that point, summarized nine additional single case reports of bipolar retarded patients; all nine had received lithium, seven had satisfactory responses, one patient had not responded, and another had become neurotoxic. The author concluded that the success of lithium treatment in mentally retarded persons made it appear that the individual's cognitive level had little effect on the basic presentation of mood disorders.

Six other patients with autism and bipolar symptomatology were separately reported on by Akuffo et al. (1986), Steingard and Biederman (1987), Linter (1987), and Kerbeshian et al. (1987). All six patients were treated with lithium, and two also received moderate to high doses of antipsychotic medication. Two of the studies specifically noted that it appeared that lithium levels of at least 1.0 mEq/L were necessary to produce clinical improvement and prevent relapse.

Lithium was also helpful in addressing clearly seasonal mood disturbance in a mildly mentally retarded woman (Arumainayagam and Kumar 1990) and three of five developmentally disabled adolescents with bipolar illness (Mc-Cracken and Diamond 1988). Finally, Reid et al. (1987) found lithium most effective, often in combination with neuroleptics, for five mentally retarded adults with bipolar disorders and flexion deformities of the fingers.

When lithium is not effective, or cannot be tolerated, anti-epileptic drugs are now alternatives for bipolar illness in mentally retarded persons. The two most commonly used alternative medications are the anticonvulsants carbamazepine (CMZ) and valproic acid (VPA), although others are also available (Silka and Hurley 1998). Reid et al. (1987) compared CMZ with placebo in a double-blind, crossover fashion in 12 "overactive" adults with severe mental retardation. Although the patients were not described as bipolar per se, those who demonstrated elevated mood and distractibility did better on CMZ that those who were only overactive. Signer et al. (1986) reported success with CMZ treatment of a moderately mentally retarded bipolar patient after thioridazine failure, and Sovner (1988) described a 21-year-old mildly mentally retarded man with chronic mania who needed combined lithium and CMZ after failing to respond to either agent separately.

Glue (1989) and Sovner (1989) were among the first to describe the treatment of "rapid-cycling" bipolar disorders in mentally retarded persons. The concept of rapid-cycling illness (based on the presence of four or more episodes of affective illness per year) had been described in non–mentally retarded persons in the mid-1970s (Dunner and Fieve 1974). Glue reported 10 rapid-cycling individuals with affective disorders who were treated sequentially, in nonblind fashion, with lithium, lithium plus CMZ, or CMZ alone. Patients progressed to the next treatment stage if they failed to respond to the previous pharmacotherapy. Three patients responded to combined therapy, and 2 others to lithium alone. None of the individuals responded to CMZ alone.

Turning to VPA, Sovner, in two reports (1989, 1990), presented nine mentally retarded adults with bipolar disorders successfully treated with VPA. Three of these patients had chronic mania, and three others had rapid-cycling disease. Several had unsuccessful trials of lithium and/or CMZ. With VPA therapy, five patients were able to have long-standing neuroleptic therapy significantly reduced or discontinued. The author concluded that VPA appeared particularly effective in the treatment of atypical bipolar syndromes in mentally retarded persons but that serum levels above that generally used in anticonvulsant regimens (above 100 micrograms/mL) may be necessary for full response.

Similarly, Kastner et al. (1990) presented three children/adolescents with severe or profound mental retardation and bipolar symptomatology. All three had previously not responded to treatment with lithium, alone and in combination with CMZ. All three patients reacted to VPA with significant resolution of mood symptoms. The authors noted that lithium side effects of tremor and incontinence may limit the utility of this drug in retarded bipolar patients and concluded that, in their experience, CMZ or VPA was preferable to lithium as the drug of choice in severe or profoundly mentally retarded children with such mood disorders. Kastner et al. (1993) then prospectively studied 21 patients with affective symptoms, including irritability, sleep disturbance, aggression/self-injurious behavior, and behavioral cycles. Each patient took VPA prospectively over a 2-year period. Of the 18 who completed the study (2 dropped out, 1 had intolerable side effects), 14 responded favorably, and 9 of the 10 patients were able to have neuroleptic medication discontinued based on the favorable response.

Pary et al. (1999a) described 6 patients with Down's syndrome and bipolar disorder (an infrequent comorbidity), 3 of whom responded to lithium alone, 1 to lithium plus CMZ, 1 to lithium plus VPA, and 1 to VPA alone. Finally, King et al. (2000) retrospectively reviewed their experience with patients with mental retardation and bipolar disorder. Only 2 from 26 were ultimately treated with lithium alone, 24 of 26 were treated with antiepileptics (CMZ and VPA alone or in combination with each other) or in combination antiepileptics with lithium. The 14 of 26 who had rapid-cycling bipolar disorder responded particularly to VPA.

The most recent developments in the treatment of bipolar disorders have been the use of newer antiepileptics (lamotrigine and gabapentin) and atypical antipsychotics (particularly clozapine) (Antonacci and de Groot 2000; Buzan et al. 1998; Mikkelsen and McKenna 1999; Pary 1994; Rubin and Langa 1995; Silka and Hurley 1998). Concerning clozapine, no specifics were available regarding treatment response, but the authors saw clozapine as safe and effective in the larger group.

■ PSYCHOTHERAPIES FOR BIPOLAR DISORDER AND MANIA

The psychotherapy of bipolar disorder and mania represents a new frontier in treatment. Recurrence of episodes of bipolar disorders is thought to occur as a result of medication noncompliance, inconsistency, or disruption of social rhythms and stressful life events. Interpersonal and social rhythm therapy has been developed as a successful treatment approach (Frank et al. 1997). Through this therapy the patient is able to discuss ongoing interpersonal problems, understand the disorder and grieve the illness, and deal with the denial that occurs in many patients.

For patients with mental retardation, especially in the severe-to-profound range, a concomitant increase in aggression and/or self-injury may coincide with cycling (Hansel et al. 1999; King and McCartney 1999; Lowry 1997, 1998; Lowry and Sovner 1992). Whereas the influence of stressful events is well appreciated in the pathogenesis of depression, it is not as well appreciated with regard to bipolar disorder. However, the support of the family and caregivers can easily be influenced to reduce stress, improve stability of daily schedule, and reduce stimulation of the patient. This may be a fertile ground for development of psychotherapeutic support for the patient. Behavioral programs to address aggression and self-injurious behavior may also be used as augmentation of pharmacotherapy and therapeutic supports (Ruedrich 1993).

■ PRAGMATICS OF TREATMENT

Gualtieri (1989a, 1989b), Day (1990), and more recently Mikkelsen and McKenna (1999), Poindexter et al. (1998), and Sovner et al. (1998), have outlined a basic paradigm to follow in order to facilitate treatment of mood disorders in mentally retarded persons. The most important factor remains the necessity of accurate diagnosis, from which all treatment decisions can flow. Day has proposed a general plan for assessing mood disorders that would include identifying the type of mood disorder, its level of severity, the presence of other psychiatric symptoms or comorbid states, any precipitating factors or events, past history of psychiatric illness and response to treatment, the premorbid personality of the patient, and, finally, other aspects of care that might affect treatment choice, such as level of mental retardation, presence of medical problems, or social circumstance. He noted the importance of fully explaining the nature of the illness and proposed treatment to the patient and his or her relatives/caregivers, and that, in general, the treatment of mood disorders is not dissimilar to that given for the same disorders in non–mentally retarded persons. Gualtieri (1989a, 1989b) agreed, highlighting the increasing utility of information regarding family history of mood disorders in determining treatment choice and emphasizing the need for clinicians to address the often deleterious life circumstances that initiate and/or aggravate mood disorders in mentally retarded persons. Both authors noted that there are really very few specific studies of pharmacologic treatment of mood disorders in groups of mentally retarded individuals.

In reviewing these issues in the area of unipolar depression, there are now at least 25 reports involving more than 200 patients, most of whom have been presented in single case reports or small open clinical trials. Although an attempt to draw specific conclusions from the above carries some risk, it also appears clear that there is a vastly larger number of depressed mentally retarded persons who have been successfully (and routinely) treated with psychotherapy, behavioral therapy, antidepressants, or ECT, but who have not been reported.

A common response in clinical medicine to a lack of methodologically sound, research-based information has been the seeking of "expert consensus." Two recent large-scale efforts in this area have produced major publications offering consensus guidelines for the psychopharmacological treatment of persons with mental retardation (Reiss and Aman 1998; Rush and Frances 2000).

In treating depressive disorders in persons with mental retardation, the recommendation by Lund (1990) regarding use of tricyclic antidepressants (TCAs) has given way to consensus favoring newer antidepressants (Rush and Frances 2000). In a recent review of the use of antidepressants for aggression and self-injurious behavior in persons with mental retardation, Mikkelsen et al. (1997) noted that fluoxetine was superior to TCAs for treating these behavioral problems but noted that, in their sample, the presence of mood symptoms did not seem to predict treatment response and that it may be that fluoxetine was not addressing a mood disorder specifically. To date there are no studies available comparing SSRIs (or other newer antidepressants) to TCAs for depression in persons with mental retardation, no studies of SSRIs with controlled methodology, and only single-case reports or small series with TCAs that have blind and placebo-controlled methodology.

We also recommend considering behavioral and cognitive psychotherapies for patients with unipolar depression. These treatments can be used as adjuncts to pharmacotherapy or can be used with patients for whom drug therapy is not a consideration. Patients of all developmental levels can be treated to reduce the overt behaviors associated with depression and for social skill deficits. Appropriate eye contact and responding to social interaction can be reinforced, for example, in even the most profoundly disabled patients.

Patients with mild mental retardation should be offered individual or group therapy to address any behaviors or thoughts contributing to depression. As with any psychotherapeutic approach, the technique must be altered to suit the patient's level of cognitive functioning (Benson 1990; Hurley 1989b). Most patients with mild levels of cognitive disability can, with assistance, perform self-monitoring of thoughts and carry out semistructured homework assignments.

Regarding pharmacologic approaches to the treatment of bipolar disorders, the literature now contains 39 reports of over 180 patients in case reports or open trials and at least 2 small studies involving blinding of researchers and/or patients and within-subject, placebo-controlled methodology. These studies, particularly the controlled series, support the apparent efficacy of lithium for both the acute treatment of mania and the prophylaxis of bipolar disorder. Pary (1991) attempted to characterize guidelines for lithium utilization. He reported that lithium is clearly indicated for bipolar illness in mentally retarded persons but probably also for the treatment of patients with aggression accompanied by a family history of mood disorders and/or behavioral problems of any type characterized by cyclic patterns.

Pary further noted that no specific literature exists differentiating the use of lithium in mentally retarded patients from that of non–mentally retarded adults and recommended similar guidelines. These include seeking lithium levels in the 0.8–1.2 mEq/L range for acute mania, 0.5–0.8 mEq/L range for bipolar prophylaxis, and continuing therapy for at least several weeks at adequate levels before considering treatment complete. He also recommended close monitoring of the patient for side effects that may necessitate discontinuing lithium, including neurotoxicity (lethargy, severe tremor, vomiting, seizures, coma), and side effects that are troublesome but can be accommodated (hypothyroidism, gastrointestinal disturbance, polyuria with incontinence, dermatitis). Although lithium neurotoxicity is known to produce seizures, there is little evidence that lithium at therapeutic doses or levels worsens preexisting epilepsy, such that a breakthrough seizure in a compensated patient need not preclude its use.

When given for the treatment of acute mania, most patients receiving lithium also required the concomitant use of neuroleptic medication, and some patients have responded to the combination of lithium and CMZ or VPA. Of interest is the relative dearth of reports of successful treatment of bipolar patients with CMZ alone. Whether this reflects a true lack of response in comparison to lithium or lack of reported efficacy is unclear. To date, there are no published reports comparing lithium to CMZ or VPA in the acute treatment or prophylaxis of bipolar disorders in mentally retarded individuals nor any study of CMZ or VPA alone or in combination with blinding or placebo control. The anecdotal reports available seem to support VPA as the first choice in patients with atypical or rapid-cycling bipolar syndromes and a second choice for more typical mania or bipolar illness in mentally retarded persons unresponsive or intolerant of lithium treatment.

Other pharmacologic approaches to the acute treatment of mania, or prophylaxis of bipolar illness in non–mentally retarded persons, have included benzodiazepines such as clonazepam, calcium channel blockers, and atypical neuroleptics (Sovner 1995). With the exception of clozapine, there have been few reports of the use of these medications in mentally retarded persons, and they cannot be recommended at this time.

Psychotherapeutically, the same approaches that are helpful for treating unipolar depression can be utilized for the depressed phase of bipolar illness.

Less information is available addressing psychotherapeutic strategies (dynamic, cognitive, or behavioral) or social skills training for patients in the manic phase. Certain techniques would appear to have therapeutic potential (e.g., using guided cognitive therapy to attempt to decrease manic behavior using demonstration of expected [nonmanic] behavior, directed practice, and feedback on performance). To date these approaches to mentally retarded manic individuals have not been described. Similarly, group psychotherapy, although difficult with manic individuals, would seem to have some possibility for success.

■ CONCLUSIONS

When treating any disorder, diagnostic accuracy is of paramount importance. Because of the sometimes insurmountable diagnostic challenge in mentally retarded patients, it is no wonder that there is little systematic research in treating affective disorders in this population. This is evident in the area of both psychotherapy and pharmacotherapy, in which most reports concerning the applicability, efficacy, safety, and long-term follow-up of treatment are case reports, uncontrolled clinical trials, and/or extrapolations from research involving the treatment of mood disorders in normal populations (Day 1990). This underrepresentation is significant in light of the more widely accepted literature documenting the prevalence of mood disorders themselves in this population and can probably be variously ascribed to the diagnostic problems noted above, as well as the ethical and scientific difficulty in mounting major research programs with disabled persons (Sovner and Hurley 1983).

Increasingly accurate diagnosis of mentally retarded persons and the advent of both safer treatments and standardized objective methodologies to monitor treatment response will continue to address these issues. At present, the treatment of mood disorders in mentally retarded persons must proceed cautiously but should proceed, given the significant relief and return of function that appropriate treatment can offer patients and their families.

■ REFERENCES

Akuffo E, MacSweeney DA, Gajwani AK: Multiple pathology in a mentally handicapped individual. Br J Psychiatry 149:377–378, 1986

American Psychiatric Association: Diagnostical and Statistical Manuel of Mental Disorders, 4th Edition, Washington, DC, American Psychiatric Association 1994

Arumainayagam M, Kumar A: Manic depressive psychosis in a mentally handicapped person; seasonality: a clue to a diagnostic problem. Br J Psychiatry 156:886–889, 1990

Beck AT, Rush AJ, Shaw BF, et al: Cognitive Therapy of Depression. New York, Guilford, 1979

Benson BA: Behavioral treatment of depression, in Depression in Mentally Retarded Children and Adults. Edited by Došen A, Menolascino FJ. Leiden, Netherlands, Logon Publications, 1990, pp 309–329

Benson BA: Psychotherapy tools: a Daily Mood Check Form for use in outpatient settings. The Habilitative Mental Healthcare Newsletter 15:91–96, 1996

Benson BA, Rice CJ, Miranti SV: Effects of anger management training with mentally retarded adults in group treatment. J Consult Clin Psychol 54:728–729, 1986

Bojanin SE, Ispanovic-Radojkovic V: Treatment of depression in mentally retarded children: a developmental approach, in Depression in Mentally Retarded Children and Adults. Edited by Došen A, Menolascino FJ. Leiden, Netherlands, Logon Publications, 1990, pp 265–280

Boyd TL, Levis DJ: Depression, in Clinical Behavior Therapy and Behavior Modification, Vol 1. Edited by Daitzman RJ. New York, Garland STPM Press, 1980, pp 54–71

Bregman S: Assertiveness training for mentally retarded adults. Ment Retard 22:12–26, 1984

Buetz MR, Bowling JB, Bliss CA: Psychotherapy with mentally retarded: a review of the literature and the implications. Professional Psychology: Research and Practice 31:42–47, 2000

Buzan RD, Dubrovski SL, Firestone D, et al: Use of clozapine in 10 mentally retarded adults. J Neuropsychiatry Clin Neurosci 10:93–95, 1998

Carlson G: Affective psychoses in mental retardates. Psychiatr Clin North Am 2(3):499–510, 1979

Clarke DJ, Gomez GA: Utility of modified DCR-10 criteria in the diagnosis of depression associated with intellectual disability. J Intellect Disabil Res 43:413–420, 1999

Cook EH, Rowlett R, Jeselkis C, et al: Fluoxetine treatment of children and adults with autistic disorder and mental retardation. J Am Acad Child Adolesc Psychiatry 31:739–745, 1992

Cutajar P, Wilson D: The use of ECT in intellectual disability. J Intellect Disabil Res 43:421–427, 1999

Dagnan D, Chadwick P: Cognitive-behaviour therapy for people with learning disabilities, in Cognitive-Behaviour Therapy for People With Learning Disability. Edited by Kroese BS, Dagnan D, Loumidis K. London, UK, Routledge, 1997, pp 110–123

Day K: Depression in moderately and mildly handicapped people, in Depression in the Mentally Retarded: Practical Issues for Diagnosis and Treatment, Proceedings of the International Symposium. Edited by Došen A, Engelen P. Leiden, PAO, Netherlands, 1988, pp 23–36

Day KA: Treatment, care and management—a general overview, in Depression in Mentally Retarded Children and Adults. Edited by Došen A, Menolascino FJ. Leiden, Netherlands, Logon Publications, 1990, pp 235–254

DiGiuseppe R: Cognitive therapy with children, in Comprehensive Handbook of Cognitive Therapy. Edited by Freeman A, Simon KM, Beutler LE, et al. New York, Plenum, 1989, pp 125–137

Dobson KS: A meta-analysis of the efficacy of cognitive therapy for depression. J Consult Clin Psychol 57:414–419, 1989

Došen A: Depression in the mentally retarded, in Depression in the Mentally Retarded: Practical Issues for Diagnosis and Treatment, Proceedings of the International Symposium. Edited by Došen A, Engelen P. Leiden, PAO, Netherlands, 1988, pp 37–57

Došen A, Menolascino FJ: Depression in Mentally Retarded Children and Adults. Leiden, Netherlands, Logon Publications, 1990

Došen A, Petry D: Treatment of depression in persons with mental retardation, in Mental Health Aspects of Mental Retardation. Edited by Fletcher RJ, Došen A. New York, Lexington Books, 1993, pp 327–349

Dunner DL, Fieve RR: Clinical factors in lithium prophylaxis failure. Arch Gen Psychiatry 30:229–233, 1974

Ellis A, Harper RA: A New Guide to Rational Living. Englewood Cliffs, NJ, Prentice Hall, 1973

Field CJ, Aman MG, White AJ, et al: A single-subject study of imipramine in a mentally retarded woman with depressive symptoms. Journal of Mental Deficiency Research 30:191–198, 1986

Fletcher RJ: Individual psychotherapy for persons with mental retardation, in Mental Health Aspects of Mental Retardation. Edited by Fletcher RJ, Došen A. New York, Lexington Books, 1993, pp 327–349

Foxx RM, McMorrow MJ, Schloss CN: Stacking the deck: teaching social skills to retarded adults with a modified table game. J Appl Behav Anal 16:157–170, 1983

Frank C, Matson JL, Ritenour A, et al: Inducing lifestyle regularity in recovering bipolar disorder patients: results from the maintenance therapies in bipolar disorder protocol. Biol Psychiatry 41:1165–1173, 1997

Gardner WI, Willmering P: Mood disorders in people with severe mental retardation, in Challenging Behavior of Persons With Mental Health Disorders and Severe Developmental Diasbilities. Edited by Wieseler NA, Hanson RH, Siperstein G, et al Washington, DC, American Association on Mental Retardation, 1999, pp 13–37

Gardner WI, Cole CL, Berry DL, et al: Reduction of disruptive behaviors in mentally retarded adults: a self-management approach. Behav Modif 7:76–96, 1983

Ghaziuddin M, Tsai L: Depression in autistic disorder. Br J Psychiatry 159:721–723, 1991

Ghaziuddin M, Tsai L, Ghaziuddin N: Fluoxetine in autism with depression. J Am Acad Child Adolesc Psychiatry 30:508–509, 1991

Glue P: Rapid cycling affective disorders in the mentally retarded. Biol Psychiatry 26:250–256, 1989

Griffiths D: The social skills game, part I. Habilitative Mental Healthcare Newsletter 9:1–5, 1990a

Griffiths D: The social skills game, part II. Habilitative Mental Healthcare Newsletter 9:9–13, 1990b

Gualtieri CT: Affective disorders, in Treatments of Psychiatric Disorders: A Task Force Report of the American Psychiatric Association. Washington, DC, American Psychiatric Association, 1989a, pp 10–13

Gualtieri CT: Antidepressant drugs and lithium, in Treatments of Psychiatric Disorders: A Task Force Report of the American Psychiatric Association. Washington, DC, American Psychiatric Association, 1989b, pp 77–84

Hamdan-Allen G: Brief report: trichotillomania in an autistic male. J Autism Dev Disord 21:79–82, 1991

Hanaway TP, Barlow DH: Prolonged depressive behaviors in a recent blinded deaf mute: A behavioral treatment. J Behav Ther Exp Psychiatry 6:43–48, 1975

Hansel TE, Johnson JEG, Harder SR, et al: Use of aggression to signal and measure depressive episodes wth a rapid cycling bipolar disorder in an individual with mental retardation. Mental Health Aspects of Developmental Disabilities 2:122–132, 1999

Hasan MK, Mooney RP: Three cases of manic-depressive illness in mentally retarded adults. Am J Psychiatry 136(8):1069–1071, 1979

Hersen M, Eisler RM, Alford GS, et al: Effects of token economy on neurotic depression: an experimental analysis. Behav Ther 4:392–397, 1973

Hollins SC: Grief therapy for people with mental handicap, in Treatment of Mental Illness and Behavioral Disorders in the Mentally Retarded. Edited by Došen A, Van Gennep A, Zwanikken G. Leiden, Netherlands, Logon Publications, 1990, pp 139–142

Hollon SD: Cognitive therapy for depression: translating research into practice. Behav Ther 7:125–127, 1984

Howland RH: Fluoxetine treatment of depression in mentally retarded adults. J Nerv Ment Dis 180(3):202–205, 1992

Hurley AD: Behavior therapy for psychiatric disorders in mentally retarded individuals, in Mental Retardation and Mental Illness: Assessment, Service and Treatment for the Dually Diagnosed. Edited by Fletcher RJ, Menolascino FJ. Lexington, MA, Lexington Books, DC Health, 1989a, pp 127–140

Hurley AD: Individual psychotherapy: a review and call for research. Res Dev Disabil 10:261–275, 1989b

Hurley AD, Sovner R: Anorexia nervosa and mental retardation: a case report. J Clin Psychiatry 40(11):480–482, 1979

James DH: Psychiatric and behavioral disorders amongst older severely mentally handicapped inpatients. Journal of Mental Deficiency Research 30:341–345, 1986

Jancar J, Gunaratne IJ: Dysthymia and mental handicap. Br J Psychiatry 164:691–693, 1994

Kastner T, Friedman DL, Plummer AT, et al: Valproic acid for the treatment of children with mental retardation and mood symptomatology. Pediatrics 86(3):467–472, 1990

Kastner T, Finesmith R, Walsh K: Long-term administration of valproic acid in the treatment of affective symptoms in people with mental retardation. J Clin Psychopharmacol 13(6):448–451, 1993

Kendall PC: Toward a cognitive-behavioral model of child psychopathology and a critique of related interventions. J Abnorm Child Psychol 13:357–372, 1985

Kendall PC, Braswell L: Cognitive behavioral self-control therapy for children: a components analysis. J Consult Clin Psychol 50:672–689, 1982

Kerbeshian J, Burd L, Fisher W: Lithium carbonate in the treatment of two patients with infantile autism and atypical bipolar symptomatology. J Clin Psychopharmacol 7(6):401–405, 1987

King R, McCartney J: Charting for a purpose: optimal treatment of bipolar disorder in individuals with developmental disability. Mental Health Aspects of Developmental Disabilities 2:50–58, 1999

King R, Fay G, Croghan P: Rapid cycling bipolar disorder in individuals with developmental disabilities. Ment Retard 38:253–261, 2000

Komoto J, Usui S: Infantile autism and affective disorder. J Autism Dev Disord 14(1):81–84, 1984

Kovacs M: The efficacy of cognitive and behavior therapies for depression. Am J Psychiatry 137:495–501, 1980

Kovacs M, Rush AJ, Beck AT, et al: Depressed outpatients treated with cognitive or pharmacotherapy: a one-year follow-up. Arch Gen Psychiatry 38:33–39, 1981

Kroese BS, Dagnan D, Loumidis K: Cognitive-Behaviour Therapy for People With Learning Disabilities. London, UK, Routledge, 1997

Laman DS, Reiss S: Social skill deficiencies associated with depressed mood of mentally retarded adults. American Journal of Mental Deficiency 92:224–229, 1987

Langee HR, Conlon M: Predictors of response to antidepressant medications. Am J Ment Retard 97(1):65–70, 1992

Lindsay WR, Howells L, Pitcaithly D: Cognitive therapy for depression with individuals with intellectual disabilities. Br J Med Psychol 66:135–141, 1993

Linter CM: Short-cycle manic-depressive psychosis in a mentally handicapped child without family history: a case report. Br J Psychiatry 151:554–555, 1987

Lowry MA: Unmasking mood disoredrs: recognizing and measuring symptomatic behaviors. The Habilitative Mental Healthcare Newsletter 16:1–6, 1997

Lowry MA: Assessment and treatment of mood disorders in persons with developmental disabilities. Journal of Developmental and Physical Disabilities 10:342–387, 1998

Lund J: Treatment of depression in mentally retarded adults: a multidimensional approach, in Depression in the Mentally Retarded: Practical Issues for Diagnosis and Treatment, Proceedings of the International Symposium. Edited by Došen A, Engelen P. Leiden, PAO, Netherlands, 1988, pp 91–99

Lund J: Psychopharmacological approaches to the treatment of depression in the mentally retarded, in Depression in Mentally Retarded Children and Adults. Edited by Došen A, Menolascino FJ. Leiden, Netherlands, Logon Publications, 1990, pp 331–339

Masi G, Marcheschi M, Pfanner P: paroxetine in depressed adolescents with intellectual disability: an open label study. J Intellect Disabil Res 41:268–272, 1997

Matson J: Treatment of the behavioral characteristics of depression in the mentally retarded. Behav Ther 13:209–218, 1982

Matson J, Dettling J, Senatore V: Treating depression of a mentally retarded adult. British Journal of Mental Subnormality 16:86–88, 1979

Mayer D: Mental handicap, psychosis and thyrotoxicosis: a demonstration of the usefulness of an integrated community and hospital service. Journal of Mental Deficiency Research 29:275–280, 1985

McClennen SE, Hoekstra R, Bryan JE: Social Skills for Severely Retarded Adults: An Inventory and Training Program. Champaign, IL, Research Press, 1980

McCracken JT, Diamond RP: Case study: bipolar disorder in mentally retarded adolescents. J Am Acad Child Adolesc Psychiatry 27(4):494–499, 1988

Menolascino FJ, Ruedrich SL, Kang JS: Mental illness in the mentally retarded: diagnostic clarity as a prelude to psychopharmacological intervention, in Mental Retardation: Developing Pharmacotherapies Program in Psychiatry Series. Edited by Ratey JJ. Washington, DC, American Psychiatric Association Press, 1991, pp 19–37

Meyers BA: Major depression in persons with moderate to profound mental retardation: clinical presentation and case illustration. Mental Health Aspects of Developmental Disabilities 1:57–68, 1998

Mikkelsen G, McKenna L: Psychopharmacologic algorithms for adults with developmental disabilities and difficult-to-diagnose behavioral disorder. Psychiatric Annals 29:302–314 , 1999

Mikkelsen EJ, Albert LG, Emens M, et al: The efficacy of antidepressant medication for individuals with mental retardation. Psychiatric Annals 27:198–205, 1997

Monfils MJ, Menolascino FJ: Modified individual and group treatment approaches for the mentally retarded–mentally ill, in Handbook of Mental Illness in the Mentally Retarded. Edited by Menolascino FJ, Stark JA. New York, Plenum, 1984, pp 155–170

Murphy GE, Simons AD, Wetzel RD, et al: Cognitive therapy and pharmacotherapy singly and together in the treatment of depression. Arch Gen Psychiatry 41:33–41, 1984

Naylor GJ, Donald JM, Le Poidevin D, et al: A double-blind trial of long-term lithium therapy in mental defectives. Br J Psychiatry 124:52–57, 1974

Nezu CM, Nezu AM, Arean P: Assertiveness and problem solving training for mildly mentally retarded persons with dual diagnoses. Research and Developmental Disabilities 12:371–386, 1991

Pary RJ: Towards defining adequate lithium trials for individuals with mental retardation and mental illness. Am J Ment Retard 95(6):681–691, 1991

Pary RJ: Clozapine in three individuals with mild mental retardation and treatment-refractori psychiatric disorders. Ment Retard 32:323–327, 1994

Pary RJ, Friedlander R, Capone GT: Bipolar disorder and Down's syndrome: six cases. Mental Health Aspects of Developmental Disabilities 2:59–67, 1999a

Pary RJ, Levitas AS, Hurley AD: Diagnosis of bipolar disorder in persons with developmental disabilities. Mental Health Aspects of Denelopmental Disabilities 2:37–49, 1999b

Poindexter AR, Cain N, Clarke DJ, et al: Mood stabilizers, in Psychotropic Medication and Developmental Disabilities: The International Consensus Handbook. Edited by Reiss S, Aman MG, Columbus, OH, Ohio State University Nisonger Center, 1998, pp 215–227

Puri BK, Langa A, Coleman RM, et al: The clinical efficacy of maintenance electroconvulsive therapy in a patient with mild mental handicap. Br J Psychiatry 161:707–709, 1992

Quinsey V, Varney S: Social skills game: a general method for the modeling and practice of adaptive behaviors. Behav Ther 2:279–281, 1977

Reid AH: Psychoses in adult mental defectives; I: manic depressive psychosis. Br J Psychiatry 120:205–212, 1972

Reid AH, Leonard A: Lithium treatment of cyclical vomiting in a mentally defective patient. Br J Psychiatry 149:316, 1977

Reid AH, Naylor GJ: Short cycle manic depressive psychosis in mental defectives: a clinical and psychological study. Journal of Mental Deficiency Research 20(1):67–76, 1976

Reid AH, Swanson JG, Jain AS, et al: Manic depressive psychosis with mental retardation and flexion deformities: a clinical and cytogenetic study. Br J Psychiatry 150:92–97, 1987

Reisinger JJ: The treatment of "anxiety-depression" via positive reinforcement and response cost. J Appl Behav Anal 5:125–130, 1972

Reiss S, Aman MG: Psychotropic Medication and Developmental Disabilities: The International Consensus Handbook. Columbus, OH, Ohio State University Nisonger Center, 1998

Reiss S, Benson BA: Psychosocial correlates of depression in mentally retarded adults; I: minimal social support and stigmatization. American Journal of Mental Deficiency 89:331–337, 1985

Reiss S, Levitan GW, Szyszko J: Emotional disturbance and mental retardation: diagnostic overshadowing. American Journal of Mental Deficiency 86:567–574, 1982

Rivinus TM, Harmatz JS: Diagnosis and lithium treatment of affective disorder in the retarded: five case studies. Am J Psychiatry 136(4B):551–554, 1979

Rubin M, Langa A: Clozapine, mental retardation and severe psychiatric illness: clinical response in the first year (letter). Harward Review of Psychiatry 3:293–294, 1995

Ruedrich SL: Treatment of bipolar mood disorder in persons with mental retardation, in Mental Health Aspects of Mental Retardation. Edited by Fletcher RJ, Dosen A. Lexington, MA, Lexington Books, 1993, pp 268–280

Ruedrich SL, Alamir S: Electroconvulsive therapy for persons with developmental disabilities: review, case report and recommendations. Mental Health Aspects of Developmental Disabilities 2:83–91, 1999

Ruedrich SL, Wilkinson L: Atypical unipolar depression in mentally retarded patients: amoxapine treatment. J Nerv Ment Dis 180(3):202–205, 1992

Rush AJ, Frances A: Expert consensus guideline series: treatment of psychiatric and behavioral problems in mental retardation. Am J Ment Retard 105:182–184, 2000

Sachs GS: Adjuncts and alternatives to lithium therapy for bipolar affective disorder. J Clin Psychiatry 50(suppl 12):31–39, 1989

Signer SF, Benson DF, Rudnick FD: Undetected affective disorder in the developmentally retarded. Am J Psychiatry 143(2):259, 1986

Silka VR, Hurley AD: Selection of antidepressant medication in persons with mental retardation. The Habilitative Mental Healthcare Newsletter 16:55–57, 1997

Silka VR, Hurley AD: New drug therapies for bipolar disorders. Mental Health Aspects of Developmental Disabilities 16:52–54, 1998

Soni S, Keave V, Soni D: Dexamethasone suppression test and response to antidepressants in depressed mentally handicapped subjects. J Intellect Disabil Res 36:425–433, 1992

Sovner R: Anticonvulsant drug therapy of neuropsychiatric disorders in mentally retarded persons, in Use of Anticonvulsants in Psychiatry. Edited by McElroy SL, Pope HG. Oxford, UK, Oxford Health Care, 1988, pp 169–181

Sovner R: The use of valproate in the treatment of mentally retarded persons with typical and atypical bipolar disorders. J Clin Psychiatry 50(suppl 3):40–43, 1989

Sovner R: Bipolar disorder in persons with developmental disorders: an overview, in Depression in Mentally Retarded Children and Adults. Edited by Došen A, Menolascino FJ. Leiden, Netherlands, Logon Publications, 1990, pp 175–197

Sovner R: Management of treatment-resistent rapid cycling bipolar disorder. The Habilitative Mental Healthcare Newsletter 14:93–94, 1995

Sovner R, Hurley AD: Diagnosing depression in the mentally retarded. Psychiatric Aspects of Mental Retardation 1:1–3, 1982

Sovner R, Hurley AD: Do the retarded suffer from affective illness? Arch Gen Psychiatry 40:61–67, 1983

Sovner R, Lowry MA: A behavioral methodology for diagnosing affective disorders in individuals with mental retardation. Habilitative Mental Healthcare Newsletter 9:7, 1990

Sovner R, Fox CJ, Lowry MJ, et al: Fluoxetine treatment of depression and associated self-injury in two adults with mental retardation. J Intellect Disabil Res 37:301–311, 1993

Sovner R, Pary RJ, Dosen A, et al: Antidepressant drugs, in Psychotropic Medication and Developmental Disabilities: The International Consensus Handbook. Edited by Reiss S, Aman MG. Columbus, OH, Ohio State University Nisonger Center, 1998, pp 179–200

Steingard R, Biederman J: Case report: lithium responsive manic-like symptoms in two individuals with autism and mental retardation. J Am Acad Child Adolesc Psychiatry 26(6):932–935, 1987

Sung H, Hawkins BA, Eklund SJ, et al: Depression and dementia in aging adults with Down's syndrome: a case study approach. Ment Retard 35:27–38, 1997

Szymanski LS, Biederman J: Depression and anorexia nervosa of persons with Down's syndrome. American Journal of Mental Deficiency 89(3):246–251, 1984

Szymanski L, Rosefsky B: Group psychotherapy with mentally retarded persons, in Emotional Disorders of Mentally Retarded Persons. Edited by Szymanski L, Tanguay P. Baltimore, MD, Baltimore University Press, 1980, pp 173–194

Thuppal M, Fink M: Electroconvulsive therapy and mental retardation. J ECT 15:140–149, 1999

Warren AC, Holroyd S, Folstein MF: Major depression in Down's syndrome. Br J Psychiatry 155:202–205, 1989

13 Treatment of Anxiety Disorders in Persons With Mental Retardation

Henry F. Crabbe, M.D., Ph.D.

Anxiety disorders are highly prevalent—they are the most common psychiatric disorder in the United States (Mosier 1973; Robins et al. 1984)—but it is uncertain how prevalent they are among persons with mental retardation (Reiss 1994). Why is this so? Perhaps diagnosticians have a penchant for mistaking such maladaptive behavior of mentally retarded persons for psychosis or affective disorders rather than straightforwardly as the physical discharge of anxiety. Given the vulnerability of the ego structure and the frail coping mechanisms of mentally retarded patients, change in the psychosocial or environmental milieu is a potent elicitor of excessive anxiety (Feinstein and Reiss 1996).

Anxiety is an emotional state of apprehension and tension that anticipates danger from an undefined source (American Psychiatric Association 1987). It is accompanied by a physiological arousal that prepares the body to "fight or flee." Of clinical significance, however, is pathological anxiety that overwhelms the organism's adaptive capacities and causes impairment in psychosocial functioning (Noyes 1986). Pathological anxiety creates a disproportionate emotional and physiological reaction to a nonthreatening environment. Table 13–1 lists the protean physical manifestations encountered in anxiety disorder syndromes.

Rosenbaum and Pollack (1987) distinguish pathological anxiety from "normal" anxiety on the basis of four criteria: 1) autonomy, 2) intensity, 3) duration, and 4) behavior. *Autonomy* means that the anxiety has taken on a "life of its own" within the patient and is thus considered endogenous. *Intensity* refers to a heightened level of anxiety, and *duration* indicates that the patient's symptoms have become persistent rather than transient. The fourth criterion, *behavior*, signifies the fact that behavioral avoidance or withdrawal is a consequence of pathological anxiety. Relevant to this final behavioral criterion is the

227

Table 13–1. Somatic manifestations of anxiety

Organ system	Symptoms	Signs
Cardiovascular	Palpitations	Tachycardia
	Substernal pressure	Elevated systolic blood pressure
	Precordial pain	Functional systolic ejection murmur
Pulmonary	Facial flushing	Hyperventilation
	Difficulty breathing	Increased frequency of sighing respiration
	Sense of suffocation	
Gastrointestinal	Epigastric distress, belching, heartburn, dyspepsia, diarrhea, constipation, anorexia, compulsive eating	
Genitourinary	Increased frequency of micturition	
	Amenorrhea, excessive menstrual flow and cramps	
	Impotence, premature ejaculation	
Nervous	Tension	Strained facial expression
	Difficulty concentrating	Stereotypic behavior
	Lightheadedness, irritability	Cold, clammy handshake
	Sleep disturbances	Pacing, restlessness, irritability
	Ill-defined fear	Fine tremor
	Fatigue	
	Headaches, poor coordination	
	Trembling, numbness, and tingling	

contribution of experimental psychology that demonstrates a diminution of task performance at levels of extreme anxiety. Hebb's inverse, U-shaped model predicts optimal on-task behavior at moderate levels of physiological arousal and a decrement in performance at high or low levels of anxiety (Hebb 1966).

Systematic research on anxiety in persons with mental retardation is limited. However, some investigations indicate that retarded individuals respond to stress with higher levels of anxiety (Cochran and Cleland 1963; Levine 1985; Ollendick et al. 1993; Reiss 1994; Stavrakaki 1999; Szymanski and King 1999). Furthermore, this higher anxiety is associated in children with a poorer performance on achievement tests with the resultant experience of failure and loss of self-esteem (Feinstein and Reiss 1996). Levine (1985) reported that unfamiliar problem-solving tasks induced more anxiety in mentally retarded adults. Furthermore, lack of employment and deficits in social skills also rendered these individuals more vulnerable to anxiety. Levine further comments that institutionalized as opposed to noninstitutionalized persons have greater degrees of fear and anxiety that may have resulted from having been sheltered from everyday stress, thereby missing opportunities for developing coping skills.

Whereas the aforementioned citations from the literature relate to individuals with mild to moderate levels of mental retardation, a conceptual framework for characterizing the elicitation of anxiety or arousal in the severely and profoundly retarded is absent.

Early research by Goldstein (1948) indicated that patients with a history of brain trauma were especially vulnerable to incoming sensory stimuli. Ordinary situations would be experienced to catastrophic proportions in which the "brain's inability to deal with the normal and ordinary contributed to a state of inner confusion and turmoil" (Sands and Ratey 1986, p. 290). Sands and Ratey (1986) refer to this state as "noise." Analogously, patients with increasing levels of mental retardation lack an adequate filtering mechanism to modulate incoming stimuli. These authors further state that a means for dealing with such intense stimuli is the lowering of the volume of noise or noxious input by such strategies as the display of a need for "sameness" by indulging in repetitive or stereotypic behavior. Alternatively, withdrawal, behavioral inhibition, or shyness can be displayed. According to Sands and Ratey, such strategies reduce the individual's internal tension and transform uncontrollable stress (or noise) into controllable stress ("attempts at reorganization"). Preclinical research (Charney et al. 1984) suggests that the perception of environmental events as uncontrollable stress will increase the neuronal firing rates of the locus coeruleus, a noradrenergic center in the brain, and will elicit anxiety. Sympathetic arousal, which is responsible for the physical symptoms of anxiety, parallels this increase in activity in the locus coeruleus. Supporting animal research demonstrates that stress reduction, attained by means of increased coping and task mastery, will reverse the increase in brain norepinephrine turnover that accompanies anxiety (Tanaka et al. 1983; Tsuda and Tanaka 1985).

Alterations in the external environment, such as changing caregivers or daily routines—or in the internal milieu, such as hunger or dental pain—can induce anxiety and arousal. Restless pacing, physical aggression, and self-injurious behavior are maladaptive responses, but they may serve to discharge the experience of internal tension or anxiety (Stavrakaki 1999). Caregivers who have bonded with their patients and are in "synch" with their internal need states may be able to modulate the anxiety by creating orderliness and familiarity. Such an intervention is consistent with the approach of tolerance, warmth, and affection utilized by John McGee in his gentle teaching paradigm (McGee 1993).

Posttraumatic stress disorder (PTSD) in persons with mental retardation is probably signifincantly underdiagnosed (Ryan 1994), and it can be presented with symptoms of panic attack, agoraphobia, and others. This disorder should be routinely considered in differential diagnosis (Szymanski and King 1999).

Obsessive-compulsive disorder is also considered as a form of an anxiety disorder that is frequently found among people with mental retardation (Szymanski and King 1999).

■ TREATMENT APPROACHES

An extensive amount of literature exists on the treatment of anxiety disorders in the psychiatric population at large. Treatment principles have been extrapolated and modified by clinicians to address the special needs of persons with mental retardation. Most of the literature on this latter subpopulation involves case study descriptions. In general, the modalities of psychotherapy, behavior therapy, relaxation training, and pharmacotherapy have been utilized to treat individuals suffering from anxiety disorders.

Psychotherapy

Psychotherapy, both individual and group, applied specifically for the treatment of anxiety has received only a meager amount of attention in the literature. There are reviews of the literature pertaining to the general use and modification of psychotherapeutic techniques that are suited for persons with mental retardation (Chandler 1989; Van Bourgandien 1989). A number of controlled investigations have indicated the superiority of behavioral techniques as opposed to psychotherapy for the treatment of phobic disorders in the nonretarded population (Noyes 1986). Consistent with this are the findings that behavioral approaches are more applicable to and effective than traditional psychotherapy with mentally retarded individuals (Davis and Rogers 1985). For example, Matson and Senatore (1981) have demonstrated the superiority of behavioral therapy over group psychotherapy in improving the interpersonal functioning of adults with mild and moderate mental retardation. Nonetheless, psychotherapy that involves education, reassurance, the heightening of self-esteem, and the provision of support during periods of stress can be considerably beneficial (see Chapters 2, 7, and 8 of this book).

Behavior Therapy

Gardner and colleagues (Gardner and Cole 1984; Gardner and Graeber 1994) have reviewed the major behavioral techniques applied in the treatment of persons with mental retardation. Such techniques include reinforcement, modeling procedures, emotional retraining, and cognitive therapy. In clinical practice, many of these approaches can be combined in a multicomponent treatment. Of particular relevance to the treatment of anxiety and phobic disorders are the procedures of systematic desensitization and contact desensitization (also known as participant modeling; see also Chapter 4 of this book).

Systematic desensitization has been defined as "gradually exposing patients (in imagination or in vivo) to a graded hierarchy of anxiety-provoking stimuli while maintaining a state of calm through deep muscle relaxation or variety of other methods applied to induce a countering relaxation" (Nemiah and Uhde 1989). Gardner and Cole (1984) affirm that the concrete presentation of anxiety-provoking stimuli in vivo would be necessary in mentally retarded individuals with limited imaginal skills. As an alternative to the use of a relaxation procedure, the anxiety-eliciting object or situation could be "counterconditioned" by a competitive activity such as eating, listening to music, or even the positive affective experience of bonding between a caregiver and patient. Frequently, in such clinical paradigms, reinforcement such as verbal praise or tokens is used to shape appropriate behavior in anxiety-provoking situations.

Several authors have reviewed case studies exemplifing the use of behavioral desensitization procedures in the treatment of phobic disorders in persons with mental retardation (Hurley and Sovner 1982; McNally and Ascher 1987). A few examples will be discussed to illustrate the behavioral techniques employed.

Mosier (1973) treated an 11-year-old boy with cerebral palsy and severe mental retardation who displayed a pathological reaction (screaming, crying, and running away) upon exposure to balloons. Boy Scout articles were used successfully as reinforcers for the sequential approaching, touching, blowing, and pricking of balloons over a period of 31 treatment sessions. Gardner and Cole (1984) classify this in vivo procedure as reinforced practice because the subject successfully approximates the appropriate approach behavior through the application of positive reinforcement. When the phobic stimulus is presented, the pleasurable experience of the desired reinforcer competes with and finally eliminates the elicitation of anxiety.

In a similar case, Freeman et al. (1976) extinguished a phobic reaction to the physical examination of a 7-year-old boy with moderate mental retardation. In this in vivo desensitization example, a positive relationship with a nurse provided the vehicle of anxiolysis in a stepwise program in which the nurse was able to conduct the physical examination. A phase of stimulus fading was then initiated whereby the physician was able to conduct parts of the examination with the nurse in attendance and eventually with the nurse absent. Generalization of the procedure took place as well—another physician was also allowed to perform the physical examination.

Matson (1981b) conducted a successful treatment study of three preadolescent girls with moderate mental retardation who displayed clinical features of social phobia. In this case description a protocol of participant modeling was used in which the parents coached the subject to engage in social behavior in the presence of unfamiliar adults. The positive nurturing support of the parents attenuated the "stranger anxiety" (of the unfamiliar adults), and verbal and tangible reinforcers were applied when appropriate social behavior was modeled by the children.

Matson (1981a) also performed a larger controlled study in which 24 phobic persons with mild and moderate mental retardation were randomly assigned to treatment versus no treatment conditions. The treatment group received in vivo desensitization involving rehearsal and participant modeling to address phobic avoidance of grocery shopping. The treatment group was significantly more effective in reducing phobic anxiety and enhancing shopping skills in the community.

In an early study of phobic desensitization procedures in 20 mildly retarded adults, Peck (1977) compared the differential efficacy of imaginal systematic desensitization and vicarious symbolic desensitization through videotape and in vivo contact desensitization. The in vivo contact desensitization with therapist modeling was the only therapeutic approach judged to be effective.

The psychiatric literature reveals that behavior therapy has selective advantages over psychotherapy in the treatment of obsessive-compulsive disorder. The specific technique of in vivo exposure, with response prevention in particular, has been recommended as a superior alternative. Little in the way of published case anecdotes about the treatment of this disorder in persons with mental retardation exists. Matson (1982), however, has described the behavioral treatment of three mentally retarded "checkers," who compulsively and ritualistically examined their body and clothes. Matson employed an in vivo exposure technique in a workshop setting where the patients' symptomatology was prominent. Differential reinforcement of noncompulsive behavior was provided by the use of tokens. When a compulsive behavior was displayed, an overcorrection procedure was implemented as a method of response prevention. This behavioral treatment was successful in suppressing the compulsions and in reducing self-reported anxiety.

Relaxation Therapy

Relaxation training as a form of behavioral therapy is characterized by its focus on self-regulation strategies for reducing physiological arousal and anxiety. Relaxation techniques have been applied in clinical counterconditioning procedures and in the treatment of a variety of psychiatric conditions including anxiety, phobias, psychosomatic illnesses, and sleep disorders (Lichstein 1988). Several review articles discuss its clinical utility in persons with mental retardation (Harvey 1979; Rickard 1986; Verberne 1989). Indeed, a few case studies describe its application to persons with mental retardation as a therapeutic adjunct to self-injurious behavior (Steen and Zuriff 1977), tantrumming (Harvey and Karen 1978), psychomotor seizures (Wells et al. 1978), and phobias (Guralnick 1973). From a more general perspective, some authors (Benson 1994; Benson and Havercamp 1999) state that relaxation training can facilitate the development of coping skills and lead to the enhancement of self-control in patients with developmental disabilities (see also Chapter 5 of this book).

Two training procedures frequently used are *progressive relaxation* (Jacobsen 1938) and *abbreviated progressive relaxation* (Bernstein and Borkovec 1973). These techniques teach the patient to alternately tense and relax certain muscle groups. However, Rickard (1986) comments on their limitations for patients with moderate, severe, and profound levels of mental retardation. Some clinicians modify these techniques by using concrete images such as squeezing and letting go of a lemon to facilitate differentiation between muscle tension and relaxation in their upper extremities. Lindsay and colleagues (1989) have developed *behavioral relaxation training*, which they have demonstrated to be more effective than abbreviated progressive relaxation for patients with moderate and severe mental retardation. This procedure teaches patients to model observable relaxed and unrelaxed behaviors of various parts of the body and to avoid reliance on internal and subjective states of tension.

A variety of other relaxation techniques including diaphragmatic breathing, imagery conditioning, and biofeedback training may be added to the anxiolytic armamentarium for persons with mental retardation. With certain patients, the creative application of music therapy, art therapy, hydrotherapy, and physical therapy might serve to facilitate anxiety reduction. In one study, the use of instrumental music showed a positive trend in diminishing anxiety during dental appointments for patients with mental retardation (Davila and Menendez 1986).

Pharmacotherapy

No systematically controlled trials have been conducted to assess the efficacy of anxiolytic medication in the treatment of anxiety disorders in persons with mental retardation. Consequently, the following section summarizes the use of these psychotropic agents in the general psychiatric population.

In patients with a diagnosis of panic disorder, treatment with tricyclic antidepressants (e.g., imipramine and clomipramine) may be effective (Werry 1998; Zitrin et al. 1983). Alternatively, the anxiolytics alprazolam (Ballinger et al. 1988), clonazepam (Rosenbaum and Tesar 1990), and lorazepam (Werry 1998) have demonstrated a panicolytic effect.

Anxiolytics (in particular benzodiazepines) are considered unsuitable for the more chronic forms of anxiety such as generalized anxiety disorder, obsessive-compulsive disorder, and PTSD, except during acute exacerbation or concurrent acute stress (Werry 1999). Sedation that is often temporary and dose-related is the most commonly noted side-effect. Potential toxic effects include ataxia and decreased motor coordination. Benzodiazepine medications should never be stopped abruptly but rather tapered gradually because of the potential for rebound anxiety and a small risk of withdrawal seizures. One caveat in the use of benzodiazepines is that the literature reports that these agents may induce behavioral disinhibition and aggressive outbursts in certain individuals (Mattes 1986; Sheard 1984). Barron and Sandman (1985) indicate that mentally retarded patients may be at a higher risk for developing paradoxical excitement in response to the administration of sedative and hypnotic medication. Thus, rigorous clinical monitoring for this potential effect is warranted.

Mild tranquilizing and antihistaminic medications such as hydroxyzine and diphenhydramine are less effective anxiolytic alternatives. Antipsychotic medications, despite their tranquilizing effects, should not be prescribed because of the higher risk of long-term side-effects such as tardive dyskinesia. The use of buspirone may be as effective as that of the benzodiazepines in the treatment of a generalized anxiety disorder. It is noteworthy that buspirone is devoid of sedating effects, and it does not have any negative influence on psychomotor performance. Several investigators (Buitelaar et al. 1998; Ratey et al. 1989, 1991), in multiple case and open studies, have successfully used buspirone in the treatment of generalized anxiety in persons with mental retardation and pervasive developmental disorders.

Clomipramine, a tricyclic psychoactive compound, has been demonstrated to possess anti-obsessional properties in a number of well-controlled clinical studies of patients with obsessive-compulsive disorder (Deveaugh-Geis et al. 1989; Rapoport 1988). Its purported mechanism of action is through serotonin reuptake blockade. Clomipramine, which is also an effective antidepressant, shares a side-effect profile that is similar to other psychoactive agents in the tricyclic class of drugs. Such adverse reactions may include sedation, anticholinergic effects (such as a dry mouth and constipation), and orthostatic hypotension.

Fluoxetine is an antidepressant drug with a dicyclic chemical structure that has been available in the United States since 1988. Fluoxetine is also a potent serotonin uptake inhibitor and has a side effect profile that is generally more favorable then other available antidepressive agents. However, it has been reported to cause nausea, vomiting, nervousness, and insomnia in some patients. Fluoxetine as well as other serotonin reuptake inhibitors have been demonstrated to be useful in obsessive-compulsive disorder, obsessional anxiety, and social phobia (Werry 1999), but they are seldom effective alone and need to be combined with other therapies (e.g., behavior therapy).

Adrenolytics like β-adrenergic blockers (e.g., propranolol and nadolol) and α-adrenergic agonists (e.g., clonidine) are also used for the treatment of anxiety disorders (Ruedrich and Erhardt 1999; Werry 1999).

■ TREATMENT OF ANXIETY INDUCED BY AKATHISIA AND TARDIVE AKATHISIA

My own clinical experience with mentally retarded patients has led me to believe that the use of neuroleptics and neuroleptic withdrawal syndromes may be important causes of organic anxiety—perhaps even the most prevalent. Akathisia is an extrapyramidal side-effect of antipsychotic drug therapy characterized by motor restlessness, pacing, and agitation and is accompanied by a feeling of intense anxiety, internal distress, and dysphoria. Akathisia, usually associated with the high-potency neuroleptics such as haloperidol, may occur within hours or may develop over several months. Unfortunately, developmentally disabled patients with minimal or no verbal skills might not be able to communicate their sense of discomfort to their caregivers. It is likely that akathisia may be the culprit responsible for such disruptive behavioral disorders as hyperactivity, aggression, noncompliance, self-injurious behavior, and insomnia. Not uncommonly, treating physicians may address the emergence of these disruptive symptoms by further increasing the dosage of antipsychotic medication, thereby leading to further deterioration of the patient's condition with an escalation of maladaptive behavior.

More recently, the clinical phenomenon of tardive akathisia has been more widely accepted as a side-effect, emerging during long-term neuroleptic therapy (i.e., greater than 6 months) or when the medication is tapered off or discontinued (Barnes and Braude 1985; Crabbe 1994; Gualtieri and Sovner 1989). Tardive akathisia is a neuroleptic withdrawal syndrome believed by investigators in the field to be a variant of tardive dyskinesia. Unlike acute akathisia, tardive akathisia may be masked by increasing the antipsychotic drug dosage. Tardive akathisia may develop when either the high-potency or low-potency antipsychotic drugs are used.

Tardive akathisia is also frequently associated with the classical abnormal involuntary movements of tardive dyskinesia. Gualtieri and Sovner (1989) have estimated the prevalence of tardive akathisia to be 14% in institutional settings. The clinical manifestations of acute akathisia are identical to those of tardive akathisia. Thus, tardive akathisia is characterized by motor restlessness, anxiety, increase in severity and frequency of maladaptive behavior, and sleep disturbance (see also Branford and Hutchins 1996; Gross et al. 1993).

Antiparkinson agents are well known to be ineffective in the treatment of acute akathisia. β-blockers such as propranolol and nadolol are recognized by most authorities to be the treatment of choice (Fleischhacker et al. 1990).

No clear guidelines for the management of tardive akathisia have been established. Yassa and colleagues (1988) provide anecdotal data from two case studies on the utility of the β-blocker propranolol in this disorder. Other authors also report beneficial effects of β-blockers (Gross et al. 1993). Zonneveld and Došen (1998) reported successful treatment with clonazepam of two mildly mentally retarded persons who suffered from tardive akathisia. Gualtieri and Sovner (1989) recommend clonazepam as a possible strategy, but supporting literature exists only for its use in the treatment of acute akathisia (Kutcher et al. 1989). Nonetheless, benzodiazepines have frequently been suggested as a palliative measure in the clinical management of tardive dyskinesia (American Psychiatric Association 1980; Gross et al. 1993; Jeste and Wyatt 1982). Consequently, if tardive akathisia is a behavioral analogue or variant of tardive dyskinesia, the selection of a benzodiazapine may be a viable option in selected cases. I have treated several cases of tardive akathisia successfully with low dosages of bromocriptine (less than 10 mg/day) (Crabbe 1994). This chemotherapeutic intervention was selected because the dopamine agonist bromocriptine preferentially stimulates presynaptic autoreceptors with the consequence of decreased dopamine synthesis and release (Jeste and Wyatt 1982). The underlying though unproven assumption in this case is that dopaminergic supersensitivity plays a central role in the pathophysiology of tardive akathisia. The literature on low-dose bromocriptine in the treatment of tardive dyskinesia has yielded mixed results (Jeste and Wyatt 1982; Jeste et al. 1983; Lenox et al. 1985). However, in my experience, the "low dose" must be individualized to the patient. A regimen of 2.5 mg of bromocriptine daily in one patient exerted positive effects, whereas a daily dosage of 10 mg exacerbated maladaptive behavior. Consequently the clinician must be mindful of the potential behavioral toxicity of bromocriptine in exacerbating tardive akathisia or precipitating psychosis (Perovich et al. 1989).

A frequent recommendation of psychopharmacological experts in mental retardation is that neuroleptic tapering should be accomplished with minimal dosages over months to years. Whereas dramatic rebound exacerbations of maladaptive behavior may be prevented, it is unfortunate that this clinical wisdom has not been empirically validated with respect to the prevention of tardive akathisia. Nonetheless, slow neuroleptic tapering with the implementation of an adjuvant psychoactive agent such as a β-blocker, benzodiazepine, or bromocriptine when a behavioral neuroleptic withdrawal syndrome occurs is a potential strategy that has not yet been clinically substantiated in controlled studies. In selected individuals, the alternative of increasing the neuroleptic dosage may be necessary.

■ Conclusions

Anxiety disorders are frequently either misdiagnosed or left undiagnosed in persons with mental retardation. The symptoms of anxiety may occur as a consequence of the stress and changes inherent in institutions and in the community. Individuals with mental disabilities are more vulnerable and, thus, react more symptomatically to the vicissitudes of daily life. Patients with mental retardation who are already at a higher risk of developing comorbid medical disorders may also develop an organically induced anxiety syndrome. Finally, other individuals might display the psychiatric symptoms of a broad spectrum of anxiety and phobic disorders.

The critical elements in this discussion are the awareness and recognition of the diverse manifestations of anxiety in medical and psychiatric illness so that an appropriate diagnosis can be established. Once the diagnostic formulation is articulated, a multimodality treatment plan—which could include behavior therapy, psychotherapy, or pharmacotherapy—can be implemented to enhance the quality of life of persons with mental retardation.

■ References

American Psychiatric Association: Tardive Dyskinesia: Task Force Report 18. Washington, DC, American Psychiatric Association, 1980

American Psychiatric Association: Diagnostic and Statistical Manual of Mental Disorders, 3rd Edition, Revised. Washington, DC, American Psychiatric Association, 1987

Ballinger JC, Burrows GD, Du Pont RL, et al: Alprazolam in panic disorder and ago-raphobia: results from a multicenter trial; I: efficacy in short-term treatment. Arch Gen Psychiatry 45:413–422, 1988

Barnes TRE, Braude WM: Akathisia variants and tardive dyskinesia. Arch Gen Psychiatry 42:874–878, 1985

Barron J, Sandman CA: Paradoxical excitement to sedative-hypnotics in mentally retarded clients. American Journal of Mental Deficiency 90:124–129, 1985

Benson BA: Anger management training: a self-control program for persons with mental retardation, in Mental Health in Mental Retardation. Edited by Bouras N. Cambridge, UK, Cambridge University Press, 1994, pp 224–232

Benson BA, Havercamp SM: Behavioural approaches to treatment: principles and practices, in Psychiatric and Behavioural Disorders in Developmental Disabilities and Mental Retardation. Edited by Bouras N. Cambridge, UK, Cambridge University Press, 1999, pp 262–278

Bernstein D, Borkovec TD: Progressive Relaxation Training. Champaign, IL, Research Press, 1973

Branford D, Hutchins D: Tardive akathisia in people with mental retardation. Journal of Developmental and Physical Disabilities 8:2:117–132, 1996

Buitelaar JK, Van Der Gaag RJ, Van Der Hoeven J: Buspirone in the management of anxiety and irritability in children with pervasive developmental disorders: results of an open-label study. J Clin Psychiatry 59(2):56–59, 1998

Chandler M: Psychotherapy, in Treatments of Psychiatric Disorders: A Task Force of the American Psychiatric Association, Vol 1. Washington, DC, American Psychiatric Association, 1989, pp 108–111

Charney DS, Heninger GR, Breier A, et al: Noradrenergic function in panic anxiety: effects of yohimbine in healthy subjects and patients with agoraphobia and panic disorder. Arch Gen Psychiatry 41:751–763, 1984

Cochran JL, Cleland CC: Manifest anxiety of retardates and normals matched as to academic achievement. American Journal of Mental Deficiency 67:539–542, 1963

Crabbe H: Pharmacotherapy in mental retardation, in Mental Health in Mental Retardation. Edited by Bouras N. Cambridge, UK, Cambridge University Press, 1994, pp 187–204

Davila JM, Menendez J: Relaxing effects of music in dentistry for mentally handicapped patients. Special Care in Dentistry 6:18–21, 1986

Davis KV, Rogers ES: Social skills training with persons who are mentally retarded. Ment Retard 23:186–196, 1985

Deveaugh-Geis J, Landau P, Katz RJ: Preliminary results from a multicenter trial of clomipramine in obsessive compulsive disorder. Psychopharmacol Bull 25:36–40, 1989

Feinstein C, Reiss AL: Psychiatric disorder in mentally retarded children and adolescents: the chalenges of meaningful diagnosis. Child Adolesc Psychiatr Clin North Am 5:827–852, 1996

Fleischhacker WW, Roth SD, Petrovic R, et al: The pharmacologic treatment of neuroleptic-induced akathisia. J Clin Psychopharmacol 10:12–21, 1990

Freeman BJ, Roy RR, Hemmick S: Extinction of a phobia of physical examination in a seven year old mentally retarded boy: a case study. Behav Res Ther 14:63–64, 1976

Gardner WI, Cole CL: Use of behavior therapy with the mentally retarded in community settings, in Handbook of Mental Illness in the Mentally Retarded. Edited by Menolascino FJ, Stark JA. New York, Plenum, 1984, pp 97–154

Gardner W, Graeber J: Use of behavioral therapies to enhance personal competency: a multimodel diagnostic and intervention model, in Mental Health in Mental Retardation. Edited by Bouras N. Cambridge, UK, Cambridge University Press, 1994, pp 205–223

Goldstein K: After Effects of Brain Injuries in War. New York, Grune & Stratton, 1948

Gross E, Hull H, Lytton G, et al: Case study of neuroleptic induced akathisia: important implications for individuals with mental retardation. Am J Ment Retard 98:156–164, 1993

Gualtieri CT, Sovner R: Akathisia and tardive akathisia. Psychiatric Aspects of Mental Retardation Reviews 8:83–88, 1989

Guralnick MJ: Behavior therapy with an acrophobia mentally retarded young adult. J Behav Ther Exp Psychiatry 4:263–265, 1973

Harvey JR: The potential of relaxation training for the mentally retarded. Ment Retard 17:71–76, 1979

Harvey JR, Karen OC: Relaxation training and cognitive behavioral procedures to reduce violent temper outbursts in a moderately retarded woman. J Behav Ther Exp Psychiatry 9:347–351, 1978

Hebb DO: A Textbook of Psychology, 2nd Edition. Philadelphia, PA, WB Saunders, 1966

Hurley AD, Sovner R: Phobic behavior and mentally retarded persons. Psychiatric Aspects of Mental Retardation Newsletter 11:41–44, 1982

Jacobsen E: Progressive Relaxation. Chicago, IL, University of Chicago Press, 1938

Jeste DV, Wyatt RJ: Understanding and Treating Tardive Dyskinesia. New York, Guilford, 1982

Jeste DV, Cutler NR, Kaufman CA, et al: Low-dose apomorphine and bromocriptine in neuroleptic-induced movement disorders. Biol Psychiatry 18:1085–1091, 1983

Kutcher S, Williamson P, Mackenzi S, et al: Successful clonazepam treatment of neuroleptic-induced akathisia in older adolescents and young adults: a double-blind, placebo-controlled study. J Clin Psychopharmacol 9:403–406, 1989

Lenox RH, Weaver LA, Saram BM: Tardive dyskinesia: clinical and neuroendocrine response to low dose bromocriptine. J Clin Psychopharmacol 5:286–292, 1985

Levine HG: Situational anxiety and every day life experiences of mildly retarded adults. American Journal of Mental Deficiency 90:27–33, 1985

Lichstein KL: Clinical Relaxation Strategies. New York, Wiley, 1988

Lindsay WR, Baty FJ, Michie AM, et al: A comparison to anxiety treatments with adults who have moderate and severe mental retardation. Res Dev Disabil 10:129–140, 1989

Matson JL: A controlled outcome study in phobias in mentally retarded adults. Behav Res Ther 19:101–107, 1981a

Matson JL: Assessment and treatment of clinical fears in mentally retarded children. J Appl Behav Anal 14:287–294, 1981b

Matson JL: Treatment of obsessive compulsive behavior in mentally retarded adults. Behav Modif 6:551–567, 1982

Matson JL, Senatore V: A comparison of traditional psychotherapy and social skills training for improving interpersonal functioning of mentally retarded adults. Behavior Therapy 12:369–382, 1981

Mattes JA: Psychopharmacology of temper outbursts: a review. J Nerv Ment Dis 174:646–670, 1986

McGee JJ: Gentle teaching for persons with mental retardation: the expression of a psychology of interdependence, in Mental Health Aspects of Mental Retardation. Edited by Fletcher R, Došen A. New York, Lexington Books, 1993, pp 350–376

McNally RJ, Ascher LM: Anxiety disorders in mentally retarded people, in Anxiety and Stress Disorders: Cognitive-Behavioral Assessment and Treatment. Edited by Michelson L, Ascher LM. New York, Guilford, 1987, pp 379–394

Mosier D: Systematic desensitization of extreme and unreasonable fear of balloons. School Applications of Learning Theory 5:9–67, 1973

Nemiah JC, Uhde TW: Obsessive-compulsive disorder, in Comprehensive Textbook of Psychiatry, 5th Edition. Edited by Kaplan HI, Sadock BJ. Baltimore, MD, Williams & Wilkins, 1989, pp 1245–1254

Noyes R: Anxiety and phobic disorders, in The Medical Basis of Psychiatry. Edited by Winokur G, Clayton P. Philadelphia, PA, WB Saunders, 1986, pp 323–341

Ollendick TH, Oswald DP, Ollendick DG: Anxiety disorders in mentally retarded persons, in Psychopathology in the Mentally Retarded. Edited by Matson J, Barrett R. Boston, MA, Allyn & Bacon, 1993, pp 41–86

Peck CL: Desensitization for the treatment of fear in the high level retardate. Behav Res Ther 15:137–148, 1977

Perovich RM, Lieberman JA, Fleishhacker WW, et al: The behavioral toxicity of bromocriptine in patients with psychiatric illness. J Clin Psychopharmacol 9:417–422, 1989

Rapoport JL: The neurobiology of obsessive-compulsive disorder. JAMA 260:2888–2890, 1988

Ratey JJ, Sovner R, Mikkelsen E, et al: Buspirone therapy of maladaptive behavior and anxiety in developmentally disabled persons. J Clin Psychiatry 50:382–384, 1989

Ratey JJ, Sovner R, Parks A, et al: Buspirone treatment of aggression and anxiety in mentally retarded patients. J Clin Psychiatry 52:159–162, 1991

Reiss S: Handbook of Challenging Behavior: Mental Health Aspects of Mental Retardation. Washington, OH, IDS Publishing, 1994

Rickard HC: Relaxation training for mentally retarded persons. Psychiatric Aspects of Mental Retardation Reviews 5:11–15, 1986

Robins LN, Helzer JE, Weissman MM, et al: Lifetime prevalence of specific psychiatric disorders in three sites. Arch Gen Psychiatry 41:934–941, 1984

Rosenbaum JF, Pollack MH: Anxiety, in Massachusetts General Hospital Handbook of General Psychiatry. Edited by Hackett TP, Cassem MH. Littleton, MA, PSG Publishing, 1987, pp 185–209

Rosenbaum JF, Tesar GE: Clonazepam and other anticonvulsants, in Clinical Aspects of Panic Disorder. Edited by Ballinger JC. New York, Wiley-Liss, 1990

Ruedrich S, Erhardt L: Beta-adrenergic blockers in mental retardation and developmental disabilities. Mental Retardation and Developmental Disabilities Research Reviews 5(4):290–298, 1999

Ryan R: Posttraumatic stress disorder in persons with developmental disabilities. Community Mental Health Journal 3(1):45–54, 1994

Sands S, Ratey JJ: The concept of noise. Psychiatry 49:290–297, 1986

Sheard MH: Clinical pharmacology of aggressive behavior. Clin Neuropharmacol 7:173–183, 1984

Stavrakaki C: Depression, anxiety and adjustment disorders in people with developmental disabilities, in Psychiatric and Behavioural Disorders in Developmental Disabilities and Mental Retradation. Edited by Bouras N. Chambridge, UK, Chambridge University Press, 1999, pp 175–187

Steen PL, Zuriff GE: The use of relaxation in the treatment of self-injurious behavior. J Behav Ther Exp Psychiatry 8:447–448, 1977

Szymanski L, King BH: Practice parameters for the assessment and treatment of children, adolescents, and adults with mental retardation and comorbid mental disorders. J Am Acad Child Adolesc Psychiatry 38(supplement 12):5–32, 1999

Tanaka M, Kohno Y, Nakagawa R, et al: Regional characteristics of stress-induced increases in brain noradrenaline release in rats. Pharmacol Biochem Behav 19:543–547, 1983

Tsuda A, Tanaka M: Differential changes in noradrenalin turnover in specific regions of rat brain produced by controllable and uncontrollable shocks. Behav Neurosci 99:802–817, 1985

Van Bourgandien ME: General counseling services, in Treatments of Psychiatric Disorders: A Task Force of the American Psychiatric Association, Vol 1. Washington, DC, American Psychiatric Association, 1989, pp 104–107

Verberne GJ: Relaxatietechnieken bij licht en matig geestelijk gehandicapten: een literatuuroverzicht. Gedragstherapie 22:205–218, 1989

Wells KC, Turner SM, Bellack AS, et al: Effects of cue-controlled relaxation on psychomotor seizures: an experimental analysis. Behav Res Ther 16:51–53, 1978

Werry JS: Anxiolytics and sedatives, in Psychotropic Medications and Developmental Disabilities: The International Consensus Handbook. Edited by Reiss S, Aman MG. Columbus, OH, The Ohio State University Nisonger Center, 1998, pp 201–214

Werry JS: Anxiolytics in MRDD. Mental Retardation and Developmental Disabilities research Riviews 5(4):299–304, 1999

Yassa R, Iskandar H, Nastase C, et al: Propranolol in the treatment of tardive akathisia: a report of two cases. J Clin Psychopharmocal 8:283–285, 1988

Zitrin CM, Klein DF, Woerner MG, et al: Treatment of phobias; I: comparison of imipramine hydrochloride and placebo. Arch Gen Psychiatry 40:125–138, 1983

Zonneveld P, Dosen A: Een overzicht van de diagnostiek en behandeling van tarddieve akathisie: is de verstandelijk gehandicapte een "geval apart." Tijdschrift voor Psychiatrie 40(6):344–355, 1998

14 Treatment of Epilepsy and Associated Disorders

Thomas P. Berney, M.B., Ch.B., D.P.M.,
F.R.C.Psych., F.R.C.P.C.H.

Epilepsy is a pervasive disorder that can become a greater burden than mental retardation. Seizure control is only one element in the wider management of a disorder that taxes all the psychiatrist's skills. Treatment must be sufficiently comprehensive to enable a patient and his or her caregivers to cope not just with the fits but with all the secondary disabilities that follow from living with a disorder that is controlled rather than cured. The epilepsy that accompanies mental retardation, being symptomatic rather than idiopathic, is frequently intractable. In this chapter, therefore, I emphasize the variety and extent of the treatments available.

■ EPIDEMIOLOGY

Epilepsy is rife in mental retardation. Prevalence rates depend on the definition employed as well as on the population selected—its age and the nature and degree of mental retardation. In the community, the frequency ranges from 8% in mild retardation to about 70% in severe retardation with concomitant physical disability or postnatal insult (Goulden et al. 1991; Shepherd and Hosking 1989). It is less frequent in Down's syndrome, and West's and Lennox-Gastaut syndromes are overrepresented although the outcome may be more benign (Stafstrom and Konkol 1994). In Down's syndrome, the frequency increases with age and eventually may herald dementia (Collacott 1993). In fragile X syndrome the overall prevalence is 26%, a figure that when adjusted for ability is probably appropriate to the degree of mental retardation (Musumeci et al. 1988). In tuberous sclerosis, epilepsy is common, often starting as neonatal seizures or infantile spasms.

Autism has a special relationship with epilepsy. First, the prevalence is high even when allowance is made for mental ability. Next, nearly 40% of the cases have an adolescent onset. Although it is uncertain whether this represents a real distinction from other forms of mental retardation of equivalent degree (Gillberg 1991), the later onset appears to be associated with higher ability (Gillberg, personal communication, 1995). It is clear that epilepsy can magnify the symptoms of autism but less certain whether subclinical ictal activity can mimic it. Assiduous investigation can find an epileptiform electroencephalogram (EEG) discharge in nearly half of the population with autism. On the other hand, it is rare for there to be a clinical response to anti-epileptic drugs (AEDs) unless there are clear clinical seizures. The report of a response to steroids draws a parallel with Landau-Kleffner syndrome (Stefanatos et al 1995).

■ PROGNOSIS

The management of epilepsy must be measured against its natural course. The frequent tendency to improve in later childhood and, after an adolescent lapse, to improve again in adulthood may be falsely attributed to treatment. The course can be divided into the *acute* (tending to early remission), the *chronic*, and the sometimes *intractable*. The latter is associated with a neurodeficit, either a neurological abnormality or mental retardation, early onset, a high seizure frequency, multiple seizure types, and initial difficulty in establishing control, all features that may indicate that the underlying epileptic process is a more malignant and intransigent one (Medical Research Council AED Withdrawal Study Group 1993). It follows that AEDs may have little effect on the long-term outcome of epilepsy (Chadwick 1995). Alternately, it may be that the occurrence of one fit predisposes the brain to subsequent fits so that early and effective seizure control would improve the prospects of long-term remission (Reynolds 1995).

By adulthood, about two-thirds of those with childhood onset epilepsy can expect to be seizure free, although often on medication. In the presence of a neurodeficit, this falls to about one-third (Annegers et al. 1979; Brorson and Wranne 1987). In Aberdeen, Scotland, the remission rate was 56% for those who were simply mentally retarded, 47% where cerebral palsy was superimposed, but only 11% where the retardation stemmed from postnatal injury (Goulden et al. 1991). Improvement continues with time, and terminal remission can occur even after 30 years of seizures (Sillanpaa 1990).

Occasionally death may come suddenly, unexpectedly, and with no clear cause (Coyle et al. 1994). It occurs in between 1:500 and 1:1,000 people with epilepsy, particularly in those with neurological abnormalities or autism— usually in sleep and frequently in association with low AED levels. Once status epilepticus and asphyxia have been excluded, cardiac arrhythmia appears to be the most likely explanation. This begs the question as to whether seizures can produce fatal arrhythmias or whether, in the longer term, they might induce cardiac changes that make the heart more vulnerable (Ansakorpi et al. 2000), an important issue as many of the AEDs might have a cardiac effect.

■ EPILEPSY AND BEHAVIOR DISORDER

An association with psychiatric disturbance is well recognized but not straightforward, relating to the lack of effective seizural control rather than to the simple presence of epilepsy (Deb and Hunter 1991a, 1991b, 1991c; Espie et al. 1989; Hunt and Stores 1994). The seizures themselves, their associated physiological changes (prodromal tension and postictal hangover), antiepileptic medication, the problems and restraints of living under the ever-present threat of a seizure, and the wider difficulties and advantages of a sick role all combine to make a person vulnerable to minor stress. However, the uncontrollable outburst of anger driven by epilepsy has to be distinguished from that of a person who, uncertain of his or her place in the world, has discovered the effectiveness of a disinhibited temper tantrum.

Ictal aggression is unusual and, when it occurs, has more to do with a misapprehension of circumstances—for example, resistive violence in response to restraint. Violence as an ictal automatism is rare (Treiman 1991), although Gedye (1989a, 1989b, 1991) forcefully argues that many of the spontaneous, short-lived, repeated episodes of self-injurious behavior might represent frontal lobe seizures, particularly when accompanied by a characteristic cluster of motor behaviors. This hypothesis lacks clinical or neurophysiological confirmation (Coulter 1991), although depth recording has brought a more general recognition that seizures may exist without concurrent change on the surface EEG. This is a development of the debate about the episodic dyscontrol syndrome. The original account was of brief episodes of aggression, of sudden onset and with little or no provocation in an otherwise even-tempered personality who showed subsequent remorse. There might have been other indications of cerebral dysfunction such as an epileptiform EEG or even frank epilepsy (Monroe 1970). The subsequent inclusion of many intemperate rages due to an abnormal background EEG widened the net to the extent of throwing doubt on the whole concept (Leicester 1982). All of this carries the danger that AEDs might replace neuroleptics as an indiscriminate, reflex response to aggression. At the same time there is some support for the wider use of AEDs from a few studies of the response to carbamazepine (Langee 1989), not always with clinical or laboratory support (Laminack 1990). Indeed, overactivity rather than epilepsy may be the identifying characteristic for success (Reid et al. 1981). The complexity of the matter is indicated by a study that found epilepsy to be one of the factors associated with a response of aggression to lithium (Tyrer et al. 1984).

Postictal disturbance is more frequent and may range from a similar resistive aggression through to a prolonged confusional state, drowsiness, irritability, depression, or anxiety, similar to an alcoholic hangover.

Disturbance might be part of a wider personality change, a Geschwind syndrome with intensified cognitive interests and emotional responses, obsessional overinclusiveness, behavioral viscosity, and altered sexuality (Benson 1991). Irritability, often with aggressive or testing undertones, may be painfully obvious but also can be subtle and overlooked. Often penumbral, disturbance has not been identified with any particular form of epilepsy and fluctuates with the degree of seizure control, responding to AEDs. This makes a sharp contrast with the hyperkinetic child who is only bearable while subdued by frequent fits. The underlying mechanism is unknown, but two factors are prominent. First, the seizures themselves can produce a general sense of malaise even if they do not have more specific sensory and psychic components. Second is the medication, in particular barbiturates and benzodiazepines, which can produce an effect akin to alcoholic irritability and disinhibition, perhaps amplified by the underlying cerebral dysfunction or damage. Irritability can be either an idiosyncratic response, as with lamotrigine, valproate, and carbamazepine, or more clearly dose dependent, as with vigabatrin.

■ DIAGNOSIS

Essential to any strategy is the recognition, first, that epilepsy is present and, second, its extent. Diagnostic criteria range from seeing every habitual chain of behavior as ictal through to an insistence on clear-cut motor episodes. Mental retardation is rich in paroxysmal episodes whether self-stimulatory, repetitive movement, stereotypy, or emotional outburst. The eye of faith can discern seizural activity in all of these, but then the same paroxysmal umbrella might be extended to include a sneeze and an orgasm. As the latter may be modified by an AED, it is clear that this is a slippery slope, and, as with the supernatural, it becomes difficult to know where to draw the line between acceptance and credulity.

The spectrum of clinical phenomena is wide, ranging from the very obvious generalized motor seizure through the tonic spasm and myoclonic jerk to the brief and subtle absences and even the transitory cognitive impairment (TCI). The last is diagnosable only when an EEG discharge highlights a coincident hiccup in clinical performance (Kasteleijn-Nolst Trenite et al. 1990); mental retardation will hamper task performance and mask the interruption.

Limited communication makes it difficult to identify subjective phenomena, hindering the diagnosis of partial complex or sensory seizures. If EEG evidence is lacking, then the diagnosis becomes especially doubt ridden. Unfortunately this is particularly likely when seizures, such as limbic and frontal lobe episodes, simulate voluntary behavior (Stores 1992). Similarly, Landau-Kleffner syndrome can be difficult to distinguish from delayed-onset autism (Appleton 1995). The EEG is central to the investigation of epilepsy although the standard scalp recording is limited in duration, circumstances, and the extent of its access. When communication and comprehension are limited, much depends on the technique and skill of the technician. With coaxing, the hyperactive patient may cooperate given the freedom of long leads or cable telemetry. A single, interictal EEG will fail to detect epilepsy in 50% of the recordings. Further recordings and the use of activation procedures such as sleep (particularly deep sleep), hyperventilation, temperature (Berney and Hewitt, unpublished observations, 1990), exercise, and the immediate postexercise recovery period (Berney et al. 1981; Kuijer 1978) will reduce this figure, but even then the records of approximately 10%–20% of the patients remain persistently negative. Confirmation may depend on prolonged recording using either radio or cable telemetry or an ambulatroy recorder. Simultaneous video recording may help although this involves ingenuity and expense for prolonged recording (Donat and Wright 1990). Even during an ictal episode, it may fail to show any epileptiform change depending on electrode placement and the site of discharge. EEG change might be expected with a generalized motor or absence seizure but is less likely for a simple partial seizure, especially with autonomic or psychic symptomatology or when the seizure arises from the mesial frontal lobe.

Epilepsy is so prevalent and communication such a barrier as to make for a bias against the recognition of nonepileptic states—such as cardiac dysrhythmia (Nousiainen et al. 1989), panic disorder, self-stimulatory and stereotypic movements, an exaggerated startle response, daydreaming, and pseudoseizure—particularly when they coexist with epilepsy.

In the end the circumstances may warrant venturing onto the quicksand of the therapeutic trial. Cases in which the episodes are clearly ictal may become a protracted experiment with a variety of AEDs being exhibited in their varied dosages and combinations. Medication may modify seizures down to a fragment of their original manifestation, making it difficult to judge when adequate control has been achieved—always remembering that the adverse effects of the medication may turn out to be worse than the seizures. Persistent pseudoseizures can also obscure this endpoint, and it may need a specialized unit to distinguish these from other paroxysmal behaviors (Holmes et al. 1983; Neill and Alvarez 1986).

Diagnostic uncertainty, in the absence of supportive laboratory evidence, can lead to several scenarios. First, an equivocal response to the early AEDs may lead to the abandonment of the trial and the assumption that the behavior is not epileptic. Next, a response to the psychogenic or placebo effects of the medication may lead to the equally false assumption that it is epilepsy. Third, a clear but temporary response to the initial AED, often seen in epilepsy, may suggest that the trial should persist. How far should this be pursued given the variety of drug and dosage? These problems are especially knotty when, lacking countable seizures, the measure is some aspect of attention, mood, or behavior. It may prove impossible to gauge the efficacy of the medication against the changeability of a stimulus-rich domestic background. At this point, a fresh start and inpatient admission may be contemplated. However, this may be may be misleading, as simply escaping from the conflict can reduce seizure frequency.

■ STATUS EPILEPTICUS

Status may be defined either as an unduly prolonged seizure or as recurrent seizures without recovery between attacks. It may be convulsive or nonconvulsive, and each may be subdivided into generalized or partial forms.

Generalized convulsive status carries a mortality rate of about 10% and may mark a turning point for the worse in an epileptic career. Treatment has been revolutionized by the introduction of rectal solutions of diazepam, clonazepam, or paraldehyde, and more recently buccal or nasal midazolam (Scott et al. 1999). This allows an effective first-aid management, but their widespread popularity carries the risk of overuse by a number of parents, unaware of the small risk of respiratory depression, who will administer the solution prematurely or inappropriately, for example, to terminate an intense and grueling tantrum. These drugs pose a special problem for many schools that are uneasy about their responsibility should there be a mishap. In the absence of a school nurse, some define the problem as one of first-aid and allow their use by suitably trained staff. Others fall back on legal safety, summoning the doctor or parent or sending the child to hospital.

Nonconvulsive status, again generalized or partial, gives a "twilight" state of altered consciousness that clinically ranges from extreme drowsiness and confusion through to more subtle states of altered responsiveness and mood. Diagnosis is confirmed by EEG and the sometimes dramatic response to intravenous diazepam (Stores 1992).

■ THE WHOLE PATIENT

With the risk of seizure come the consequent restrictions as well as the problems of medication, overprotection, and prejudice. Treatment should aim at developing a sense of self-respect and confidence in spite of these. It must encompass the attitudes of caregivers, friends, teachers, and employers, all of whom will influence, and be influenced by, the patient's attitude (Espie et al. 1998).

The development of the caregivers' attitudes depends on three elements. First is their degree of self-confidence, which will depend on the combination of their personalities and their relationships. Nothing is as likely to make a mother or nurse overcautious and overprotective as to be told repeatedly that whatever she did was wrong or that it could have been done better. Second are the attitudes to illness in general, and seizures in particular, that they have acquired in their own development. Parental early example is modified by the flood of information and advice they then receive, either through formal teaching and training or informally from the media and friends, the psychiatrist becoming the latest recruit to this advisory host. The third element is the extent and availability of support. It is easier for caregivers to be confident in the midst of a well-developed network of care, readily accessed by telephone, than to be isolated and unable to share the sense of responsibility. Frequent appointments may add to a family's burden, but they may also be seen as evidence of the doctor's continuing interest and care.

Few moments match the one at which the diagnosis is presented, and vivid images can mask the extent to which perception is blurred or distorted. The presence of a friend, community nurse, or key worker is invaluable, as are further appointments for follow-up points that were overlooked or misunderstood. A diagnosis of epilepsy can be terrifying, carrying fears of madness and death (particularly when asleep or in status epilepticus) as well as inadequacy when faced with the first aid of fits. Later comes the difficulty of balancing overprotection with rejection of the disability. Instruction needs to be practical and reassuring. A videotaped collection of seizures may help to desensitize both the patient (who may have fantasies about the repulsiveness of his or her fits) and the caregiver. It can also help them to recognize the full range of seizures.

Unfortunately, epilepsy may prove to be too much for those parents who, with effort, have allowed their mentally retarded child some autonomy. Everyday routines and restrictions should be reviewed. There should be no blanket rules, but any regimen must take into account the severity and circumstances of the seizures as well as the degree of supervision. Water and heights present specific hazards that can be minimized by routine (e.g., arranging for a caregiver to be within earshot during showering). The reduction of open fires and unguarded stoves has virtually eliminated the epileptic hallmark of burns. Everyday life carries some risk: epilepsy tempts caregivers to try to create a life substantially safer than their own, imposing a secondary layer of handicap on both themselves and the patient and imprisoning the patient in a claustrophobic cocoon. In adulthood, in which a combination of mental retardation and high levels of unemployment can make work hard to find, epilepsy can be the final, backbreaking straw. Unemployment erodes confidence further and the resultant boredom is epileptogenic.

Better seizure control often improves disturbance. However, family and behavioral work are often necessary to remedy the habitual patterns that have developed over time and that, if left untreated, will keep the disturbance running.

Associated states such as anxiety and depression should be treated. Phenothiazines, tricyclic antidepressants (Toone and Fenton 1977), and lithium (Julius and Brenner 1987) can induce seizures, but when the patient's epilepsy is well controlled with AEDs, their use is safe provided they are introduced gradually and are in moderate dosage (James 1986; Ojemann et al. 1987). Indeed, a paradoxical improvement in seizure control has been reported with prochlorperazine (Carter 1959) and thioridazine (Baldwin and Kenny 1966). These may be the result of a pharmacokinetic effect, simply altering the amount of free drug available, but may also be more direct and parallel the anticonvulsant effect of imipramine.

Seizure threshold is altered by a great variety of environmental factors, both internal and external, although associations are usually inconsistent (Verduyn et al. 1988). General physical health is significant, and infections, particularly in their early stages, often have an adverse effect although the occasional patient may improve. Probable factors are fever and toxins: although not reflected in routine liver function tests, interferon-inducing agents can impair hepatic enzymes to raise AED levels (Jann and Fidone 1986). There is a popular belief that constipation can lower seizure threshold, and enemas are a frequent resort. A study of this found a positive association in only 3 of 14 patients (Livingston and Berney 1992). Emotional state alters the threshold although this may be an indirect effect mediated through missed medication, sleep deprivation, or hyperventilation (Mattson 1991). There is merit in regularity.

■ ANTI-EPILEPTIC DRUGS (AEDS)

Details of specific AEDs are given in a variety of texts, although this fast-changing scene is best served by frequently updated formulary.

Considering the variety of neurotransmitters, the differing neuroreceptors, and the complexity of counterbalanced neuronal interaction, it is to be expected that a large number of agents will affect seizure control. Although guided by the theoretical, therapy must follow the empiric "what works for this patient," for the evidence is often flimsy. First, there are a large number of conditions to be assessed, and often it is unclear whether the relevant distinction is the type of seizure, type of epilepsy, or underlying neurological process. Next, although many drugs are better used on their own, some are enhanced by adjuvants or combination. As dosage is also a significant variable, it is to be expected that experience is varied. There are relatively few comparative trials, particularly with regard to populations with mental retardation. Much of the evidence is from open case series, often with a selection bias toward nonresponders compounded by a publication bias toward positive results. In the end, it is difficult to estimate how many patients are going to remain unresponsive to all drugs compared with those who will respond only to a few specific and unusual AEDs. Only trial and error will show where an individual belongs, but time and the newer AEDs should whittle down the first group.

At what point should experimentation halt? The ideal goal is absolute seizure control without any toxicity and on a single daily dosage. In practice there is often a compromise between an acceptable number of seizures and further changes in AED. What is "acceptable" will depend on the individual— drop attacks may become tolerable when a bruising crash to the floor has been modified to a gentle slide.

Rationalization of medication means a careful review of therapy with the elimination of the more sedative drugs as well as an overall reduction (Collacott et al. 1989). In one study (Alvarez 1989), complete withdrawal was achieved and sustained for 8 years in 48% of the adults studied. Success was related neither to the degree of mental retardation nor to the duration of the seizure disorder but was most likely in those who had had only a few seizures, were on low levels of medication, and were free of neurological deficits. Relapse was predicted by a deterioration in the EEG rather than prewithdrawal abnormality. Seizure recurrence was evenly spread over the first 3 years, and after that only 20% recurred.

Rationalization is often taken to mean a change to monotherapy, an ideal that has been insufficiently explored in the past, is economic, and makes for a more ready understanding of the clinical effects and side effects (Shorvon et al. 1977). The reports of improved well-being and diminished seizure frequency are alluring (Beghi et al. 1987; Fischbacher 1982), so that there sometimes is a dogmatic disbelief in the reasons for multiple drug usage. Relapse is frequent, even in the third year of follow-up (Alvarez 1989), and many studies stop short of this. Next, certain drugs (such as ethosuximide) are seizure specific so that the presence of several seizure types can require several drugs. Finally, our knowledge of the additive effects of different AEDs is very limited, and in some circumstances the interaction of two drugs might produce a better therapeutic effect for lesser toxicity. Examples are the combination of valproate with ethosuximide (Bourgeois 1988a; Rowan et al. 1983), carbamazepine (Bourgeois 1988b), and lamotrigine, but not the traditional blend of phenobarbitone and phenytoin (Bourgeois 1986). In practice, the transition from one drug to the next means that, for a while, the patient is on two drugs and withdrawal of the first drug sometimes results in deterioration. The withdrawal of barbiturates and benzodiazepines has to be especially slow, requiring months to avoid withdrawal fits, although Tennison and colleagues (1994) suggest that such weaning might equally well be accomplished in 6 weeks. Such forces can result in a regimen frozen on multiple AEDs until a further deterioration in seizure control forces a more radical overhaul. Rationalization requires the determined persistence of the patient as well as the therapist.

It needs some skill to gauge the speed at which dosage and drug should be changed. Too fast means more adverse effects and the response overshot, too slow and the patient tires of the lack of progress. Thus the pace depends on the drug—lamotrigine and topiramate are particularly prone to adverse effects if introduced rapidly; vigabatrin can take weeks to develop its full effect. Much also depends on the frequency of the seizures, for it is difficult to appraise progress when they come in occasional clusters or as rare episodes of status. Seizures may not occur with random regularity but take on a pattern that reflects an underlying biological rhythm (Balish et al. 1991), and an apparent response may have more to do with this rhythm than any change in medication.

In some AEDs, the serum levels are relevant to their clinical effect. However, the therapeutic range is an individual property, and the well-publicized statistical norms are so crude a guide that the value of assay has been questioned. This is particularly because the usual assay includes the inactive, bound drug and, secondly, ignores the metabolites that may be more active than the drug itself (Chadwick 1987; Meijer 1991). Circumstances are different in mental retardation, in which communication is limited, seizures take unusual forms, and it is a recurrent question whether the patient's aberrant behavior, especially drowsiness, is the result of uncontrolled epilepsy or excessive medication. Serum levels are essential in the use of phenytoin, whose pharmacokinetics mean that a small change in dosage can result in an upward rush to toxic blood levels. They are also necessary to prevent the insidious upward creep of the longer acting drugs such as ethosuximide, barbiturates, and bromide. Next, they may be the only way of teasing out the tangled effects of polypharmacy. The interactions between drugs, through interference with protein binding and metabolism and by enzyme induction, mean that after a change in dosage, it is simpler to measure drug levels rather than to guess the outcome. Salivary estimates can provide a guide to free carbamazepine and phenytoin (McAuliffe et al. 1977). Levels also give reassurance in those cases in which heroic dosages are needed to produce adequate drug levels in the face of malabsorption or well-induced enzymes. Finally, they can be a guide to compliance—often a problem when a caregiver is faced with a patient who is stronger willed or simply stronger. Diurnal fluctuation requires that several levels be taken to appreciate the full variation from peak to trough and will depend as much on the preparation as on the drug itself. For example, a sugared syrup will be absorbed more rapidly and reach an earlier and higher peak than a tablet. The pattern is modified further by the frequency and timing (especially relative to meals) of dosage. In some cases these routines can alter the exquisite balance between the therapeutic and toxic effects of an AED, but in most, the dosage is crude, fine-tuning is irrelevant, and the medication can be given twice (and occasionally even once) a day. All AEDs come with their complement of adverse effects. They are used from an early age, over long periods of time, in varying combinations with each other, and with different forms of disability. Consequently, chronic effects are frequent and are often missed because of their insidious nature and the camouflage of multiple disability. Long recognized in well-established drugs such as the barbiturates and phenytoin, we are now beginning to discern the complications of newer, apparently cleaner drugs such as carbamazepine and valproate. Most florid is a rare, confusional pseudodementia. It is important to appreciate that all AEDs can exacerbate epilepsy, and this reaction may be dose-dependent or idiosyncratic and specific to that patient. However, at the milder end of the spectrum, caregivers frequently comment on the increased alertness and cheerfulness that follow a drug reduction.

Lamotrigine (Smith et al. 1993; Wallace 1994), topiramate (Glauser 1999), and valproate (Forsythe et al. 1991) are powerful, broad-spectrum anti-epileptics that appear to have little adverse effect on cognition. In addition there may be an improvement in mood (Kastner et al. 1993), which, in the case of lamotrigine, may come within days (see Table 14–1).

Carbamazepine has been reputed to be specific to partial onset seizures, although there is an increasing awareness that it can sedate and can impair learning even to the extent that some patients fare better on phenobarbitone (Mitchell and Chavez 1987). As with phenytoin, there is a therapeutic U-curve (the Goldilocks effect) present here where either too large or too small a dosage can produce an increase in seizure frequency. In the case of carbamazepine, which stimulates the secretion of anti-iuretic hormone, the U may well represent the outcome of an anti-epileptic effect being undermined by water intoxication (Perucca et al. 1978). Water restriction (Stubbe-Teglbjaerg 1936) and furosemide (Ahmad et al. 1976) have been shown to be effective anti-epileptics. Although acetazolamide has been deemed ineffectual in its own right, it is a very effective adjuvant to carbamazepine (Forsythe et al. 1981) with the sub-

Table 14–1. Anti-epileptic drugs: an approximate treatment sequence for epilepsy in mental retardation

Lamotrigine

Valproate

   (+ Ethosuximide when myoclonic phenomena prominent)

Carbamazepine (but may exacerbate myoclonic phenomena)

   + Imipramine (low dose)

   + Calcium blockers (cinnarizine/flunarizine/nifedipine/amlodipine)

   + Clobazam

   + Diuretics (acetazolamide/chlorthalidone)

Topiramate

Tiagabine

Gabapentin

Phenytoin

Barbiturate-primidone/phenobarbitone

Bromide

Note. 1. The sequence requires a gradual phased shift from one drug to the next until satisfactory seizure control is attained. In practice the sequence for an individual will be determined by the efficacy, toxicity, and availability of a drug. 2. The sequence assumes that epilepsy is secondary to the condition producing the mental retardation. If myoclonic phenomena are present they may require separate consideration. +=in combination with.

stitution of chlorthalidone should depression or tolerance develop.

Myoclonic phenomena (myoclonic jerks, atypical absences, atonic-akinetic seizures, and tonic spasms) can be exacerbated by carbamazepine, gabapentine, and tiagabine but respond to valproate and the succinimides, notably ethosuximide and methsuximide; the latter may control complex partial seizures as well (Tennison et al. 1991). They also respond to benzodiazepines, and clonazepam has been singled out, although clobazam and nitrazepam also have their place. Clonazepam's propensity to increase and thicken secretions makes it unsuitable for those with a more severe physical disability with whom respiratory infections are a major concern. Benzodiazepines, like barbiturates and alcohol, may produce a paradoxical disinhibition that greatly increases a patient's irritability and hyperactivity, testing all limits. The frequent development of tolerance to the antiepileptic effect within weeks or months further limits their utility, although they can provide a temporary crutch to cope with an episode of infection or a cluster of seizures. With clobazam, which is used as an adjunct, tolerance may be less frequent or only partial, but, unfortunately, mental retardation may mean an ill-sustained response for complex partial seizures (Canadian Clobazam Cooperative Group 1991; Heller et al. 1989).

Imipramine has the same suppressant effect on cortifugal inhibition as ethosuximide and trimethadione. A clinical trial, using doses of up to 200 mg/day, found it to be effective in the control of absence, myoclonic, and akinetic seizures, as well as improving mood and attention, although generalized motor and complex partial seizures were made worse if not covered by another AED. Although 75% of the cases responded initially, the effects were sustained in only 20% (Fromm et al. 1972). As an adjuvant in lower dosage (10–20 mg/day), it occasionally produces a dramatic improvement in both groups of seizures and a safe and well-established drug with a rapid onset of effect, it warrants early trial.

Calcium blockers are being tried in a variety of conditions, including migraine, dementia, Tourette's syndrome, bipolar affective disorder, and epilepsy. The focus has been on the piperazine group of calcium overload blockers (flunarizine, cinnarizine) because of their potency to enter the brain (Overweg et al. 1986). However, both the dihydropyridine (nifedipine, amlodipine) and phenylalanine (verapamil) calcium channel blockers are also effective. This begs the question as to whether some seizures have a vascular underlay—an issue similar to that raised by the response to oligoallergenic diets. As yet, calcium blockers have been used only as adjuvants, and their place has yet to be established.

Vigabatrin may be effective in West and Lennox-Gastaut syndromes (Chiron et al. 1990) as well as have a sustained effect in about one-third of mentally disabled adults (Matiainen et al. 1989; Pitkanen et al. 1993). Adverse effects appear to be related to dosage as well as to incompatibility with other drugs. After an initial drowsiness, its major limitations appear to be an increase in irritability and psychiatric disturbance, but this rarely amounts to psychosis (Sander et al. 1991). Although a gradual introduction as well as the reduction of other AEDs will often avoid these unwanted effects, the discovery that it can reduce the visual fields (not easy to detect in someone with mental retardation) severely restricts its use.

Phenytoin is well tried and effective but, because of its pharmacokinetics, is prone to unwitting overdosage. It has given way to newer drugs, such as valproate and carbamazepine, which are perceived as having fewer adverse effects, although much of phenytoin's reputation is rooted in chronic overdosage. Of particular concern is the possibility that phenytoin might be associated with a chronic encephalopathy affecting both cognition and cerebellar function (Besag 1988). The effects of hirsuties and coarsened features are also underrated. Although short stature has been ascribed to this drug (McGowan 1983), this has not been supported by a study following children up to puberty (Tada et al. 1986). Barbiturates (e.g., phenobarbitone and primidone) are well established, well tested, and well known, yet their side effects, particularly depression, paradoxical excitement, and irritability, still pass unrecognized (Poindexter et al. 1993). As with phenytoin, their use is limited by cognitive and mood impairment.

Potassium bromide was introduced by Locock in 1857 to suppress seizures induced by masturbatory hyperexcitability. Although its use started to decline from the advent of phenobarbitone in 1912, it is not yet redundant (Ramsay and Slater 1993) and has the advantage of being cleared through the kidney. Drowsiness and acneiform skin eruptions are the main adverse effects but reputedly less so in childhood. Serum monitoring should forestall the creep to the higher levels and the more severe effects such as psychosis and neurological abnormality.

Other AEDs are being developed and other treatments evaluated. High-dosage, parenteral γ-globulin can produce a lasting change in some (Ariizumi et al. 1983; Bedini et al. 1985; Sandstedt et al. 1984), which may be limited to those with a deficit of IgG2 (Duse et al. 1986). Other reports, such as of the effectiveness of naloxone (Turner and Stewart 1991), reinforce the idea that epilepsy is a heterogeneous condition that presents itself in various forms and requires various responses.

Enzyme induction lowers folate levels and these should be monitored. It is doubtful that supplementation helps phenytoin-induced gingival hyperplasia (Backman et al. 1989; Brown et al. 1991) or disturbance (Deb 1994). An uncontrolled, open trial suggested that the combination of folate with vitamin B_{12} produces a general improvement in fit frequency, mood, and behavior (Neubauer 1970). Enzyme induction, malabsorption, a suboptimal diet, and little exposure to sunlight can result in vitamin D deficiency. When present, it is usually subclinical and may be more a characteristic of institutionalized people with mental retardation (Deb et al. 1985). Serum calcium and alkaline phosphatase might be monitored, the bone iso-enzyme being assayed only when clinical osteomalacia is suspected.

■ DIET

Ketogenic Diet

The ketogenic diet, high in fat and low in carbohydrate, followed from the observation that starvation stopped seizures. The mechanism is unknown, and factors such as the level of ketosis or of acidosis only apply to some. Livingstone (1972) gives details of the classical diet, although the fat content, together with the vitamin supplements, not only is unpalatable but also can cause nausea, abdominal discomfort, and diarrhea. In addition, the reduction in carbohydrate is so restrictive that wholehearted consent to treatment is important. Poor compliance led to the use of medium-chain triglycerides (MCTs) as an alternative to some of the fat; being more ketogenic, the diet is less restrictive of carbohydrate intake—Clark and House (1987) provide a recipe. An emulsion may be more acceptable than oil (Sills et al. 1986), although palatability is an idiosyncratic characteristic and many enjoy the cream and butter of the classical diet. Given compliance, the variants seem equally effective (Schwarz et al. 1989). The very restrictive diet is an ideal focus for a food battle, and although some centers report a high level of success, both initial and sustained, this may say as much about their enthusiasm and charisma as about the diet.

Oligoallergenic Diet

Epilepsy has been associated with immunological anomalies, and a large number of reports link seizures or EEG abnormalities with allergic disorders. The oligoallergenic diet removes most varieties of foodstuff, certainly those to which reactions have been frequently reported, for several weeks. Egger et al. (1989) found that in cases in which there was a coexistent migraine, such a diet gave a global response, improving both the epilepsy and the migraine. The migraine may be the trigger for an otherwise latent epilepsy in that when the migraine persisted, the epilepsy did, too.

■ SURGERY

Until now surgery has been largely reserved for epilepsy that has not responded to medication. Some of the results, with improvements not only in seizure control but also in behavior, personality, and intelligence, suggest that it should be considered more readily, particularly in childhood (Lindsey et al. 1984). More extensive reviews are provided by Polkey and Binnie (1993) and Devinsky and Pacia (1993).

The best tried and most successful approach is resection of the offending area of the brain (usually a temporal lobectomy), which ranges from removal of a carefully circumscribed area of cortex through to stripping a hemisphere. The seizures must originate from a single area, and if a mirror focus has developed in the other hemisphere, it must not be sufficiently independent to continue generating seizures on its own. There are encouraging early results from subpial transection—a grid is cut in the offending cortex. This prevents the cortex from generating paroxysmal activity by cutting horizontal fibers while preserving physiological function by sparing the vertical fibers.

The second approach is to interrupt the neural pathways by which the epileptic discharge is spread and amplified. This can be done with a stereotactically placed lesion in a variety of sites, including the thalamus, globus pallidus, or amygdala. When a single discrete focus cannot be identified, an alternate approach is to section fiber connections such as those of the temporal lobe or corpus callosum, the latter being particularly effective for atonic seizures. Limited, staged surgery has reduced the risk of a devastating disruption of psychological function such as in the disconnection syndromes. The third approach is that of neural stimulation. This is complex and requires the tuning of a large number of variables, including the electrode site, size and the length, shape, frequency, and current of the pulse as well as its timing, whether continuous, intermittent, or reflex. Cerebellar stimulation, as much art as science, was discredited by controlled trials (Wright et al. 1985), but the vagus nerve is more accessible and its stimulation holds promise (Vagal Stimulation 1990).

Whatever the approach, success depends on careful investigation and subject selection. The level of experience and skill required limit surgery to specialist centers. The battery of investigations alone can be a sufficient ordeal not to be undertaken lightly, particularly when the ability to give consent is an issue. Any conclusions about success must include long-term (at least 5 years) outcome.

■ CONCLUSIONS

Epilepsy is a major component of the practice of mental retardation psychiatry, with a substantial proportion of patients being considered intractable. Nevertheless, time heals or at least improves, and medication should be rationalized regularly. Specialists must be aware of the breadth and novelty of the range of available treatments as new AEDs are released and surgery becomes more practicable. However, the management of epilepsy requires more than simply stopping fits; it includes helping the patient and his or her caregivers to enjoy their lives fully.

■ REFERENCES

Ahmad S, Clarke L, Hewett AJ, et al: Controlled trial of furosemide in focal epilepsy. Br J Clin Pharmacol 3:621–625, 1976

Alvarez N: Discontinuance of antiepileptic medications in patients with developmental disability and diagnosis of epilepsy. Am J Ment Retard 93(6):593–599, 1989

Annegers JF, Hauser WA, Elveback LR, et al: Remission of seizures and relapse in patients with epilepsy. Epilepsia 20:729–737, 1979

Ansakorpi H, Korpelainen JT, Svominen K, et al: Interictal cardiovascular autonomic responses in patients with temporal lobe epilepsy. Epilepsia 41:42–47, 2000

Appleton RE: The Landau-Kleffner syndrome. Arch Dis Child 72(5):386–387, 1995

Ariizumi M, Shiiara H, Hibio S, et al: High dose gammaglobulin for intractable childhood epilepsy. Lancet 2:162–163, 1983

Backman N, Holm A-K, Hanstrom L, et al: Folate treatment of diphenylhydantoin-induced gingival hyperplasia. Scandanavian Journal of Dental Research 97:222–232, 1989

Baldwin RW, Kenny TJ: Thioridazine in the management of organic behavior disturbances in children. Current Therapeutic Research 8:373–377, 1966

Balish M, Albert PS, Theodore WH: Seizure frequency in intractable partial epilepsy: a statistical analysis. Epilepsia 32:642–649, 1991

Bedini R, de Feo MR, Orano A, et al: Effects of g-globulin therapy in severely epileptic children. Epilepsia 26:98–102, 1985

Beghi E, Bollini P, Di Mascio R, et al: Effects of rationalizing drug treatment of patients with epilepsy and mental retardation. Dev Med Child Neurol 29:363–369, 1987

Benson E: The Geschwind syndrome, in Neurobehavioral Problems in Epilepsy: Advances in Neurology, Vol 55. Edited by Smith DB, Treimann DM, Trimble MR. New York, Raven, 1991, pp 190–205

Berney TP, Osselton JW, Kolvin I, et al: Effect of discotheque environment on epileptic children. BMJ 282:180–182, 1981

Besag FMC: Cognitive deterioration in children with epilepsy, in Epilepsy, Behavior and Cognitive Function. Edited by Trimble MR, Reynolds EH. Chichester, UK, Wiley, 1988, pp 79–91

Bourgeois BFD: Antiepileptic drug combinations and experimental background: the case of phenobarbital and phenytoin. Arches of Pharmacology 333:406–411, 1986

Bourgeois BFD: Combination of valproate and ethosuximide: antiepileptic and neurotoxic interaction. J Pharmacol Exp Ther 247:1128–1132, 1988a

Bourgeois BFD: Anticonvulsant potency and neurotoxicity of valproate alone and in combination with carbamazepine or phenobarbital. Clin Neuropharmacol 11:348–359, 1988b

Brorson LO, Wranne L: Long-term prognosis in childhood epilepsy: survival and seizure prognosis. Epilepsia 28:324–330, 1987

Brown RS, Di Stanislao PT, Beaver WT, et al: The administration of folic acid to institutionalized epileptic adults with phenytoin-induced gingival hyperplasia: a double-blind, randomized, placebo-controlled, parallel study. Oral Surgery, Oral Medicine, and Oral Pathology 71(5):565–568, 1991

Browne TR, Dreifuss FE, Dyken PR, et al: Ethosuximide in the treatment of absence (petit mal) seizures. Neurology 25:515–524, 1975

Canadian Clobazam Cooperative Group: Clobazam in treatment of refractory epilepsy: the Canadian experience—a retrospective study. Epilepsia 32:407–416, 1991

Carter CH: Prochlorperazine in emotionally disturbed, mentally defective children. South Med J 52:174–178, 1959

Chadwick DW: Overuse of monitoring of blood concentrations of antiepileptic drugs. BMJ 294:723–724, 1987

Chadwick DW: Do anticonvulsants alter the natural course of epilepsy? Case for early treatment is not established. BMJ 310:177–178, 1995

Chiron C, Dulac O, Luna D, et al: Vigabatrin in infantile spasms. Lancet 335:363–364, 1990

Clark BJ, House FM: Medium chain triglyceride oil ketogenic diets in the treatment of childhood epilepsy. J Human Nut 32:111–116, 1987

Collacott RA: Epilepsy, dementia and adaptive behavior in Down's syndrome. J Intellect Disabil Res 37:153–160, 1993

Collacott RA, Dignon A, Hauck A, et al: Clinical and therapeutic monitoring of epilepsy in a mental handicap unit. Br J Psychiatry 155:522–525, 1989

Coulter DL: Frontal lobe seizures: no evidence of self-injury. Am J Ment Retard 96:81–85, 1991

Coyle HP, Baker BN, Brown SW: Coroners' autopsy reporting of sudden unexplained death in epilepsy (SUDEP) in the UK. Seizure 3(4):247–254, 1994

Deb S: Effect of folate metabolism on the psychopathology of adults with mental retardation and epilepsy. Am J Ment Retard 98(6):717–723, 1994

Deb S, Hunter D: Psychopathology of people with mental handicap and epilepsy; I: maladaptive behavior. Br J Psychiatry 159:822–826, 1991a

Deb S, Hunter D: Psychopathology of people with mental handicap and epilepsy; II: psychiatric illness. Br J Psychiatry 159:826–830, 1991b

Deb S, Hunter D: Psychopathology of people with mental handicap and epilepsy; III: personality disorder. Br J Psychiatry 159:830–834, 1991c

Deb S, Cowie VA, Tsanaclis LM, et al: Calcium homeostasis in mentally handicapped epileptic patients. Journal of Mental Deficiency Research 29:403–410, 1985

Devinsky O, Pacia S: Epilepsey surgery. Neorologic Clinics 11:951–971, 1993

Donat JF, Wright FS: Episodic symptoms mistaken for seizures in the neurologically impaired child. Neurology 40:156–157, 1990

Duse M, Tiberti S, Plebani A, et al: IgG2 deficiency and intractable epilepsy of childhood. Monogr Allergy 20:128–134, 1986

Egger J, Carter CM, Soothill JF, et al: Oligoantigenic diet treatment of children with epilepsy and migraine. J Pediatr 114:51–58, 1989

Espie CA, Pashley AS, Bonham KG, et al: The mentally handicapped person with epilepsy: a comparative study investigating psychosocial functioning. Journal of Mental Deficiency Research 33:123–135, 1989

Espie CA, Paul A, Graham M, et al: The Epilepsy Outcome Scale: the development of a measure for use with carers of people with epilepsy plus intellectual disability. J Intelect Disabil Res 42:90–96, 1998

Fischbacher E: Effect of reduction of anticonvulsants on well-being. BMJ 285:423–424, 1982

Forsythe I, Butler R, Berg I, et al: Cognitive impairment in new cases of epilepsy randomly assigned to carbamazepine, phenytoin and sodium valproate. Dev Med Child Neurol 33:524–534, 1991

Forsythe WI, Owens JR, Toothill C: Effectiveness of acetazolamide in the treatment of carbamazepine-resistant epilepsy in children. Dev Med Child Neurol 23:761–769, 1981

Fromm GH, Amores CY, Thies W: Imipramine in epilepsy. Arch Neurol 27:198–204, 1972

Gedye A: Episodic rage and aggression attributed to frontal lobe seizures. Journal of Mental Deficiency Research 33:369–379, 1989a

Gedye A: Extreme self-injury attributed to frontal lobe seizures. Am J Ment Retard 94(1):20–26, 1989b

Gedye A: The self-injury hypothesis: addressing a neurologist's concerns. Am J Ment Retard 96:85–94, 1991

Gillberg C: The treatment of epilepsy in autism. J Autism Dev Disord 21(1):61–77, 1991

Gluaser TA: Topiramate. Epilepsia 40:71–80, 1999

Goulden KJ, Shinnar S, Koller H, et al: Epilepsy in children with mental retardation: a cohort study. Epilepsia 32:690–697, 1991

Heller AJ, Ring HA, Reynolds EH: Clobazam for chronic epilepsy: factors relating to a dramatic response, in Chronic Epilepsy: Its Prognosis and Management. Edited by Trimble MR. London, Wiley, 1989, pp 163–185

Holmes GL, McKeever M, Russman BS: Abnormal behavior or epilepsy? Use of long-term EEG and video monitoring with severely to profoundly mentally retarded patients with seizures. American Journal of Mental Deficiency 87(4):456–458, 1983

Hunt A, Stores G: Sleep disorder and epilepsy in children with tuberous sclerosis: a questionnaire-based study. Dev Med Child Neurol 36:108–115, 1994

James DH: Neuroleptics and epilepsy in mentally handicapped patients. Journal of Mental Deficiency Research 30:185–189, 1986

Jann MW, Fidone GS: Effect of influenza vaccine on serum anticonvulsant concentrations. Clinical Pharmacology 5:817–820, 1986

Jay GW, Leestma JE: Sudden death in epilepsy. Acta Neurol Scand 63(suppl 82):1–66, 1981

Julius SC, Brenner RP: Myoclonic seizures with lithium. Biol Psychiatry 22:1184–1190, 1987

Kasteleijn-Nolst Trenite DGA, Smit AM, Velis DN, et al: On-line detection of transient neuropsychological disturbances during EEG discharges in children with epilepsy. Dev Med Child Neurol 32:46–50, 1990

Kastner T A, Finesmith R, Walsh K: Long-term administration of valproic acid in the treatment of affective symptoms in people with mental retardation. J Clin Psychopharmacol 13(6):448–451, 1993

Kuijer A: Epilepsy and exercise. Doctoral thesis, University of Amsterdam, 1978

Laminack L: Carbamazepine for behavioral disorders. Am J Ment Retard 94:563–564, 1990

Langee HR: A retrospective study of mentally retarded patients with behavioral disorders who were treated with carbamazepine. Am J Ment Retard 93:640–643, 1989

Leicester J: Temper tantrums, epilepsy and episodic dyscontrol. Br J Psychiatry 141:262–266, 1982

Lindsey J, Glaser G, Richards P, et al: Developmental aspects of focal epilepsies of childhood treated by neurosurgery. Dev Med Child Neurol 26:574–587, 1984

Livingston M, Berney TP: Bowel function and epilepsy (abstract). Seizure 1(suppl A):P4/03, 1992

Livingstone S: Comprehensive Management of Epilepsy in Infancy, Childhood, and Adolescence. Springfield, IL, Charles C Thomas, 1972

Matilainen R, Pitkanen A, Ruutiainen T, et al: Vigabatrin in epilepsy in mentally retarded patients. Br J Clin Pharmacol 27:113s–118s, 1989

Mattson RH: Emotional effects on seizure occurrence, in Neurobehavioral Problems in Epilepsy: Advances in Neurology, Vol 55. Edited by Smith DB, Treimann DM, Trimble MR. New York, Raven, 1991, pp 71–83

McAuliffe JJ, Sherwin AL, Leppik IE, et al: Salivary levels of anticonvulsants: a practical approach to drug monitoring. Neurology 27:409–413, 1977

McGowan MEL: Final adult height of patients with epilepsy. Dev Med Child Neurol 25:591–594, 1983

Medical Research Council AED Withdrawal Study Group: Prognostic index for recurrence of seizures after remission of epilepsy. BMJ 306:1374–1378, 1993

Meijer JW: Knowledge, attitude and practice in antiepileptic drug monitoring. Acta Neurol Scand 82(suppl 134):1–128, 1991

Mitchell WG, Chavez JM: Carbamazepine versus phenobarbitone for partial onset seizures in children. Epilepsia 28:56–60, 1987

Monroe R: Episodic Behavioural Disorders: A Psychodynamic and Neurophysiologic Analysis. Cambridge, MA, Harvard University Press, 1970

Musumeci SA, Colognola RM, Ferri R, et al: Fragile-X syndrome: a particular epileptogenic EEG pattern. Epilepsia 29:41–47, 1988

Neill JC, Alvarez N: Differential diagnosis of epileptic versus pseudoepileptic seizures in developmentally disabled persons. Applied Research in Mental Retardation 7:285–298, 1986

Neubauer C: Mental deterioration in epilepsy due to folate deficiency. BMJ 2:759–761, 1970

Nousiainen U, Mervaala E, Uusitupa M, et al: Cardiac arrhythmias in the differential diagnosis of epilepsy. J Neurol 236:93–96, 1989

Ojemann LM, Baugh-Bookman BS, Dudley DL: Effect of psychotropic medications on seizure control in patients with epilepsy. Neurology 37:1525–1527, 1987

Overweg J, Ashton D, de Beukelaar F, et al: Add-on therapy in epilepsy with calcium blockers. Eur Neurol 25(suppl 1):93–101, 1986

Perucca E, Garratt A, Hebdige S, et al: Water intoxication in epileptic patients receiving carbamazepine. J Neurol Neurosurg Psychiatry 41:713–718, 1978

Pisani F, Oter IG, Russo M, et al: The efficacy of valproate-lamotrigine co-medication in refractory complex partial seizures: evidence for a psychodynamic interaction. Epilepsia 40:1141–1146, 1999

Poindexter AR, Berglund JA, Kolstoe PD: Changes in antiepileptic drug prescribing patterns in large institutions: preliminary results of a five-year experience. Special issue: epilepsy and mental retardation. American Journal on Mental Retardation 98(suppl):34–40, 1993

Polkey CE, Binnie CD: Neurosurgical treatment of epilepsy, in A Textbook of Epilepsy. Edited by Laidlaw J, Richens A, Chadwick D. London, Churchill Livingstone, 1993, pp 561–612

Ramsay RE, Slater JD: Bromides, in The Treatment of Epilepsy. Edited by Wyllie E. Philadelphia, PA, Lea & Febiger, 1993, pp 955–958

Reid AH, Naylor GJ, Kay DSG: A double-blind, placebo controlled, crossover trial of carbamazepine in overactive, severely mentally handicapped patients. Psychol Med 11:109–113, 1981

Reynolds EH: Do anticonvulsants alter the natural course of epilepsy? Treatment should be started as early as possible. BMJ 310:176–177, 1995

Rowan AJ, Meijer JWA, Beer de-Pawlikokwski N, et al: Valproate-ethosuximide combination therapy for refractory absence seizures. Arch Neurol 40:797–802, 1983

Sander JWAS, Hart YM, Trimble MR, et al: Vigabatrin and psychosis. J Neurol Neurosurg Psychiatry 54:435–439, 1991

Sandstedt P, Kostulas V, Larsson LK: Intravenous gammaglobulin for post-encephalitic epilepsy. Lancet 2:1154–1155, 1984

Schwarz RH, Eaton J, Bower BD: Ketogenic diets in the treatment of epilepsy: short-term clinical effects. Dev Med Child Neurol 31:145–151, 1989

Scott R, Besag F, Neville B: Buccal midazolam and rectal diazepam for teatment of prolonged seizures in childhood and adolescence: a randomised trial. Lancet 353(2): 623–626, 1999

Shepherd C, Hosking G: Epilepsy in school children with intellectual impairments in Sheffield: the size and nature of the problem and the implications for service provision. Journal of Mental Deficiency Research 33:511–514, 1989

Shorvon SD, Chadwick D, Galbraith AW, et al: One drug for epilepsy. BMJ 1:474–476, 1977

Sillanpaa M: Children with epilepsy as adults: outcome after 30 years of follow-up. Acta Paediatrica Scandinavica Supplement 368:1–78, 1990

Sills MA, Forsythe WI, Haidukewych D, et al: The medium chain triglyceride diet and intractable epilepsy. Arch Dis Child 61(12):1168–1172, 1986

Smith D, Chadwick D, Baker G, et al: Seizure severity and the quality of life. Epilepsia 34(5):S31–S35, 1993

Stafstrom CE, Konkol RJ: Infantile spasms in children with Down syndrome. Dev Med Child Neurol 36:576–585, 1994

Stefanatos GA, Grover W, Geller E: Case study: corticosteroid treatment of language regression in pervasive developmental disorder. J Am Acad Child Adolesc Psychiatry 34:1107–1111, 1995

Stores G: Types of childhood epilepsy misdiagnosed as psychiatric disorder. European Journal of Child and Adolescent Psychiatry 1(4):222–226, 1992

Stubbe-Teglbjaerg HP: Investigations on epilepsy and water metabolism. Acta Psychiatrica et Neurologica Scandinavica 9:1–247, 1936

Tada H, Wallace SJ, Hughes IA: Height in epilepsy. Arch Dis Child 61:1224–1226, 1986

Tennison MB, Greenwood MD, Miles MV: Methsuximide for intractable childhood seizures. Pediatrics 87:186–189, 1991

Tennison M, Greenwood R, Lewis D, et al: Discontinuing antiepileptic drugs in children with epilepsy: a comparison of a six-week and a nine-month taper period. N Engl J Med 330(20):1407–1410, 1994

Toone BK, Fenton GW: Epileptic seizures induced by psychotropic drugs. Psychol Med 7:265–270, 1977

Treiman DM: Psychobiology of ictal aggression, in Neurobehavioral Problems in Epilepsy: Advances in Neurology, Vol 55. Edited by Smith DB, Treiman DM, Trimble MR. New York, Raven, 1991, pp 325–336

Turner M, Stewart M: Reversal of unconsciousness by use of naloxone in a profoundly mentally handicapped epileptic. Journal of Mental Deficiency Research 35:81–84, 1991

Tyrer SP, Walsh A, Edwards DE, et al: Factors associated with a good response to lithium in aggressive mentally handicapped subjects. Prog NeuroPsychopharmacol Biol Psychiatry 8:751–755, 1984

Vagal stimulation. Epilepsia 31(suppl 2), 1990

Verduyn CM, Stores G, Missen A: A survey of mothers' impressions of seizure precipitants in children with epilepsy. Epilepsia 29:251–255, 1988

Wallace SJ: Lamotrigine: a clinical overview. Seizure 3(suppl A):47–51, 1994

Wright GDS, McLellan DL, Brice JG: A double-blind trial of chronic cerebellar stimulation in twelve patients with severe epilepsy. J Neurol Neurosurg Psychiatry 47:769–774, 1985

15 Mood and Affect as Determinants of Psychotropic Drug Therapy

*Response in Mentally Retarded Persons
With Organic Mental Syndromes*

Robert Sovner, M.D.
Michael Lowry, Ph.D.

In mentally retarded persons, central nervous system (CNS) dysfunction is considered to be an important factor in the genesis and maintenance of maladaptive behaviors such as self-injury, aggression, and stereotypy (Jancar 1979; Lewis and McLean 1982; Menolascino et al. 1986; Reid 1982; Reid et al. 1984; Roberts 1986). Shortly after the introduction of chlorpromazine in the mid-1950s, antipsychotics became the principal form of pharmacotherapy for the management of these organic mental syndromes[1] despite the lack of clearly demonstrated efficacy and the potential for these drugs to produce serious adverse reactions (see review by Lipman et al. 1978). It has been only during the past decade that neuropsychiatry has begun to refine response predictors and develop innovative (and nonneuroleptic) drug interventions (Baumeister and Sevin 1990; Gualtieri 1991; Ratey 1991).

---

[1]We have used the term *organic mental syndrome* from the DSM-III-R (American Psychiatric Association 1987) to refer to any disturbance in behavior or psychological function related to CNS disease irrespective of whether or not the etiology is known. (ICD-9 [Kramer et al. 1979] uses the term *organic psychotic conditions* to describe the same clinical phenomena.) In our opinion, the DSM-IV (American Psychiatric Association 1994) category of *mental disorders due to a general medical condition* does not deal with the issue of perinatal CNS dysfunction because it assumes that all "organic" disorders begin later in life (Sovner 1992).

A major problem in the pharmacological management of organic mental syndromes is drug selection. What criteria should be used to select specific psychotropic agents? We believe that overt behavior such as aggression and self-injury are too nonspecific to predict drug response. In this chapter, we propose that disruptions in the psychological operations that maintain and regulate mood and affect can be used instead of behavior to predict drug response. In particular, irritability, overarousal, excitement, and rage attacks are common drug-responsive manifestations of CNS dysfunction.

■ NEUROPSYCHIATRIC ASPECTS OF IRRITABILITY, OVERAROUSAL, EXCITEMENT, AND RAGE

Irritability

Clinical Characteristics

Irritability can be defined as a state of excessive, easily provoked anger, annoyance, or impatience (Goldenson 1984). The irritable individual is hostile and prone to explosive outbursts (e.g., tantrums in the developmentally disabled). Factor I of the Aberrant Behavior Checklist (irritability, agitation, and crying), for example, describes a variety of irritability-related behaviors: self-injury, aggression, temper tantrums, inappropriate crying and screaming, and demands that must be met immediately (Aman et al. 1985).

In addition to its association with both depression and mania (American Psychiatric Association 1994), irritability is a common sequela of traumatic brain injury (Silver et al. 1987), pre-ictal states (Fenwick 1989), dementia (Yudofsky et al. 1990), encephalitis (Hierons et al. 1978), Tourette's disorder (Goldman 1988), and metabolic disorders such as Wilson's disease (Dening and Berrios 1989). Reid et al. (1978), in a survey of 100 randomly selected mentally retarded persons with severe or profound disabilities, found that 32% were irritable. Matin and Rundle (1980) found that 15 of 17 (88%) severely mentally retarded individuals, who had been identified as having significant self-injurious behavior (SIB), were also irritable. On the other hand, Ballinger et al. (1991) reported that only 9% of their sample was irritable. This lower figure probably reflects that their sample included individuals with mild disabilities as well as those with more severe ones.

Irritability appears to be associated with alterations in CNS levels of serotonin (Coccaro 1989). Both animal and clinical research suggest that deficits in serotonergic inhibition of nigrostriatal dopaminergic activity mediate irritability (see reviews by Cloninger 1987 and Coccaro 1989).

Treatment

If pathological irritability reflects an imbalance between serotonergic and dopaminergic neuronal activity with a shift toward the latter (see previous discussion), then drugs that increase CNS serotonergic activity (e.g., fluoxetine, trazodone, lithium) or decrease dopaminergic activity (neuroleptics) should be useful in its management. Sheard (1984), for example, observed that both lithium and carbamazepine are effective for those conditions in which irritability was a primary feature, irrespective of diagnosis; both drugs affect serotonergic activity (Coccaro 1989).

Irritability can be an underlying determinant of SIB, which occurs in demand situations. Therefore, recent reports of the successful treatment of SIB with serotonergic agents may be due to a reduction in irritability (Sovner 1990b; Sovner et al. 1993). Markowitz (1992) used fluoxetine to treat SIB in eight mentally retarded persons with severe or profound disabilities. All patients were receiving concomitant neuroleptic drug therapy and one was also receiving lithium. Improvement was considered marked in five patients, moderate in one, and mild in the remaining two. A diet high in serotonin-containing foods was successfully used by Gedye (1990) to treat a 26-year-old woman with Down's syndrome and profound mental retardation who also had severe, chronic, and treatment-resistant SIB.

In mentally retarded persons, neuroleptic agents have been used to moderate irritability associated with temper tantrums (Sovner 1988) and aggression/SIB (Gualtieri and Schroeder 1989). Carbamazepine has been reported to be effective for treating combativeness and irritability in nondisabled patients with Alzheimer's disease (Gleason and Schneider 1990; Marin and Greenwald 1989; Patterson 1987).

Proposal for an Organic Irritability Syndrome

Irritability may be a primary feature of a distinct organic mental syndrome, which we have termed organic irritability syndrome (Sovner 1990b). Reid et al. (1978), in their cluster analysis, identified 8 residents who had in common a triad of features, including irritability with or without overactivity, chaotic sleep pattern, and severe maladaptive behavior. Matin and Rundle (1980) also found that irritability and a sleep disturbance were much more likely to occur in a group of 17 residents with severe or profound disabilities and severe SIB than in a control group of 14 with similar disabilities, but not SIB. In addition, there have been four published case reports that are consistent with this syndrome. Sovner (1988) presented treatment data for a 25-year-old woman with severe disabilities associated with congenital rubella (associated with irritability and disrupted sleep) who responded to carbamazepine with normalization of her sleep and a marked decrease in maladaptive behavior related to irritability. Sovner and Hurley (1989) described a 44-year-old woman with severe mental retardation secondary to congenital syphilis whose chronic overactivity, interrupted sleep, tantrums, and self-injury responded to lithium. O'Neil et al. (1986) treated a 22-year-old man with Cornelia de Lange syndrome who presented disrupted sleep, aggression, temper tantrums, and self-injurious behavior. The patient responded to a combination of trazodone 200 mg qhs and L-tryptophan 23 gm qd. (This patient had low pretreatment whole blood serotonin levels.) Kastner et al. (1990) used valproic acid to treat a 13-year-old girl with profound mental retardation secondary to a congenital rubella infection and a 7-year history of hyperactivity, irritability, aggressiveness, and self-injurious behavior associated with a sleep disturbance. Lastly, Welch and Sovner (1992) successfully treated with dextromethorphan (which acts as a presynaptic reuptake blocker of serotonin) a 25-year-old man with congenital rubella and a lifelong history of overactivity, irritability, a "chaotic" sleep pattern, self-injury, and aggression.

Our diagnostic criteria for this proposed organic mental syndrome are listed in Table 15–1. The absence of true hyposomnia and an excited/euphoric mood argues against this disorder being a variant of a manic illness. Organic irritability syndrome would correspond to Blumer et al.'s (1990) irritable-impulsive disorder in their classification of the "neurobehavioral disorders of epilepsy," which they believed could also serve as a more general taxonomy of psychiatric disorders related to CNS dysfunction.

Organic irritability syndrome may reflect limbic system dysfunction. In their study of limbic encephalitis, Hierons et al. (1978) described a patient with childhood onset viral encephalitis associated with developmental disabilities, irritability, overactivity, and aggression. Autopsy findings included virtually the complete destruction of her right temporal lobe. Rabies, which also affects the limbic system, can produce a behavioral syndrome suggestive of our proposed syndrome (Papez 1937).

Overarousal

Clinical Characteristics

Overarousal can be defined as a state of inappropriate alertness and readiness for action (Goldenson 1984). Overaroused individuals are in a state of hypervigilance associated with autonomic activation (i.e., a state of readiness for flight or fight activities). Behavioral concomitants include agitation (i.e., increased motor activity associated with a state of tension), distractibility, and impulsivity.

Overarousal may be a pathological phenomenon associated with attention-deficit/hyperactivity disorder (Voeller 1991) or brain-stem dysfunction in

Table 15–1.   Diagnostic criteria for proposed organic irritability syndrome

All of the following are required:

A. A persistent mood state characterized by irritability that may manifest itself by tantrums, self-injury, or aggression
B. Persistent sleep disturbance characterized by an irregular sleep pattern with at least 25% of nights per month with less than 4 hours of total sleep time
C. Onset during childhood or infancy
D. Evidence of an organic factor such as brain injury or the presence of moderate or greater developmental disabilities
E. Absence of another mental disorder such as rapid-cycling bipolar disorder

An associated feature may be pervasive overactivity.

such conditions as delirium. In mentally retarded persons, especially those with a pervasive developmental disorder, repetitive motor behavior and social withdrawal can be associated with overarousal and may represent adaptive responses to this state (Walters et al. 1990). There are little data on the prevalence of overarousal in this population, but high levels of arousal are considered to be a characteristic feature of atypical pervasive developmental disorders (Cohen et al 1987), fragile X syndrome (Hagerman and Sobesky 1989), and Cornelia de Lange syndrome (O'Neil et al. 1986).

Arousal is associated with increased activity in the locus coeruleus and ascending noradrenergic system possibly due to subsensitivity of α_2 autoreceptors or loss of GABAergic- and/or serotonergic-mediated inhibition of adrenergic function (Charney and Henninger 1986; Charney et al. 1990; Paul 1988).

Treatment

Antiadrenergic agents such as clonidine (Bond 1986) and β-blockers (Lader 1988) have been reported to be effective in modulating arousal. In mentally retarded persons, most of the research has been with the latter. Both uncontrolled (Ratey et al. 1987) and controlled (Ratey and Lindem 1991) drug trials have demonstrated that β-blocker therapy can decrease SIB and aggression in autistic adults, probably by decreasing arousal.

Buspirone may also be effective in the treatment of arousal-mediated behavior (Ratey et al. 1989, 1991), possibly via serotonergic mechanisms (Eison 1990). Another possible intervention may be naltrexone. Preliminary results from a controlled trial by Campbell et al. (1990) and a case report by Walters et al. (1990) suggest that opiate antagonists may exert their decelerative effect on stereotypic SIB via a downregulation of arousal by altering the endogenous opiate modulation of noradrenergic activity (Charney and Henninger 1986).

Excitement

Clinical Characteristics

Excitement is a mood state characterized by a readiness for precipitous action (i.e., impulsivity) (Goldenson 1984; Wohlman 1991). The excited individual is restless and searching for highly stimulating activities. Excitement is often a concomitant of a manic state. For example, the Inpatient Multidimensional Psychiatric Scale defines *excitement* as an excess and acceleration of the individual's speech and motor activities and also as a lack of restraint in the expression of emotions and feelings. Mood level and self-esteem are usually high (National Institute of Mental Health 1973). The prevalence of excitement in mentally retarded persons is unknown. Sovner (1990a) has proposed that excitement rather than euphoria is the typical mood state observed in profound and severely disabled persons with mania.

Alterations in mesolimbic dopaminergic activity appear to be involved in mediating excitement (Goodwin and Jamison 1990). Also, Cloninger (1987) has proposed that an excess of dopaminergic activity underlies the personality dimension of behavioral activation/novelty seeking, characterized by excitability and impulsivity.

Treatment

There have been several reports describing a chronic maniclike illness in individuals with severe and profound disabilities. Reid et al. (1978), in a cluster analysis of the behavior of 100 such residents of a mental retardation hospital, identified 6 individuals with a longstanding history of hyperactivity associated with elation and/or distractibility. In a subsequent report (Reid et al. 1981), individuals with this profile were reported to be more likely to respond to carbamazepine than a group of overactive residents without elation or overactivity. Sovner (1990a) successfully used divalproex (a valproic acid derivative) to treat a severely handicapped man with the childhood onset of boisterous/excited mood, overactivity, and decreased sleep time associated with severe SIB and aggression.

Excitement and Chronic Mania

We believe that individuals with chronic overactivity, boisterous/excited mood, a sleep disturbance, and distractibility may be suffering from chronic mania, a bipolar variant. It is probably a variant of organic mood syndrome, and the antimanic anticonvulsants (i.e., carbamazepine and valporic acid) may be effective for this disorder (Sovner 1991). This disorder would be subsumed under mood disorders in Blumer et al.'s classification (1990).

Rage

Clinical Characteristics

Rage can be defined as a state of precipitous anger characterized by a "blindly furious impulse to violence and destruction" (Adams and Victor 1986). Rage attacks are a concomitant of brain damage, particularly a sequela of closed head injury. There are little data on the prevalence of rage-associated behavior in persons with mental retardation, but this problem is often the focus of attention in drug therapy (Ruedrich et al. 1990). In the absence of the signs and symptoms of another psychiatric disorder, patients with rage attacks as the primary psychiatric disturbance are usually considered to have a personality change due to a general medical condition, aggressive type, in DSM-IV (American Psychiatric Association 1994; corresponding to organic personality disorder, explosive type, in DSM-III-R [American Psychiatric Association 1987]). This disorder overlaps with the organic aggression syndrome proposed as a distinct disorder by Yudofsky et al. (1990). It is characterized by rage attacks precipitated by minor provocations. The behavior is intermittent, and the patient usually perceives a loss of control during the aggressive acts.

Rage attacks are believed to be mediated via a disinhibition of hypothalamic, amygdaloid, and septal nucleus activity due to cortical dysfunction (Bear 1991; Donovan 1988), possibly mediated via disturbances in adrenergic activity (Leavitt et al. 1990).

Treatment

Rage attacks typically respond to β-blocker therapy (Lader 1988; Ruedrich et al. 1990). The effect of these agents may be twofold: they may have a specific CNS effect of suppressing rage attacks and also moderate nonspecific arousal. The latter action would serve to minimize the aversive effects of stress. Irritability and arousal, for example, tend to lower the threshold for the occurrence of rage attacks.

■ A PSYCHOLOGICAL OPERATIONS–BASED APPROACH TO PSYCHOTROPIC DRUG THERAPY

Our psychotropic drug therapy paradigm is based on the premise that disruptions of regulation of mood- and affect-associated CNS dysfunction can alter the motivational properties of a wide range of environmental stimuli and events by changing the emotional state of the individual. This change, in turn, affects an individual's adaptive responses. The role of affect in organizing cognition and behavior has been reviewed by others (Bradley 1990; Ciompi 1991) and is relevant to this discussion.

Thus, in our treatment model, pharmacotherapy is not directed at maladaptive behavior, per se, but at the dysfunctions in psychological operations. We deal mainly with the role of abnormal mood states in the mediation of maladaptive behavior, but the principles would also apply to other disturbances such as the regulation of attention.

One implication of this approach is that both diagnosis and treatment require mood state assessments. Although maladaptive behavior is an important outcome measure, the measurement of affective responses may also need to be objectively monitored because the behavior in question may serve a variety of functions. Aggression, for example, may be associated with irritability and, at the same time, be a means of nonverbal communication for the affected person.

State-Dependent Learning and Behavior

Evidence in support of our strategy comes from the study of rapid-cycling bipolar disorder in mentally retarded persons. This affective disorder provides a naturally occurring model for the impact of pathological mood states on behavior. Case reports of such patients demonstrate that some maladaptive behavior can be a state-dependent phenomenon of a specific mood state. Reid and Leonard (1977) have described a patient with depression-dependent vomiting, and Lowry and Sovner (1992) have described a case of mania-dependent aggression and one of depression-dependent SIB. These cases argue that biologically mediated alterations in mood can significantly affect a mentally retarded person's adaptive behavioral responses.

The principle of affect-dependent behavior also applies to chronic mood disturbances associated with organic brain disease. To the individual with pathological irritability secondary to CNS dysfunction, for example, many everyday events (simple requests to dress, participate in activities, wait before beginning an activity) become aversive. If SIB or aggression results in the termination or postponement of such aversive irritants, they may become part of the individual's adaptive style via mechanisms of positive and negative reinforcement. Thus, the perception of the aversive nature of a stimulus results in a behavior initiated to manage it (e.g., SIB to modulate an unpleasant affective experience and/or prompt caregivers to remove the stimulus). Pharmacologically decreasing the neurobiological substrate mediating chronic irritability should decrease the individual's level of irritability and, therefore, decrease maladaptive responses because the same events are no longer experienced as aversive.

Role of Neuroleptics

In this chapter, we have deemphasized the role of neuroleptics in the treatment of emotional and behavioral problems associated with CNS dysfunction. We concur with Gualtieri (1991) that the risk-benefit ratio for this drug class is far too low for it to be considered as a first-choice treatment for a behavior associated with an organic mental syndrome.

Use of Multidrug Regimens

In some cases, it may be appropriate to use two or more drugs, each with specific pharmacological actions, to treat behavioral disturbances when more than one psychobiological dysfunction are present (Yudofsky 1991). Thus, one drug for irritability (e.g., a serotonergic antidepressant) and a second one for rage attacks (e.g., a β-blocker) may be required. A summary of some possible treatments of specific mood dysfunctions is provided in Table 15–2.

Value of a Mood and Affect Dysregulation Drug Therapy Strategy

The value of our approach to the use of psychotropic drug therapy to treat organic mental syndromes is threefold:

1. **It provides a way to integrate neurobiological and behavioral concepts.** On the one hand, operant behavioral formulations provide mechanisms of action (i.e., ways to understand the adaptive role of seemingly dysfunctional behavior), but they cannot explain why the individual has had to resort to such responses. On the other hand, neurobiological formulations, which do not take into account the influence of psychosocial factors on brain function, cannot be used as the basis for drug selection. For example, primate research involving the aggressive effects of subcortical stimulation in animals living in naturalistic settings has demonstrated that the electrical stimulation of specific sites will only produce complex aggressive behavior in high-ranking and dominant animals (see discussion by Reynolds 1990). The idea that there is a direct correlation between alterations in neurotransmitter activity and specific behaviors is too simplistic to be of value in drug selection (Hughes et al. 1988).

2. **It facilitates the assessment of whether a specific behavior is drug-responsive and how to treat it.** Determining whether or not a

Table 15–2. Proposed drug therapy options for the treatment of mood and affect disturbances associated with organic brain disease in mentally retarded persons

Psychological dysfunction	Possible behavioral presentation	Psychopharmacological intervention	Comments
Excitement	Aggression, overactivity, self-injury	Carbamazepine, lithium, valproate	May be a reflection of an organic mood syndrome, especially when associated with a sleep disturbance and overactivity.
Irritability	Tantrums with self-injury, aggression	Carbamazepine, lithium, low-dose neuroleptic therapy, serotonergic antidepressants	A sleep disturbance is often present and represents difficulty in regulating sleep-wake cycles rather than an affective disorder.
Overarousal	Aggression, self-injury	Buspirone, β-blockers, clonidine	Usually a problem in autistic individuals and those with fragile X syndrome.
Rage	Aggression, self-injury, swearing	β-blockers	May occur in the absence of other psychopathology.

Note. This table assumes that the indicated behaviors are present in the absence of a classic psychiatric illness such as bipolar disorder. In such cases, treatment should be directed at the underlying condition.

disturbance in one or more psychological operations is present should be an important part of any neuropsychiatric assessment of a developmentally disabled person manifesting clinically significant maladaptive behavior. We believe that evaluating an individual's perceptions, mood state, affect regulation, and other neuropsychological functions is a powerful clinical tool for pharmacotherapy because demonstrating a relationship between behavior and a disturbance in one or more psychological operations provides a way to differentiate drug-responsive subtypes of behavior. We subscribe to Powers's contention that "[o]nce one has identified what the [person] is controlling . . . the relationship of a whole family of seemingly unrelated responses to a whole family of seemingly unrelated stimuli becomes completely predictable (1973, p. 153)."

Unfortunately, the complex interactions between various CNS neurotransmitter systems and the multiple CNS effects of the psychotropic agents, whose therapeutic effects we have described, limit the significance of any discussions of differential efficacy. At this time, however, we believe our approach has heuristic value in selecting possible treatments.

3. **It provides a rationale for selecting subjects for drug studies.** In general, most of the pharmacotherapy research studies in mentally retarded people have focused on the treatment of behavior—the use of lithium to treat aggression exemplifies this research strategy. In general, results have been equivocal and have failed to determine clear-cut response predictors (Craft et al. 1987; Dale 1980; Luchins and Dojka 1989; Spreat et al. 1989; Tyrer et al. 1984; Worrall et al. 1975). We suggest that behavior is too nonspecific to be used in such studies as the principal inclusion criteria.

Subject selection in these studies should take into account the presence of underlying disturbances in psychological operations. Only then can relatively homogeneous populations be studied and hypotheses such as irritability-mediated aggression, for example, be tested.

■ CONCLUSIONS

The treatment of "behavior" in mentally retarded persons, irrespective of the specific modality being considered, must be based on rigorous diagnostic assessment and the recognition that behavior is a final common pathway that can express a multiplicity of biopsychosocial dysfunctions. It seems unlikely to us that, in the near future, drug selection will be based solely on neurochemical assays or tests of neurophysiological function. The choice of specific pharmacological agents (in both mentally retarded persons and their nondisabled counterparts with CNS dysfunction) will continue to depend on rigorous clinical assessments and a drug selection strategy that focuses on the underlying psychobiological state of the individual, not his or her overt behavior alone. Therefore, even when working with profound and severely mentally retarded persons, there must be an appreciation of the subjective aspects of psychological life.

■ REFERENCES

Adams RD, Victor M: Principles of Neurology. New York, McGraw-Hill, 1985

Aman MG, Singh NN, Stewart AW, et al: The Aberrant Behavior Checklist: a behavior rating scale for the assessment of treatment effects. American Journal of Mental Deficiency 89:485–491, 1985

American Psychiatric Association: Diagnostic and Statistical Manual of Mental Disorders, 3rd Edition, Revised. Washington, DC, American Psychiatric Association, 1987

American Psychiatric Association: Diagnostic and Statistical Manual of Mental Disorders, 4th Edition. Washington, DC, American Psychiatric Association, 1994

Ballinger BR, Ballinger CB, Reid AH, et al: The psychiatric symptoms, diagnoses and care needs of 100 mentally handicapped patients. Br J Psychiatry 158:251–254, 1991

Baumeister AA, Sevin JA: Pharmacologic control of aberrant behavior in the mentally retarded: towards a more rational approach. Neurosci Biobehav Rev 14:253–262, 1990

Bear D: Neurological perspectives on aggressive behavior. Journal of Neuropsychiatry 3:S3–S8, 1991

Blumer D, Neppe V, Benson FD: Diagnostic criteria for epilepsy-related mental changes. Am J Psychiatry 145:676–677, 1990

Bond WS: Psychiatric indications for clonidine: the neuropharmacologic and clinical basis. J Clin Psychopharmacol 6:81–87, 1986

Bradley SJ: Affect regulation and psychopathology: bridging the mind-body gap. Can J Psychiatry 35:540–547, 1990

Campbell M, Anderson LT, Small AM, et al: Naltrexone in autistic children: a double-blind and placebo-controlled study. Psychopharmacol Bull 26:130–135, 1990

Charney DS, Henninger GR: Alpha 2-adrenergic and opiate receptor blockade. Arch Gen Psychiatry 43:1037–1041, 1986

Charney DS, Woods SW, Nagy LM, et al: Noradrenergic function in panic disorder. J Clin Psychiatry 51(suppl A):5–11, 1990

Ciompi L: Affects as central organizing and integrating factors. Br J Psychiatry 159:97–105, 1991

Cloninger CR: A systematic method for clinical description and classification of personality variants. Arch Gen Psychiatry 44:573–588, 1987

Coccaro EF: Central serotonin and impulsive aggression. Br J Psychiatry 155(suppl 8):52–62, 1989

Cohen DJ, Paul R, Volkmar FR: Issues in classification of pervasive developmental disorders and associated conditions, in Handbook of Autism and Pervasive Developmental Disorders. Edited by Cohen DJ, Donnellan AM. New York, Wiley, 1987, pp 20–40

Craft M, Ismail IA, Krishnamuirti JH, et al: Lithium in the treatment of aggression in mentally handicapped patients. Br J Psychiatry 150:685–689, 1987

Dale PG: Lithium in aggressive mentally subnormal patients. Br J Psychiatry 137:469–474, 1980

Dening TR, Berrios GE: Wilson's disease: psychiatric symptoms in 195 cases. Arch Gen Psychiatry 46:1126–1134, 1989

Donovan BT: Humors, Hormones, and the Mind. Chicago, IL, Year Book Medical Publishers, 1988

Eison MS: Serotonin: a common neurobiologic substrate in anxiety and depression. J Clin Psychopharmacol 10(suppl 3):26S–30S, 1990

Fenwick P: The nature and management of aggression in epilepsy. Journal of Neuropsychiatry 1:418–425, 1989

Gedye A: Dietary increase in serotonin reduces self-injurious behavior in a Down's syndrome adult. Journal of Mental Deficiency Research 34:195–203, 1990

Gleason RP, Schneider LS: Carbamazepine treatment of agitation in Alzheimer's outpatients refractory to neuroleptics. J Clin Psychiatry 51:115–118, 1990

Goldenson RM (ed): Longman Dictionary of Psychology and Psychiatry. New York, Longman, 1984

Goldman JJ: Tourette syndrome in severely behavior disordered mentally retarded children. Psychiatr Q 59:73–78, 1988

Goodwin FK, Jamison RK: Manic Depressive Illness. New York, Oxford University Press, 1990

Gualtieri CT: TMS: a system for prevention and control, in Mental Retardation: Developing Pharmacotherapies. Edited by Ratey JJ. Washington, DC, American Psychiatric Press, 1991, pp 35–50

Gualtieri CT, Schroeder SR: Pharmacotherapy for self-injurious behavior: preliminary tests of the D1 hypothesis. Psychopharmacol Bull 25:364–371, 1989

Hagerman RJ, Sobesky WE: Psychopathology in fragile-x syndrome. Am J Orthopsychiatry 59:142–152, 1989

Hierons R, Janota I, Corsellis JAN: The late effects of necrotizing encephalitis of the temporal lobes and limbic areas: a clinico-pathological study of 10 cases. Psychol Med 8:21–42, 1978

Hughes JR, Higgins ST, Bickel WK: Behavioral "properties" of drugs. Psychopharmacology 96:557–567, 1988

Jancar J: Organic causes of mental illness in the mentally retarded, in Psychiatric Illness and Mental Handicap. Edited by James FE, Snaith RP. London, Gaskell Press, 1979, pp 115–124

Kastner T, Friedman DL, Plummer AT: Valproic acid for the treatment of children with mental retardation and mood symptomatology. Pediatrics 86:467–472, 1990

Kramer M, Sartorious N, Jablensky A, et al: The ICD-9 classification of mental disorders: a review of its development and contents. Acta Psychiatr Scand 59:242–262, 1979

Lader M: β-adrenoceptor antagonists in neuropsychiatry: an update. J Clin Psychiatry 49:213–223, 1988

Leavitt ML, Yudofsky SC, Maroon JC, et al: Effect of intraventricular nadolol infusion on shock-induced aggression in 6-hydroxydopamine-treated rats. J Neuropsychiatry 1:167–172, 1990

Lewis MH, McLean WE Jr: Issues in treating emotional disorders, in Psychopathology in the Mentally Retarded. Edited by Matson J, Barrett RP. New York, Grune & Stratton, 1982, pp 1–36

Lipman RS, DiMascio A, Reatig N, et al: Psychotropic drugs and mentally retarded children, in Psychopharmacology: A Generation of Progress. Edited by Lipton MA, DiMascio A, Killam KF. New York, Raven, 1978, pp 1437–1449

Lowry MA, Sovner R: The functional significance of problem behavior: a key to effective treatment. The Habilitative Mental Healthcare Newsletter 10:59–63, 1991

Lowry MA, Sovner R: Severe behavior problems associated with rapid cycling bipolar disorder in two adults with profound mental retardation. Journal of Mental Deficiency Research 36:269–281, 1992

Luchins DJ, Dojka D: Lithium and propranolol in aggression and self-injurious behavior in the mentally retarded. Psychopharmacol Bull 25:372–375, 1989

Marin DB, Greenwald BS: Carbamazepine for aggressive agitation in demented patients during nursing care. Am J Psychiatry 146:805–807, 1989

Markowitz PI: Effect of fluoxetine on self-injurious behavior in the developmentally disabled: a preliminary study. J Clin Psychopharmacol 12:27–31, 1992

Matin MA, Rundle AT: Physiological and psychiatric investigations into a group of mentally handicapped subjects with self-injurious behavior. Journal of Mental Deficiency Research 24:77–83, 1980

Menolascino FJ, Levitas A, Greiner C: The nature and types of mental illness in the mentally retarded. Psychopharmacol Bull 22:1060–1071, 1986

National Institute of Mental Health: Handbook of Psychiatric Rating Scales, 2nd Edition. Rockville, MD, U.S. Department of Health and Human Services, 1973

O'Neil M, Page N, Adkins WN, et al: Tryptophan-trazodone treatment of aggressive behavior. Lancet 2:859–860, 1986

Papez JW: A proposed mechanism of emotion. Archives of Neurology and Psychiatry 27:725–743, 1937

Patterson JF: Carbamazepine for assaultive patients with organic brain disease. Psychosomatics 28:579–581, 1987

Paul SM: Anxiety and depression: a common neurobiological substrate. J Clin Psychiatry 49(suppl 10):13–16, 1988

Powers WT: Behavior: The Control of Perception. New York, Aldine De Gruyter, 1973

Ratey JJ (ed): Mental Retardation: Developing Pharmacotherapies. Washington, DC, American Psychiatric Press, 1991

Ratey JJ, Lindem KJ: β-blockers as primary treatment for aggression and self-injury in the developmentally disabled, in Mental Retardation: Developing Pharmacotherapies. Edited by Ratey JJ. Washington, DC, American Psychiatric Press, 1991, pp 51–82

Ratey JJ, Mikkelsen E, Sorgi P, et al: Autism: the treatment of aggressive behaviors. J Psychopharmacol 7:35–41, 1987

Ratey JJ, Sovner R, Mikkelsen E, et al: Buspirone therapy for maladaptive behavior and anxiety in developmentally disabled persons. J Clin Psychiatry 50:382–384, 1989

Ratey JJ, Sovner R, Parks A, et al: Buspirone treatment of aggression and anxiety in mentally retarded patients: a multiple baseline, placebo lead-in study. J Clin Psychiatry 52:159–162, 1991

Reid AH: The Psychiatry of Mental Handicap. London, Blackwell Scientific Publications, 1982

Reid AH, Leonard A: Lithium treatment of cyclical vomiting in a mentally defective patient. Br J Psychiatry 130:316, 1977

Reid AH, Ballinger BR, Heather BB: Behavioral syndromes identified by cluster analysis in a sample of 100 severely and profoundly retarded adults. Psychol Med 8:399–412, 1978

Reid AH, Naylor GJ, Kay DSG: A double-blind, placebo controlled crossover trial of carbamazepine in overactive severely mentally handicapped patients. Psychol Med 11:109–113, 1981

Reid AH, Ballinger BR, Heather BB, et al: The natural history of behavioral symptoms among severely and profoundly mentally retarded patients. Br J Psychiatry 145:289–293, 1984

Reynolds EH: Structure and function in neurology and psychiatry. Br J Psychiatry 157:481–490, 1990

Roberts JKA: Neuropsychiatric complications of mental retardation. Psychiatr Clin North Am 9:647–657, 1986

Ruedrich SL, Grush L, Wilson J: Beta adrenergic blocking medications for aggressive or self-injurious mentally retarded persons. Am J Ment Retard 95:110–119, 1990

Sheard MH: Clinical pharmacology of aggressive behavior. Clin Neuropharmacol 7:173–183, 1984

Silver JM, Yudofsky SC, Hales RE: Neuropsychiatric aspects of traumatic brain injury, in Textbook of Neuropsychiatry. Edited by Hales RE, Yudofsky SC. Washington, DC, American Psychiatric Press, 1987, pp 235–250

Sovner R: Behavioral psychopharmacology: a new psychiatric subspecialty, in Mental Retardation and Mental Health: Classification, Diagnosis, Treatment, Services. Edited by Stark JFJ, Menolascino FJM, Albarielli M, et al. New York, Springer Verlag, 1988, pp 229–242

Sovner R: Bipolar disorder in persons with developmental disorder: an overview, in Depression in Mentally Retarded Children and Adults. Edited by Dosen S, Menolascino FJ. Leiden, Netherlands, Logon Publications, 1990a, pp 175–198

Sovner R: Psychotropic drug prescribing principles for mentally retarded persons, in Treatment of Mental Illness and Behavioral Disorder in the Mentally Retarded. Proceedings of the International Congress, Amsterdam, Netherlands, May 3–4, 1990. Edited by Došen A, Van Gennnep A, Zwanikken GJ. Leiden, Netherlands, Logon Publications, 1990b, pp 91–102

Sovner R: Use of anticonvulsant agents for treatment of neuropsychiatric disorders in developmentally disabled persons, in Mental Retardation: Developing Pharmacotherapies. Edited by Ratey JJ. Washington, DC, American Psychiatric Press, 1991, pp 97–101

Sovner R: Classification of organic mental disorders (letter). Am J Psychiatry 149:1617, 1992

Sovner R, Hurley AD: The management of chronic behavior disorders in mentally retarded adults with lithium carbonate. J Nerv Ment Dis 169:191–195, 1989

Sovner R, Fox CJ, Lowry MJ, et al: Fluoxetine treatment of depression and associated self-injury in two adults with mental retardation. J Intellect Disabil Res 37:301–311, 1993

Spreat S, Behar D Reneski B, et al: Lithium carbonate for aggressive mentally retarded persons. Compr Psychiatry 30:505–511, 1989

Tyrer SP, Walsh A, Edwards DE, et al: Factors associated with a good response to lithium in aggressive mentally handicapped subjects. Prog Neuropsychopharmacol Biol Psychiatry 8:751–755, 1984

Voeller KS: What can neurological models of attention, intention, and arousal tell us about attention deficit-hyperactivity disorder? J Neuropsychiatry 3:209–216, 1991

Walters AS, Barrett RP, Feinstein C, et al: A case report of naltrexone treatment of self-injury and social withdrawal in autism. J Autism Dev Disord 20:169–176, 1990

Welch L, Sovner R: The treatment of a chronic organic mental disorder with dextromethorphan in a man with severe mental retardation. Br J Psychiatry 161:118–120, 1992

Wohlman BB (ed): Dictionary of Behavioral Science, 2nd Edition. New York, Academic Press, 1991

Worrall EP, Moody JP, Naylor GJ: Lithium in non-manic depressives: antiaggressive effect and red blood cell lithium values. Br J Psychiatry 126:4464–4468, 1975

Yudofsky SC: Psychoanalysis, psychopharmacology, and the influence of neuropsychiatry. Journal of Neuropsychiatry 3:1–5, 1991

Yudofsky SC, Silver JM, Hales RE: Pharmacologic management of aggression in the elderly. J Clin Psychiatry 5(suppl 10):22–28, 1990

Treatment of Behavior Disorders

16 Pharmacotherapy in Aggressive and Auto-Aggressive Behavior

Willem M.A. Verhoeven, M.D., Ph.D.
Sigfried Tuinier, M.D., Ph.D.

Aggressive spectrum disorders, particularly self-injurious behavior (SIB), are common in institutionalized mentally retarded populations. The estimated prevalence rate of SIB is 8%–14% in institutional populations and retarded persons and 1.7%–2.6% in the community (Griffin et al. 1987; Ricketts 1986). Similar differences between community-based samples and selective samples are reported for aggressive behavior. These contrasting figures raise doubts about the intrinsic relationship between behavioral disorders and mental retardation. Moreover, a considerable overlap is found between aggressive and auto-aggressive behavior in most if not all clinical studies (Nyhan 1976; Sovner 1990; Stone et al. 1989).

Aggression and auto-aggression occur frequently in clinical psychiatry. The prevalence rate of violent behavior of any kind in psychiatric patients is at least as high as that in mentally retarded subjects and varies between 7%–10% for assaults (Tardiff and Sweillam 1982) and 3%–4% for self-mutilation (Simpson 1976). Furthermore, it should be emphasized that violent behavior is not a symptom of a single disorder but may occur in the context of a broad spectrum of disorders such as psychiatric and general medical diseases and mental retardation (Rojahn et al. 1993). Thus, careful neuropsychiatric examination is necessary in mentally retarded subjects to determine whether the aggressive behavior is a symptom of an underlying neuropsychiatric disorder or a variable belonging to the mental retardation per se, in order to apply goal-directed pharmacotherapy.

Self-injurious behavior is defined as a chronic repetitive behavior causing external trauma on a mechanical basis and occurring mostly in a cognitively impaired patient and is often part of a spectrum of maladaptive behavior reflecting higher levels of disordered psychobiological function (Rojahn

1986). Sometimes SIB is considered to be a unitary behavioral entity, although it is well known that SIB can be a key symptom of neuropsychiatric disorder. Many different etiological factors may underlie SIB, and some of them may implicate specific treatments (Gualtieri 1989). SIB occurs frequently in mentally retarded subjects with or without psychiatric comorbidity. It is often associated with, or preceded by, stereotyped behavior that suggests the existence of a common denominator that may originate in a lack of normal peer interaction as is repeatedly demonstrated in animal experiments with primates (Kraemer and Clarke 1990; Kraemer et al. 1991). SIB may be a developmental disorder or a symptom of an underlying somatic or neuropsychiatric disorder, and this differentiation is important.

The first step in the diagnosis of aggression and SIB is to assess the level of development and behavioral repertoire and to collect data on the occurrence of behavioral problems, using specific targets such as the number of aggressive and auto-aggressive outbursts or time in or out of restraints. Secondly, it has to be established whether aggression and SIB are symptoms of general medical, neurologic, or psychiatric disorders or can be considered as an idiopathic phenomenon. It is important to exclude the possibility that (auto-)aggressive behavior is the consequence of undetected physical disorders, such as migraine, peptic ulcer, and hypoglycemia, or the result of toxicity from sedatives, anticonvulsants, or neuroleptics. In addition, it should be noted that recurring severe behavioral disorders may be associated with the menstrual cycle of mentally retarded females (Colella et al. 1992; Taylor et al. 1993). Paroxysmal aggression and/or SIB may sometimes be a seizure equivalent for which adequate treatment with anticonvulsants, like carbamazepine or valproic acid, may be indicated.

Finally, a differentiation should be made between traditional major psychiatric diagnoses with an unfamiliar clinical presentation and psychiatric syndromes specific to mentally retarded subjects. Aggression and SIB in mentally retarded patients are associated with schizophrenia, major affective disorder, panic disorder, Tourette's syndrome, cycloid psychosis, and delirious states. In these cases, appropriate treatment of the primary condition should result in a substantial reduction in aggression or auto-aggression. In such cases, a successful response to the specific treatment confirms the psychiatric disorder retrospectively (Tuinier and Verhoeven 1994).

Before considering pharmacological approaches, it is necessary to decide whether aggression or SIB should be treated at all. Treatment is obviously indicated when the behavior places the patient at the risk of life, limb, or sensory organ damage. Mostly, however, aggressive symptomatology requires treatment because the behavior can interfere directly with a patient's performance rather than because of injury concerns. Regarding the treatment, two strategies can be followed: medication or behavior modification. Positive findings have been reported with behavior modification, although most studies are case reports, highly labor-intensive, and lack a well-designed long-term follow-up (Favell et al. 1982; Tarnowski et al. 1989; see also Chapter 18 of this book).

With respect to pharmacotherapy, representatives of all classes of compounds have been administered to patients with aggression and/or auto-aggressive behavior. None have been studied sufficiently enough to recommend them unequivocally (Aman 1993; Singh and Millichamp 1985; Verhoeven et al. 1993). In this chapter, the neurochemical hypotheses that are under investigation at present as well as some possible psychopharmacological approaches will be discussed.

■ NEUROCHEMICAL HYPOTHESES

Dopamine

Lesch-Nyhan syndrome (LNS) is a developmental disorder in which an inborn error of purine metabolism (deficiency of hypoxanthine-guanine-phosphoribosyl-transferase [HGPRT]) results in massive overproduction of uric acid and is characterized by choreoathetoid movements, hypertonicity, opisthotonos, and compulsive self-biting (Lesch and Nyhan 1964). Autopsy has demonstrated a central deficiency of dopamine (DA). Because this deficiency in LNS was accompanied by reduction of synthesizing enzymes such as tyrosine hydroxylase and dopa decarboxylase in terminal areas, the reduction in DA is believed to be the result of a loss of DA-ergic terminals (Lloyd et al. 1981). The possible association between SIB and a specific biochemical-deficit LNS has given impetus to animal experiments in an attempt to clarify the neurochemical substrate of the behavior abnormality.

A promising animal model for SIB was developed by Breese and colleagues (1984, 1986, 1989, 1990), who induced a neonatal destruction of DA-containing fibers in the rat brain by treatment with 6-hydroxydopamine (6-OHDA). Treatment of these animals as adults with L-dopa results in a dose-dependent increase of SIB that can be blocked with the D_1-DA blocker *cis*-flupenthixol but not by the D_2-DA antagonist haloperidol. These observations suggest that the pharmacological basis of SIB in the neonatal 6-OHDA-treated rat may be a D_1-DA-receptor supersensitivity state. Goldstein and colleagues (Goldstein 1989, 1990) hypothesized that the mechanism of the development of striatal supersensitive DA receptors is somehow related to the deficiency of HGPRT activity in LNS, because their results indicate that HGPRT is localized on intrastriatal neurons that are known to contain D_1- and D_2-DA receptors.

These findings suggest that in these neurons the DA receptor might be regulated by nucleotide levels arising from the salvage pathway. The abnormal regulation of affinity states of the DA receptors by the guanine nucleotides might be involved in the pathology of LNS. It is therefore conceivable that D_1-DA-receptor supersensitivity is related to the occurrence of SIB, although the data from the neonatal 6-OHDA-lesioned rat model do not allow conclusions concerning whether activation of DA receptors is the mechanism by which self-biting is induced in LNS. Although it seems likely that the increased susceptibility for self-biting in LNS is the result of the reduced neonatal DA function, mechanisms other than the release of DA may be responsible. The data collected in the model of DA deficiency in LNS suggest that SIB, particularly self-biting, could be related to a neonatal deficiency of DA, even in the absence of HGPRT deficiency as observed in LNS.

If D_1-DA-receptor supersensitivity is mediating SIB, then patients with SIB but without LNS can possibly also be treated effectively with a compound that blocks the D_1-DA receptor. Based on this hypothesis, Gualtieri and Schroeder (1989) treated 15 severely to profoundly mentally retarded subjects with a long history of SIB and refractory to alternative treatments with the neuroleptic fluphenazine (FPZ). FPZ was chosen because it antagonizes both D_1- and D_2-DA receptors, but preferentially D_1 (Seeman 1981). The starting dose of FPZ was 0.5 mg twice daily, increasing weekly until optimal response was achieved or until side effects developed, up to a maximum of 15 mg per day. In 11 of the 15 patients, some degree of favorable response was observed as measured by number of SIB attempts, number of tantrums during which SIB occurred, and time in or out of restraints. It appeared that a low dose of FPZ (range 1.5–8 mg daily) was effective and that in most cases higher doses were accompanied by symptoms of akathisia, which actually made the SIB worse after an initial favorable response.

From these limited data the tentative conclusion may be drawn that the efficacy of low dosages of FPZ is consistent with the D_1-DA-receptor supersensitivity hypothesis. Because FPZ is not a pure D_1-DA-receptor antagonist, it does not, however, confirm this hypothesis. Research with a genetic mouse model, using the selective D_1-DA-receptor agonist SKF 38393 challenges the supersensitivity hypothesis (Jinnah et al. 1992). Moreover, the results of other animal studies suggest that severe forms of SIB can also be provoked by long-term isolation (Jones 1982) and social deprivation during development (Kraemer and Clarke 1990; Kraemer et al. 1991) or indicate that SIB may serve a de-arousal function as can be concluded from the amphetamine stereotypy model (Mittleman et al. 1991).

Thus, further studies are warranted to elucidate the involvement of DA pathways in SIB, using more selective D_1-DA-blocking compounds such as *cis*-flupenthixol, clozapine, or SKF 38393 and applying other animal models. These investigations will possibly yield more information about the relationship between SIB and a dysfunction of DA neuronal systems.

Serotonin

The serotonin hypothesis of aggression and SIB is based on the observations made by several investigators that patients with diverse kinds of violent, impulsive, or (auto-)destructive behavior show significantly lower cerebrospinal fluid (CSF) concentrations of the main serotonin metabolite 5-hydroxyindoleacetic acid (5-HIAA). Moreover, an inverse relationship has been demonstrated between the levels of CSF 5-HIAA and a life history of aggressive/impulsive behavioral disorders (for a review and references, see Brown et al. 1990; Roy and Linnoila 1990; Tuinier et al. 1996). In a study of patients with behavioral disorders, Greenberg and Coleman (1973, 1976) reported a relationship between patterns of behavioral problems, including SIB, and depressed plasma 5-HIAA levels. In these patients the elevation of serotonin levels into the normal range, by administration of a variety of psychoactive agents, appeared to be associated with an improvement of the behavioral disturbances. O'Neal et al. (1986) described a patient with Cornelia de Lange's syndrome whose SIB was significantly reduced by treatment with the serotonin reuptake blocker trazodone and the serotonin precursor L-tryptophan, which additionally markedly increased his abnormally low peripheral serotonin levels. Primeau and Fontaine (1987) found a decrease of SIB associated with obsessive-compulsive disorder in two patients treated with the serotonergic antidepressant clomipramine. Gualtieri (1989) reported a dramatic therapeutic response in aggressive symptomatology upon treatment with the specific serotonin reuptake inhibitor fluoxetine in combination with L-tryptophan.

Promising research in the 1970s mentioned the elimination of SIB symptoms like head banging, self-biting, and self-mutilation by administering serotonin-enhancing medication (e.g., 5-hydroxytryptophan [5-HTP] in subjects with mental retardation and SIB due to different etiologies). As can be inferred from Table 16–1, favorable responses to treatment with 5-hydroxytryptamine (5-HT) were sometimes demonstrated in patients with LNS. These results, however, have to be interpreted carefully because it is well-known that 5-HTP influences both 5-HT and catecholaminergic systems, whereas tryptophan selectively increases the 5-HT turnover (Van Praag 1983; Van Praag et al. 1990). Raleigh (1987) examined the effects of the serotonin reuptake inhibitor fluoxetine in animals and the catecholamine reuptake inhibitor desmethylimipramine (DMI) or tryptophan and 5-HTP on inducing behavioral changes. Tryptophan produced dose-dependent reductions in

Table 16–1.   Clinical trials with 5-hydroxytryptophan (5-HTP) in self-injurious behavior (SIB)

Authors	Clinical diagnosis, N	Design	Treatment	Effects on SIB
Perry and Tischler 1964	Phenylketonuria, 2	Double-blind, placebo-controlled	50 mg twice daily orally for 3½ months	None
Mizuno and Yugari 1975	Lesch-Nyhan, 4	Open	1–8 mg/kg/day orally during 36 weeks	Complete disappearance during active treatment; induction of tolerance after initial effectiveness
Nyhan 1976	Lesch-Nyhan, 1	Open	Dosage unknown	Decrease followed by tolerance
Frith et al. 1976	Lesch-Nyhan, 1	Double-blind, placebo-controlled	100 mg daily orally during 7 fortnightly treatment blocks	None
Anderson et al. 1976	Lesch-Nyhan, 4	Double-blind, placebo-controlled, crossover	4 mg/kg/day orally for 2 weeks	None
Ciaranello et al. 1976	Lesch-Nyhan, 1	Open	5–50 mg/kg/day orally during 30 days	None (reduced irritability)
Anders et al. 1978	Lesch-Nyhan, 1	Double-blind, placebo-controlled, crossover	5–50 mg/kg/day orally for 30 days	None
Castells et al. 1979	Lesch-Nyhan, 1	Open	48–96 mg daily orally up to 18 months	Temporary reduction followed by tolerance

Note.   For references, see Verhoeven et al. 1993.

aggression, vigilance, and locomotion and increases in eating. In contrast, 5-HTP increased aggression and vigilance and did not affect locomotion or eating. Fluoxetine produced effects identical to tryptophan, whereas DMI resulted in dose-dependent increases in aggression, vigilance, and locomotion. These results suggest that the effect of 5-HTP on catecholaminergic systems may underlie the differential behavioral effects of tryptophan and 5-HTP, especially with regard to aggression. Recently, Geyde (1990) reported reduced SIB in a Down's syndrome patient by means of increased dietary serotonin availability. In a study of people with Tourette's syndrome, lower CSF 5-HIAA concentrations were reported (Young et al. 1987). In addition, Volavka et al. (1990) found tryptophan to be effective in the treatment of aggressive psychiatric inpatients, in that it significantly reduced the need for injections of antipsychotics and sedatives.

In summary, some evidence is available that disturbances in central serotonergic mechanisms, as reflected in lowered 5-HIAA CSF concentrations, are involved in violent, impulsive, and (auto-)destructive behavior. Most data have been obtained from clinical studies with non–mentally retarded psychiatric subjects (for a review, see Brown et al. 1990; Tuinier et al. 1996). A considerable co-occurrence of aggression and auto-aggression in both nonretarded and mentally retarded subjects has been reported, although the mechanisms underlying the direction of this behavior are not well understood as yet (Plutchik and Van Praag 1990). Future research could focus on the therapeutic efficacy of serotonin-enhancing compounds in aggression and SIB. One possible strategy may be the administration of serotonin receptor–agonistic compounds such as azaperone (Blier and De Montigny 1990) or eltoprazine (Rasmussen et al. 1990).

Concerning the azaperones, several studies have been performed using buspirone, most of which followed a nonblind design. In the only placebo-controlled study, a decrease of aggression was found in five out of six patients treated with 15–40 mg buspirone for 11 weeks (Ratey and Lindem 1991). In recent reviews (Ricketts et al. 1994; Verhoeven and Tuinier 1999a), it was concluded that buspirone generates a mixed but generally favorable response in controlling intractable self-injury. However, confirmative data from well-controlled studies are required before this compound can be regarded as a therapeutic agent for this condition.

With respect to eltoprazine, a compound that pharmacologically closely resembles buspirone, preclinical research demonstrated specific inhibition of offensive components of agonistic interactions without material effects on flight, defense, and social capabilities, suggesting potential specific anti-aggressive effects (Mak et al. 1995). Three studies, including a total of 24 mentally retarded subjects with aggressive and self-injurious behavior, have been reported. In a study by Tiihonen et al. (1993), six subjects were treated with 30–60 mg eltoprazine orally per day following an open design for 12 weeks. In three of the six subjects, some improvement was noticed in that outward-directed aggression was reduced. Kohen (1993) reported no effect on aggression and SIB in five subjects during treatment with 20 mg eltoprazine daily for 6 weeks following a double-blind placebo-controlled design. Of the original eight subjects, three had to be excluded for various reasons. In our own study (Tuinier et al. 1995), the effects of eltoprazine with a daily oral dosage up to 60 mg were investigated in 10 mentally retarded male subjects on symptoms of behavioral disinhibition, mainly SIB. A therapeutic response was observed in 5 patients, starting in the second week of active treatment, that gradually disappeared in the subsequent 8 weeks. The response was characterized by a significant decline in frequency and/or intensity of SIB and/or need for restraints. In addition some patients showed other marked behavioral changes such as elevation of mood, increased activity and alertness, and enhanced social correctability. Apart from dose-related sleep disturbances, no major side effects occurred. Thus, treatment strategies with 5-HT$_1$ agonistic compounds seem to open some promising vistas. Because the clinical development of eltoprazine has recently been discontinued, this interesting pathway cannot be investigated further.

Although the beneficial effects of 5-HT agonistic agents are thought to be generated via the 5-HT neuronal systems, other monoaminergic pathways may be involved as well. Accumulating evidence is available suggesting that 5-HT subsystems are functional in a behavioral restraint system in which septo-hippocampal 5-HT structures inhibit behavior under circumstances of stress, anxiety, and uncertainty, whereas mesolimbic dopaminergic (sub)systems are involved in mobilizing and orientating goal-directed behaviors and the associated locomotion (Depue and Spoont 1986; Van Praag et al. 1990). Thus, the serotonin and dopamine hypotheses of aggressive behavior cannot be considered to be mutually exclusive.

Endogenous Opioids

The discovery that biologically active neuropeptides such as adrenocorticotropin/melanotropin-stimulating hormone (ACTH/MSH) and β-endorphin are colocated in a single precursor peptide proopiomelanocortin (POMC) has given impetus to hypotheses about the interaction of neuropeptides in behavior and brain function. In the late 1970s, Watson and colleagues presented the first evidence that biologically active neuropeptides derived from POMC were localized in brain cells (Watson et al. 1979). Since then, a vast amount of research has been performed focusing on the influences of neuropeptides on brain development, plasticity, and functioning (for overviews, see De Wied

1990; Sandman and O'Halloran 1986; Van Ree et al. 1990). Concerning SIB, it has been hypothesized that this disorder may be due to functional disturbances in the endogenous opioid system. There are two primary biological hypotheses. The first is the so-called addiction hypothesis stating that SIB may be considered a symptom of addiction to endogenous opioid neuropeptides. According to this hypothesis, the release of endorphins is stimulated by SIB-inducing addiction behavior to endogenous opioids (Van Ree 1987). The second, the so-called pain hypothesis, deals with opioid overactivity that may be responsible for maintaining a relatively tonic level of pain insensitivity (Sandman 1988). Support for this opioid overactivity hypothesis comes from animal as well as from human studies. Animal studies indicate that, in contrast to the effects of opiate antagonists, compounds with an affinity for opiate receptors may induce stereotyped behavior, including self-mutilation symptoms. Opiate antagonists appeared to reverse these effects (Herman and Goldstein 1981). In human studies Gillberg et al. (1985) found higher concentrations of fractions I and II opioid concentrations in the CSF of 24 autistic children compared with normal control subjects. They demonstrated a positive correlation between fraction II levels and decreased sensitivity to pain as well as a weak correlation between fraction I levels and SIB. Fraction II levels were significantly increased in the group of children with SIB as compared with those without self-destructiveness. Subsequently, two studies were published reporting elevated plasma β-endorphin levels in patients with SIB or stereotypy (Sandman 1988; Sandman et al. 1990). Recently, we have confirmed these findings.

Early in the 1980s, several case studies were published demonstrating some of the beneficial effects of parenteral administration of the opiate antagonist naloxone (for review and references, see Verhoeven et al. 1993). Since 1987, there have been 13 controlled studies with the orally administered opiate antagonist naltrexone (see Table 16–2). As can be inferred from the table, the two large-scale studies by Campbell et al. (1993) and Willemsen-Swinkels et al. (1995) did not reveal any beneficial effect on SIB. Summing up, 17 patients responded, whereas 46 did not. These results do not support the hypothesis that opiate-receptor blockade can be used in the treatment of SIB and are inconsistent with theories suggesting a role of endogenous opioids in the etiology of SIB and stereotypy. Interestingly, Leboyer et al. (1993), Campbell et al. (1993), and Willemsen-Swinkels et al. (1995) reported that naltrexone significantly reduced hyperactivity and irritability. Whether these observations can be attributed to side effects of naltrexone is not as yet elucidated.

In spite of these negative conclusions about the effectiveness of naltrexone in the treatment of SIB and stereotypy, it is still likely that endogenous opioids are involved in the etiology of this type of aberrant behavior. Animal experi-

Table 16–2. Controlled clinical trials with the opiate antagonist naltrexone in self-injurious behavior (SIB)

Authors	Number of patients	Age (years)	Daily dosage and duration of treatment	Effects on SIB
Bernstein et al. 1987	1	18	12.5–50 mg; 14 days	Dose-dependent decrease for several days
Szymanski et al. 1987	2	21 and 29	50 mg; 3 weeks	None
Herman et al. 1987	3	10, 17, and 17	0.5, 1.0, 1.5, 2.0 mg/kg; once weekly	Dose-dependent decrease
Sandman 1988	4	23–26	25, 50, 100 mg; once weekly	Dose-dependent decrease in 3 patients
Barrett et al. 1989	1	12	50 mg; 12 days (2 periods)	Decrease to zero ratio during 22 months after experimental period
Kars et al. 1990	6	15–23	50 mg; 3 weeks	Temporary decrease in 2 patients
Walters et al. 1990	1	14	50 mg daily; 3 weeks	Decrease
Taylor et al. 1991	1	20	0.5, 1.0, 2.0 mg/kg; 12 days	Decrease
Scifo et al. 1991	2 (12)	Unknown	0.5, 1.0, 1.5 mg/kg; 15 days	Clinically relevant reduction in 1
Leboyer et al. 1992	4	4–19	0.5, 1.0, 2.0 mg/day; 3 weeks	Decrease, but not at ≤1.0 mg/kg
Campbell et al. 1993	21 (41)	3–8	0.5–1.0 mg/kg; 3 weeks	None
Zingarelli et al. 1992	8	19–39	50 mg; 17 weeks	None
Willemsen-Swinkels et al. 1994	9 (12)	18–46	100 mg; 1 week 50 or 150 mg; 4 weeks	None

Note. For references, see Verhoeven et al. 1993 and Willemsen-Swinkels et al. 1995.

ments have revealed data suggesting that stereotypies can be antagonized by opiate antagonists during an early stage of their development only, probably with a temporary and coinciding increase of β-endorphin plasma levels (Kennes et al. 1988; Wiepkema and Schouten 1992). It is questionable whether this mechanism can be studied adequately in humans.

■ PHARMACOLOGICAL APPROACHES

As can be inferred from the previous discussion, pharmacotherapy based on a clear pathogenetic concept has so far not led to a rational and effective treatment for behavioral disorders associated with aggression in mentally retarded subjects. In addition, some other pharmacological approaches have been applied in subjects with aggressive spectrum behavior and will be mentioned briefly (Verhoeven and Tuinier 1999b).

Lithium

Lithium is interesting because it is a pharmacological class in itself. Concerning its mode of action, some evidence is available that lithium treatment alters 5-HT function in animals as well as humans (Price et al. 1989). Because it is effective in treating mania, it has been used with repeated success for aggressive behavior and, subsequently, for auto-aggressive behavior (Dale 1980; Dostal 1972; Tyrer et al. 1984). From a review of the use of lithium carbonate in mentally retarded subjects, it cannot be concluded that the compound is effective in reducing aggression and SIB but rather that aditional controlled studies are needed before a definitive statement can be made (Sovner and Hurley 1981). In two clinical studies in which the use of lithium was analyzed retrospectively, the results indicated a clear therapeutic effect for both aggression and SIB in the majority of the subjects (Luchins and Dojka 1989; Spreat et al. 1989). However, caution in the interpretation of these studies has to be taken because they assume implicitly that SIB and aggression are drug-responsive behaviors, irrespective of their causes, whereas both forms of behavior may be the result of pathological states, including impulsivity, irritability, and anxiety, in the context of mood disorders. In a study by Spreat et al. (1989), evidence was provided that hyperactivity (extreme stimulus sensitivity) may be the mediating variable in predicting lithium responsiveness, supporting data reported previously (for references, see Stewart et al. 1990). In addition, Craft et al. (1987) reported the results of a double-blind trial lasting 4 months with 42 mentally retarded patients in which treatment with lithium carbonate (serum levels 0.7–1.25 mmol/L) was compared with a placebo. A reduction in aggressiveness was observed in three-quarters of the patients following treatment with lithium. There was a statistically significant difference between the treatment groups in terms of the weekly mean aggression scores and the weekly counts of aggressive episodes during the experimental period. Classic side effects were noted in about one-third of the patients in the lithium group, but they were mainly short-lived and in no case necessitated discontinuation of lithium. In summary, only equivocal data exist suggesting a place for lithium as a potentially useful agent in the management of mentally retarded patients with aggressive behavior.

β-Blocking Agents

β-adrenergic–blocking medications, like propranolol, have been used for a variety of neuropsychiatric disorders (Lader 1988). Volavka (1988) and Yudofsky et al. (1988) concluded from their studies that enough preliminary evidence exists to support the use of β-blockers in the treatment of aggression. There are a limited number of single case studies or nonblind open trials describing the use of β-blockers in the treatment of aggression and SIB in the mentally retarded (Ruedrich et al. 1990; Thibaut and Colonna 1993). Summarizing these data, it was found that a substantial number of patients involved in these studies showed a moderate to marked response to propranolol administered in an average dose of 120 mg daily. In one double-blind, placebo-controlled study, the β-blocking agents pindolol and nadolol were used and produced a moderate reduction of SIB and aggression (Ratey and Lindem 1991). The absence of randomized, double-blind, placebo-controlled trials of β-blocking agents in mentally retarded patients necessitates skepticism about the results obtained so far. The mechanism through which β-adrenergic–blocking medications exert their effect on aggression or SIB remains unclear. Most probably, they induce decreased somatic anxiety or hyperarousal via a peripheral effect, resulting in decreased aggression and SIB. However, there are some indications that propranolol enhances 5-HT transmission, which might explain its antiaggression effects (Scheinin et al. 1984).

Selective Serotonin Reuptake Inhibitors (SSRIs)

Since the single case report by O'Neal and colleagues in 1986 of the use of trazodone in combination with tryptophan, there has been a growing of reports on the use of the SSRI fluoxetine in mentally retarded subjects with comorbid psychiatric disorders. Warnock and Kestenbaum (1992) described the successful treatment with relatively high doses of fluoxetine of two patients with the Prader-Willi syndrome who displayed the repetitive self-mutilating behavior of skin picking (for references, see Tuinier and Verhoeven 1994). Sovner et al. (1993) reported the beneficial effects of fluoxetine on SIB symptoms associated with major depression in two subjects taking 20–40 mg for more than 1 year. Ricketts et al. (1993) described four cases of patients with SIB without a clear psychiatric codiagnosis who were treated with fluoxetine for at least 1 year in a dosage varying between 20 and 60 mg daily. A moderate to marked beneficial effect on SIB was observed in all subjects. In addition, Bodfish and Madison (1993) treated 16 mentally retarded subjects, 10 of whom met the criteria for obsessive-compulsive disorder. All exhibited aggressive and/or self-injurious behavior. Fluoxetine was administered in a dosage up to 80 mg daily for 5–6 months. All subjects who responded had compulsive behavior disorders and SIB as main symptoms. In the 7 responders a substantial reduction in level and amount of variability of target behavior was observed. The SSRI sertraline was administered successfully at a dose of 50 mg daily in 1 patient with a possible diagnosis of obsessive-compulsive disorder (Wiener and Lamberti 1993). Finally, Garber et al. (1992) reported a substantial reduction in target symptoms such as SIB and stereotypy in 10 of 11 mentally retarded subjects treated with 25–125 mg clomipramine per day.

These studies suggest that behavioral disorders coinciding with psychiatric syndromes involving anxiety and mood disturbances can be treated effectively with such antidepressant compounds. Whether these compounds can be used in behavioral disorders sui generis is so far unclear.

Neuroleptics and Anticonvulsants

For a long time, the most commonly administered agents for the treatment of aggressive mentally retarded patients were the neuroleptics, with the majority of studies using thioridazine or haloperidol. Although neuroleptics in low doses are reported to be effective in the treatment of aggression, tardive dyskinesia and withdrawal dyskinesia occur in approximately one-third of the mentally retarded patients, and exacerbation of seizure disorders, behavioral toxicity, and impairment of cognitive function are observed frequently (Breuning et al. 1983; Lipman 1986; Platt et al. 1984; Tuinier and Verhoeven 1994). Although the antiaggressive effects of neuroleptics are behaviorally nonspecific (Miczek et al. 1994), being secondary to sedation and motor retardation, these compounds should be used with caution in the treatment of (auto-)aggressive behavior unless there is strong evidence suggesting a neuroleptic-responsive psychiatric disorder. The administration of neuroleptics should further be weighed against their risk of inducing anticholinergic delirious states (Tuinier and Verhoeven 1994) and akathisia (Gross et al. 1993). Vanden Borre et al. (1993) reported the effects of the combined dopamine-serotonin antagonist risperidone on behavioral disturbances in mentally retarded subjects. The results suggest that risperidone may be beneficial in the regulation of behavioral dyscontrol without inducing extrapyramidal symptoms.

Anticonvulsants like carbamazepine and valproic acid have also been used in the treatment of aggression. Reid et al. (1981) demonstrated, in a placebo-controlled crossover study, the effectiveness of carbamazepine in a group of 12 hyperactive, aggressive, mentally retarded patients, independent of any history of seizures or EEG abnormality. Similar findings were reported by Rapport et al. (1983) in one mentally retarded subject. Other studies using carbamazepine or valproic acid were not directed at its effect on aggression but designed to delineate hidden cases of bipolar disorder (Glue 1989; Kastner et al. 1993). Thus, very limited data are available with regard to the specific anti-aggressive effect of anticonvulsants. The beneficial effects as reported in the literature seem to be mostly related to the effectiveness on episodic violent behavior due to either bipolar disorders or a cerebral dyscontrol syndrome.

Other Compounds

Benzodiazepines have also been used. Their effects on aggression and SIB are most likely secondary to muscle relaxation and sedation. Generally, benzodiazepines should be used restrictively because of their risk of inducing paradoxical effects, including an increase in aggression (Barron and Sandman 1985). The same holds for barbiturates, now considered obsolete, especially since they may exacerbate SIB (Mayhew et al. 1992).

■ CONCLUSIONS

In spite of extensive efforts, no rational pharmacological treatment for aggression and SIB has yet been found for mentally retarded subjects, with the exception of those cases in which behavioral disinhibition is a part of a treatable psychiatric disorder.

It should be emphasized that behavioral approaches have been successfully applied in the treatment of aggressive spectrum behavior disorders and that there is no need to dichotomize between pharmacological and behavioral approaches, particularly because it is well known that these behavior disorders may be induced or worsened by environmental factors. Thus, attention should be paid to combining the two treatment strategies as recommended by several investigators (Durand 1982).

There are several explanations for the apparent lack of specific pharmacological treatment regimens. First, it is virtually impossible to collect sufficient data representative of biologically homogeneous groups. A major impediment in this respect is the complete absence of reliable diagnostic tools to enable adequate grouping of subjects. Thus, all studies dealing with therapeutic programs are difficult to interpret because they comprise subjects with a totally heterogeneous etiology and symptomatology. In fact, only cumulative single-case ($N = 1$) studies with a methodologically correct design can be applied, after which the data can be pooled. Second, most if not all studies applying pharmacological approaches in mentally retarded subjects are heavily biased by the assumption that behavioral routines that have existed for a long time can be changed in the course of a relatively short drug trial. Experience in clinical psychiatry has demonstrated that anxiety-related behavior, for example, can only be treated adequately and with a persistent therapeutic effect if pharmacotherapy is supplemented with behavior modification techniques. Third, it should be emphasized that symptoms of behavior disinhibition, such as stereotypy, aggression, and SIB, may originate within the framework of a disturbed stress responsivity. If this hypothesis could be further substantiated with biological data, the primary pharmacological goal would be the reduction of exaggerated stress vulnerability and responsivity. So far, only azaperones like buspirone seem to influence the neurobiological structures involved in this responsivity. Finally, following a research strategy using specific pharmacological agents, it might become possible to construct a nosology of aggressive symptomatology, especially if certain clinical characteristics that typify individual patient groups can be identified.

In conclusion, no specific and rational pharmacological treatment regimes are available as yet. Future research should therefore be guided by the "functional orientation" that attempts to correlate biological variables with psychological dysfunctions such aggression or auto-aggression. In this approach, behavioral disorders are not specific for any nosological entity but rather are related to psychopathological dimensions.

■ REFERENCES

Aman MG: Efficacy of psychotropic drugs for reducing self-injurious behavior in the developmental disabilities. Ann Clin Psychiatry 5:171–188, 1993

Barron J, Sandman CA: Paradoxical excitement to sedative-hypnotics in mentally retarded clients. American Journal of Mental Deficiency 90:124–129, 1985

Blier P, De Montigny C: Differential effect of gepirone on presynaptic and postsynaptic serotonin receptors: single-cell recording studies. J Clin Psychopharmacol 10:13S–20S, 1990

Bodfish JW, Madison JT: Diagnosis and fluoxetine treatment of compulsive behavior disorder of adults with mental retardation. Am J Ment Retard 98:360–367, 1993

Breese GR, Baumeister AA, McCown TJ, et al: Behavioral differences between neonatal and adult 6-hydroxy-dopamine-treated rats: relevance to neurological symptoms in clinical syndromes with reduced dopamine. J Pharmacol Exp Ther 231:343–354, 1984

Breese GR, Mueller RA, Napier TS, et al: Neurobiology of D_1-dopamine receptors after neonatal-6-OHDA-treatment: relevance to Lesch-Nyhan disease. Adv Exp Med Biol 204:197–215, 1986

Breese GR, Croswell HE, Duncan GE, et al: Dopamine deficiency in self-injurious behavior. Psychopharmacol Bull 25:353–357, 1989

Breese GR, Croswell HE, Mueller RA: Evidence that lack of brain dopamine during development can increase the susceptibility for aggression and self-injurious behavior by influencing D_1-dopamine receptor function. Prog Neuropsychopharmacol Biol Psychiatry 14:S65–S80, 1990

Breuning SE, Ferguson DG, Davidson NA, et al: Effects of thioridazine on the intellectual performance of mentally retarded drug responders and nonresponders. Arch Gen Psychiatry 40:309–313, 1983

Brown GL, Linnoila M, Goodwin FK: Clinical assessment of human aggression and impulsivity in relationship to biochemical measures, in Violence and Suicidality. Edited by Van Praag HM, Plutchnik R, Apter A. New York, Brunner/Mazel, 1990, pp 184–217

Campbell M, Anderson LT, Small AM, et al: Naltrexone in autistic children: behavioral symptoms and attentional learning. J Am Acad Child Adolesc Psychiatry 32:1283–1291, 1993

Colella RF, Ratey JJ, Glaser AI: Paramenstrual aggression in mentally retarded adult ameliorated by buspirone. Int J Psychiatry Med 22:351–356, 1992

Craft M, Ismail IA, Krishnamurti D, et al: Lithium in the treatment of aggression in mentally handicapped patients: a double-blind trial. Br J Psychiatry 150:685–689, 1987

Dale PG: Lithium therapy in aggressive mentally subnormal patients. Br J Psychiatry 137:469–471, 1980

Depue RA, Spoont MR: Conceptualizing a serotonin trait: a behavioral dimension of constraint. Ann N Y Acad Sci 99(1):47–62, 1986

De Wied D: Effects of peptide hormones on behavior, in Neuropeptides: Basics and Perspectives. Edited by De Wied D. Amsterdam, Netherlands, Elsevier, 1990, pp 1–44

Dostal T: Antiaggressive effect of lithium salts in mentally retarded adolescents, in Depressive States in Childhood and Adolescence. Edited by Annell A. Stockholm, Sweeden, Almquist & Wiksell, 1972, pp 491–498

Durand VM: A behavioral/pharmacological intervention for the treatment of severe self-injurious behavior. J Autism Dev Disord 12:243–251, 1982

Favell JE, Azrin NH, Baumeister AA, et al: The treatment of self-injurious behavior. Behavior Therapy 13:529–554, 1982

Garber HJ, McGonigle JJ, Slomka GT, et al: Clomipramine treatment of stereotypic behaviors and self-injury in patients with development disabilities. J Am Acad Child Adolesc Psychiatry 31:1157–1160, 1992

Geyde A: Dietary increase in serotonin reduces self-injurious behavior in a Down's syndrome adult. Journal of Mental Deficiency Research 34:195–203, 1990

Gillberg C, Terenius L, Lunnerholm G: Endorphin activity in childhood psychosis. Arch Gen Psychiatry 42:780–783, 1985

Glue P: Rapid cycling affective disorders in the mentally retarded. Biol Psychiatry 26:250–256, 1989

Goldstein M: Dopaminergic mechanisms in self-inflicting biting behavior. Psychopharmacol Bull 25:349–352, 1989

Goldstein M: Dopamine agonist induced dyskinesias, including self-biting behavior in monkeys with supersensitive dopamine receptors, in Violence and Suicidality. Edited by Van Praag HM, Plutchnik R, Apter A. New York, Brunner/Mazel, 1990, pp 316–323

Greenberg AG, Coleman M: Depressed whole blood serotonin levels associated with behavioral abnormalities in the Lange syndrome. Pediatrics 51:720–724, 1973

Greenberg AG, Coleman M: Depressed 5-hydroxyindole levels associated with hyperactive and aggressive behavior: relationship to drug response. Arch Gen Psychiatry 33:331–336, 1976

Griffin JC, Ricketts RW, Williams DE, et al: A community survey of self-injurious behavior among developmentally disabled children and adolescents. Hospital and Community Psychiatry 9:959–963, 1987

Gross EJ, Hull HG, Lytton GJ: Case study of neuroleptic-induced akathisia: important implications for individuals with mental retardation. Am J Ment Retard 98:156–164, 1993

Gualtieri CTh: The differential diagnosis of self-injurious behavior in mentally retarded people. Psychopharmacol Bull 25:358–363, 1989

Gualtieri CTh, Schroeder SR: Pharmacotherapy for self-injurious behavior: preliminary tests of the D_1 hypothesis. Psychopharmacol Bull 25:364–371, 1989

Herman BH, Goldstein A: Cataleptic effects of dynorphin-(1-13) in rats made tolerant to a mu opiate receptor agonist. Neuropeptides 2:13–22, 1981

Jinnah HA, Langlais PJ, Friedman T: Functional analysis of brain dopamine systems in a genetic mouse model of Lesch-Nyhan syndrome. J Pharmacol Exp Ther 263:596–607, 1992

Jones IH: Self-injury: toward a biological basis. Perspect Biol Med 26:137–150, 1982

Kastner T, Finesmith R, Walsh K: Long-term administration of valproic acid in the treatment of affective symptoms in people with mental retardation. J Clin Psychopharmacol 13:448–451, 1993

Kennes D, Odberg FO, Bouquet Y, et al: Changes in naloxone and haloperidol effects during the development of captivity-induced jumping stereotypy in bank voles. Eur J Pharmacol 153:19–24, 1988

Kohen D: Eltoprazine for aggression in mental handicap. Lancet 341:628–629, 1993

Kraemer GW, Clarke AS: The behavioral neurobiology of self-injurious behavior in rhesus monkeys. Prog Neuropsychopharmacol Biol Psychiatry 14:141–168, 1990

Kraemer GW, Ebert MH, Schmidt DE, et al: Strangers in a strange land: a psychobiological study of infant monkeys before and after separation from real or inanimate mothers. Child Dev 62:548–566, 1991

Lader ML: β-adrenoceptor antagonists in neuropsychiatry: an update. J Clin Psychiatry 49:213–223, 1988

Leboyer M, Bouvard MP, Launay JM, et al: Une hypothèse opiacée dans l'austisme infantile? Encephale 19:95–102, 1993

Lesch M, Nyhan WL: A familial disorder of uric acid metabolism and central nervous system function. Am J Med 36:561–570, 1964

Lipman RA: Overview of research in psychopharmacological treatment of the mentally ill/mentally retarded. Psychopharmacol Bull 22:1046–1054, 1986

Lloyd KG, Hornykiewicz O, Davidson L, et al: Biochemical evidence of dysfunction of brain neurotransmitters in the Lesch-Nyhan syndrome. N Engl J Med 305:1106–1111, 1981

Luchins DJ, Dojka D: Lithium and propranolol in aggression and self-injurious behavior in the mentally retarded. Psychopharmacol Bull 25:372–375, 1989

Mak M, Koning P de, Mos J, et al: Preclinical and clinical studies on the role of 5-HT_1 receptors in aggression, in Impulsivity and Aggression and Disorders of Impulse Control. Edited by Hollander E, Stein D. New York, Wiley, 1995, pp 289–372

Mayhew LA, Hanzel TE, Ferron FR, et al: Phenobarbital exacerbation of self-injurious behavior. J Nerv Ment Dis 180:732–733, 1992

Miczek KA, Weerts E, Haney M: Neurobiological mechanisms controlling aggression: preclinical developments for pharmacotherapeutic interventions. Neurosci Biobehav Rev 18:97–110, 1994

Mittleman G, Jones GH, Robbins TW: Sensitization of amphetamine stereotypy reduces plasma corticosterone: implications for stereotypy as a coping response. Behavioral and Neural Biology 56:170–182, 1991

Nyhan WL: Behavior in the Lesch-Nyhan syndrome. Journal of Autism and Childhood Schizophrenia 3:235–252, 1976

O'Neal M, Page N, Atkins WN, et al: Tryptophan-trazodone treatment of aggressive behavior. Lancet 2:859–860, 1986

Platt JE, Campbell M, Green WH, et al: Cognitive effects of lithium carbonate and haloperidol in treatment-resistant aggressive children. Arch Gen Psychiatry 41:657–662, 1984

Plutchik R, Van Praag HM: Psychosocial correlates of suicide and violence risk, in Violence and Suicidality. Edited by Van Praag HM, Plutchnik R, Apter A. New York, Brunner/Mazel, 1990, pp 37–65

Price LH, Charney DS, Delgado PL, et al: Lithium treatment and serotonergic function. Neuroendocrine and behavioral responses to intravenous tryptophan in affective disorder. Arch Gen Psychiatry 46:13–19, 1989

Primeau F, Fontaine R: Obsessive disorder with self-mutilation: a subgroup responsive to pharmacotherapy. Can J Psychiatry 32:699–700, 1987

Raleigh MJ: Differential behavioral effects of tryptophan and 5-hydroxytryptophan in velvet monkeys: influence of catecholaminergic systems. Psychopharmacol 93:44–50, 1987

Rapport MD, Sonis WA, Fialkov MJ, et al: Carbamazepine and behavior therapy for aggressive behavior: treatment of a mentally retarded, postencephalitic adolescent with seizure disorder. Behav Modif 7:255–265, 1983

Rasmussen DL, Olivier B, Raghoebar M, et al: Possible clinical applications of serenics and some implications of their preclinical profile for their clinical use in psychiatric disorders. Drug Metabol Drug Interact 8:159–186, 1990

Ratey JJ, Lindem KJ: β-blockers as primary treatment for aggression and self-injury in the developmentally disabled, in Mental Retardation: Developing Pharmacotherapies. Edited by Ratey J. Washington, DC American Psychiatric Press, 1991, pp 5–81

Reid AH, Naylor GJ, Kay DS: A double-blind, placebo-controlled, cross-over trial of carbamazepine in overactive, severely mentally handicapped patients. Psychol Med 11:109–113, 1981

Ricketts RW: Self-injurious behavior: a community based prevalence survey. Self-Injurious Behavior 2:1–2, 1986

Ricketts RW, Goza AB, Ellis CR, et al: Fluoxetine treatment of severe self-injury in young adults with mental retardation. J Am Acad Child Adolesc Psychiatry 32:865–869, 1993

Ricketts RW, Goza AB, Ellis CR, et al: Clinical effects of buspirone on intractable self-injury in adults with mental retardation. J Am Acad Child Adolesc Psychiatry 33:270–276, 1994

Rojahn J: Self-injurious and stereotypic behavior of non-institutionalized mentally retarded people: prevalence and classification. American Journal of Mental Deficiency 91:268–276, 1986

Rojahn J, Borthwick-Duffy SA, Jacobson JW: The association between psychiatric diagnoses and severe behavior problems in mental retardation. Ann Clin Psychiatry 5:163–170, 1993

Roy A, Linnoila M: Monoamines and suicidal behavior, in Violence and Suicidality. Edited by Van Praag HM, Plutchnik R, Apter A. New York, Brunner/Mazel, 1990, pp 141–183

Ruedrich SL, Grush L, Wilson J: Beta adrenergic blocking medications for aggressive or self-injurious mentally retarded persons. Am J Ment Retard 95:110–119, 1990

Sandman CA: β-endorphin disregulation in autistic and self-injurious behavior: a neurodevelopmental hypothesis. Synapse 2:193–199, 1988

Sandman CA, O'Halloran JP: Pro-opiomelanocortin, learning, memory and attention, in Encyclopeida on Pharmacology and Therapeutics. Edited by De Wied D, Gispen WH, Van Wimersma Greidanus JHB. New York, Pergamon, 1986, pp 397–420

Sandman CA, Barron JL, Chicz-Demet A, et al: Plasma β-endorphin levels in patients with self-injurious behavior and stereotypy. Am J Ment Retard 95:84–92, 1990

Scheinin M, Van Kammen DP, Ninan PT, et al: Effect of propranolol on monoamine metabolites in cerebrospinal fluid of patients with chronic schizophrenia. Clin Pharmacol Ther 36:33–39, 1984

Seeman P: Brain dopamine receptors. Psychol Rev 32:229–313, 1981

Simpson MA: Self mutilation. British Journal of Hospital Medicine 16:430–440, 1976

Singh NN, Millichamp CJ: Pharmacological treatment of self-injurious behavior in mentally retarded persons. J Autism Dev Disord 15:257–267, 1985

Sovner R: Developments in the use of psychotropic drugs. Current Opinion in Psychiatry 3:606–612, 1990

Sovner R, Hurley A: The management of chronic behavior disorders in mentally retarded adults with lithium carbonate. J Nerv Ment Dis 169:191–195, 1981

Sovner R, Fox CJ, Lowry MJ, et al: Fluoxetine treatment of depression and associated self-injury in two adults with mental retardation. J Intellect Disabil Res 37:301–311, 1993

Spreat S, Behar D, Reneski B, et al: Lithium carbonate for aggression in mentally retarded persons. Compr Psychiatry 30:505–511, 1989

Stewart JT, Myers WC, Burket RC, et al: A review of the pharmacotherapy of aggression in children and adolescents. J Am Acad Child Adolesc Psychiatry 29:269–277, 1990

Stone RK, Alvarez WF, Ellman G, et al: Prevalence and prediction of psychotropic drug use in California developmental centers. Am J Ment Retard 93:627–632, 1989

Tardiff K, Sweillam A: Assaultive behavior among chronic inpatients. Am J Psychiatry 139:212–215, 1982

Tarnowski KJ, Rasnake LK, Mulick JA, et al: Acceptability of behavioral interventions for self-injurious behavior. Am J Ment Retard 93:575–580, 1989

Taylor DV, Rush D, Betrick WP, et al: Self-injurious behavior within the menstrual cycle of women with mental retardation. Am J Ment Retard 92:659–664, 1993

Thibaut F, Colonna L: Efficacité antiaggressive des beta-bloquants. Encephale 19:263–267, 1993

Tiihonen J, Hakola P, Paanila J, et al: Eltoprazine for aggression in schizophrenia and mental retardation (abstract). Lancet 341:307, 1993

Tuinier S, Verhoeven WMA: Pharmacological advances in mental retardation; a need for reconceptualization. Current Opinion in Psychiatry 7(5):380–386, 1994

Tuinier S, Verhoeven WMA, Van Praag HM: Serotonin and disruptive behavior: a critical evaluation of clinical data. Human Psychopharmacology 11:469–482, 1996

Tuinier S, Verhoeven WMA, van den Berg Y, et al: Modulation of serotonin metabolism in self-injurious behavior, an open study with the 5-HT1 agonist eltoprazine in mental retardation. European Journal of Psychiatry 9:226–237, 1995

Tyrer SP, Walsh A, Edwards DE, et al: Factors associated with a good response to lithium in aggressive mentally handicapped subjects. Prog Neuropsychopharmacol Biol Psychiatry 8:751–755, 1984

Vanden Borre R, Vermote R, Buttiëns M, et al: Risperidone as add-on therapy in behavioral disturbances in mental retardation: a double-blind placebo-controlled cross-over study. Acta Psychiatr Scand 87:167–171, 1993

Van Praag HM: In search of the mode of action of antidepressants: 5-HT-tyrosine mixtures in depressions. Neuropharmacology 22:433–440, 1983

Van Praag HM, Asnis GM, Kahn RS, et al: Monoamines and abnormal behavior: a multi-aminergic perspective. Br J Psychiatry 157:723–734, 1990

Van Ree JM: Reward and abuse: opiates and neuropeptides, in Brain Reward Systems and Abuse. Edited by Engel J, Oreland L. New York, Raven, 1987, pp 75–88

Van Ree JM, Jolles J, Verhoeven WMA: Neuropeptides and psychopathology, in Neuropeptides: Basics and Perspectives. Edited by De Wied D. Amsterdam, Netherlands, Elsevier, 1990, pp 313–351

Verhoeven WMA, Tuinier S: Serotonin agonist buspirone in disruptive behavior. Acta Psychiatrica Belgica 99:80–91, 1999a

Vehoeven WMA, Tuinier S: The psychopharmacology of challenging behaviours in developmental disabilities, in Psychiatric and Behavioural Disorders in Developmental Disabilities and Mental Retardation. Edited by Bouras N. Cambridge, UK, Cambridge University Press, 1999b, pp 295–316

Verhoeven WMA, Tuinier S, Sijben NES: Biological aspects and pharmacological treatment of self-injurious behavior in persons with mental retardation, in Mental Health Aspects of Mental Retardation: Progress in Assessment and Treatment. Edited by Fletcher RJ, Došen A. New York, Lexington Books, 1993, pp 291–333

Volavka J: Can aggressive behavior in humans be modified by beta-blockers? J Postgrad Med (Feb 29):163–168, 1988

Volavka J, Crowner M, Brizer D, et al: Tryptophan treatment of aggressive psychiatric inpatients. Biol Psychiatry 28:728–732, 1990

Warnock JKB, Kestenbaum T: Pharmacological treatment of severe skin picking behavior in Prader-Willi syndrome. Arch Dermatol 128:1623–1625, 1992

Watson SJ, Akil A, Berger PHA, et al: Some observations on the opiate peptides and schizophrenia. Arch Gen Psychiatry 36:35–41, 1979

Wiener K, Lamberti JS: Sertraline and mental retardation with obsessive-compulsive disorder. Am J Psychiatry 150:1270, 1993

Wiepkema PR, Schouten WGP: Stereotypies in sows during chronic stress. Psychother Psychosom 57:194–199, 1992

Willemsen-Swinkels SHN, Buitelaar JK, et al: Failure of noltrexone hydrochloride to reduce self-injurious and autistic behavior in mentally retarded adults. Arch Gen Psychiatry 52:766–773, 1995

Young JG, Halparin JM, Loven LI, et al: Developmental neuropharmacology: clinical and neurochemical perspectives on the regulation of attention, learning and movement, in Handbook of Psychopharmacology. Edited by Svensen LL, Svensen SD, Snyder SD. New York, Plenum, 1987, pp 59–122

Yudofsky SC, Silver JM, Schneider SE: The use of beta-blockers in the treatment of aggression. Psychiatry Letter 15–23, 1988

17 Strategic Behavioral Interventions in Aggression

Dorothy Griffiths, Ph.D.

Aggression to self, property, or others is one of the most challenging behaviors to deal with effectively because of the complexity of the causes. As such it cannot be treated as a single phenomenon that can be easily treated with any one intervention (Sovner and DesNoyers Hurley 1986). In this chapter, I will address aggression from a number of diagnostic and intervention approaches as it pertains to persons with developmental disabilities.

Persons with developmental disabilities often exhibit more disruptive and dangerous behavior than their nondisabled peers (Carr 1977; Favell et al. 1982). It has been estimated that severe behavior problems, such as self-injury or aggression, may be displayed by 12%–15% of individuals with developmental disabilities (Altmeyer et al. 1987; Oliver et al. 1987).

Until the past 15 years, behavior reduction strategies, often of a highly intrusive nature, were considered to be the most effective techniques for the management of aggression and other severe behavior problems (Favell et al. 1982; Lennox et al. 1988). However there is a distinction between "effective treatment" and "symptom management" (Gardner and Cole 1987). Treatment conditions are characterized by 1) producing enduring effects across time and situations, 2) providing socially appropriate alternative skills, and 3) altering how the individual responds to previous antecedents for the behavior (Gardner and Cole 1987). In contrast, management strategies provide a temporary suppression of the problem behavior, which is likely to return to the preintervention level when the intervention conditions are removed (Gardner and Cole 1987).

When aggression is displayed by a person with developmental disabilities, caregivers typically respond by suppressing or restraining the behavior, either chemically or physically. These management strategies work through negative reinforcement by providing escape from an unpleasant or undesired situation. However, the precipitating factors that prompted the problem behavior still exist, as does the individual's need to control these factors. Suppression of the behavior through punishment or control fails to address why the behavior occurred and whether the individual has the capacity of handling a similar situation in the future.

In contrast to the management approach that involves responding to aggression, strategic behavioral intervention is based on performing a complex differential assessment to determine the meaning or cause of the aggression. The goal of assessment is to determine the biopsychosocial events that are correlated with the occurrence of the aggression (Gardner 1998).

Typically, behavioral assessments were limited to an antecedent-behavior-consequence analysis. This type of assessment provides information about the antecedent events that frequently preceded the problem behavior and the consequences that frequently followed the behavior that appeared to be correlated with the behavior. However, in recent years a multimodal behavioral support model has gained acceptance as "best practice" (Gardner 1998; Griffiths et al. 1998). This multicomponent approach includes a comprehensive assessment of biomedical and environmental influences on maladaptive behavior (Feldman and Griffiths 1997) that typically rely on indirect (e.g., informant interview) and descriptive functional assessment (O'Neill et al. 1997), and determination of stimulus control events (Touchette et al. 1985) to generate hypotheses. Although experimental (analog) functional analysis methodology is often used in research settings to confirm hypotheses, it is generally not feasible in most clinical settings (Feldman and Griffiths 1997).

It has been hypothesized that the combination of these assessment areas would lead to effective treatment for even the most severe behavior, such as aggression (Axelrod 1987; Iwata et al. 1982).

■ COMPREHENSIVE ASSESSMENT AND TREATMENT COMPONENTS

The key to effective strategic behavior intervention is the assessment of the basis of the behavior. Aggression can be a reaction to internally or externally precipitated distress, a response to current or previously conditioned events, or serve a specified function. Behaviors, such a aggression, can be analyzed in terms of being reactive, responsive, or functional. However, most complex behaviors are not singularly determined but are influenced by a number of factors that interplay to produce the aggressive behavior. By conducting a comprehensive analysis of a variety of potential influences, a differential diagnosis of the behavior can be achieved. As illustrated in Figure 17–1, in order to make the differential diagnosis of aggressive behavior, there must be an investigation at multiple levels.

It should be noted that the levels of analysis suggested below are for descriptive purposes. Often, and more often than not, cases of severe aggression

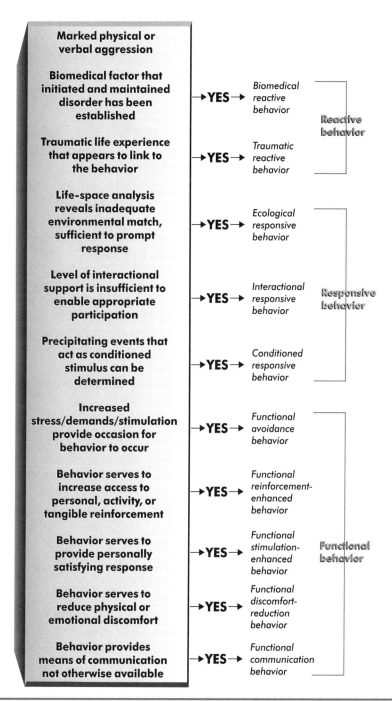

Figure 17–1.   Differential diagnosis of aggressive behavior.

and self-injury are found to be influencing factors at several levels of the assessment process, and the existence of certain conditions at one level can interact with conditions at other levels to produce a compound effect.

■ REACTIVE BEHAVIORS

Sovner and DesNoyers Hurley (1986) suggest that "any psychiatric or medical disorder which can produce emotional distress can cause aggressive behavior" (p. 17). Aggressive behavior has been observed in some cases to be a direct or indirect reaction to a state of internal distress caused by some biomedical disturbance or traumatic event. Gardner and Sovner (1994) caution that in most cases behaviors are not directly caused by a psychiatric or biomedical state, but rather the state renders the individual more vulnerable to psychological and environmental influences that then trigger the aggression.

Biomedical Reactive Behavior

Aggression can sometimes be explained as a manifestation of a biomedical state that is physical, medication induced, or psychiatric in nature. In some cases the aggression can be caused by the biomedical condition, such as some types of seizure disorders. However, as stated previously, in most cases the biomedical state preconditions the individual to be more "vulnerable" to events in the environment (Gardner and Sovner 1994).

Physical Disorder

Partial complex seizure disorders and the resultant personality changes have been shown to be associated with aggressive behavior (Devinsky and Bear 1984). In addition there are a number of conditions that are associated with an increased risk of behavior problems (e.g., Lesch-Nyhan, Rett's, fragile X, Prader-Willi, fetal alcohol, traumatic brain injury, and posttraumatic stress disorder [PTSD]) (Feldman and Griffiths 1997). Because of the communication problems of many individuals with disabilities, aggression has also been seen as being a means of indicating discomfort from a variety of medical conditions, such as migraines, dental problems, hypoglycemia, or a blocked shunt. If an underlying physical condition can be determined for the aggression and that condition is treatable medically, then appropriate medical intervention would be advised as the treatment of first choice.

Medication Reaction

Aggression can result from drug therapy, which may produce a mental state in which the person may be more predisposed to act aggressively (Sovner and

Des Noyers Hurley 1986). The medication reaction may result from a side effect of the medication, such as akathisia, disinhibition, excitability, and disorientation, or at the time of drug withdrawal.

Psychiatric/Emotional Disorder

Aggression is a defining characteristic in some psychiatric disorders listed in DSM-IV (American Psychiatric Association 1994). Aggression is often associated with schizophrenia, mania, agitated depression, generalized anxiety, or borderline and antisocial personality disorders (Sovner and DesNoyers Hurley 1986). Persons with developmental disabilities experience the same range of emotional and psychiatric disorders as nondisabled persons (Menolascino and McCann 1983), although these disorders are frequently overlooked (Reiss et al. 1982) or misdiagnosed (Sovner and Des Noyers Hurley 1986).

Sovner and DesNoyers Hurley (1989) have suggested that psychiatric disorders, when experienced by persons with developmental disabilities, can often appear as maladaptive behavior. Determining that there is a biomedical condition associated with the aggression does not necessarily determine causality but may predispose the individual to be more vulnerable to other external conditions. It has been suggested that "the more severe the disabilities, the more likely it is that the individual will express his or her discomfort in a nonspecific way such as hitting out" (Sovner and DesNoyers Hurley 1986, p. 17). Regardless of whether the discomfort is caused by physical or psychological states, persons with disabilities are more likely to express the problem behaviorally (Sovner and DesNoyers Hurley 1989).

The person whose behavior is a reaction to a psychiatric condition may well respond to medication to relieve symptoms of the disorder; however, this does not necessarily preclude the need for behavioral intervention or changes in the environment.

Although medication may be the first step in the therapeutic process when there is a clearly diagnosable medication-responsive condition, lifestyle changes and behavioral programming may be concurrently recommended. For example, research on depression with individuals with developmental disabilities has shown that although medication is advised, concurrent intervention to reduce insularity and to teach social skills is often recommended (Benson et al. 1985).

Traumatic Reactive Behavior

Wolpe (1973) suggested that the function of some behaviors is to indicate distress or a need for help from some traumatic situation. Recently, it has been identified that a high incidence of traumatic experiences in the life of persons with disabilities may be a contributing factor to severe behavioral manifestations, including aggression (Ryan 1990). These experiences are primarily, but not limited to, sexual and physical abuse.

International advocacy groups such as the Association for Persons With Severe Handicaps (TASH) have identified a number of human rights violations and allegations of cruel and unusual punishment of persons with developmental disabilities. Recent research has revealed that people with disabilities are 150% more likely to be sexually abused, assaulted, or exploited than nondisabled persons (Sobsey 1988). It is therefore more likely that persons with a developmental disability may experience posttraumatic stress disorder (PTSD), which until recently has not been diagnosed nor treated in persons with disabilities. According to DSM-IV, outbursts of anger are one of the persistent symptoms of increased arousal associated with PTSD.

Ryan (1994) suggests a treatment regime for PTSD that includes the judicious use of medication, identification, and treatment of medical problems; minimization of iatrogenic complications; psychopathology; habilitative change to control triggers; and education for support staff. The systematic application of this intervention approach has been reported to result in positive changes in both the functioning of the individual and their reports of well-being.

■ RESPONSIVE BEHAVIORS

Aggression has most probably evolved as a defensive response (Scott 1970). Behaviors such as aggression may be responsive to factors that occur prior to the behavior and set the occasion for the behavior to occur. These factors could be events related to the environment or social ecology, interactional variables, or events that have been previously conditioned to elicit aggression. It has been demonstrated that by altering the care environment to provide a highly structured and organized program and by altering the interactional nature to increase reinforcement for appropriate behaviors, it is possible to reduce problem behaviors (Myers et al. 1991).

Ecological Responsive Behavior

The social and physical environment is an important variable in the assessment of behavior. Behavior can be a response to specific aspects of the environment (Boe 1977; Rago et al. 1978). In recent years, educators have developed a life-space analysis to evaluate if the environment provides adequate physical space and appropriate habilitative programming and is suitable for individual preferences and needs.

Cataldo and Risley (1974) defined the quality of a setting by the degree to which the clients are stimulated by the environment (exhibit movement, vocalization, and attention to external stimulation), interact with the environment, and are encouraged to participate in activities. Research has shown that when an environment is enriched, aggression to self and property can be significantly reduced (Levy and McLeod 1977). Unfortunately, the physical environment of many persons with disabilities is enormously sparse, characterized by a limited number of environments, a lack of meaningful activities, and minimal engagement with the environment and others. If the environment is experientially limited or without sufficient involvement to keep the person participating appropriately, then behavior problems are more likely to occur. Aggression toward self, others, or property is often an adaptive means to increasing stimulation, interest, and changes in an unenriched environment.

Social disorganization is also a major cause of destructive violence (Scott 1970). Gilson and Levitas (1987) noted that individuals with developmental disabilities experience a number of developmental milestones that are marked by emotional turmoil. The crisis effect results from the interplay of physical and social influences experienced by persons with disabilities (Webster 1970). For example, the placement of a person with disabilities out of the home can mark the achievement of a personal goal of emancipation and maturation; however, too often the person has little to say with regard to when and where he or she will be relocated (Gilson and Levitas 1987).

All too often persons with disabilities are faced with disruption in their social conditions, such as institutionalization; deinstitutionalization; repeated home, job, staff, or roommate changes; or programming changes, over which they have little choice or determination. The neurological difficulties and limited coping skills of many persons with developmental disabilities may make it more difficult for them to adjust to these changes. It has been suggested that common stress experiences, such as the death of a parent or environmental changes, may be sufficient in persons with developmental disabilities to precipitate a PTSD reaction (Crabbe 1991).

Transitional stressors may be exhibited as a loss of adaptive skills, referred to as "cognitive disintegration," or a rapid or exaggerated acceleration of more primitive coping strategies, described as "baseline exaggeration" of typical coping patterns (Sovner and DesNoyers Hurley 1986). However, there have been documented reports of individuals who, when subjected to repeated changes in their environments over short periods of time, may experience "relocation syndrome," characterized by weight loss, depression, and even death (Cochran et al. 1977). It has been suggested that the systematic and graduated change of stimulus events during major transitions, such as deinstitutionalization, would reduce the incidence of transitional problems (Cochran et al. 1977). In a follow-up review of the process of deinstitutionalization of Pine Ridge Center in Ontario, Canada, it was reported that 86% of the residents demonstrated successful social and developmental progress in the year that followed the community placement (Griffiths 1985). The individuals who experienced difficulty adjusting to the transition were not necessarily those who were predicted to have a higher risk of developing problems. Many individuals who were expected to experience major difficulty in transition showed adequate to excellent adjustment. Thus it was concluded that the best predictor of success of community adjustment was the environment's ability and commitment to supporting the individual rather than any factors related to the individual (Griffiths 1985).

Interactional Responsive Behavior

The interactional quality and quantity of the person's life are crucial areas to examine. Despite the richness of the setting, all people, and perhaps in particular persons who are disabled, need support to be able to interact appropriately in life. Many people with developmental disabilities are not afforded appropriate quality or quantity of personal care or personal contact so as to ensure that they can effectively interact in all aspects of daily life. A lack of interactional richness, evaluated as loneliness and social isolation, has been shown to contribute to depression in persons with developmental disabilities (Benson et al. 1985).

In agencies or services, we assume that interactional quality is measured by staff ratio. Staff ratios alone are insufficient indicators of interactional richness; one must examine how much time staff spend on paperwork, housekeeping without clients, or in staff discussions compared with direct or parallel client interaction. The caregiving approach, including level of attention, disapproval, and demands, has been shown to relate directly to behavior (respectively, Carr and Durand 1985; Mace et al. 1986; Carr et al. 1980). Similarly, peer modeling and taunting have been shown to affect aggressive behavior (Cole et al. 1985; Talkington and Altman 1973).

Conditioned Responsive Behavior

Where and when does the behavior occur? Does it occur randomly across people, activities, and times, or are there identifiable persons, environments, interactions, materials, or routines in which the behavior frequently or infrequently occurs? Establishing the prompting and discriminate stimuli that are associated with a behavior can be systematically accomplished using a "scatter plot" (Touchette et al. 1985).

A scatter plot is a method of data collection that traces the pattern of the behavior to the person's daily routine to identify problem-eliciting and problem-free events. Using the scatter plot, it is possible to evaluate whether a problem behavior is associated with time of day, certain people, specific activities, physical conditions, or a combination of these and other variables. Managing aggression involves the systematic change of events that prompts the problem behavior and events that could prevent the behavior. Touchette et al. (1985) demonstrated that by using the "scatter plot," situations in which the behavior was very likely to occur and those in which it was least likely to occur could be identified. The environment was then rearranged so that situations in which the behavior was least likely to occur were maximized and situations in which the behavior was most likely to occur were minimized. Once the pattern was established, the life space was altered to minimize events that were likely to prompt the problem and maximize events that were likely to be problem free. The objective of this stimulus change was to create a "zero baseline," or the reduction of the problem behavior to as close to zero as possible (Touchette et al. 1985).

Severe aggressive behaviors were able to be reduced to a zero baseline level by identifying and then eliminating the environmental conditions that were associated with the assaultive behavior (Touchette et al. 1985). Bailey (1989) refers to the manipulation of events, to prevent problem behavior or to reduce or eliminate its occurrence, as "passive behavior management."

The removal of the prompting stimuli for a period of time has been demonstrated to be sufficient to alter the stimulus-response pattern that previously existed (Touchette 1990). This experience creates a "vacation tolerance effect," which occurs when the withdrawal of the provoking stimuli for a sufficiently long period of time allows a sufficient vacation from the provoking stimuli such that the individual is no longer provoked or has a greater tolerance to the prompting stimuli. However, it has not been demonstrated that removal of the prompting stimuli will always alter the tolerance level.

Many stimulus changes are complex and cannot realistically be maintained indefinitely. However, stimulus change techniques can serve as an effective crisis intervention approach until the effect of functional replacement training can be realized. Under these conditions, stimulus change methods do not serve a therapeutic purpose, which is to make long-term changes that free the individual from ongoing intervention, but serve as crisis management, which is the temporary reduction of the behavior until more therapeutic strategies can be employed.

■ FUNCTIONAL BEHAVIOR

Aggression can serve a variety of social functions (Scott 1970). Aggressive behavior exists and continues to exist because it receives reinforcement. The reinforcement theory, based on operant principles, has substantial support (Carr 1977; Favell et al. 1982; Frankel and Simmons 1976; Iwata et al. 1982). According to this theory, behavioral disorders are learned patterns of responding to contingencies of reinforcement that are present in the person's past or current environments.

The main source of motivation for behavior is either positive or negative reinforcement (Carr 1977). Problem behaviors exist and persist because they have a reinforcement value for the individual. There is value in the problem behavior, no matter what its form; it pays off for the person in his or her natural environment and interactions.

A behavior can be motivated by more than one form of reinforcement (Iwata et al. 1982) or serve multiple functions. The same behavior may be used at some times to gain attention while at other times to escape from demands. The assessment of conditions under which maladaptive behaviors occur is often referred to as a "functional assessment" (Axelrod 1987; Iwata et al. 1982). Functional assessment involves identifying the contingencies of reinforcement, either positive or negative, that are maintaining the behavior (Axelrod 1987). This is accomplished through interviews, naturalistic observations of the antecedents and consequences that surround a behavior, and/or experimental manipulation of events using a functional analysis (Durand and Crimmins 1988; O'Neill et al. 1997).

There are five basic functions that behavior has been demonstrated to serve: reinforcement enhancement, avoidance, stimulation enhancement, discomfort reduction, and communication.

Reinforcement Enhancement

Self-injury and aggression in persons with developmental disabilities have been demonstrated to be motivated to gain attention (Lovaas et al. 1967) or material needs, such as food or tangible items (Lovaas and Simmons 1969).

Stimulation Enhancement

Sensory reinforcement has been identified as the motivation for behaviors such as self-injury, aggression, and stereotypy (Favell et al. 1982; Rincover and Devany 1982; Rincover et al. 1979).

Avoidance

Aggressive behavior can be motivated by negative reinforcement, to avoid or escape an unpleasant situation (Carr 1977; Carr et al. 1980; Donnellan et al. 1985), or when frustrated or experiencing extinction of a previously available reinforcement.

Discomfort Reduction

Hutt and Hutt (1965) demonstrated that behaviors could be motivated to terminate an overly stimulating situation from which the person could not escape. Environmental engineering has been shown to have a dramatic influence in reducing aggression induced by factors affecting physical discomfort (Levy and McLeod 1977; Rago et al. 1978).

Communicative Skills

DSM-IV states that a lack of communication skills in persons with mental retardation may predispose them to disruptive and aggressive behaviors that substitute for communicative language. Carr and Durand (1985) hypothesized that behaviors such as crying, tantrums, aggression, noises, intimidations, facial responses, or social distance served a communicative function. However, it has been further suggested that each motivational function could be interpreted as a means to communicate a request for attention/interaction or an object or help, a protest to routines or the termination of a desired activity, a declaration of needs, or to encourage another to do something (Donnellan et al. 1985).

The functional assessment may reveal several conditions that are responsible for prompting the problem behavior. Based on the functional assessment, the individual is taught a functional replacement behavior, which is an alternative means to aggression to achieve the desired outcome (e.g., Carr 1988; Evans and Meyer 1985). Functional replacement training involves the following:

- Identifying of an alternative behavior that can be taught or strengthened to serve as a replacement for the inappropriate behavior
- Increasing the probability of the replacement behavior's being elicited (Horner et al. 1991; Mace et al. 1988)
- Providing reinforcement for an appropriate replacement behavior that is functionally equivalent to the inappropriate behavior (Favell and Reid 1988)
- Providing functional extinction for the inappropriate expression of achieving the desired function by no longer providing the previous reinforcement that maintained the behavior (Carr et al. 1980; Mazalwski et al. 1993; Rincover and Devany 1982)

Caution should to be taken in ensuring that the functional replacement skills are established as an alternate means of achieving the desired function so that the possible side effects of extinction, such as extinction bursts and extinction-induced aggression, are minimized (Sulzer-Azaroff and Mayer 1972).

There is a growing body of research that has demonstrated that behavior enhancement techniques based on a functional analysis are effective strategies for reducing aggressive behaviors in persons with severe disabilities (National Institute of Health 1991). In a review of 23 studies on the treatment of severe aggression and self-injury, Freeman (1993) reported that functional analyses were conducted in more than half the studies, and that when these analyses were used to direct treatment, the problem behavior was suppressed by more than 79%.

Communication training is one of the most common skills taught as a replacement for a number of problem behaviors (Bird et al. 1989; Carr and Durand 1985; Durand and Carr 1987; Horner and Budd 1985). Carr and Durand (1985) showed that teaching alternative communicative behavior that can serve the same function provides an effective strategy for decreasing problem behavior.

There is a range of behavior enhancement programs that can be implemented, depending on the function of the behavior. They could include social skills, tolerance training, self-care training, problem solving, leisure skills, and relaxation training. For example, aggression can be reduced by teaching an incompatible relaxation response to the arousal. Relaxation training programs have been successfully employed with persons with developmental disabilities (Cautela and Grodin 1978; Harvey et al. 1978). However, experience has shown that some individuals with developmental disabilities demonstrate difficulty in identifying the physiological arousal necessary to apply the relaxation in a preventative manner. It is also important to determine if the arousal is the result of anxiety that is responsive to relaxation techniques or if there is a condition that requires biomedical intervention.

In anger management training, persons with disabilities are taught social problem-solving skills as alternative strategies to their aggression (Benson 1986). In this training, participants are taught that anger is a signal that there is a problem to be solved. They are taught a four-step plan to solve problems: 1) identify the problem, 2) generate possible solutions, 3) select the best solution, and 4) implement the chosen solution (Benson 1986).

■ CONCLUSIONS

The National Institute of Health (NIH) (1991) published a report, "Treatment of Destructive Behavior in Persons With Developmental Disabilities." The report identified three major classes of intervention: behavior enhancement techniques, behavior reduction methods, and pharmacological treatment. They concluded that the most effective treatments would involve multiple components of intervention. The components may include medical/

psychiatric aspects, social-ecological factors, and behavioral influences. However, the NIH report findings suggest that intervention that includes functional analysis of skills and setting events appeared most effective. They further noted that when behaviors were precipitated by multiple factors, intervention based on a combination of approaches was useful.

The strategic intervention for aggression is based on a comprehensive client-specific analysis of biomedical, environmental, and functional variables acting to instigate the aggression. It has been suggested that "the goal of research should not be to determine which techniques work in any circumstance, but whether an appropriate combination of treatments can be identified following an assessment of the multiple variables which influence the target behavior" (Freeman 1993, p. 22). Based on the differential diagnosis of the aggressive behavior, intervention can take on many forms.

Therapeutically, there is increasing evidence to support the efficacy of treatment procedures selected on the basis of client-specific diagnostic information and designed to teach alternative coping skills to replace aggressive behavior. Comprehensive and habilitative procedures for treating aggressive behaviors are more socially and ethically acceptable and avoid the potential negative side effects associated with behavior control strategies.

■ REFERENCES

Altmeyer BH, Locke BJ, Griffin JC, et al: Treatment strategies for self-injurious behavior in a large service-delivery network. American Journal of Mental Deficiency 91:333–340, 1987

American Psychiatric Association: Diagnostic and Statistical Manual of Mental Disorders, 4th Edition. Washington, DC, American Psychiatric Association, 1994

Axelrod S: Functional and structural analyses of behavior: approaches leading to reduced use of punishment procedures. Res Dev Disabil 8:165–178, 1987

Bailey J: Behavioral diagnostic. Article presented at the State of the Art Strategic Behavior Intervention Conference, Toronto, Ontario, Canada, June 1989

Benson BA: Anger management training. Psychiatric Aspects of Mental Retardation Reviews 5:51–55, 1986

Benson BA, Reiss S, Smith DC, et al: Psychosocial correlates of depression in mentally retarded adults; II: poor social skills. American Journal of Mental Deficiency 6:657–659, 1985

Bird F, Dores PA, Moniz D, et al: Reducing severe aggressive and self-injurious behaviors with functional communication training. Am J Ment Retard 94:37–48, 1989

Boe RB: Economical procedures for the reduction of aggression in a residential setting. Ment Retard 15:25–28, 1977

Carr EG: The motivation of self-injurious behavior: a review of some hypotheses. Psychol Bull 84:800–816, 1977

Carr EG: Functional equivalence as a mechanism of response generalization, in Generalization and Maintenance: Life-Style Change in Applied Settings. Edited by Horner R, Dunlop G, Koegel R. Baltimore, MD, Paul H Brookes, 1988, pp 54–72

Carr EG, Durand VM: Reducing behavior problems through functional communication training. J Appl Behav Anal 18:111–126, 1985

Carr EC, Newsom CD, Binkoff JA: Escape as a factor in the aggressive behavior of two retarded children. J Appl Behav Anal 13:101–117, 1980

Cataldo MF, Risley TR: Evaluation of living environments: the MANIFEST description word activities, in Evaluation of Social Programs in Community Residential and School Settings. Edited by Davidson PO, Clark FW, Hamerlynch LA. Champaign, IL, Research Press, 1974, pp 159–168

Cautela J, Grodin J: Relaxation: A Comprehensive Manual for Adults, Children, and Children With Special Needs. Champaign, IL, Research Press, 1978

Cochran WE, Sran PK, Varano GA: The relocation syndrome in mentally retarded individuals. Ment Retard 4:10–12, 1977

Cole CL, Gardner WI, Karan OC: Self-management training of mentally retarded adults presenting severe conduct difficulties. Applied Research in Mental Retardation 6:337–347, 1985

Crabbe H: A neuropsychiatric overview of anxiety disorders in persons with mental retardation. Article presented at the 8th Annual Conference of National Association for the Dually Diagnosed. Denver, CO, December 1991

Devinsky G, Bear D: Varieties of aggressive behavior in temporal lobe epilepsy. Am J Psychiatry 141:651–656, 1984

Donnellan AM, Mirenda P, Mesaros RA, et al: Analyzing the communicative functions of aberrant behavior. Journal of the Association for Persons With Severe Handicaps 9:201–212, 1985

Durand VM, Carr EG: Social influences on self-stimulatory behavior: analysis and treatment application. J Appl Behav Anal 20:119–132, 1987

Durand VM, Crimmins DB: Identifying the variables maintaining self-injurious behavior. J Autism Dev Disord 18: 99–117, 1988

Evans IM, Meyer LH: An Educative Approach to Behavior Problems: A Practical Decision Model for Intervention With Severely Handicapped Learners. Baltimore, MD, Paul H Brookes, 1985

Favell JE, Reid DH: Generating and maintaining improvement in problem behavior, in Generalization and Maintenance: Lifestyle Changes in Applied Settings. Edited by Horner R, Dunlop G, Koegel R. Baltimore, MD, Paul H Brookes, 1988, pp 171–196

Favell JE, McGimsey JF, Schell RM: Treatment of self injury by providing alternative sensory activities. Analysis and Intervention in Developmental Disabilities 2:83–104, 1982

Feldman M, Griffiths D: Comprehensive assessment of behavior problems with persons with developmental disabilities, in Treatment of Severe Behavior Problems: Models and Methods. Edited by Singh NN. Pacific Grove, GA, Brooks/Cole, 1997, pp 23–48

Frankel F, Simmons JQ: Self-injurious behavior in schizophrenic and retarded children. American Journal of Mental Deficiency 80:512–522, 1976

Freeman N: Treatment strategies for aberrant behaviors in people with developmental disabilities: a review of recent literature. Toronto, Ontario, Canada, Ontario Mental Health Foundation, December 1993

Gardner WI: Initiating the case formulation process; in Behavioral Supports: Individual Centered Interventions. Edited by Griffiths D, Gardner WI, Nuget JA. Kingston, NY, NADD Press, 1998, pp 17–66

Gardner WI, Cole CL: Behavior treatment, behavior management, and behavior control: needed distinction. Behavioral Residential Treatment 237–253, 1987

Gardner WI, Sovner R: Self-Injurious Behaviors: Diagnosis and Treatment—A Multimodal Functional Approach. Willow Street, PA, Vida Publishing, 1994

Gilson SF, Levitas AS: Psychosocial crises in the lives of mentally retarded people. Psychiatric Aspects of Mental Retardation Reviews 6(6):27–31, 1987

Griffiths D: Pine Ridge: A Follow Up Study. Toronto, Ontario, Canada, The Ontario Association for the Mentally Retarded, 1985

Griffiths D, Gardner WI, Nuget JA: Creating habilitatively appropriate environments, in Behavioral Supports: Individual Centered Interventions. Edited by Griffiths D, Gardner WI, Nuget JA. Kingston, NY, NADD Press, 1998, 99–132

Harvey JR, Karan OC, Bhargava D, et al: Relaxation training and cognitive behavioral responses to reduce violent temper outbursts in a moderately retarded woman. J Behav Ther Exp Psychiatry 9:347–351, 1978

Horner RH, Budd CM: Teaching manual sign language to a nonverbal student: generalization of sign use and collateral reduction of maladaptive behavior. Education and Training of the Mentally Retarded 20: 39–47, 1985

Horner RH, Day M, Sprague R, et al: Interspersed requests: A nonaversive procedure for reducing aggression and self-injury during instruction. J Appl Behav Anal 24:265–278, 1991

Hutt C, Hutt S: Effects of environmental complexity on stereotyped behavior of children. Animal Behavior 13:1–12, 1965

Iwata BA, Dorsey MF, Slifer KJ, et al: Toward a functional analysis of self-injury. Analysis and Intervention in Developmental Disabilities 2:3–20, 1982

Lennox DB, Miltenberger RG, Spengler RE, et al: Decelerative treatment practices with persons who have mental retardation: a review of five years of the literature. Am J Ment Retard 92:492–510, 1988

Levy E, McLeod W: The effects of environmental design on adolescents in an institution. Am J Ment Retard 15:28–32, 1977

Lovaas OI, Simmons JG: Manipulation of self-destruction in three retarded children. J Appl Behav Anal 2:143–157, 1969

Lovaas OI, Frietag C, Gold VJ, et al: Experimental studies in childhood schizophrenia: analysis of self-destructive behavior. J Exp Child Psychol 2:67–84, 1967

Mace FC, Page TJ, Ivancic MT, et al: Analysis of environmental determinants of aggression and disruption in mentally retarded children. Applied Research in Mental Retardation 7:203–221, 1986

Mace FC, Hock ML, Lalli JS, et al: Behavioral momentum in the treatment of noncompliance. J Appl Behav Anal 21:123–141, 1988

Mazalwski JL, Iwata BA, Vollmer TR, et al: Analysis of the reinforcement and extinction components in DRO contingencies with self injury. J Appl Behav Anal 26:143–156, 1993

Menolascino FJ, McCann BM: Mental Health and Mental Retardation: Bridging the Gap. Baltimore, MD, University Park Press, 1983

Myers AM, Richards T, Huff J: "Time-In": a two year project for the reduction of severe maladaptive behaviours in a center for persons with developmental disabilities. Behavioral Residential Treatment 6:119–144, 1991

National Institute of Health: Treatment of Destructive Behaviors in Persons With Developmental Disabilities. Bethesda, MD, National Institute of Health, 1991

Oliver C, Murphy GH, Corbett JA: Self-injurious behavior in people with mental handicap: a total population study. Journal of Mental Deficiency Research 31:147–162, 1987

O'Neill RA, Horner RH, Albin RW, et al: Functional Analysis of Problem Behavior: A Practical Guide. Sycamore, IL, Sycamore Press, 1997

Rago WV, Parker RM, Cleland CC: Effect of increased space on the social behavior of institutionalized profoundly retarded adult males. American Journal of Mental Deficiency 82:554–558, 1978

Reiss S, Levitan GW, Szysko J: Emotional disturbance and mental retardation: diagnostic overshadowing. American Journal of Mental Deficiency 86:567–574, 1982

Rincover A, Devany J: Using sensory reinforcement and sensory extinction principles in the treatment of self-injury. Analysis and Intervention in Developmental Disabilities 2:67–81, 1982

Rincover A, Cook R, Peoples A, et al: Sensory extinction and sensory reinforcement principles for programming multiple adaptive behavior change. J Appl Behav Anal 12: 221–233, 1979

Ryan R: Posttraumatic stress syndrome: assessing and treating the aftermath of sexual assault. NADD Newsletter 1(3):5–7, 1994

Scott JP: Biology and human aggression. Am J Orthopsychiatry 40(4):568–576, 1970

Sobsey D: Sexual offenses and disabled victims: research and practical implications vis-a-vis: a national newsletter on family violence. Ottawa, Canada, Canadian Council on Social Development 6:4, 1988

Sovner R, DesNoyers Hurley A: Four factors affecting the diagnosis of psychiatric disorders in mentally retarded persons. Psychiatric Aspects of Mental Retardation Reviews 5(9):45–49, 1986

Sovner R, DesNoyers Hurley A: Ten diagnostic principles for recognizing psychiatric disorders in mentally retarded persons. Psychiatric Aspects of Mental Retardation Reviews 8(2):9–13, 1989

Sulzer-Azaroff B, Mayer GR: Applying Behavior Analysis With Children and Youth. New York, Holt, Rinehart, & Winston, 1972

Talkington LW, Altman R: Effects of film-mediated aggressive and effectual models on behavior. American Journal of Mental Deficiency 77:420–425, 1973

Touchette PE: Stimulus control. Paper presented at the State of the Art Strategic Behavior Intervention Conference. Toronto, Ontario, Canada, June 1990

Touchette PE, MacDonald RF, Langer SN: A scatter plot for identifying stimulus control of problem behavior. J Appl Behav Anal 18(4):343–351, 1985

Webster TG: Unique aspects of emotional development in mentally retarded children, in Psychiatric Approaches to Mental Retardation. Edited by Menolascino FJ. New York, Basic Books, 1970, pp 1–54

Wolpe J: The Practice of Behavior Therapy, 2nd Edition. Elmsford, NY, Pergamon, 1973

18 Self-Injurious Behaviors

Multimodal Contextual Approach to Treatment

William I. Gardner, Ph.D.
Janice L. Graeber-Whalen, Ph.D.
Debby R. Ford, Ph.D.

■ INTRODUCTION

Self-injurious behaviors (SIBs) refer to those repetitive and chronic stereo-typed acts that either result in direct physical damage or potentially endanger the physical well-being of the person displaying the behavior. SIBs include such acts as self-striking; biting various body parts; cutting and burning the skin; pulling, poking, or scratching various body parts; teeth grinding; and inserting objects in body cavities such as ears and nose. Among those who exhibit SIBs, head banging, self-biting, self-striking, and scratching occur with the greatest frequency. It is estimated that over 50% of those engaging in SIBs exhibit more than one form (e.g., head banging, self-biting, and self-pinching) (Benson and Aman 1999; Gardner and Sovner 1994; Luiselli et al. 1992).

SIBs are significant not only because the person is placed in serious jeopardy of physical harm (e.g., tissue damage, amputation, fractures, loss of vision) but also because frequent and intense episodes of self-injurious acts interfere with efforts at providing positive social and educational experiences for the person. As a result, the development of the person's social, emotional, intellectual, and adaptive behavior characteristics is impeded. In addition, the physical and chemical procedures frequently used for managing and protecting the person may interfere significantly with habilitative program efforts. The cost of care and treatment of severe cases requiring residential placement can run as high as $100,000 per year. Finally, the prolonged use of various physical and/or chemical restraints as a means of managing or minimizing the frequency and intensity of SIBs may result in permanent

---

Ms. Graeber-Whalen died in early 2000, shortly after beginning her professional career. This chapter is dedicated to her.

physical and/or neurological damage to the person (Favell 1982; Schroeder et al. 1990).

Individual Differences in Type and Severity

Marked individual differences are evident in the type, frequency, severity, and duration of self-injurious episodes. In some persons, SIBs may be stereotyped and occur hundreds of times and in numerous situations throughout the day, as illustrated by an individual who repetitively bangs his fist against his head for extended periods. Other forms of SIBs may be relatively nonrepetitive (e.g., eye gouging and rectal digging) and may occur only in certain situations or at certain times. Some individuals may display only a single SIB such as hand biting, head banging, cutting or burning the skin, or face and head slapping; others may display multiple forms of SIBs. The majority of individuals who engage in self-injury demonstrate other stereotyped behaviors such as repetitive screaming and body rocking. In addition, in some persons, SIBs occur in a sequence or chain of other aberrant behaviors such as aggression or destruction of property (Davidson et al. 1996; Lewis et al. 1995; Rojahn 1994; Schroeder et al. 1990; Winchel and Stanley 1991).

Comorbidity: Risk Factors

Although SIBs may occur among individuals with mild and moderate levels of mental retardation, the greatest frequency and severity are observed among individuals with severe and profound mental retardation, communication deficits (especially those reflecting receptive skills that are more advanced than expressive skills), sensory disabilities, and lengthy histories of institutional living as well as with diagnoses of brain injury, seizure disorders, pervasive developmental disorder with associated severe social impairment, and specific medical disorders such as fragile X, Lesch-Nyhan, Prader-Willi, and Tourette's syndromes. In addition, some forms of SIBs may co-occur with various mental disorders such as borderline personality disorders, psychoses, major depression, compulsions, autistic disorder, and stereotypic movement disorder. Such acts of self-injury as cutting and burning the skin and sticking objects under the skin, when observed, occur typically among those with mild cognitive impairments and the accompanying psychiatric impairments. Although few of these disorders or conditions would be viewed as primary causes of the SIBs, they may be viewed as risk or predisposing factors that increase the likelihood of initiation and recurrence of SIBs when other instigating conditions are present (Bodfish et al. 1995; Došen 1993; Gardner and Sovner 1994; Mace and Mauk 1999; McLean et al. 1994; Oliver and Head 1990; Sovner and Fogelman 1996; Sovner and Pary 1993).

Prevalence of SIBs

Although reported to occur in all age groups, the relationship of SIBs to age represents a curvilinear one. Adolescents and adults have a higher prevalence of SIBs than young children and the elderly. Typically, the lower the person's IQ level, the more frequent, severe, and treatment resistant the SIBs are likely to be. Various studies report rates ranging from 8% to over 20% of the individuals with mental retardation living in public residential facilities and from 2% to 11% of those living in community settings. Females have a slightly lower rate of occurrence than males (Borthwick-Duffy 1994; Rojahn 1986, 1994).

Developmental Nature of Onset of SIBs

Specific biomedical or psychological conditions seldom result directly in SIBs. An exception may be seen in cases of involuntary self-injurious movements associated with seizure disorders (Gedye 1989). In most instances chronic self-injury may be viewed as representing learned behaviors that have been shaped and strengthened gradually by contingent reinforcing consequences (Iwata et al. 1994; Shore and Iwata 1999).

The reinforcement view of the development of chronic self-injury offers two hypotheses relating to the initial onset of self-injury, namely, the overarousal hypothesis and the homeostatic hypothesis. In the *overarousal hypothesis* model of initial onset, SIBs may reflect a rage, fear, or overarousal reaction to various painful or stressful circumstances. The SIBs represent attempts to reduce the high arousal level arising from the fear, anxiety, or other sources of discomfort such as an inner ear infection. The SIBs may result in reduction or termination of the arousal-inducing condition and also produce social feedback, reinforcement being provided by these consequences. This reinforcement adds to the likelihood of recurrence of SIBs at a future time under similar stimulus conditions. In this manner, self-injury becomes a coping (functional) behavior. The second learning view of the conditions giving rise to the initial onset of self-injury reflects a *homeostatic theory*. From this perspective, stereotypy occurs in understimulating environments as a means of regulating a desired level of arousal. The intensity of the stereotypic movements may be shaped inadvertently by contingent social feedback to the point that the behavior becomes self-injurious. The person gradually learns that the more intense forms of the rhythmic movements (SIBs) most reliably produce reinforcing social feedback (Guess and Carr 1991).

Prevalent Intervention

Various studies report that 30%–50% of the individuals with SIBs receive psychotropic medication to manage these problem behaviors. In fact, recent data indicate that, next to aggression and related agitated/disruptive behaviors, SIBs are the most commonly recorded behaviors of persons receiving psychotropic medication. This widespread use of psychotropic medication is very prevalent even though the general treatment efficacy of these drugs for SIBs has not been established. Although there is currently no successful pharmacotherapy for SIBs, in those instances in which SIBs reflect the secondary influence of various physical or mental illnesses or disorders, treatment of these underlying disorders may result in the reduction of SIBs (Gardner and Sovner 1994; Mace and Mauk 1999). In addition, evolving theoretical biochemical models offer possible pharmacological agents that may prove valuable in selective cases of chronic SIBs (Lewis et al. 1996; Schroeder and Tessel 1994; Thompson et al. 1994; Werry and Aman 1999). Various behavioral interventions have demonstrated efficacy in selected instances; however, these are not available to many persons with chronic SIBs due to the professional skill level and time required for adequate implementation. As a consequence of the current knowledge base and limited availability of resources, severe SIBs are typically managed by the use of medication and such protective devices as helmets and mechanical restraining devices such as cuffs, straps, splints, and vests (Baumeister and Sevin 1990; Gualtieri 1989).

■ MULTIMODAL CONTEXTUAL ANALYTIC APPROACH

As is evident, self-injury is a complex phenomenon and represents the effects of a variety of biomedical and psychosocial influences. To reflect the multiple and complex factors involved in the instigation and maintenance of self-injury, a multimodal contextual diagnostic and intervention model (described in Chapter 4 of this book) is offered to guide the practitioner in developing initial diagnostic-intervention formulations that translate into an integrated set of biomedical and psychosocial interventions (Gardner and Sovner 1994; Gardner et al. 1996; Mace and Mauk 1999).

In brief, this multimodal contextual analytic model represents a biopsychosocial view of self-injury. The initial step in devising an intervention program consists of developing a set of interrelated diagnostic and treatment formulations reflecting relevant biomedical, psychological, and socioenvironmental influences. Such formulations are necessary as self-injury is best viewed as a "final common pathway" reflecting an individual's adaptation to environmental demands and physical discomfort as well as to disturbances in neurochemical and physiological function. In view of the potential for multiple factors to contribute to the functionality of SIBs, there can be no single biomedical or psychosocial intervention. Self-injury associated with rage attacks, for example, may respond favorably to β-adrenergic receptor blocker therapy (e.g., propranolol), whereas SIBs associated with manic irritability will not. Self-injury representing an attempt to escape from an aversive task demand may not respond to an intervention tactic of increased staff attention. In sum, interventions must address the person-specific complex of instigating and maintaining conditions if enduring change in a person's SIBs is to be realized. Although this chapter addresses psychosocial interventions, the reader is reminded that, in most cases of severe and chronic SIBs, these will represent only one component of a more comprehensive multimodal intervention program (Gardner and Sovner 1994).

■ PSYCHOLOGICAL MODELS AND RELATED INTERVENTIONS

Although psychodynamic theories have drawn some attention to the factors that, following initial onset, result in the habitual recurrence of self-injury, these theories provide minimal direction for specific treatments of this problem behavior. One promising exception is the integrative developmental psychiatric approach described by Došen (1993). Currently, the major empirical contributions have come from learning models that view self-injury as learned behavior maintained by its consequences (Carr 1977; Iwata et al. 1994; Mace and Mauk 1999). These models also suggest a variety of intervention procedures for use in reducing or eliminating these aberrant behaviors. The following sections provide illustrations of the range of specific psychosocial interventions for self-injury that have been used successfully with persons with developmental disabilities. Consistent with the individualized diagnostic and program prescriptive emphasis of the multimodal contextual model, selection of any one or a combination of these and similar procedures should be based on the functional hypotheses derived from the study of each person. Additionally, when diagnostically indicated, these psychosocial interventions are closely interfaced with biomedical and environmental interventions. Interventions may address instigating and/or vulnerability antecedent influences and/or focus on presumed maintaining conditions (Carr et al. 1996; Gardner and Sovner 1994; Gardner et al. 1996; Griffiths et al. 1998).

As the level of health risk associated with self-injury varies from patient to patient, the selection of intervention approaches is influenced somewhat by the severity and specificity of the self-injury and related collateral behaviors. Suppressive procedures are used by some therapists to inhibit health-threatening self-injury and combined with therapy procedures to develop and maintain alternative skills of 1) gaining valued sensory and social stimulation and 2) coping with various aversive conditions (Linscheid 1992).

▓ REINFORCEMENT-MOTIVATED SIBS

After initial onset, SIBs may occur with consistency under specific instigating stimulus conditions because these result in valued social activity or tangible consequences. In addition, some persons with severe and profound levels of mental retardation, with limited social behaviors and/or with sensory and neurological difficulties, may resort to SIBs to obtain valued visual, auditory, proprioceptive, tactile, or other sensory stimulation. This view represents the *reinforcement-motivated hypothesis* of self-injury and provides direction in the selection of specific intervention procedures designed to alter the influence of these controlling conditions (Gardner and Sovner 1994; Mace and Mauk 1999; Oliver and Head 1990; Sprague and Horner 1999).

Antecedent Stimulus Events

In this approach to reducing self-injury, the stimulus conditions that initiate a person's self-injury are modified or replaced by conditions that mark the occasion for alternative adaptive responding. Systematic reinforcement of the resulting alternative behaviors may be provided to ensure maintenance of these new functional behaviors.

Enriched Stimulus Condition

Favell et al. (1982) observed that the eye poking, hand mouthing, and pica SIBs of young adults with profound mental retardation occurred primarily when they were socially isolated and unoccupied. An intervention program—based on the assumption that the SIBs were maintained by the resulting visual or gustatory sensory reinforcement—altered the antecedent stimulus conditions by providing toys that set the occasion for an appropriate alternative to SIBs. Under these enriched conditions, the adults had an opportunity to engage in toy play that provided sensory reinforcement similar to that associated with SIBs. An added component of external reinforcement of more appropriate conventional toy play resulted in further reduction. In each case, the self-stimulation produced by the toys involved the same sensory modality as that associated with SIBs (i.e., patients who eye-poked used toys to produce visual self-stimulation; those who engaged in hand mouthing and pica began chewing the toys).

Alternative Stimulation via Gross Motor Activities

Lancioni et al. (1984) and Baumeister and MacLean (1984) used a similar program approach of providing alternative means of gaining sensory stimulation. To illustrate, Lancioni et al. (1984) were successful in reducing the infrequent but severe self-injurious tantrums of three adolescents with multiple disabilities by providing daily periods of gross motor activities designed to provide a variety of sensory input. The gross motor activities were selected on the assumption that the self-injurious tantrums were being maintained by the resulting sensory consequences.

Functionally Equivalent Behavioral Alternatives to SIBs

Functional equivalence training, based on the assessment of instigating and maintaining conditions, is designed to teach functionally equivalent and socially appropriate behavioral replacements for the self-injury. The new skills may involve motor responses or communicative behaviors of a nonverbal or verbal nature.

Motor Responses

Functional diagnostics of the chronic self-injurious mouthing and biting of a severely multiply disabled 8-year-old boy indicated that these behaviors were likely to occur at a high rate under solitary conditions (toileting and positioning). Based on the hypothesis that the SIBs served a self-stimulatory function, an alternative functional motor response producing valued sensory stimulation was taught and remained dominant over the SIBs at the 6-month follow-up (Steege et al. 1989).

Nonverbal Communication Skills

In individuals with severe cognitive impairment, limited communication skills, and few social behaviors, SIBs may represent forms of communicating wishes, concerns, and physical/psychological states such as pain or dysphoria. This communication hypothesis of self-injury, using communication as a metaphor, suggests the program strategy of replacing the SIBs with alternative functionally equivalent forms of communicative skills to ensure that individually relevant positive consequences are obtained or that aversive conditions are reduced, terminated, or avoided (Carr and Durand 1985; Carr et al. 1994; Durand 1990). Durand and Kishi (1987) taught young adults—with severe/profound mental retardation and dual sensory impairments—who engaged in self-injury either to sign or to present a token as a means of communicating their requests for staff attention or access to favorite objects. Functional diagnostics indicated that SIBs were serving these communicative functions. Following training, significant reductions in SIBs were observed in those instances in which the staff consistently responded to the communicative requests.

Verbal Communication Skills

Carr and Durand (1985) demonstrated through functional diagnostics that children in an educational setting engaged in SIBs as a nonverbal means of communicating a desire for teacher attention. A verbal communication response, "Am I doing good work?" was taught as an alternative means of gaining teacher attention. This communicative inquiry resulted in prompt teacher feedback including verbal praise, smiles, and physical approval. Self-injury and other disruptive behaviors were reduced to infrequent occurrence as the newly acquired verbal communication skills replaced the function served previously by the problem behaviors.

Competing Behaviors

In those instances in which an appropriate behavior becomes self-injurious due to its excessive occurrence, the person may be taught an alternative incompatible behavior. McNally et al. (1988) selected this procedure to successfully reduce polydipsia in a young woman with severe mental retardation who presented a history of multiple hospitalizations for emergency medical treatment for water intoxication.

Extinction

In reinforcement-motivated extinction, consequences such as social attention, access to materials and activities, or increase in sensory stimulation are no longer provided on a contingent basis following SIBs. Rincover and Devany (1982), in the treatment of young children with profound mental retardation whose self-injury appeared to be self-stimulatory and thus presumed to be maintained by the sensory stimulation produced, demonstrated the value of a sensory extinction procedure in immediately and substantially reducing SIBs. The sensory stimulation associated with the specific SIB of each child was removed. In illustration, one boy who engaged in head banging was provided a helmet that attenuated the tactile sensory consequences of the SIB. Another child, who engaged in self-injurious face scratching, was required to wear thin rubber gloves. Blankenship and Lamberts (1989) reported a rapid and significant reduction in self-injurious cheek gouging and face slapping in two women with profound mental retardation through reducing contingent sensory input. The results were maintained at low levels over a 6-month maintenance period.

Noncontingent Reinforcement

Vollmer et al. (1993) demonstrated the value of noncontingent reinforcement (NCR) in reducing the chronic and severe SIBs of three female adults. Assessment suggested social attention as a potential maintaining consequence. During NCR treatment, social attention was provided on a fixed-time schedule in which the person's SIBs did not influence the frequency of reinforcement. The procedure was highly effective in reducing self-injury.

■ ESCAPE-MOTIVATED SIBs

The escape/avoidance hypothesis suggests that self-injury initially becomes a functional means of escape from current aversive conditions. After successful escape experiences, SIBs may then become functional in completely avoiding these aversive events (Iwata et al. 1990). In some instances, SIBs may become functional in reducing aversive stimulus conditions arising from biomedical conditions. As examples, the distress associated with an ear infection or a dysphoric mood state may be temporarily attenuated by ear hitting or head hitting or other forms of self-injury (Rincover and Devany 1982).

Aversive Antecedent Conditions

After establishing that the SIBs of a young adult in a residential treatment program occurred principally during the late afternoon and evening hours and was associated with the staff person assigned, the afternoon activities, and the number of peers present, Touchette et al. (1985) altered these antecedents. A reversal of A.M. and P.M. staff assignments correlated with a total reversal of the times during which the self-abuse occurred. In this instance, the therapists were able to manage the SIBs by identifying and removing the correlated instigating conditions.

Aversive Qualities of Antecedent Conditions

Weeks and Gaylord-Ross (1981) demonstrated the value of altering the escape-producing antecedent stimuli by reducing or eliminating the aversive and discriminative properties of these antecedents for reducing self-injury. The self-injurious hand biting and finger biting behaviors of a 13-year-old girl with diagnoses of severe mental retardation and autism varied with the difficulty level of instructional tasks presented in a day school program. Difficult task presentation was changed to an errorless learning procedure using a stimulus-fading sequence. Low rates of SIBs were observed under this revised teaching condition.

Extinction and Compliance Training

In using an escape-motivated extinction procedure, the SIBs become nonfunctional as these do not result in escape from or avoidance of the aversive stimulus events. To illustrate, if SIBs occur following an instructional directive, the person is physically guided to engage in the behaviors requested while SIBs are either ignored or blocked. Full physical guidance is faded into physical prompts as permitted by progress. Physical prompts are replaced by a firm verbal directive and faded further into the typical verbal directive.

Reinforcement, provided for task completion and during initial training for compliance, has two beneficial effects, namely, the strength of instruction following increases and the aversiveness of the tasks is reduced through pairing with the preferred reinforcer.

Iwata et al. (1990) initially selected children whose SIBs occurred in an instructional setting as various task demands were presented. Compliance was socially reinforced; if SIBs occurred, the child was physically guided through task completion. Following implementation of this extinction plus physical guidance, SIBs decreased to zero or near-zero, and compliance increased noticeably. A maintenance and generalization program was implemented in each child's ongoing instructional programs and consisted of continued use of the extinction plus physical guidance procedure combined with reinforcement.

Functionally Equivalent Behaviors

Nonverbal Communication Skills

Bird et al. (1989) used functional communication training (FCT) to treat the high levels of several SIBs of a 27-year-old male with diagnoses of autistic disorder and profound mental retardation. The SIBs had resulted in the detachment of both retinas. Expressive language skills were limited to approximately 15 one-word utterances that were seldom spontaneous and often difficult to interpret. A range of medical and behavioral interventions had been attempted with only minimal success.

Assessment suggested an escape-from-task-demands hypothesis. An FCT was successful in teaching an alternative nonverbal (exchanging a plastic token) but functionally equivalent means of obtaining a break from task demands presented in the work training program. An immediate and substantial reduction in self-injurious episodes was obtained. These results were maintained with the introduction of successive task demands of increasing difficulty and duration and generalized across three teachers. A concurrent increase was observed in 1) spontaneous verbal requests to initiate work even during periods of time when he had an opportunity to avoid work demands completely, and 2) spontaneous verbal requests for food, a behavior that seldom occurred prior to the training program.

Verbal Communication Skills

After demonstrating that children with developmental disabilities attending a day school program engaged in SIBs when presented difficult instructional tasks, Carr and Durand (1985) taught a verbal response as a means of soliciting teacher assistance. This FCT consisted of three stages. The child initially was prompted by the teacher to say "I don't understand." Following consistent correct imitation of this verbal behavior, the child was presented with a difficult task. When an error was made, the teacher said "That's not correct!" and added "Do you have any questions? Say, 'I don't understand.'" When correctly imitated, the teacher replied "O.K. I'll show you" and, through use of gestures and verbal statements, demonstrated the correct response. In the final training stage, the teacher's verbal prompts were faded until the child responded correctly to the inquiry "Do you have any questions?"

Following FCT, SIBs and other disruptive behaviors decreased to infrequent occurrence. Through learning an alternative verbal response that resulted in adult assistance on difficult tasks, the children experienced less failure. The reduced aversiveness of the tasks was presumed to remove the motivation for the SIBs.

FCT, Extinction, and Punishment

In noting that sources of reinforcement may be unclear in a substantial number of cases involving self-injury, Fisher et al. (1993) suggested a multicomponent treatment package involving use of FCT, extinction, and punishment to obtain maximum effects. After determining that FCT was not sufficient to produce a clinically significant reduction in destructive behaviors, these therapists added a mild punishment procedure and obtained generalized and enduring treatment effects. These results are consistent with those reported by Wacker et al. (1990). In sum, in those patients who do not respond to FCT with a clinically acceptable reduction of their self-injurious and related destructive behaviors, it may be useful to add a mild punishment contingency to increase their motivation to select the alternative communicative response as an alternative to the SIBs.

Response Efficiency of Functionally Equivalent Behaviors

A critical factor in the successful application of functional equivalence training is that of response efficiency (Bird et al. 1989; Wacker et al. 1990).

Horner and Day (1991) examined the role of the following three components of response efficiency relative to the acquisition and maintenance of functionally equivalent behaviors: 1) the physical effort required to perform the equivalent response, 2) the schedule of reinforcement, and 3) the delay in time between presentation of the discriminative stimulus for a target response and the delivery of the reinforcer for that response.

"Paul," a 12-year-old boy with severe mental retardation and a 6-year history of severe aggression (hitting, kicking, scratching) and self-injury (severe self-hits to his head), was used to evaluate the physical effort component. Functional assessment suggested that Paul's aberrant responding was maintained by escape from difficult tasks. He initially was taught the American Sign Language signs for "I want to go please." During the presentation of training in self-care skills, the use of the sentence resulted in an immediate 30- to 45-second break from task demands. During initial sessions, destructive behaviors decreased noticeably as Paul was using the functionally equivalent sentence to request a break. These gains were short-lived, however, as attempts to use the sentence declined and destructive behaviors showed a dramatic increase. Paul was next taught to sign "break" that required considerably less physical effort on his part. Under this condition, the destructive responding decreased substantially and remained low. Additionally, even though Paul had an opportunity to escape the demand on each presentation of a task directive, he averaged 80% attempts to comply with directives during the training sessions. After learning the word sign, Paul made no further attempts to use the functionally equivalent sentence of "I want to go please."

The efficiency component of the schedule of reinforcement was evaluated with "Peter," a 14-year-old adolescent with profound mental retardation and an 11-year history of severe self-injury. Functional analysis indicated that the aberrant behavior was functional in obtaining trainer assistance when he was provided difficult tasks. Initially, Peter was taught to sign "help" as a functionally equivalent means of soliciting staff assistance. During a difficult picture-matching task, Peter was provided staff assistance immediately after he signed "help" three times. Although an initial reduction in self-injury occurred, Peter's use of signing gradually decreased to near zero, and his SIB returned to 95%–100% of trials. After booster training to reestablish the "help" response, Peter was then provided assistance following each request. Under this reinforcement schedule, he signed for help on nearly every trial, attempted it, and engaged in no SIBs.

The final component of response efficiency, delay of reinforcement, was demonstrated with "Mary," a 27-year-old with a 5-year history of severe self-injury and aggression. Assessment implicated escape motivation as the maintaining condition. Initially, Mary was taught to hand the trainer a card with the word *BREAK* on it. A 1-second delay and a 20-second delay in providing a break from task demands were contrasted. Initially, a 20-second delay was imposed from the time Mary handed the card to the trainer until she was provided a break from task demands. Destructive behavior increased under this condition as Mary quickly discovered that she could escape from task demands faster through using her aberrant behaviors. After a change to a 1-second delay, destructive acts decreased to low levels.

These results clearly demonstrate that newly taught equivalent behaviors will be used as substitutes for aberrant responding in escaping from or in gaining assistance in dealing with aversive tasks only if these are as efficient as (or more efficient than) the aberrant response in gaining reinforcement. The most desirable results are obtained when each of these three components—physical effort, schedule of reinforcement, and delay between the functionally equivalent response and the reinforcement—considered in designing a training program.

■ MULTIPLY MOTIVATED SIBS

Often the functional analysis of SIBs yields not one but several instigating and/or maintaining factors (e.g., functional diagnostics may indicate that SIBs are reinforcement motivated on some occasions and escape motivated on other occasions). In such cases, although addressing one factor may lead to decreases in self-injury, this effect may not be sustained or clinically significant to a sufficient degree until additional contributing factors are targeted. This is illustrated by Heidorn and Jensen (1984) in their successful treatment of the severe and chronic SIBs of a 27-year-old male diagnosed as profoundly developmentally delayed. Because of the severity of the SIBs (rubbing his head on walls, floors, and other objects and digging his fingernails into his forehead and nose), the man was placed in restraints almost 17 hours daily and provided various psychotropic medications. Previous SIBs of eye poking had resulted in blindness in both eyes.

Contextual analysis implicated both reinforcement- and escape-motivated SIBs. When left alone during free time, SIBs and screaming would occur until someone talked to him or touched him. Treatment involved extinction and differential reinforcement. When placed in situations requiring the man's cooperation or compliance, SIBs would occur until demands were removed. Treatment involved response prevention or redirection as the trainer guided the patient through to task completion. Upon task completion, edibles, verbal praise, and physical contact were provided, and the demand situation was terminated. A relaxation procedure was implemented when the patient attempted to hit or pinch the trainer. When calm, he was returned to the task and prompted to complete it. These procedures were implemented in various settings and with various tasks in order to enhance generalization and maintenance.

■ ADDITIONAL INTERVENTION STRATEGIES

Although they are not diagnostically established as being related to the functionality of a patient's SIBs, a number of approaches involving differential reinforcement, relaxation training, and punishment contingencies may be useful in reducing self-injury. These treatment effects are best maintained, nonetheless, if they are combined with interventions that do address the specific instigating and maintaining conditions.

Differential Reinforcement

The procedure of differential reinforcement involves providing frequent and valued consequences for appropriate behaviors or for the nonoccurrence of the self-injurious acts during specific periods of time. Lovaas et al. (1965) reduced the high rate of self-hitting behaviors of a 9-year-old boy to a near-zero level after systematically reinforcing the child for clapping his hands to music—an appropriate use of hands that replaced the SIBs. Tarpley and Schroeder (1979), in the treatment of three adults with profound mental retardation, found the procedure of providing reinforcement following periods of play activity and no SIBs to be effective in reducing head banging. Tierney (1986), working with a 14-year-old male with profound mental retardation, reported a significant reduction in episodes of self-slapping, punching, and hitting accompanied by screaming, jumping, running, and/or clinging to the nearest person. This reduction coincided with reinforcement of an incompatible behavior of sitting calmly in a chair with hands resting on his knees. A 12-month follow-up revealed maintenance of treatment gains.

Differential Reinforcement and Self-Management

Grace et al. (1988) demonstrated the successful application of self-management and related reinforcement procedures in reducing the SIBs of a 14-year-old boy with diagnoses of Lesch-Nyhan syndrome and moderate mental retardation. During most of 9 years of institutional living, the patient's legs and hands had been physically restrained due to frequent and recurring hand and finger biting. His front teeth had been removed in an attempt to limit his self-injury. During the initial phase of treatment, the boy was initially taught to self-assess occurrence or nonoccurrence of his hand biting SIBs by nodding or pointing to a pictorial happy or sad face. Verbal reprimands were used at occurrences of SIBs, and verbal praise was provided for no self-biting at the time of staff-prompted self-assessment. The time period between self-assessment was gradually increased to 1-hour intervals. Treatment, initially provided in the dayroom, produced an immediate reduction in SIBs; SIBs were completely eliminated after 3 days of the self-management program. After treatment was expanded to include the bedroom, there was an immediate elimination of SIBs in that setting, too. SIBs in both settings were maintained at a zero level during a 19-week follow-up.

Differential Reinforcement and Physical Interruption

Azrin and colleagues (1982, 1988) reported a reduction in the severe and chronic SIBs of adolescents and adults with severe and profound mental retardation to near-zero levels in both school and living settings. This was accomplished through providing reinforcement following periods of no self-injury and the occurrence of play, social, or other appropriate behaviors. This reinforcement procedure was combined with interrupting each self-injurious episode and requiring the person's hands to rest in his or her lap for 2 minutes.

Relaxation Training

In a novel approach to producing alternatives to SIBs, Schroeder et al. (1977) demonstrated that the relaxation training of two adolescents with severe mental retardation and chronic high-rate head banging resulted in a physiological state that was incompatible with the occurrence of self-injury. The effects were short-lived, however, suggesting the need for a more comprehensive intervention program for effective and durable results. Steen and Zuriff (1977) used relaxation training with a 21-year-old woman with profound mental retardation who had been in full restraint for 3 years as a means of managing severe biting and scratching. Intervention consisted of training the woman to relax her hand and arm while providing her with a continuous schedule of reinforcement—food, praise, and physical contact. Restraints were gradually removed during 115 sessions; self-injury ceased and a follow-up of 1 year revealed a continued low rate of SIBs.

Punishment Procedures

Punishment procedures, consisting of contingent removal of positive reinforcers or contingent presentation of aversive conditions, may be useful in reducing SIBs even though no attempt is made to alter the instigating or maintaining conditions. Undesired side effects (increase in agitation, tantrum-like behaviors, aggression) that occasionally accompany the presentation of aversive conditions, however, may have unacceptable deleterious effects. Because of the controversy over the use of operant punishment procedures as treatment for SIBs, the reader is encouraged to consult the National Institutes of Health's Consensus Development Conference Statement on Treatment of Destructive Behaviors in Persons With Developmental Disabilities (1989), Repp and Singh (1990), and the critical review by Linscheid (1992) for a balanced discussion of the issues involved.

■ MAINTENANCE AND GENERALIZATION OF TREATMENT EFFECTS

The primary objective of a psychosocial intervention program for SIBs is to obtain treatment effects that hold under conditions and settings differing from those involved in treatment. Although only minimal systematic research has specifically addressed the problem of generalization and maintenance following the treatment of self-injury, some promising guidelines are evolving from recent studies based on the functional analytic model. These suggest that generalization and maintenance of treatment effects may be enhanced under the following conditions. For SIBs maintained by positive reinforcement, 1) establish the functionality of the SIB, 2) eliminate the functionality through extinction, 3) provide equivalent positive reinforcement for alternative prosocial behaviors, and 4) ensure that the reinforcement schedule and type are equal to or exceed the ones previously associated with SIBs (Heidorn and Jensen 1984). As a second approach, 1) establish the functionality of the SIBs, 2) teach a functionally equivalent response as an alternative to the SIBs, and 3) provide reinforcement consistency to ensure that this alternative behavior is as effective and efficient as the SIBs in gaining maintaining reinforcers (Carr and Durand 1985; Durand and Kishi 1987; Steege et al. 1989).

For SIBs maintained by negative reinforcement, 1) establish the functionality of the SIBs, 2) eliminate this functionality through extinction and compliance training, and 3) provide positive reinforcement for compliance and related substitute behaviors (Heidorn and Jensen 1984; Iwata et al. 1990). As a second approach, 1) establish the functionality of SIBs, 2) teach a functionally equivalent response as an effective and efficient alternative, and 3) ensure continued reinforcement of this substitute behavior by various persons in various settings (Bird et al. 1989; Carr and Durand 1985).

■ CONCLUSIONS

Multiple factors representing biopsychosocial influences underlie the development and persistent recurrence of SIBs. A multimodal contextual diagnostic and intervention model is offered as best reflecting this complexity. Psychosocial interventions derived from diagnostic hypotheses about relevant instigating and maintaining influences offer promise of reducing or eliminating the SIBs and replacing these with prosocial functional alternatives.

■ REFERENCES

Azrin NH, Besalel VA, Wisotzek IE: Treatment of self-injury by a reinforcement plus interruption procedure. Analysis and Intervention in Developmental Disabilities 3:105–113, 1982

Azrin NH, Besalel VA, Jamner JP, et al: Comparative study of behavioral methods of treating severe self-injury. Behavioral Residential Treatment 3:119–152, 1988

Baumeister AA, MacLean WE Jr: Deceleration of self-injurious and stereotypic responding by exercise. Applied Research in Mental Retardation 5:385–393, 1984

Baumeister AA, Sevin JA: Pharmacologic control of aberrant behavior in the mentally retarded: toward a more rational approach. Neurosci Biobehav Rev 14:253–262, 1990

Benson BA, Aman MG: Disruptive behavior disorders in children with mental retardation, in Handbook of Disruptive Behavior Disorders. Edited by Quay HC, Hogan AE. New York, Plenum, 1999, pp 559–578

Bird F, Dores PA, Moniz D, et al. Reducing severe aggressive and self-injurious behaviors with functional communication training. Am J Ment Retard 94:37–48, 1989

Blankenship MD, Lamberts F: Helmet restraint and visual screening as treatment for self-injurious behavior in persons who have profound mental retardation. Behavioral Residential Treatment 4:253–265, 1989

Bodfish JW, Crawford TW, Powell S, et al: Compulsions in adults with mental retardation: prevalence, phenomenology, and co-morbidity with stereotypy and self injury. Am J Ment Retard 100:183–192, 1995

Borthwick-Duffy SA: Prevalence of destructive behaviors, in Destructive Behavior in Developmental Disabilities: Diagnosis and Treatment. Edited by Thompson T, Gray DB. Thousand Oaks, CA, Sage Publications, 1994, pp 3–23

Carr EG: The motivation of self-injurious behavior: a review of some hypotheses. Psychol Bull 84:800–816, 1977

Carr EG, Durand VM: Reducing behavior problems through functional communication training. J Appl Behav Anal 18:111–126, 1985

Carr EG, Levin L, McConnachie G, et al: Communication-Based Intervention for Problem Behavior. Baltimore, MD, Paul H Brookes, 1994

Carr EG, Reeve CE, Magito-McLaughlin D: Contextual influences on problem behavior in people with developmental disabilities, in Positive Behavioral Supports: Including People With Difficult Behaviors in the Community. Edited by Koegel LK, Koegel RL, Dunlap G. Baltimore, MD, Paul H Brookes, 1996, pp 403–423

Davidson PW, Jacobson J, Cain NN, et al: Characteristics of children and adolescents with mental retardation and frequent outwardly directed aggressive behavior. Am J Ment Retard 101:244–255, 1996

Došen A: Self-injurious behavior in persons with mental retardation: a developmental psychiatric approach, in Mental Health Aspects of Mental Retardation. Edited by Fletcher RJ, Došen A. New York, Lexington Books, 1993, pp 141–168

Durand VM: Severe Behavior Problems: A Functional Communication Training Approach. New York, Guilford, 1990

Durand VM, Kishi G: Reducing severe behavior problems among persons with dual sensory impairments: an evaluation of a technical assistance model. Journal of the Association for Severely Handicapped 12:2–10, 1987

Favell JE: The treatment of self-injurious behavior. Behavior Therapy 13:529–554, 1982

Favell JE, McGimsey JF, Schnell RM: Treatment of self-injury by providing alternate sensory activities. Analysis and Intervention in Developmental Disabilities 2:83–104, 1982

Fisher W, Piazza C, Cataldo M, et al: Functional communication training with and without extinction and punishment. J Appl Behav Anal 26:23–36, 1993

Gardner WI, Sovner R: Self-injurious Behaviors: Diagnosis and Treatment. Willow Street, PA, Vida Press, 1994

Gardner WI, Graeber JL, Cole C: Behavior therapies: a multimodal diagnostic and intervention model, in Manual of Diagnosis and Professional Practice in Mental Retardation. Edited by Jacobson JW, Mulick JA. Washington,DC, American Psychological Association, 1996, pp 355–370

Gedye A: Extreme self-injury attributed to frontal lobe seizures. Am J Ment Retard 94:20–26, 1989

Grace N, Cowart C, Matson JL: Reinforcement and self-control for treating a chronic case of self-injury in Lesch-Nyhan syndrome. Journal for Multihandicapped Persons 1:53–59, 1988

Griffiths D, Gardner WI, Nuget JA: Behavioral Supports: Individual Centered Interventions. Kingston, NY, NADD Press, 1998

Gualtieri CT: The differential diagnosis of self-injurious behavior in mentally retarded people. Psychopharm Bull 25:358–363, 1989

Guess D, Carr D: Emergence and maintenance of stereotypy and self-injury. Am J Ment Retard 96:299–320, 1991

Heidorn SD, Jensen CC: Generalization and maintenance of the reduction of self-injurious behaviors maintained by 2 types of reinforcement. Behav Res Ther 22:581–586, 1984

Horner RH, Day HM: The effects of response efficiency on functionally equivalent competing behaviors. J Appl Behav Anal 24:719–732, 1991

Iwata BA, Pace GM, Kalsher MJ, et al: Experimental analysis and extinction of self-injurious escape behavior. J Appl Behav Anal 23:11–27, 1990

Iwata BA, Pace GM, Dorsey MF, et al: The functions of self-injurious behavior: an experimental-epidemiological analysis. J Appl Behav Anal 27:215–240, 1994

Lancioni GE, Smeets PM, Ceccarani PS, et al: Effects of gross motor activities on the severe self-injurious tantrums of multihandicapped individuals. Applied Research in Mental Retardation 5:471–482, 1984

Lewis MH, Silva J, Silva S: Cyclicity of aggression and self-injurious behavior in individuals with mental retardation. Am J Ment Retard 99:436–444, 1995

Lewis MH, Bodfish JW, Powell SB et al: Clomipramine treatment for self-injurious behavior of individuals with mental retardation: a double-blind comparison with placebo. Am J Ment Retard 100:654–665, 1996

Linscheid TR: Aversive stimulation, in Self-injurious Behavior: Analysis, Assessment, and Treatment. Edited by Luiselli JK, Matson JL, Singh NN. New York, Springer-Verlag, 1992, pp 137–154

Lovaas O, Freitag G, Gold V, et al: Experimental studies in childhood schizophrenia: Analysis of self-destructive behavior. J Exp Child Psychol 2:67–84, 1965

Luiselli JK, Matson JL, Singh N (eds): Self-injurious Behavior: Analysis, Assessment, and Treatment. New York, Springer-Verlag, 1992

Mace FC, Mauk JE: Biobehavioral diagnosis and treatment of self-injury, in Functional Analysis of Problem Behavior. Edited by Repp AC, Horner RH. Belmont, CA, Wadsworth Publishing, 1999, pp 78–97

McLean WE, Stone WL, Brown WH: Developmental psychopathology of destructive behavior, in Destructive Behavior in Developmental Disabilities. Edited by Thompson T, Gray DB. Thousand Oaks, CA, Sage Publications, 1994, pp 68–79

McNally RJ, Calamari JE, Hansen PM, et al: Behavioral treatment of psychogenic polydipsia. J Behav Ther Exp Psychiatry 19:57–61, 1988

National Institutes of Health: Consensus Development Conference Statement on Treatment of Destructive Behaviors in Persons With Developmental Disabilities. Washington, DC, National Institutes of Health, 1989

Oliver C, Head D: Self-injurious behavior in people with learning disabilities: determinants and interventions. International Review of Psychiatry 2:101–116, 1990

Repp AC, Singh NN (eds): Perspectives on the Use of Nonaversive and Aversive Intervention for Persons With Developmental Disabilities. Sycamore, IL, Sycamore Publishing, 1990

Rincover A, Devany J: The application of sensory extinction procedures to self-injury. Analysis and Intervention in Developmental Disabilities 2:67–81, 1982

Rojahn J: Self-injurious and stereotypic behavior of noninstitutionalized mentally retarded people: prevalence and classification. American Journal of Mental Deficiency 91:268–276, 1986

Rojahn J: Epidemiology and topographic taxonomy of self-injurious behavior, in Destructive Behavior in Developmental Disabilities: Diagnosis and Treatment. Edited by Thompson T, Gray D. Thousand Oaks, CA, Sage Publications, 1994, pp 49–67

Schroeder SR, Tessel R: Dopaminergic and serotenergic mechanisms in self-injury and aggression, in Destructive Behavior in Developmental Disabilities: Diagnosis and Treatment. Edited by Thompson T, Gray D. Thousand Oaks, CA, Sage Publications, 1994, pp 198–210

Schroeder SR, Mulick JA, Schroeder CS: Self-injurious behavior, in Handbook of Behavior Modification With the Mentally Retarded, 2nd Edition. Edited by Matson JL. New York, Plenum Press, 1990, pp 141–180

Schroeder SR, Peterson CR, Solomon LJ, et al: EMG feedback and the contingent restraint of self-injurious behavior among the severely retarded: two case illustrations. Behavior Therapy 8:738–741, 1977

Shore BA, Iwata BA: Assessment and treatment of behavior disorders maintained by nonsocial (automatic) reinforcement, in Functional Analysis of problem Behavior. Edited by Repp AC, Horner RH. Belmont, CA, Wadsworth Publishing, 1999, pp 117–146

Sprague JR, Horner RH: Low frequency high-intensity problem behavior: toward an applied technology of functonal assessment and intervention, in Functional Analysis of Problem Behavior. Edited by Repp AC, Horner RH. Belmont, CA, Wadsworth Publishing, 1999, pp 98–116

Sovner R, Fogelman S: Irritability and mental retardation. Seminars in Clinical Neuropsychiatry 1:105–114, 1996

Sovner R, Pary RJ: Affective disorders in developmentally disabled persons, in Psychopathology in the Mentally Retarded, 2nd Edition. Edited by Matson J, Barrett RP. Needham Heights, MA, Allyn & Bacon, 1993, pp 87–147

Steege MW, Wacker DP, Berg WK, et al: The use of behavioral assessment to prescribe and evaluate treatment for severely handicapped children. J Appl Behav Anal 22:23–33, 1989

Steen PL, Zuriff GE: The use of relaxation in the treatment of self-injurious behavior. J Behav Ther Exp Psychiatry 8:447–448, 1977

Tarpley HD, Schroeder SR: Comparison of DRO and DRI on rate of suppression of self-injurious behavior. American Journal of Mental Deficiency 84:188–194, 1979

Thompson T, Engli M, Symons F, et al: Neurobehavioral mechanisms of drug action in developmental disabilities, in Destructive Behavior in Developmental Disabilities. Edited by Thompson T, Gray DB. Thousand Oaks, CA, Sage Publications, 1994, pp 133–180

Tierney DW: The reinforcement of calm sitting behavior: a method used to reduce the self-injurious behavior of a profoundly retarded boy. J Behav Ther Exp Psychiatry 17:47–50, 1986

Touchette PE, MacDonald RF, Langer SN: A scatter plot for identifying stimulus control of problem behavior. J Appl Behav Anal 18:343–351, 1985

Vollmer TR, Iwata BA, Zarcone JR, et al: The role of attention in the treatment of attention-maintained self-injurious behavior: noncontingent reinforcement and differential reinforcement of other behavior. J Appl Behav Anal 26:9–21, 1993

Wacker DP, Steege MW, Northup J, et al: A component analysis of functional communication training across three topographies of severe behavior problems. J Appl Behav Anal 23:417–429, 1990

Weeks M, Gaylord-Ross R: Task difficulty and aberrant behavior in severely handicapped students. J Appl Behav Anal 14:449–463, 1981

Werry JS, Aman MG: Anxiolytics, sedatives, and miscellaneous drugs, in Practitioner's Guide to Psychoactive Drugs for Children and Adolescents, 2nd Edition. Edited by Werry JS, Aman MG. New York, Plenum, 1998, pp 433–469

Winchel RM, Stanley M: Self-injurious behavior: a review of the behavior and biology of self-mutilation. Am J Psychiatry 148:306–317, 1991

19 Group Therapy for Mentally Retarded Sex Offenders

Diane Cox-Lindenbaum, A.C.S.W.

Group therapy is a viable treatment option for the mentally retarded sex offender. Obstacles to treatment must be overcome in order for effective treatment to occur. The attitudes and values of professionals must be evaluated so that the assessment and treatment of the offender are not overshadowed by the presence of mental retardation. In this chapter, I will identify the key components of treatment and provide guidelines for creating a therapeutic alliance with this challenging population.

A multimodal group therapy process is recommended as a prime modality. The group psychodynamic processes described in this chapter create an opportunity to break the cycle of isolation, alienation, and discrimination that is inherent in the personality profile of the sex offender. Through the use of cognitive modules and experiential processes, members of the group will develop a heightened sense of awareness of their internal stressors and environment triggers that will assist them in reducing the opportunity to reoffend. Through the therapeutic process and peer support, each member of the group will be able to choose to create a life situation that manages the acting out and replaces it with responsible behavior in his or her interactions with others. In this chapter, I will describe how this is accomplished through group therapy.

◼ OBSTACLES TO TREATMENT

Traditionally, the clinical treatment of the mentally retarded sex offender has focused primarily on the offense rather than the developmental and psychodynamic issues involved—often taking the form of confining the patient to a restrictive environment with no recourse for therapeutic intervention other than sex education programs.

A major obstacle to treatment has been a failure on the part of the professional community to recognize a sexual disorder in a mentally retarded person and to distinguish it from a sexually inappropriate learned behavior. Often, sexually violent acts such as rape, child molestation, sexual masochism, sexual sadism, and exhibitionism were assumed to be the result of the mental retardation rather than severe clinical dysfunction and personality deficits. This process of "diagnostic overshadowing" (Reiss et al. 1982) often results in the person not being appropriately diagnosed and not receiving the necessary clinical services. With the focus being primarily on the descriptive aspects of the sexually coercive incidents such as the sexuality, the violence, and the legality issues, the opportunity for clinical treatment may be missed and the person falls through the gap in the service delivery system.

Another obstacle has been the professional's own value judgments and attitudes, which may bias and limit treatment options for the mentally retarded sex offender. As Emily Coleman states, "Our attitude does this population a grave injustice by belittling them as people, absolving them of responsibility, and incorrectly assuming treatment will not be effective" (Haaven et al. 1990). Haaven (1993) indicates that barriers to treatment are manifest in the attitudes of a society that fails to address a person with a disability as a whole person who is sexually functional as well as sexually dysfunctional. According to Haaven, society continues to associate an adult with disabilities as childlike and therefore innocent of crimes. The clinician often colludes with the mentally retarded sex offender by denying and minimizing the trauma of sexual abuse, especially when the victim is also mentally retarded, thereby negating "client-to-client" abuse.

Our history of not advocating sexual expression for mentally retarded people leaves us guilt-ridden and tentative in our ability to support the sex offender, and to pursue and develop the unique treatment that the offender needs. Advocates' and professionals' concern about labeling a person "sex offender" often takes precedence over actually treating the complex pathology. All of these factors can interfere with and diffuse the energy needed to establish a treatment that is based on the clinical needs of the mentally retarded sex offender. Szymanski and Tanguay (1980) have indicated that mentally retarded people are vulnerable to mental disorders, yet few clinicians in the field have acknowledged this in their treatment. Traditional service provision has focused only on the cognitive or on sex education programs, the assumption being that the "sexual misconduct" was due to a lack of sexual information, poor opportunities for sexual interaction, and unavailable sexual counseling. Through the process of deinstitutionalization and community living, it has become clear that some mentally retarded people who have recurrent and persistent levels of sexual dysfunctioning and who are repetitive sexual offenders have received comprehensive sex education programs but have not been able to integrate this information or modify their sexually violent behavior. Mentally retarded sex offenders require a more comprehensive clinical treatment approach.

■ PERSONALITY PROFILE AND CHARACTERISTICS OF MENTALLY RETARDED SEX OFFENDERS

The clinical work of Menolascino (1984) indicates that a person with an intellectual disability is already "at risk" for emotional disturbance based on deficits in the area of interpersonal relations. Therefore, there are unique emotional challenges in working with this population. These challenges can be caused by internal (pathological) or external (familial/environmental) factors. The mental illness is not part of the mental retardation but rather emerges out of the vulnerability that the mental retardation brings to the person and his or her ability to master and control an otherwise nonresponsive world. This awareness of the presence of a dual diagnosis sets the stage for treatment.

Offenses committed by intellectually disabled sex offenders generally parallel those of nondisabled offenders (Knopp and Lackey 1987), although the manifestation of the acting-out behaviors may differ. The majority of sex offenders, including those who are mentally retarded, are not psychotic, nor are they misbehaving sexually. Instead, they have serious psychological differences that handicap them in social-sexual relationships under stress; they act out sexually (Groth 1979). Violent aggressive acting-out behaviors such as rape, child molestation, and exhibitionism are in fact "pseudo" sexual acts. As Groth has found, they are acts of hostility rather than acts of passion; they are always symptoms of psychological dysfunctioning. These deficits make it difficult, if not impossible, to establish and maintain adult relationships that could lead to a bond with an adult partner. Kohut (1994) states that perversions are often driven by enactments with figures or symbols that give them the feeling of being wanted, alive, or powerful. He also states that youthful offenders often repeat acts through which they can demonstrate to themselves an escape from the realization that they feel devoid of any real sense of sustained self-confidence.

Characteristically, the most prominent feature of paraphiliacs in general, whether they are cognitively impaired or not, is the visible absence of an ability to form close emotional relationships with others. They lack warmth, trust, companionship, and empathy for others. Clinically, they are not motivated for treatment. In fact, they often do not appreciate the seriousness of the offense, nor do they recognize that they have a problem. Given the fear of legal consequences, they are apt to withhold any information about their involvement in sexual offenses.

Becker and Hunter (1993) state that early life experiences of abuse and deprivation appear to leave youthful offenders angry, bitter, and cynical. These offenders' ability to form attachments to others is impaired, and there seems to be a distinct fear or disdain of interpersonal intimacy. Intimacy may be synonymous with vulnerability and exploitation.

Mentally retarded sex offenders manifest the following personality deficits, which are similar to those found in paraphiliacs who have normal cognitive functioning (Griffiths et al. 1987; Kempton 1988):

1. Low self-esteem, a sense of worthlessness
2. A learned helplessness, a sense of powerlessness regarding daily living functioning
3. An inability to form close relationships with peers (separate self from other mentally retarded patients)
4. Poor impulse control
5. Poor anger management skills
6. High anxiety levels (agitated depression/altered mood states)
7. Resistance to treatment
8. A focus on unavailable partners (enhances rejection cycle)
9. Poor adaptive use of sexual knowledge
10. Poor social skills (loner, withdrawn)
11. Denial of mental retardation disability, alienation from peers
12. Moderate-mild mental retardation, borderline intellectual functioning
13. Poor coping methods
14. Emotional difficulties in accepting change, rigidity in approach to daily living
15. History of family violence
16. History of early childhood deprivation and neglect; history of physical/sexual abuse
17. Suicidal ideations or gestures that may lead to suicide attempts
18. Sexual acting out manifested in adolescence

The clinician working with a mentally retarded sex offender is presented with an individual who has learned to use sex dysfunctionally through violence and who possesses deficits in personality development, social/sexual skills, and life management skills, and who also has experienced significant childhood trauma. By understanding these personality deficits and characteristics of this disorder, clinicians will be less likely to engage in countertransferential control issues with the patients in treatment. By isolating those personality traits that are dysfunctional, the clinical team can develop treatment plans that are focused on assisting the patient in the therapeutic process. Becker and Hunter

(1993) emphasize the importance of linking prior victimization experiences and one's own emotional pain and suffering with antecedent sexual acting-out behaviors.

■ DIAGNOSTIC EVALUATION AND ASSESSMENT

The assessment process is an integral part of the clinical treatment of the mentally retarded sex offender. It is an ongoing process that needs constant review. The assessment process is a tool to be utilized by the clinician to assist him or her in identifying the psychological deficits of the patient and the distortions that the patient possesses that lead to sexual acting-out behaviors. The information accumulated should be used for treatment and placement planning. A major issue for the clinical team is the immediacy of supervision, both short term and in the future. A recommendation for a more restrictive placement may be part of the initial assessment so as to keep the patient and others safe from any continued destructive behaviors.

The evaluation and assessment process of mentally retarded offenders should adhere to basic principles. The setting should be private and conducive to encouraging openness and honesty. Risk factors need to be evaluated and safety rules must be the priority at all times. Assessment tools using picture indexes are useful in obtaining information. Mentally retarded individuals require time for the framing and reframing of questions so that they can answer them adequately. The use of the patient's slang words can be of help in acquiring information and can assist in the comprehension of the questions being asked. Having knowledge of any particular communication deficits may be of use when phrasing the questions. The comprehensive assessment should use historical clinical data, determine risk factors, incorporate the strengths/needs into the treatment plan, and provide direction for treatment, placement, monitoring, and follow-up.

An assessment tool should measure gender identification, sexual knowledge, recognition of social cues, ego-dystonic and ego-syntonic sexual expressions, sexual deductions experienced and seductions used, coercion experienced and coercion used, distortions regarding consenting sexuality, and age-appropriate sexuality and distortions regarding violence and coercion.

According to the National Task Force on Sexual Offending Behaviors (National Council of Juvenile and Family Court Judges 1988), a comprehensive assessment should also include the following:

1. Family background, educational background
2. Progression of sexually aggressive behavior over time
3. Dynamics/process of victim selection

4. Intensity of sexual arousal prior to offense
5. Use of force
6. Spectrum of injury
7. Sadism
8. Deviant sexual fantasies
9. Deviant nonsexual history
10. History of assaultive behaviors
11. Sociopathy
12. Personality disorders (affective disorder)
13. Attention deficits
14. Behavioral warning signs
15. Identifiable triggers
16. Ability to accept responsibility
17. Denial or minimization
18. Understanding of wrongdoing
19. Victim empathy
20. Family's denial
21. Substance abuse
22. History of sexual victimization
23. Family dysfunction
24. Parental separation and loss
25. Masturbating patterns
26. Impulse control
27. Mental status, degree of mental retardation
28. Organicity

A major contribution of the assessment instrument is its ability to identify the perceptual distortions of the patient that lead to acting out sexual behaviors. Usually patients are unable to discriminate deviant from nondeviant behaviors. When mildly retarded patients are shown drawings of rape scenes, they often identify the act as "sexual." They often cannot identify the violence in the drawing, although they can describe and define coercions for a sex education program. Patients who display pedophiliac behaviors can explain the legal ramifications of a molestation but will often believe they are only being affectionate when they are in a child's presence. They do not see their interactions as being coercive. Traditionally, these perceptual distortions have been thought to be the result of the mental retardation rather than of serious psychological dysfunctioning. The ability to identify the distortion that the patient possesses can give the clinician an opportunity to enable the patient to work with the distortion in group treatment through the feedback obtained in cognitive restructuring. Patients can have a heightened awareness and accept that they have distortions in those areas of sexual coercion, age-appropriate sexuality, or what is sexually violent and what is not, as in the following example:

> Frank is a high-functioning male with mental retardation living in a community residence. Although he could articulate the legal implications if he had sex with children, when asked if a 12-year-old child approached him and asked for directions, his interpretation of a normal appropriate conversation became interpreted as a sexual provocation from the child. As the evaluation explored this interpretation further, distortions regarding age-appropriate sexual behavior emerged.

Hayashino et al. (1995) state that child molesters have higher cognitive distortions and continue to endorse a system of beliefs that regulates the appropriateness of having sex with children. Based on the assessment of mentally retarded sex offenders, the results often indicate that they possess poor social skills, poor judgment, deficits in impulse control, dysfunctional family backgrounds, deficits in sex education, and distortions regarding consent, violence, and age-appropriate sexuality. The diagnostic purpose of the assessment process is to understand these dysfunctions for the individual and to formulate a treatment plan that will address both the cognitive deficits of a mentally retarded person and the underlying emotional issues that lead to consequent dysfunctional sexual acting-out behaviors. Breaking down these areas into workable and treatable clinical goals enables the clinician to formulate a treatment plan with a vision toward managing violent behavior.

■ GROUP THERAPY

Group therapy is one part of the required treatment process for reducing and managing sexually deviant behaviors. Individual therapy, psychopharmacological intervention, masturbatory satiation programs, behavior management, and family therapy all contribute to comprehensive care and treatment. In their work with sexualized children, Gil and Johnson (1993) emphasize the group as the treatment of choice and in coordination with adjunctive modalities. They stress that the greatest learning for children comes from being with other children. They cite the importance of learning to manage behaviors through the modality of the peer group process.

Group treatment as described in this chapter is a clinical intervention comprising cognitive modules and experiential processes. The cognitive modules are not classroom instruction but rather the presentation of material and the integration of this material through an interpersonal dynamic group process. This process fosters a therapeutic alliance that needs to be created to treat this complex disorder. The entire program stresses commitment, involvement, and responsibility on the part of all participants, both members and facilitators. Through the bonding process each member will learn to identify stressors and patterns of self-destructive behaviors and to explore more responsible alternatives. Because the most prominent personality deficit of a mentally retarded sex offender is his or her inability to form an intimate, warm, sympathetic relationship with an adult peer, the prime modality for treatment is the group. The process addresses the issue of one's inability to bond with peers and provides a support system for managing destructive sexual behaviors as well.

The treatment presented can be used for all levels and aspects of sexually deviant behavior (rape, child molestation, exhibitionism, self-mutilation). The group therapy program has been used for patients at both inpatient and outpatient treatment facilities. The setting must provide an area of privacy/confidentiality and integrate safety features for both group members and facilitators. The sessions should be held weekly and be consistent with regard to the day, place, time, and duration of the session. As the group begins to take on a life of its own, such consistency often lends substantial and reliable support in providing structure to individuals whose lives are often in turmoil. The group process is and must reflect a microcosm for life experiences. Therefore, the group process must be an organized, reliable treatment modality.

Group treatment can be inherently stressful, given that patients need to disclose painful memories and experiences (sexual offenses) in front of strangers. Patients must also listen to detailed accounts of their own distorted thinking, which often increases their own anxiety, anger, and resentment. Also, concurrent individual psychotherapy may be useful not only to reinforce newly acquired appropriate learning but also to assist the patient in dealing with the emotional experiences as his or her defenses of denial and resistance are broken down. The psychotherapeutic aspects of treatment and group therapy are best used when adjunctive psychotherapies are available.

■ ORGANIZATION OF TREATMENT

Treatment is organized into three stages. Stage I consists of feelings identification, relaxation training, and anger management. Stage II consists of social skills training and cognitive restructuring/relapse prevention. Stage III is transition planning, termination, and aftercare.

Stage I

Stage I is characterized by two processes: the cognitive/didactic process and the experiential process. The first stage of treatment is highly structured, and the leader is very active and direct. The main task in the initial stage is to establish a group with clear goals, purposes, expectations, and guidelines for functioning. All participants create and contribute to establishing a contract in the group. Issues of trust, confidence, and responsibilities are highlighted. The process of contracting is typically lengthy but necessary for establishing treatment goals. Early defenses in therapy with mentally retarded persons generally include massive denial of problems, use of projection, and affective isolation. These defenses tend to make a sex offender very resistant to group membership. Engaging these patients in a therapeutic alliance is the utmost challenge, and group facilitators need to present a clear purpose and rationale of the benefits of a group accompanied by excellent engaging and bonding skills.

The cognitive modules in stage I involve feelings identification, relaxation training, and anger management. The appropriate labeling of feelings is essential to the understanding and identification of the antecedents to sexually aggressive behaviors. Many mentally retarded people are taught not to express feelings but rather to deny them. Ability to identify, label, and recognize feelings becomes an integral part of identifying antecedents to the expression of sexually violent behaviors. Feeling logs such as Benson's anger management program (Benson et al. 1986) and those found in "Pathways" (Kahn 1990) can be adapted and utilized in assisting patients to work with feelings and feeling exploration. At this early stage of treatment, resistance to treatment may be manifested by the patient's failure to use the logs as an assignment. Immediately, the clinician must address this issue and work with the patient in involvement in treatment. The group facilitator should be very active together with the patient in identifying what responsible and irresponsible group behaviors are. A direct and matter-of-fact attitude should be adopted in referring back to agreed-upon guidelines and for establishing a procedural and structural framework for group processes.

Groth (1979) and others have stated that violent sexual behavior is an acting out of the person's inability to handle the stress and responsibilities of daily living. Relaxation training addresses this issue by preparing the patient for the application of new coping mechanisms for daily life stresses. Group members are directed to use various methods in order to reach a state of relaxation. Deep breathing, music, and imagery become a part of each group session. Patients learn to apply spontaneously these relaxation techniques in stressful life situations. Each participant begins by identifying the internal and external stressors that go hand in hand with the daily regime of living. The patient participates actively by intervening in the stressful aspects of his or her life. The patient learns to discern the emotional and environmental triggers that activate the destructive patterns of behavior that often lead to sexually deviant acting out. The participant accepts the responsibility of actively intervening in this process. Each patient begins to develop a stress reduction plan that must become integrated into daily life. Here is an example:

> Ken is a pedophiliac who is a high-functioning, mildly retarded man who was participating in overnight Special Olympics. He was accompanied by a supervisor. The hotel he was residing in was populated with young children who were also participants in the Special Olympics event. Ken, anxious with fear that he would act out sexually, clung to the bed all night, breathing deep and playing his relaxation tapes, although the staff was unaware of what was happening and assumed he was hallucinating. With assistance, Ken related his overstimulation and through counseling efforts chose to return to his group home. Totally unprepared to deal with so many children, he related in the group how his learned relaxation techniques "got him through the night."

Anger management training is the third part of stage I of treatment. An adapted version of Benson's anger management program can be utilized. Through the process of assertiveness training, self-instruction, and the understanding of one's own antecedent behaviors and the feelings and events that lead to anger and rage, the patient learns to control his or her emotions and find more appropriate and responsible ways of expressing feelings. Group members practice the recognition of the physical body cues that lead to anger states as well as adjunctive mood states that trigger rage. Feelings of embarrassment, humiliation, shyness, fear, panic, and insecurity often lead to an outburst of uncontrolled destructive behaviors. Once they understand the impact these emotions have on their daily life functioning, patients can begin to use supportive interventions to redirect rage and acting-out behaviors. Nonsexual incidents such as feeling humiliated, belittled, or condescended to at work can lead to serious acting-out episodes involving sexual coercion. Understanding antecedent triggers, sexual or not, may be of assistance in managing anger and raising the patient's awareness of his or her internal state that may lead to destructive sexual behaviors.

During this period of group work, patients begin to identify sources of rage that are unique to mentally retarded sex offenders. The expression of discomfort and anger regarding their own cognitive limitations (mental retardation, learning disability, physical disability) emerges. The family's approach to these limitations is often explored, and feelings of rage and pain emerge regarding placement issues. The patient's family's dysfunctioning and the patient's own victimization (physical, psychological, and/or sexual abuse) become apparent (Abel 1984). As patients begin to share life experiences, the identified similarity among members, and how they have had to cope with growing up as mentally retarded persons, becomes an engaging and bonding factor. The emotional alienation and denial of who one is become replaced by feelings of belonging.

The group facilitators are very focused on exploring issues and their impact on negative cycle behavior. Focused feedback, pointing out how one's rage affects one's cycle of abuse, is used. Facilitators need to employ empathic, sensitive listening while addressing realities. The final aspects of stage I of treatment are important to the group process as members present issues that are real to them and contribute to the group having a life of its own.

As stage II of treatment is approached, each member's demonstration of involvement, commitment, and responsibilities for treatment needs to be evaluated. Each member is required to discuss progress and needs, and this self-evaluation is reviewed by the group as a whole with peer feedback. Integration of the feedback from peers is then reframed as the goals for stage II of the treatment.

Stage II

Stage II of treatment uses social skills training and cognitive restructuring/relapse prevention. According to Abel and Becker (1984), 40.8% of child molesters and 46.9% of rapists have poor social skills. In addition, mentally retarded offenders are seemingly more deficient in heterosexual skills. This deficit probably is a major causative factor in sexual acting-out behavior. Benson et al. (1985) have found that poor social skills lead to low levels of social experiences. Given the impact of poor social skills development on mentally retarded people in general and sex offenders in particular, social skills training is one of the most important forms of treating major personality deficits in the mentally retarded sex offender. Appropriate social modeling is presented and introduced by facilitators as treatment begins and is presented and integrated in all stages of treatment. In stage II, however, social skills training is refined and presented as a cognitive module.

In social skills training, the sense of fear and anxiety regarding peer interaction manifests itself, as do the patients' conflicts regarding their own sexual identity. The goals of treatment are to develop communicative skills, to enhance interpersonal relationships with peers, to give and receive constructive feedback, and to train assertiveness. Practical appropriate verbal and gestural greetings (eye contact, handshake) are integrated into the group process. All levels of social communication presently used by group members are reviewed by members and, when they are inappropriate, replaced by more socially acceptable behaviors.

Training in assertiveness techniques and skills ("I" statements, eye contact, appropriate voice control and volume) are practiced. Increased focus on enhancing listening skills and interpersonal communication styles are modeled. Role modeling is practiced to teach appropriate skills for confrontation and conflict resolution and for giving and receiving constructive feedback. Direct instruction, modeling, and social reinforcement are used to enhance appropriate social group interaction. Minor impolite gestures such as belching, burping, and noise making are all addressed in treatment and evaluated for social appropriateness. The facilitators are very active during this process, addressing inappropriate behaviors directly, firmly, and humanely while remaining respectful to the members.

In the course of treatment, the group members' conflicts in male/female relationships emerge, manifesting themselves through withdrawal or bravado. Members share their anxieties in social situations, exploring feelings of insecurity and of being "found out" (cognitive limitations), or if their disabilities are physical, they express their fear of rejection. Issues of low self-esteem present themselves, and personal defense mechanisms that may be repulsive to others are addressed and explored by group members, as in the following example:

> John initially came to the group sassy and provocative with verbalizations and gestures (eye winking). He was confronted with his behaviors as being obnoxious and distasteful, encouraging rejection rather than contact. It was suggested through role modeling that a firm handshake/eye contact and a strong hello replace the old behavior; it took John several weeks to feel secure and overcome his shyness. He explained that he used his bravado to counteract his feelings of being short and physically deformed. Through practice and supportive reinforcement by group members, his lewd staring and sexual verbalizations discontinued.

Very often, sexually lewd, inappropriate behaviors (verbal and gestural) are a learned cover-up to mask the inadequacies mentally retarded persons experience internally. This internal anxiety needs to be dealt with directly and replaced with socially appropriate behaviors that can lead to more socially appropriate interactions.

The purpose of social skills training is to provide the patient with a set of behaviors that will enhance the patient's ability to encourage positive/reinforcing relationships so that the use of force and coercion is not necessary for human contact.

Stage II of treatment also includes cognitive restructuring/relapse prevention. In cognitive restructuring, focused feedback is used in the interactions among the group members and becomes part of the interpersonal communication style. Patients continue to explore their own self-destructive cycles and perceptual distortions. This phase addresses their emerging sense of depression and loss, and their alienation and rejection of peers as an expression of their own self-hate. The goal is to explore perceptual distortions and the self-destructive style, increase awareness, and accept responsibility for their own sexual behavior through self-examination and feedback.

Through cognitive restructuring, the group begins to break into each patient's faulty belief system. Their denials of irresponsible sexual and nonsexual behaviors are confronted. They are encouraged to discuss behaviors/incidents more extensively so that distortions will be more visible and can be challenged. Through this sensitive process, the patients will begin to identify emotional and attitudinal precipitants to sexually offensive behaviors, and to develop an increased awareness of their own emotional and psychological processes that led to their victimizing others. They slowly begin to have an understanding of the impact of their sexual abuse on others, given the exploration of their own sexual abuse and exploitation, and some awareness of emotional and attitudinal precipitants of sexual offending behavior that are unique to a mentally retarded person.

This process is a very sensitive/emotional one for both group members and facilitators. The facilitator is very active, direct, and empathic. By this time, peers can assist in pointing out distorted thinking and are better able to engage in reality testing. The group facilitator can guide the members in direct self-evaluation and in observations of offending behaviors.

Generally, this stage of treatment can be typified by the overpowering feelings of rage expressed by patients who are being confronted with irresponsible behaviors as well as by intense feelings of depression that are experienced by patients trying to accept their dual disability of being not only cognitively impaired but also sexually deviant. This acceptance of the self is often riddled with self-hate, which may be manifested in suicidal ideations, gestures, or attempts.

The cofacilitators must be engaging, firm, and empathic to the painstaking efforts the patients make during this phase of treatment. Treatment has often been termed "tough and tender" or "a kick and a hug." The emotional aspects of treatment involve managing the patient's feelings of depression, loss, anxiety, and rejection. As the patient passes through this growth cycle, he or she can enter into self-examination and a new yearning for continued treatment.

In the process of relapse prevention, members review patterns of abusive behaviors and replace these with patterns of coping behaviors and strategies that avoid relapse. Haaven (1993) simplifies the process of relapse prevention by teaching group members to identify and label "setups" (thoughts/feelings/actions) and replace them with "what to dos" (coping strategies) that intervene in destructive patterns of behavior.

Stage III

The final stage of treatment involves transition planning/termination/aftercare. During this stage of treatment, the patient is helped to identify coping strategies, recognize safety cues, recognize and overcome distortions, accept dependency issues, and utilize supportive peer interactions in a positive way. The ability to accept one's dual diagnosis and commitment to manage it through participation in the treatment process become the focus of the after-care program. The prevention of any relapse is an integral part of the transitional planning process in the group.

Movement into this stage of treatment is accompanied by fears, dependency, and hopefulness. Members have an increased ability to bond with peers and leaders. They use the group to work through daily life issues and integrate behavioral vulnerabilities to avoid relapse. They have an increased awareness of the safety cues necessary for not acting out. They rely less on external indicators (supervision) and spontaneously recognize other members' distortions and realities. They are better able to apply coping strategies to situations in which their cycle of destructive behavior can begin again. They are better able to accept responsibility for their actions.

One of the goals of the group is to recognize that sexually deviant behavior cannot be "cured." Participants need to accept their disabilities and manage them. Accepting the need for ongoing therapeutic support and treatment is an indicator of the progress the member has made; such maintenance counseling assists in continuing the goal of self-activization (Ingusal and Patton 1990).

■ CONCLUSIONS

One of the major obstacles to treatment has been the failure of the professional community to accept a sexual disorder in a mentally retarded person. We have learned that a mentally retarded person who exhibits violent sexual behaviors is capable of being involved in straightforward comprehensive treatment once the sexual disorder is identified. Treatment needs to address the cognitive limitations of the person as well as the underlying emotional issues. Throughout this chapter I have focused on some of the cognitive modules presented in treatment and how the psychotherapeutic group process enables the patient to integrate the educational material. Further studies and basic research will provide better insight into how we can best refine our treatment of this complex disorder.

■ REFERENCES

Abel G, Becker M: Treatment of Child Molestation. Los Angeles, CA, California University Press, 1984

Becker J, Hunter J: Aggressive sex offenders. Child Adoles Psychiatr Clin North Am 2:477–485, 1993

Benson B, Reiss S, Smith DC, et al: Psychosocial correlates of depression in mentally retarded adults; II: poor social skills. American Journal of Mental Deficiency 6:657–659, 1985

Benson BA, Rice CJ, Miranti S: Effects of anger management training with adults in group treatment. J Consult Clin Psychol 154:728–729, 1986

Gil E, Johnson CT: Sexualized Children. New York, Launch Press, 1993

Griffiths D, Verna Q, Hingsberger D, et al: Changing Inappropriate Sexual Behavior: Community Based Treatment of Developmentally Disabled Individuals Displaying Inappropriate Sex Behaviors. New York, Central, 1987

Groth N: Men Who Rape. New York, Plenum, 1979

Haaven J: An Introduction to the Treatment of Intellectually Disabled Sex Offenders. Brandon, VT, Safer Society Press, 1993

Haaven J, Little R, Petre-Miller R: Treating Intellectually Disabled Sex Offenders. Brandon, VT, Safer Society Press, 1990

Hayashino DS, Wirtele SK, Klebe KJ: Child molesters: an examination of cognitive factors. Interpersonal Violence 10:106–117, 1995

Ingusol S, Patton S: Treating Perpetrators of Sexual Abuse. Lexington, MA, Lexington Books, 1990

Kahn T: Pathways. Orwell, VT, Safer Society Press, 1990

Kempton W: Sex Education for Persons With Disabilities That Hinder Learning. Santa Monica, CA, Stanfield Company, 1988

Knopp FH, Lackey S: Sexual Offenders Identified as Intellectually Disabled. Orwell, VT, Safer Society Press, 1987

Kohut H: Self Deficits and Addiction: The Dynamics and Treatment of Alcoholism: Essential Papers. Northvale, NJ, Jason Aranson, 1994

Menolascino F: Promising Practices in Knowledge/Technique and Strategies in Meeting the Need of Persons With Dual Diagnosis. Suffern, NY, University of Nebraska, 1984

National Council of Juvenile and Family Court Judges: Juvenile and Family Court Journal 39(2), 1988

Reiss S, Levitan GW, Szyszko J: Emotional disturbances and mental retardation: diagnostic overshadowing. American Journal of Mental Deficiencies 86:567–574, 1982

Szymanski L, Tanguay M: Emotional Disorders of Mentally Retarded Persons. Baltimore, MD, University Park Press, 1980

20 Treatment and Care of Mentally Retarded Offenders

Kenneth Day, M.B., Ch.B., F.R.C.Psych., D.P.M.

Offending behavior is uncommon in mentally retarded people. Studies reveal a point prevalence of 0.5%–1%, a lifetime risk of between 3% and 5%, and a prevalence of 1%–2% in the United Kingdom and 1%–10% in the United States in remanded and convicted prisoners. Some increase is to be anticipated in coming years as implementation of ordinary life policies exposes more mentally retarded people to greater temptations and opportunities for offending and the hidden offenses that occur regularly in institutions become more visible. A hint of this is provided by Lund's (1990) finding of a significant increase from 1973 to 1989 in mentally retarded offenders in Denmark receiving their first sentence. The typical mentally retarded offender is a young male functioning in the mild to borderline intellectual range from a poor urban environment with a history of psychosocial deprivation, behavior problems, and personality disorder, and who is likely to have spent substantial periods in residential care and to have a family history of criminality. As in the general population, the most common offenses are acquisitive and technical, but sex offenses and arson are considerably overrepresented. Recidivism is common, and there is a tendency for the mentally retarded to commit a wider spectrum of offenses than their nonretarded counterparts. Female offenders are rare, and although their offense behavior tends to be trivial, they are invariably grossly disturbed individuals who present a wide range of behavioral difficulties and who are extremely difficult to help. (For a more detailed account of the prevalance and the characteristics and offense behavior of mentally retarded offenders, see Day 1990a, 1993, 1997.)

It is generally agreed that mentally retarded offenders require treatment and care in the health and welfare services rather than punishment in the criminal justice system. This principle is embodied to a greater or lesser degree in the service philosophy and provision and mental health legislation in

359

most countries. Mentally retarded offenders are unable to adjust to prison regimes; are victimized, abused, and manipulated by more able prisoners; exhibit emotional and behavioral problems and self-mutilation; and tend to go unidentified and unhelped (Finn 1992; Hall 1992; Reichard et al. 1982; Smith et al. 1990). Attempts to introduce special treatment and rehabilitation programs to improve staff training in prisons have proved difficult, if not impossible, to achieve because of conflicting missions and cultures (Hall 1992).

The vulnerability of mentally retarded people in the criminal justice system, particularly their ability to comprehend a police caution on arrest and their suggestibilty when making a statement, is recieving increasing attention (Gudjonnson et al. 1993; Murphy and Clare 1998). This has led to a number of initiatives including the publication in the United Kingdom of simple guidelines for mentally retarded people who find themselves under arrest or on trial (Hollins et al 1997a, 1997b).

■ LEGAL BASIS FOR TREATMENT

It is essential that mentally retarded offenders cooperate in their care and treatment, and in the majority of cases some form of legal restraint is necessary, at least in the early stages. Legislation differs from country to country, but there are common elements (see Bluglass and Bowden 1990). In England and Wales, for example, the Criminal Justice Acts have provisions for offenders found unfit to plead or suffering from a mental disorder (which includes mental retardation), a range of options for disposal under the Mental Health Act of 1983, and the power to make a probation order, which includes a condition of either inpatient or outpatient psychiatric treatment for up to 3 years. The Mental Health Act of 1983 provides for remand to a hospital for assessment or treatment, admission to a hospital for treatment, guardianship in the community, and transfer of a prisoner suffering from a mental disorder to a hospital. The court may impose a restriction order in the case of dangerous patients, but in all other cases the offender is treated as if he or she were on a civil order under the act (see Gostin 1986 for more detail). There is an increasing trend toward diversion of mentally disordered offenders from the criminal justice system to the mental health services (Department of Health and Home Office 1992), although this appears not to be much used in the case of mentally retarded offenders (Cooke 1991; Joseph and Potter 1993).

The choice of legal disposal depends on the nature of the offense, the needs of the individual, and the treatment and management goals; each has its advantages and disadvantages (Ashworth and Gostin 1985; Day 1990a). For minor offenses in the absence of gross psychopathology and where general care and management needs are being satisfactorily cared for, conventional punishments such as a fine or conditional discharge may be an appropriate means of helping the individual to feel accountable for his or her actions.

There is a tendency, particularly when the offense is a trivial one, not to report or prosecute (Day 1994), and sometimes the police and the victim need to be persuaded that prosecution is in the best long-term interests of the offender. Failure to prosecute can lead to a negative learning situation. This may be partly compensated for by the issuing of an informal warning from the police and requiring a formal apology to the victim and restitution of articles stolen or a token payment toward the cost of any damage done (Day 1990a). The treatment approaches described in this chapter apply equally to mildly mentally retarded people who have engaged in antisocial behavior but have not been before the courts or convicted as they do to convicted offenders.

■ TREATMENT APPROACHES

Offending in the mentally retarded population usually occurs in the context of undersocialization, poor internal controls, and faulty social learning compounded by educational underachievement, lack of social and occupational skills, and poor self-image. The principal aims of the treatment, therefore, are to assist maturation; facilitate the development of adequate levels of self-control; establish acceptable social mores; improve social, occupational, and educational skills; and instill a sense of personal worth and personal responsibility (Day 1988). Offense-specific measures also need to be addressed. Sex offenders, for example, will need sex education programs, interpersonal skills training, and specific programs related to their sex offending. Fire-setters will need interaction skills and assertiveness training, and violent offenders will need training in anger management and possibly medication to reduce explosivity.

■ TREATMENT SETTING

The majority of mentally retarded offenders can be treated in the community. This offers the best opportunities for socialization skills and other training, provided that an adequate range of services is available. Many are able to remain with their families, attending community facilities and being supported by social workers, community nurses, and probation officers with psychiatric oversight as necessary. Others may require a community-based residential placement because of the nature of their offense, their personal need for structure and support, or their family situation. A full weekly occupational and training program is essential and helps to fill unstructured time, reducing the risk of further offending. A guardianship or probation order needs to be considered when problems of cooperation are anticipated. White and Wood (1988; Wood and White 1992) have described a highly successful community-based service involving a combined approach from the mental retardation and probation services and an intensive treatment program that incorporates all of the components described below.

Treatment in a specialist hospital unit is indicated in the following circumstances:

- The offense is a serious one that would in the normal course of events have attracted a custodial sentence.
- The offender is deemed to pose a significant danger to the public—not necessarily in terms of the current offense but because of his or her antecedent history and other factors.
- The offender has a general need for care, training, supervision, and control of a degree that cannot be provided in the community.
- An in-depth assessment is required that cannot be carried out in the community.
- There have been persistent multiple offenses that have proved unresponsive to other treatment approaches even though the offenses themselves may be trivial.
- It is not possible to meet the offender's general and specific treatment needs within the community due to lack of specialist personnel and facilities or factors in the offender's social background.

■ ASSESSMENT

A comprehensive assessment of the individual and his or her offending behavior forms the basis of the treatment plan (Campbell 1990; Day 1990a), the key elements of which are listed in Table 20–1. The current offense, the context in which it occurred, and any triggering events or contributory factors should be thoroughly explored, and statements from the offender, his or her victim(s), and any witnesses as well as photographic or other evidence should be carefully scrutinized. Full details of all previous offenses including disposal and outcome should be obtained. Particular regard should be paid to any factors pertaining to offending behavior, including evidence of brain damage, family psychopathology, offender typology, and subcultural factors. Information should be collected from as many sources as possible, including the patient, his or her relatives, care workers, the probation service, and previous medical and social records. Medical examination should cover minor as well as major physical defects, level of mental retardation, psychiatric illness, personality features, and the offense-related issues. Particular attention should be

Table 20–1. Examination of the mentally retarded offender: essential elements

History

Current offense — Nature, circumstances, solitary/joint, planned/impulsive, motive, associated factors (e.g. alcohol, emotional upset, level of support/supervision, life events)

Previous offense(s) — Dates, nature, disposal (include offenses not prosecuted)

Neuropsychiatric disorder — Other conduct/behavior disorder, mental illness, epilepsy, with details

Personality disorder — Friends, interests, relationships, status, gang membership

Family and social background — Upbringing, family structure and psychodynamics including status of offender in family, schooling, employment/occupation, socioeconomic status, neighborhood crime

Family psychopathology — Family history of mental illness, mental handicap, delinquency, criminality, or other psychopathology

Examination

Mental state — Intellectual status, degree of literacy, superadded psychiatric illness, personality disorder, attitude toward offense (shame, remorse, concern for victim, concept of right and wrong), fitness to plead, attitude toward examiner, dangerousness

Physical state — Minor and major defects

Investigations

Psychometry: IQ, educational attainments, personality, structured analysis of offense cycle

EEG studies as indicated

Chromosome studies as indicated

Adapted with permission from Day K: "Mental Retardation: Clinical Aspects and Management," in *Principles and Practice of Forensic Psychiatry*. Edited by Bluglass R, Bowden P. Edinburgh, UK, Churchill Livingstone, 1990a, pp. 399–418.

paid to the offender's attitude toward the offense, concern for the victim and the victim's family, concern for the offender's family, understanding of the offense's seriousness and the possible consequences, and the offender's concept of right and wrong. Psychological assessment should include IQ assessment, educational attainments, adaptive behavior, personality, and an in-depth exploration of specific offense-related issues, including sexual knowledge, attitude to offense, offense cycle, etc. If brain damage or epilepsy is suspected, EEG studies should be undertaken. Chromosome studies may be indicated to exclude a genosomal abnormality.

Dangerousness

An assessment of dangerousness and the likelihood of further offending are crucial in shaping treatment recommendations, assessing progress, and making the eventual decision to discharge. Currently, this assessment lacks scientific rigor and is more an art than a science (Prins 1993). Thoroughness and persistence in data collection and the pursuance of clues and cues about dangerous behavior (Scott 1977), careful and detailed analysis of the offense and associated factors, and a healthy skepticism at all times (Prins 1993) are essential. Key factors to be considered include the nature and circumstances of the offense and its apparent motivation, personality features, attitude toward the offense, and an assessment of the likelihood of response to treatment (Duggan 1997; Hamilton and Freeman 1982; Maden 1996; Prins 1990; Scott 1977; Vinestock 1996). There are no specific studies relating to the mentally retarded population, but poor self-control, low frustration tolerance, unpredictability, emotional coldness, attitude toward and understanding of the offense, indifference to the victim, and any specific contributory or precipitating factors (including offender typology and the level of support and supervision at the time of the offense) would seem to be particularly important in assessment of dangerousness (Day 1990a, 1997). A past history of offending behavior is also relevant and is the best predictor of the form and frequency of future offending. A record of at least two previous offenses of serious violence or sexual molestation has been shown to be associated with a high probability of committing further similar offenses (Day 1988, 1994; Gibbens and Robertson 1983; Payne et al. 1974; Soothill and Gibbens 1978). Assessments of readiness for discharge should take account not only of patient characteristics but also of the environmental and situational contexts in which the patient will be functioning on discharge, including the availability of necessary support services. Prins (1993) gives a useful list of factors to be considered, including current capacity for coping with provocation, the extent to which the patient has come to terms with what he or she did, the nature of the offense, responsiveness to and compliance with drugs and other treatment, and the level of personality disorder.

■ THE TREATMENT PACKAGE

A properly formulated treatment program with explicitly stated goals is essential. All professionals involved with the offender should work together to reach an agreed-on strategy and meet regularly to monitor progress and review the treatment program. The successful implementation of the treatment package requires experienced and skilled staff, an adequate range of appropriate hospital and community-based facilities, and good multidisciplinary working relationships and close liaison with the courts, probation service, generic mental retardation services, and voluntary agencies. The key elements of the treatment program are listed in Table 20–2. The relative role of each component and the nature of any offense-specific intervention will depend on the specific needs of the individual.

Socialization Programs

Socialization programs aim to link personal behavior with its consequences, using token economy principles to reinforce socially desirable behavior and penalties for undesirable behavior. Successful implementation requires a controlled environment, a high staff/patient ratio, well-trained and experienced personnel, and intensive support from a multiprofessional team. These programs are, therefore, only suitable for use in specialized residential treatment units.

A number of institution-based socialization programs have been described (Burchard 1967; Day 1988, 1990b, 1997; Denkowski and Denkowski 1984; Denkowski et al. 1984; Fidura et al. 1987; Sandford et al. 1987; Santamour and Watson 1982). They all use the systematic issuing of tokens or points contingent on appropriate behavior that can be exchanged for a range of backup reinforcers from cigarettes or sweets to attendance at social events and outings. The programs have been applied to all aspects of behavior (Burchard 1967; Day 1988, 1990b) or differentially targeted at antisocial behavior (Denkowski and Denkowski 1984; Sandford et al. 1987). In some schemes, tokens or points are issued immediately following a behavioral event (Denkowski and Denkowski 1984; Fidura et al. 1987), whereas in others rewards are received on a daily or weekly basis (Day 1988, 1990b; Sandford et al. 1987). The programs have all been developed as part of a comprehensive treatment program that includes individualized packages of social and personal skills training, counseling, and offense-specific treatments and a phased progression, from closed units to eventually a halfway hostel as a final preparation for discharge, once set goals have been satisfactorily achieved. Good results with sustained positive behavioral changes during the treatment period (Burchard 1967; Day 1988; Denkowski and Denkowski 1984; Sandford et al. 1987) and at up to 5 years' follow-up (Day 1988; Sandford et al. 1987) have been reported.

Table 20–2. Treatment program key components

Legal framework

Life skills training
Personal
Interpersonal
Social
Occupational
Educational
Recreational
Sex education

Counseling and supportive psychotherapy

Treatment/amelioration of physical disabilities and mental illness

Socialization programs

Psychological treatments
Self-management strategies
Relaxation therapy
Anger management
Assertiveness
Coping strategies
Recognition/avoidance of risk situations
Escape strategies
Offense specific
Sex behavior management
Program for fire-setters

Drug therapy
Mood-stabilizing medication
Antilibidinal medication

Family and caregiver support

Rehabilitation, aftercare, relapse prevention

Training in Life Skills

Most mentally retarded offenders show marked deficiencies in life skills and have failed to achieve their educational potential. A package of personal, social, occupational, and recreational skills training and further education are essential components of the treatment program (Day 1988, 1990b; Fidura et al. 1987). Life skills training should focus on those areas—work habit, personal care and hygiene, basic literacy and numeracy, constructive use of leisure, hobbies, etc.—that will enable the individual to better cope and integrate with society. A key component is training in interpersonal skills, which are frequently poorly developed and often a factor in offending behavior.

Life skills training is best carried out in a peer group situation as part of a structured weekly program, although hobbies can be tackled individually. It is important that activities are enjoyable, are seen as relevant by the offender, and provide opportunities for personal achievement. A proper balance must be struck between work activity, social training, and further education. Recreational training and the development of hobbies should take place in the evenings and on weekends.

The principal aim is to improve competencies, develop skills, and increase self-confidence and independence. Life skills training also facilitates the development of social awareness, personal responsibility, and self-control. Work situations, special projects, and sporting activities all provide valuable opportunities for learning about the needs and feelings of others, teamwork, motivation and persistence, and for experiencing achievement, ownership, and personal worth.

Counseling and Supportive Psychotherapy

Group or individual counseling and supportive psychotherapy should deal with specific problems such as attitudes about offending, personal relationships, and sex, alcohol, and drug abuse. Counseling should be kept simple and use concrete examples arising from everyday experience. The depth of interpretation can be varied according to the ability and receptiveness of the individual concerned, but elaborate explanations should be avoided. In group settings, topics usually suggest themselves, common examples being absconding, attitudes to staff, relationships within the group, bullying, thieving, and the need for rules and regulations. Role-play and psychodrama are potentially useful but underused techniques for teaching how to handle difficult situations and personal feelings; facilitating an appreciation of the rights and feelings of others; and training in more complex social skills like handling an interview for group home accommodation, work, or occupational placement. Specific offense-related group and individual work are considered later.

Working With Families

The problems and management of families of mentally retarded offenders are a neglected area in clinical practice and so far have not been addressed in the research literature. Families need help to enable them to understand their son's or daughter's problems and needs and why the offense was committed. The initial response of many families is shame and censure and a fear that a relatively minor sex offense, for example, is the first indication that their son is en route to becoming a sex monster, a situation that calls for sensitive handling and a careful explanation. Families may also need help in dealing with the reaction of the local community, particularly if the victim is an immediate neighbor or if the offense is a particularly serious one. The whole family can become ostracized and subject to threats and actual violence.

Family cooperation with the treatment program is crucial, especially when the offender continues to live at home. Relatives sometimes view residential treatment as a period of punishment ("serving time") and have difficulty, along with the offender, in understanding the purpose of and cooperating with what is essentially an open-ended period of residential care and treatment. Good communication, a full explanation of the aims and purpose of the treatment program, involvement in case reviews, and frequent informal contact all help to resolve problems and improve cooperation. A clear distinction should be made between allowable "treats" and the requirements of the treatment program.

Some families are so dysfunctional and show such a high level of psychopathology that only limited and controlled contact with the offender is desirable. Many have features that have generated the offending behavior in the first instance. In these cases a decision has to be made, based on a knowledge of the family and an assessment of their ability to cooperate and respond, whether to engage them in some form of family therapy. In families in which this is clearly not possible or has proved unsuccessful in the past, the treatment program should focus on insulating the mentally retarded offender from the adverse influences of his or her family and the wider subculture in which he or she lives.

Medical and Psychiatric Problems

Active mental illness is very rarely a causative factor in offending. Day (1994), for example, found that only 3 of 191 sex offenses/incidents committed by 47 men occurred in the presence of active mental illness (mild hypomania in 2 cases and early arteriosclerotic dementia in 1 case). However, about a third of the mentally retarded offenders have a history of mental illness (Day 1988, 1994; Isweran and Bardsley 1987; Tutt 1971), and the possibility of an underlying mental illness should always be thoroughly explored and, if present, treated appropriately. Very occasionally the offender will be found to be suffering from Asperger's syndrome and require a highly specific approach to management.

A high percentage of mentally retarded offenders show evidence of minor but highly visible physical disabilities such as squint, obesity, speech and hearing defects, or poorly controlled epilepsy (Day 1988, 1994). These contribute to the alienation of the individual from society, impede social integration and the processes of socialization and social learning, give rise to feelings of inferiority, and may be a factor instigating criminal behavior (Hunter 1979; Maberly 1950). They should be thoroughly assessed and corrected as far as possible. Adjustment issues should be addressed through counseling and supportive psychotherapy. Improved seizure control has been shown to make a substantial difference to the longer term course of offending (Milne and O'Brien 1997).

Offense-Specific Treatments/Interventions

Offense-specific interventions for mentally retarded offenders are still in their infancy but include behavioral programs, group therapy, and social skills training for sex offenders (Cox-Lindenbaum and Lindenbaum 1994; Foxx et al. 1986; Griffiths et al. 1989; Haaven et al. 1990; Knopp 1984; Lund 1992; Swanson and Garwick 1990); interaction skills and assertiveness training for arsonists (Clare et al. 1992); and self-management techniques including anger management and relaxation therapy (Benson 1992; Cullen 1993). Antilibidinal medication has been successfully used as an adjunct to treatment in sex offenders (Clarke 1989; Cooper 1995) and neuroleptics, lithium, and anticonvulsants have been used in those displaying abnormal aggression (see Chapter 3 of this book).

■ SEX OFFENDERS

Sex offenders are considerably overrepresented in the mentally retarded offender population and form between one-third to one-half of those admitted to residential treatment units. Mentally retarded sex offenders differ significantly from other sex offenders, and this has considerable relevance to treatment, risk assessment, and prevention. These offenders show a much lower specificity for offense type and victim characteristics (e.g., the victim's age and sex being more a matter of circumstance and opportunity than an indication of sexual preference or orientation; heterosexual offenses rarely occur in the context of an established or developing relationship; alcohol is seldom a predisposing factor; and true sexual deviancy is rare) (Day 1994; Gilby et al. 1989; Murrey et al. 1992). Sexual naivete, inability to understand normal sexual relationships, lack of relationship skills, difficulties in mixing with the opposite sex, poor impulse control, and susceptibility to the influence of others are prominent features (Day 1994; Gebhard et al. 1965; Gilby et al. 1989; Hingsburger 1987; Radzinowicz 1957). Sex abuse during childhood features in the background of a significant proportion of these offenders (Beail and Warden 1995; Day 1994; Gilby et al. 1989).

A recent study identified two principal groups of mentally retarded sex offenders distinguished by whether or not they had committed other types of offenses (Day 1994). The sex offenses–only group were typically shy, immature, and sexually naive individuals with a low prevalence of psychosocial pathology and who tended to commit a high percentage of minor or nuisance offenses. Their sex offending appeared to be a consequence of crude attempts to fulfill normal sexual impulses in the context of lack of opportunities, poor impulse control, and poor adaptive behavior skills, suggesting that treatment measures should be directed at sex education and counseling, relationship skills, and improvement of self-image and self-confidence (Craft 1987; Sovner and Hurley 1983). These individuals can usually be treated quite safely and satisfactorily in the community. The second group who had committed both sex and other offenses were more markedly damaged individuals who showed a high degree of sociopathy, psychosocial deprivation, and brain damage. Their sex offending was part of a wider tapestry of offending and other antisocial behavior indicative of undersocialization, poor parental models, and poor impulse control. They tended to become persistent offenders and to commit serious sex offenses. This group requires highly specialized assessment and treatment on an inpatient basis. A third, much smaller group are the true sexual deviants who require specialized interventions.

In dealing with mentally retarded sex offenders, it is important to recognize that their sex offending often occurs in the context of a wide range of problems including deficits in adaptive behavior skills and other disturbed behaviors that may require behavioral or environmental intervention (Day 1997; Murphy et al. 1983). Specific interventions include sex education, psychological treatments, antilibidinal drugs, and, in rare cases, treatment for deviant sexual behavior. Murphy et al. (1983) have developed a useful scheme for the behavioral assessment and treatment of sex offenders. Progress should be judged on a global basis including improvements in general behavior, level of self-control, personal responsibility, and social awareness as well as sexual behavior.

Sex Education and Sociosexual Skills

The majority of mentally retarded sex offenders are sexually naive and have usually been denied access to knowledge normally acquired in the process of growing up. A sex education program should address the following specific areas:

- Basic sexual knowledge
- Issues of male and female sexuality

- Sociosexual skills—relationships, awareness, and courtship skills
- The laws and social codes governing appropriate or inappropriate sexual behavior including age appropriateness of partners, consensual relationships, interpretation of cues, and rejecting sexual contact

Sex education programs are best carried out in small groups. Explicit photographic and other material may need to be employed as mentally retarded people find fantasizing difficult. A major problem is putting theoretical skills into practice, and opportunities to meet a peer group of the opposite sex in appropriate social situations is desirable although often difficult to achieve. There are a number of excellent sex education packages available (Craft 1987; Johnson 1984; Kempton 1988; Lindsay et al. 1992), and innovative programs on the laws and social rules of sexual behavior (Charman and Clare 1992) and relationship and courtship skills (Forchuk et al. 1995; Valenti-Hein and Mueser 1990) have been developed (see Chapter 5 in this book for a more detailed account of the assessment and sociosexual skills training). Sex education programs alone are insufficient to modify or decrease sex offending. They must be combined with more specialized treatment programs.

Psychological Treatments

A number of psychological treatment programs have been developed specifically for mentally retarded sex offenders based on techniques used in the treatment of nonretarded sex offenders (Cox-Lindenbaum and Lindenbaum 1994; Griffiths et al. 1989; Haaven et al. 1990; Hingsburger 1987; Knopp 1984; Lund 1992; Swanson and Garwick 1990; see also Chapter 19 of this book). Employing a range of behavioral, cognitive, and psychodynamic measures, these programs utilize the confrontation and peer pressure of group therapy to

- Assist the offender to recognize, acknowledge, and accept responsibility for his or her problem
- Change the offender's attitude to his or her sexual behavior and rectify any cognitive distortions
- Teach the offender to gain control over and modify his or her behavior through understanding its causes and his or her offense cycle
- Assist the offender to recognize the danger signals and develop coping strategies to gain control over his or her sexual behavior

The majority of programs involve a phased approach over several years, commencing with a desensitization process to enable the offender to work within a group setting and assist effective communication, followed by an indepth exploration of personal issues, emotional attitudes, and difficulties aimed at heightening personal awareness and appreciation of the moral dimensions of offending behavior and its practical consequences, including the effects on the victim, and finally to an understanding of the offense cycle and the teaching of coping strategies including the recognition of high-risk situations and how to avoid them and escape strategies such as verbal self-regulation. Relaxation therapy and anger management may be employed at any stage to assist the patient to control his or her emotions and find more appropriate ways of expressing them. The overall aim is to replace sex offending with private, relatively safe, and nonprosecutable sexual behavior.

Patients must be carefully chosen for their ability to participate in the group and to cope with self-revelation, must have a reasonable ability to communicate, and must have the potential for change (Cox-Lindenbaum and Lindenbaum 1994). Swanson and Garwick (1990) stress the importance of a realistic appraisal of the intellectual strengths and weaknesses of the offender as part of this process. Good results have been reported by most programs. Swanson and Garwick (1990) utilized goal attainment scaling and further sex offending to measure progress and report success rates of 50% and 90%, respectively, in their group. Reconviction rates of 12.5% during a 3- to 5-year follow-up were reported by Day (1988), 37.5% over a 2-year follow-up by Lund (1992), 23% over a 10-year follow-up period by Haaven et al. (1990), and 0 over a 5-year follow-up period by Griffith and colleagues (1989).

Antilibidinal Drugs

Antilibidinal drugs reduce the intensity of sex drive, improve the patient's capacity for self-control, relieve intrusive obsessional erotic fantasies, and may obviate the need for institutional care (Myers 1991). They are indicated in the following circumstances:

- As a short-term measure while a detailed assessment is being undertaken and other treatment approaches are being explored and developed or to provide additional control at times of particular stress
- As an adjunct to other treatment approaches when they may help to facilitate concurrent therapy or obviate the need for residential treatment
- As the principal treatment in those patients who fail to respond to other treatment approaches and continue to pose serious problems
- To control sexually deviant impulses and provide relief from intrusive fantasies in paraphilias

Dosage should be titrated according to the desired result. It is not always necessary to completely eliminate the sex drive, the aim in most cases being to reduce it to a level that the patient can control. In patients undergoing psychological treatments, it is necessary to retain a certain level of sex drive; otherwise, the program cannot proceed. In many cases a lengthy period of treatment with antilibidinal medication is required, with a gradual reduction of dosage leading to eventual withdrawal, depending on improvements in the patient's behavior and the efficacy of other treatment approaches. With patients in residential care a decision has to be made as to whether the drug should be withdrawn prior to discharge.

Cyproterone acetate (Androcur) in doses of 100–300 mg daily is currently the drug of choice in the United Kingdom. Compliance is not usually a problem, but when it is, usually as a consequence of forgetfulness, a depot injection of 300 mg intramuscularly every 10–14 days is available. In the United States, medroxyprogesterone acetate is used in a usual daily dose of 100–400 mg intramuscularly every 7–10 days. Both are highly effective in reducing sex drive in the mentally retarded population. Another useful antilibidinal drug is goserelin. It has not been specifically developed as an antilibidinal agent and is not licensed as such in many countries. Nevertheless, it has undoubted efficacy and is valuable in the event of a poor response to cyproterone acetate or medroxyprogesterone acetate and continuing serious problems. (For more information about the use of antilibidinal drugs in the mentally retarded population, the reader is referred to recent review articles by Clarke [1989] and Cooper [1995] and Chapter 3 of this book.) Specific consent for the use of antilibidinal drugs should always be obtained from the patient and discussed with his or her family prior to commencing treatment. The majority of mentally retarded sex offenders are capable of giving informed consent and ususally willing to undertake treatment.

Treatment of Deviant Sexual Behavior

The small number of sex offenders who show true sexual deviancy require specialized treatment programs using techniques used in the treatment of sexual deviancy in the nonretarded population and aimed at reducing deviant sexual arousal and increasing appropriate sexual arousal. There has been little work with the mentally retarded in this area. Foxx and colleagues (1986) critically reviewed 13 research reports on the behavioral treatment of maladaptive sexual behavior in the mentally retarded and concluded that although high success rates were reported, the majority of studies did not employ sufficiently rigorous experimental designs to permit an unequivocal evaluation of their findings. Murphy et al. (1983), Griffiths et al. (1989), Swanson and Garwick (1990), Myers (1991), Murphy and Clare (1991), and Clare (1993) have reported positive results in the use of orgasmic reconditioning, satiation, and covert sensitization in the mentally retarded. Good results have been reported with the use of antilibidinal drugs in cases of pedophilia, exhibitionism, and fetishism in the mentally retarded (Collacott and Cooper 1995; Murphy et al. 1983; Myers 1991).

■ FIRE-SETTERS

Fire-setting is an offense committed by both male and female mentally retarded people, and clinical experience and anecdotal evidence indicate a high recidivism rate (Day 1993). Like their nonretarded counterparts, mentally retarded fire-setters show a high incidence of aggression to property (other than arson), self-mutilation, attempted suicide, sexual problems (in the case of females), and psychotic overlay and a low incidence of aggression to others and sex offenses (in males) (McKerracher and Dacre 1966; O'Sullivan and Kelleher 1987; Tennent et al. 1971). Geller and Bertsch (1985) suggest that fire-setting is used as a communicative vehicle by those with poor verbal skills, and O'Sullivan and Kelleher (1987) have hypothesized that this might be the explanation in many cases of arson committed by the mentally retarded. McKerracher and Dacre (1966) suggest that arson can be a form of displaced aggression in passive, inadequate individuals who are incapable of interacting at an emotional level with others. Conflict or stress is frequently associated with episodes of arson, and in many instances the fire is started in the immediate living area of the patient (Clare et al. 1992; Yesevage et al. 1983). In some patients it is difficult to identify a motive, but sometimes feelings of power and excitement generated by fire-setting and its consequences appear to be the explanation (Day 1990a; Murphy and Clare 1996).

Psychological Approaches to Treatment

Using functional analysis, Jackson et al. (1987) have advanced a developmental model of recidivistic arson as a basis for treatment. They hypothesize that personal and environmental disadvantage, dissatisfaction with self and/or life, and actual or perceived ineffective social interaction are the key contextual elements in which fire-setting might take place; that special factors such as previous exposure to fire-setting behavior in an acquaintance direct the arsonist toward fire-setting; and that the absence of a "person target" in situations in which the arsonist feels powerless to change trigger the fire-setting episodes. They recommend that management strategies should therefore focus upon helping the arsonist to develop alternative and successful methods of affecting social influence through the development of interaction skills and training in appropriate assertiveness. Clare et al. (1992) have reported the successful treatment of a mildly mentally retarded male arsonist using this approach involving cosmetic surgery, social skills and assertiveness training, alternative coping strategies, assisted covert sensitization, and a "helpline." Stewart (1993) and Murphy and Clare (1996) recommend adopting a relapse prevention model approach, in which the arsonist is helped to understand his or her offense cycle and the emotional and other antecedents to his or her fire-setting. Treatment should focus on the teaching of coping strategies including escape from and avoidance of high-risk situations and training in self-management techniques such as relaxation, self-talk, and cognitive restructuring.

General Measures

The management of the fire-setter poses special problems because of the risk of repetition and the potentially serious consequences to life and property. Deliberate fire-setting is usually an indication for treatment in a residential setting under close supervision and conditions of security. The needs of the individual must be balanced against minimizing the risk of further episodes, and a complete ban on personal matches and lighters, close supervision in situations in which incendiary materials are available, supervised smoking, and regular searches are all essential in the early stages of treatment. Such a regime can impose considerable strain on both the nursing staff and the patient and cause potentially explosive situations. It should therefore be reviewed frequently and relaxed gradually according to progress of the patient. Duration of inpatient treatment will depend on the progress of the individual and an assessment of the risk of further fire-setting episodes. As with all dangerous offenders, risk to the community should be the paramount consideration.

■ THE AGGRESSIVE MENTALLY RETARDED OFFENDER

Although violent offenses are uncommon (Day 1990a, 1993), a substantial number of mentally retarded offenders display low frustration tolerance and explosivity, often in association with underlying organic brain damage. This impairs their ability to cooperate satisfactorily with treatment programs, renders them potentially dangerous to themselves and others, and therefore requires specific therapeutic interventions, both behavioral and pharmacological.

Recent prospective studies suggest that mentally retarded males and females are significantly more likely to commit a violent offense than the normal population (Hodgins 1992; Hodgins et al. 1996). Evidence is emerging to suggest that violent behavior may be a particular feature of Asperger's syndrome (Mawson et al. 1985).

Anger management training, pioneered with the mildly mentally retarded by Benson (1992, 1994), is a key therapeutic intervention. (For a review and discussion of the use of this and other self-control procedures in mentally retarded offenders, see Chapter 5 of this book and Cullen 1993.) The neuroleptics lithium and certain anticonvulsants have been shown to be effective mood stabilizers in reducing explosivity and increasing frustration tolerance in the mentally retarded, particularly in those with evidence of underlying organic brain damage. They are indicated in the aggressive mentally retarded offender

- As an initial strategy while other treatment approaches are being introduced
- As part of an overall treatment plan to control explosivity and facilitate cooperation with psychological and other treatments
- As a major intervention in seriously aggressive individuals in the absence of success of other treatment approaches

For guidance on the selection and use of these drugs, see Chapters 3 and 16 of this book. Duration of pharmacotherapy will vary with the individual and its purpose. Drug therapy should not be withdrawn abruptly or discontinued during potentially vulnerable periods such as discharge from hospital, transfer between agencies, or other life events.

■ PROPERTY AND TECHNICAL OFFENSES

Petty theft, robbery, burglary, delinquency, acts of vandalism, and vehicle offenses are the most common forms of offending by the mentally retarded. They are frequently rooted in faulty upbringing with poor parental models and criminal behavior in other family members compounded by delinquent contamination, status seeking, poor supervision, and a lack of self-control. Offenses are often committed jointly, frequently with chronologically younger but intellectually superior peers, with the not infrequent consequence that the mentally retarded offender is erroneously regarded as the ringleader. Solitary delinquent acts are usually a consequence of poor self-control or sometimes an overreaction to frustration or occasionally blind panic in situations that the individual cannot understand or handle (Day 1990a).

The majority of offenders in this category can be managed in the community where they require no more than an infrastructure of services, including support personnel, day and residential services, and structured leisure activities. More serious or persistent offenders require a period of specialized treatment in a residential unit. Although they usually do well in the structured and stable setting of such a program, the prognosis of further offending is poor if they return to the family or neighborhood that produced their delinquent behavior in the first place (Day 1988).

The principal treatment goals are improved self-control and insulation against adverse environmental factors. Some workers advocate a constructional approach that focuses on proactive rather than reactive strategies, the function of which is to establish attractive, acceptable alternative repertoires to antisocial behavior (Cullen 1993; Dana 1993; Donnellan et al. 1988). Cole and colleagues (1985) have described the successful use of self-regulation techniques involving self-monitoring, self-evaluation, and coping strategies akin to anger management, and relaxation therapy to increase self-control in this population.

■ REHABILITATION AND AFTERCARE

Return to the community after a period of residential treatment should be a carefully phased process beginning with a lessening of restrictions within the unit with progression through a graduated range of less restrictive treatment settings and progressing through weekend and longer leaves to eventual discharge (Day 1988, 1990b). Periods of extended leave help to test the offender's willingness and ability to cooperate with the aftercare program and enable a quick return to the treatment unit should the situation break down. A comprehensive aftercare package, comprising domiciliary support, occupational placement, residential placement where required, and leisure activities, is essential if social breakdown and drift back into offending are to be avoided (Craft 1984; Day 1988; Hunter 1979; Walker and McCabe 1973). Intensive support is required during the immediate postdischarge period when the risk of breakdown is the highest (Day 1988). Families must be properly prepared for a return home, and staff in community day and residential placements should be fully informed about the offender's problems and needs. Involvement from an early state in the planning of rehabilitation and aftercare packages is the best way of achieving this. Regular occupational and residential services for mentally retarded people are not geared to meeting the continuing need of offenders for structure and supervision, and specialized provision is required in the early stages of rehabilitation for the majority and on a longer term basis for some (Day 1988; Murphy and Clare 1991).

The importance of properly planned rehabilitation and aftercare for all groups of mentally disordered people has been recognized in the development of the care program and key worker approach (NHS Executive 1994). In the United Kingdom, the Mental Health Act 1983 contains the requirement for a properly developed aftercare plan. Supervision registers have recently been introduced for patients deemed as being particularly dangerous to themselves or others, and supervised discharge for those patients in whom marked lack of cooperation with treatment and aftercare is anticipated (NHS Executive 1994).

■ PROGNOSIS AND OUTCOME

Follow-up studies show that between 40% and 60% of the hospitalized mentally retarded offenders are reconvicted and nearly a third rehospitalized or imprisoned following discharge, but that very few commit serious offenses (Craft 1969, 1984; Day 1988; Gibbens and Robertson 1983; Walker and McCabe 1973). The majority reoffend during the first year, but in one 15-year follow-up study (Gibbens and Robertson 1983), 20% of the patients did not reoffend until 4 years or more after discharge. Reconviction rates alone paint an unduly pessimistic picture, and global assessments indicate a slightly better outcome. Day (1988), for example, found that whereas 55% of his offender group were reconvicted following discharge (40% more than once), nearly 70% were rated as being well adjusted or reasonably well adjusted at the last follow-up contact using a range of social adjustment measures.

Factors shown to be associated with a good outcome include a duration of 2 or more years', inpatient treatment (Day 1988; Lindsay and Smith 1998) and stable residential placement, regular daytime occupation, and regular supervision and support in the community—emphasizing the crucial importance of the quality of aftercare (Craft 1984; Day 1988). Poor outcome is associated with a history of previous convictions (Gibbens and Robertson 1983; Payne et al. 1974), a past history of behavior problems (Lund 1990), and a poor response to inpatient treatment (Day 1988). There is some evidence that offenders against the person have a better prognosis than property offenders (Day 1988; Payne et al. 1974). This may reflect real differences between the two groups—offenses against the person being essentially problems of poor self-control and immaturity with the potential to respond to treatment, whereas property offenses are more a function of overall lifestyle and subcultural influences to which the offender so frequently returns on discharge (Day 1988). Long-term studies show a low but persistent tendency toward recidivism in sex offenders (Day 1994; Haaven et al. 1990; Soothill and Gibbens 1978).

■ SERVICE PROVISION

Mentally retarded offenders differ significantly from other mentally disordered offenders in the origin, nature, and presentation of their offending behavior and in their care and treatment needs. They are disadvantaged and vulnerable in generic forensic psychiatry settings where they do not mix well with other mentally disordered offenders. In these settings, it is difficult to meet their special treatment and rehabilitation needs, and the staff lack the necessary expertise and experience in care and management. Treatment in small multipurpose units along with mentally ill and behaviorally disturbed mentally retarded patients is equally counterproductive and detrimental to all groups (Day 1983, 1988, 1993, 1995). Specialist forensic psychiatric services are required, the key components of which are

- Secure residential treatment units for dangerous offenders
- Open treatment units for less serious offenders and the initial rehabilitation of dangerous offenders
- Long-stay secure facilities for continuing care
- Rehabilitation services
- Community-based services, including support teams and specialist residential care, occupation and leisure activities for aftercare, continuing care, and community support
- Specialist treatment programs
- Appropriately trained and experienced professional staff

A comprehensive service model based on services in the United Kingdom, together with estimates of bed requirements, is shown in Table 20–3.

Secure provision is essential for more dangerous offenders for the protection of the public. In the United Kingdom, four levels of secure provision (see Table 20–3) have been developed to reflect different levels of need, and a policy of treatment in the least restrictive environment is necessary (Department of Health and Home Office 1992). The extent to which physical containment and locked facilities are required in low secure provision is currently the subject of debate. It is suggested that this can be avoided by the judicious use of highly experienced staff, high staffing levels, and careful regimes (Murphy et al. 1991; Smith 1988). It is the author's view that perimeter security improves the therapeutic atmosphere within a unit; reduces the need for close supervision and high staff presence, which can have a deleterious effect; allows greater opportunities to learn appropriate social behavior within a safe environment; and reduces the likelihood of spurious and misleading conformity (see Spring 1996).

Specialist treatment units must be therapeutically and economically viable and able to provide a comprehensive range of care and treatment programs from admission to rehabilitation. Provision needs to be made for continuing care on a long-term basis under conditions of minimum security for a small minority of offenders. Numerous specialist treatment units have been described that vary in size, scope, and treatment philosophy (Cumella and Sansom 1994; Denkowski and Denkowski 1984; Fidura et al. 1987; Hoare and O'Brien 1991; Isweran and Bardsley 1987; Isweran and Brener 1990; Johnson et al. 1993; Mayor et al. 1990; Murphy et al. 1991; Santamour and Watson

Table 20–3.   Services for mentally retarded offenders in the United Kingdom

Level	Facility	Role	Number of places
National	Special hospitals	High security	5/million population[a]
		Medium to long stay	
Regional	Medium secure units	Medium security	10/million population[b]
		Medium stay	
		Direct admissions	
		Rehabilitation of special hospital patients	
Subregional	Low secure units	Low security	40/million population[c]
	Open units	Short, medium, and long stay	
		Direct admissions	
		Rehabilitation of special hospital and medium secure unit patients	
Local community services	Specialized day and residential care services	Rehabilitation	
	Multiprofessional specialist support teams	Aftercare	
	Regular mental retardation services	Continuing care	

Table 20–3. Services for mentally retarded offenders in the United Kingdom (*continued*)

Level	Facility	Role	Number of places
Local community services		Assessment	
		Treatment	
		Support	
		Continuing care and support	

[a]Existing provision.
[b]Department of Health and Home Office 1992.
[c]Day 1983.

Source. Adapted with permission from Day K: "Crime and Mental Retardation: A Review," in *Clinical Approaches to the Mentally Disordered Offender.* Edited by Howells K, Hollin CR. Chichester, UK, Wiley, 1993, pp. 111–144. Adapted by permission of John Wiley & Sons, Ltd.

1982; Smith 1988; White and Wood 1988, Wood and White 1992). One of the most comprehensive is that developed at Northgate Hospital (Day 1983, 1988, 1990b, 1995), which provides a range of secure and open residential settings for the assessment, treatment, rehabilitation, and continuing care of male and female offenders, together with a range of specialist treatment programs and interventions.

Regular community facilities for the mentally retarded are not geared to meeting the continuing need of mentally retarded offenders for structure, control, and supervision, and specialized rehabilitation and aftercare facilities are required. This is a major gap in current provision in most services with consequent unnecessary hospital admissions, longer duration of stay, and greater chance of breakdown and return to offending on discharge to the community.

A single organizational responsibility for the key elements of the service is desirable and has the advantages of flexibility and readily available backup between the various elements of the service and facilitates a smooth transition from one phase of treatment to the next, thereby enhancing the chances of therapeutic success.

■ PREVENTION

As in the general population, much offending in the mentally retarded is associated with a range of adverse psychosocial factors. In these circumstances primary prevention depends on breaking the "cycle of deprivation" and insulating the potential offender against these adverse influences, a difficult task and essentially a social policy issue. At service level, however, the potential for preventative intervention in problem families has yet to be fully exploited and supervised.

The potential impact of community care policies on increasing the incidence of offending by the mentally retarded has already been referred to. If this is to be minimized, it is essential that community care programs are properly set up and researched and individuals adequately supported and supervised.

There is room for some optimism in relation to sex offenses. More enlightened attitudes on the sexuality of the mentally retarded and their rights to sexual expression, coupled with better sex education and a more normal lifestyle with opportunities for developing sexual relationships, should substantially reduce the incidence of offenses in this category in the future.

Tertiary prevention depends on effective intervention, and this requires adequate provision of specialist services. Positive action should be taken at the first sign of antisocial behavior even if the offense is considered to be trivial. Early identification is crucial, but the fact that a defendant is mentally retarded is frequently missed by the judicial system (Conley et al. 1992). Better training for the police, lawyers, and the judiciary is required. Screening has a role, and a short checklist for use by the police and other criminal justice personnel has recently been developed in the United Kingdom (Gudjonsson et al. 1993).

Simple, sensible precautions in the management of known offenders can help minimize the risk of further offending. For example sex offenders should not be left unsupervised in situations with potential vulnerable victims (Day 1997).

■ CONCLUSIONS

Mentally retarded offenders are one of a number of groups of mentally retarded people whose special needs are being increasingly highlighted by the shift from institutional to community care. Regular mental retardation services, forensic psychiatry, and the penal services are unsuitable and unable to cater to their special needs. Specialized services, both hospital and community based, organized and staffed by properly trained and experienced doctors, nurses, and other staff are required. An appropriate legislative framework is necessary. There is a need for more research into offender characteristics, the etiology of offending behavior, treatment methods, and treatment outcomes.

■ REFERENCES

Ashworth A, Gostin L: Mentally disordered offenders and the sentencing process, in Secure Provision. Edited by Gostin L, London, Tavistock Publications, 1985, pp 211–235

Beail N, Warden S: Sexual abuse of adults with learning disabilities. J Intellect Disabil Res 39:282–287, 1995

Benson B: Teaching Anger Management to Persons With Mental Retardation. Worthington, OH, IDS Publishing, 1992

Benson B: Anger management training: a self-control programme for persons with mild mental retardation, in Mental Health in Mental Retardation. Edited by Bouras N, Cambridge, UK, Cambridge University Press, 1994, pp 224–232

Bluglass R, Bowden P: Principles and Practice of Forensic Psychiatry. London, UK, Churchill Livingstone, 1990

Burchard JD: Systematic socialisation: a programmed environment for the rehabilitation of antisocial retardates. Psychosocial Record 17:461–476, 1967

Campbell L: Impairment, disabilities and handicaps: assessment for court, in Principles and Practice of Forensic Psychiatry. Edited by Bluglass R, Bowden P. Edinburgh, UK, Churchill Livingstone, 1990, pp 419–424

Charman T, Clare I: Education about the laws and social rules relating to sexual behavior: an education group for male sex offenders with mild mental handicaps. Mental Handicap 20:74–80, 1992

Clare ICH: Issues in the assessment and treatment of male sex offenders with mild learning disabilities. Sexual and Marital Therapy 8:276–280, 1993

Clare ICH, Murphy JH, Cox D, et al: Assessment and treatment of fire setting: a single case investigation using a cognitive behavioral model. Criminal Behavior and Mental Health 2:253–268, 1992

Clarke DJ: Antilibidinal drugs and mental retardation: a review. Med Sci Law 29:136–148, 1989

Cole CL, Gardener WI, Karan OC: Self-management training of mentally retarded adults presenting severe conduct difficulties. Applied Research in Mental Retardation 6:337–347, 1985

Collacott RA, Cooper SA: Urine fetish in a man with learning disabilities. J Intellect Disabil Res 39:145–147, 1995

Conley RW, Lucaxasson R, Bonthicet GJ: The Criminal Justice System and Mental Retardation: Defendants and Victims. Baltimore, MD, Paul H Brookes, 1992

Cooke DJ: Treatment as an alternative to prosecution: offenders diverted for treatment. Br J Psychiatry 153:636–644, 1991

Cooper AJ: Review of the role of two antilibidinal drugs in the treatment of sex offenders with mental retardation. Can J Psychiatry 33:42–48, 1995

Cox-Lindenbaum D, Lindenbaum L: A modality for the treatment of aggressive behaviors and sexual disorders in people with mental retardation, in Mental Health in Mental Retardation. Edited by Bouras N, Cambridge, UK, Cambridge University Press, 1994, pp 244–254

Craft A (ed): Mental Handicap and Sexuality: Issues and Perspectives. Tunbridge Wells, UK, Costello Press, 1987

Craft M: The moral responsibility for Welsh psychopaths, in The Mentally Abnormal Offender. Edited by de Reuck AVS, Porter R. London, Churchill, 1969, pp 91–94

Craft M: Should one treat or gaol psychopaths, in Mentally Abnormal Offenders. Edited by Craft M, Craft A. London, Balliere Tindall, 1984, pp 384–396

Cullen C: The treatment of people with learning disabilities who offend, in Clinical Approaches to the Mentally Disordered Offender. Edited by Howells K, Hollin CR. Chichester, UK, Wiley, 1993, pp 145–163

Cumella S, Sansom D: A regional mental impairment service. Mental Handicap Research 7:257–272, 1994

Dana L: Treatment of personality disorder in persons with mental retardation, in Mental Health Aspects of Mental Retardation. Edited by Fletcher RJ, Dosen A. New York, Lexington Books, 1993, pp 281–290

Day K: A hospital based psychiatric unit for mentally handicapped adults. Mental Handicap 11:137–140, 1983

Day K: A hospital based treatment programme for male mentally handicapped offenders. Br J Psychiatry 153:635–644, 1988

Day K: Mental retardation: clinical aspects and management, in Principles and Practice of Forensic Psychiatry. Edited by Bluglass R, Bowden P. Edinburgh, UK, Churchill Livingstone, 1990a, pp 399–418

Day K: Treatment of antisocial behavior, in Treatment of Mental Illness and Behavior Disorders in the Mentally Retarded. Edited by Došen A, van Gennep A, Zwanikken GJ. Leiden, Netherlands, Logon Publications, 1990b, pp 103–122

Day K: Crime and mental retardation: a review, in Clinical Approaches to the Mentally Disordered Offender. Edited by Howells K, Hollin CR. Chichester, UK, Wiley, 1993, pp 111–144

Day K: Male mentally handicapped sex offenders. Br J Psychiatry 165:630–639, 1994

Day K: Specialist psychiatric services for mentally retarded offenders, in Proceedings of the International Congress 11 on the Dually Diagnosed. Edited by Fletcher R, McNiells D, Fusaro L. New York, National Association for the Dually Diagnosed, 1995, pp 102–106

Day K: Sex offenders with learning disabilities, in Psychiatry in Learning Disability. Edited by Read SG. London, Saunders, 1997, pp 278–306

Denkowski GC, Denkowski KM: Community based residential treatment model for mentally retarded adolescent offenders, in Perspectives and Progress in Mental Retardation Vol 2. Edited by Berg JM, Baltimore, MD, University Park Press, 1984, pp 303–311

Denkowski GC, Denkowski KM, Mabli J: A residential treatment model for MR adolescent offenders. Hospital and Community Psychiatry 35:279–281, 1984

Department of Health and Home Office: Review of Health and Social Services for mentally disordered offenders and others requiring similar services. Final Summary Report, CM2088, London, HMSO, 1992

Donnellan AM, LaVigna GW, Negri-Shoultz N, et al: Progress Without Punishment: Effective Approaches for Learners With Behavior Problems. New York, Teachers College Press, 1988

Duggan C: Assessing risk in the mentally disordered. Br J Psychiatry 170(suppl 32):1–3, 1997

Fidura JC, Lindsey ER, Walker GR: A special behavior unit for treatment of behavior problems of persons who are mentally retarded. Ment Retard 25:107–111, 1987

Finn MA: Prison misconduct among mentally retarded inmates. Criminal Behavior in Mental Health 2:287–299, 1992

Forshuk C, Martin ML, Griffiths M: Sexual knowledge interview schedule reliability. J Intellect Disabil Res 39:35–39, 1995

Foxx RM, Bittle RG, Bechtel DR, et al: Behavioral treatment of the sexually deviant behavior of mentally retarded individuals. International Review of Research in Mental Retardation 14:291–317, 1986

Gebhard PH, Gagnon JH, Pomeroy WB, et al: Sex Offenders: An Analysis of Types, London, Heinemann, 1965

Geller JL, Bertsch G: Fire setting behavior in the histories of a state hospital population. Am J Psychiatry 142:464–468, 1985

Gibbens TCN, Robertson G: A survey of the criminal careers of hospital order patients. Br J Psychiatry 143:362–369, 370–375, 1983

Gilby R, Wolfe L, Goldberg B: Mentally retarded adolescent sex offenders: a survey and pilot study. Can J Psychiatry 34:542–548, 1989

Gostin L: Mental Health Services: Law and Practice. London, Shaw & Sons, 1986

Griffiths DM, Quinsey UL, Hingsburger D: Changing Inappropriate Sexual Behavior: A Community Based Approach for Persons With Developmental Disabilities. Baltimore, MD, Paul H Brookes, 1989

Gudjonsson G, Clare I, Rutter S, et al: Persons at Risk During Interviews in Police Custody: The Identification of Vulnerabilities. London, UK, Her Majesty's Stationary Office, 1993

Haaven S, Little R, Petre-Millder D: Treating Intellectually Disabled Sex Offenders: A Model Residential Programme. Orwell, VT, Safer Society Press, 1990

Hall NJ: Correctional services for inmates with mental retardation: challenge or catastrophe, in The Criminal Justice System and Mental Retardation. Edited by Conley RW, Luckasson R, Bouthilet GN. Baltimore, MD, Paul H Brookes, 1992, pp 167–190

Hamilton JR, Freeman H (eds): Dangerousness: Psychiatric Assessment and Management. London, Gaskell, 1982

Hingsburger D: Sex counselling for the developmentally handicapped: the assessment and management of seven critical problems. Psychiatric Aspects of Mental Retardation Reviews 6:41–45, 1987

Hoare S, O'Brien G: The impact of the Mental Health (Amendment) Act 1983 on admissions to an interim regional secure unit for mentally handicapped offenders. Psychiatric Bulletin 15:548–550, 1991

Hodgins S: Mental disorder, intellectual deficiency and crime: evidence from a birth cohort. Arch Gen Psychiatry 49:476–483, 1992

Hodgins S, Mednick SA, Brennan YA, et al: Mental disorder and crime: evidence from a Danish birth cohort. Arch Gen Psychiatry 53:489–496, 1996

Hollins S, Clare ICH, Murphy G, et al: You're Under Arrest. London, UK, Gaskell Press, 1997a

Hollins S, Clare ICH, Murphy G, et al: You're on Trial. London, UK, Gaskell Press, 1997b

Hunter H: Forensic psychiatry in mental handicap, in Psychiatric Illness and Mental Handicap. Edited by James FE, Snaith RP. London, Gaskell Press, 1979, pp 141–146

Isweran MS, Bardsley EM: Secure facilities for mentally impaired patients. Bulletin of the Royal College of Psychiatrists 11:52–54, 1987

Isweran MS, Brener N: Psychiatric disorders in mentally retarded patients and their treatment in a medium secure unit, in Treatment of Mental Illness and Behavioral Disorders in the Mentally Retarded. Edited by Dosen A, van Gennep A, Zwanikken GJ. Leiden, Netherlands, Logon Publications, 1990, pp 429–436

Jackson HF, Glass C, Hope S: A Functional Analysis of Recidivistic Arson. Br J Clin Psychol 26:175–185, 1987

Johnson C, Smith J, Stainer G, et al: Mildly mentally handicapped offenders: an alternative to custody. Psychiatric Bulletin 17:199–201, 1993

Johnson PR: Community based sexuality programmes for developmentally handicapped adults, in Prospective Progress in Mental Retardation, Vol 1. Edited by Berg JM, Baltimore, MD, University Park Press, 1984, pp 313–321

Joseph PLA, Potter M: Diversion from custody; 1: psychiatric assessment at the magistrates court. Br J Psychiatry 162:325–330, 1993

Kempton W: Life Horizons (Sex Education for Persons with Special Needs). Santa Monica, CA, James Stanfield, 1988

Knopp FH: Retraining Adult Sex Offenders: Methods and Models. Orwell, VT, Safer Society Press, 1984

Lindsay WR, Smith AWH: Responses to treatment for sex offenders with intellectual disability: a comparison of men with 1 and 2 year probation sentences. J Intellect Disabil Res 42:346–353, 1998

Lindsay WR, Bellsbaw E, Culross G, et al: Increases in knowledge following a course of sex education for people with intellectual disabilities. J Intellect Disabil Res 36:531–539, 1992

Lund J: Mentally retarded criminal offenders in Denmark. Br J Psychiatry 156:726–731, 1990

Lund J: Long term treatment of sexual behavior problems in adolescent and adult developmentally disabled adults. Annals of Sex Research 5:5–31, 1992

Lyall I, Holland A, Collins S, et al: Incidence of persons with a learning disability detained in police custody: a needs assessment for service development. Science, Medicine, and the Law 35(1):61–71, 1995

Maberly A: Delinquency in handicapped children. British Journal of Delinquency 1:125–128, 1950

Maden A: Risk assessment in psychiatry. British Journal of Hospital Medicine 56:78–82, 1996

Mayor J, Bhate M, Firth H, et al: Facilities for mentally impaired patients: 3 years experience of a semi-secure unit. Psychiatric Bulletin 14:333–335, 1990

Mawson DC, Grounds A, Tantum D: Violence and Asperger's syndrome: a case study. Br J Psychiatry 147:566–569, 1985

McKerracher DW, Dacre AJI: A study of arsonists in a special security hospital. Br J Psychiatry 112:1151–1154, 1966

Milne E, O'Brien G: Epilepsy in learning disabled offenders: prevalance, diagnosis and impact on treatment. Epilepsia 38(suppl 3):111, 1997

Murphy GH, Clare ICH: A service option for people with mild mental handicap and challenging behavior or psychiatric problems; 2: psychological assessment and treatment, outcome for service users and service effectiveness. Mental Handicap Research 4:180–206, 1991

Murphy GH, Clare ICH: Analysis of motivation in people with mild learning disabilities (mental handicap) who set fires. Psychology, Crime, and Law 2:153–168, 1996

Murphy GH, Clare ICH: People with learning disabilities as offenders or alleged offenders on the UK criminal justice system. J R Soc Med 21:178–182, 1998

Murphy G, Holland A, Fowler P: MIETS: A service option for people with mild mental handicaps and challenging behavior or psychiatric problems; 1: philosophy, service and service users. Mental Handicap Research 4:41–66, 1991

Murphy WD, Coleman EM, Haynes MR: Treatment and evaluation issues with the mentally retarded sex offender, in The Sex Aggressor: Current Prospectives on Treatment. Edited by Greer JG, Stuart IR. New York, Van Nostrand Reinhold, 1983, pp 22–41

Murrey JG, Briggs D, Davis MS: Psychopathic disordered mentally ill and mentally handicapped sex offenders: a comparative study. Med Sci Law 32:331–336, 1992

Myers BA: Treatment of sexual offences by persons with developmental disabilities. Am J Ment Retard 95:563–569, 1991

NHS Executive: Guidance on the discharge of mentally disordered offenders and their continuing care in the community, HSG (94) 27, Health Publications unit, Heywood, Lancs, UK, Natural Health Service Executive, 1994

O'Sullivan GH, Kelleher MJ: A study of fire setters in south west of Ireland. Br J Psychiatry 151:818–823, 1987

Payne C, McCabe S, Walker N: Predicting offender patients reconvictions. Br J Psychiatry 125:60–64, 1974

Prins H: Dangerousness: a review, in Principles and Practice of Forensic Psychiatry. Edited by Bluglass R, Bowden P. Edinburgh, UK, Churchill Livingstone, 1990, pp 499–505

Prins H: Service provision and facilities for the mentally disordered offender, in Clinical Approaches to the Mentally Disordered Offender. Edited by Howells K, Hollin CR. Chichester, UK, Wiley, 1993, pp 35–67

Radzinowicz L: Sexual Offences: Report of the Cambridge Department of Criminal Science. London, MacMillan, 1957

Reichard SG, Spencer J, Spooner F: The mentally retarded defendant offender, in The Retarded Offender. Edited by Santamour M, Watson P. New York, Praegar, 1982, pp 121–139

Sandford DA, Elzinga RH, Grainger W: Evaluation of a residential behavioral programme for behaviorally disturbed mentally retarded young adults. American Journal of Mental Deficiency 91:431–444, 1987

Santamour MB, Watson PS (eds): The Retarded Offender. New York, Praeger, 1982

Scott PD: Assessing dangerousness in criminals. Br J Psychiatry 131:127–142, 1977

Smith C, Algozzine B, Schmid R, et al: Prison adjustment of youthful inmates with mental retardation. Ment Retard 28:177–181, 1990

Smith J: An open forensic unit for borderline mentally impaired offenders. Bulletin of the Royal College of Psychiatrists 12:13–15, 1988

Soothill KL, Gibbens TCN: Recidivism of sexual offenders: a reappraisal. British Journal of Criminology 18:267–276, 1978

Sovner R, Hurley AD: Treatment of sexual deviation in mentally retarded persons. Psychiatric Aspects of Mental Retardation 2:4–7, 1983

Spring M: In safe keeping: medium secure unit architecture. Building, May 3, 1996, pp 42–46

Stewart LA: Profile of female fire setters; implications for treatment. Br J Psychiatry 163:248–256, 1993

Swanson CK, Garwick GB: Treatment for low functioning sex offenders; group therapy and interagency co-ordination. Ment Retard 28:155–161, 1990

Tennent G, McQuaid A, Lougmane T: Female arsonists. British Journal of Criminology 9:4–21, 1971

Tutt NS: The subnormal offender. British Journal of Subnormality 17:42–47, 1971

Valenti-Hein D, Mueser K: The Dating Skills Programme: Teaching Sociosexual Skills to Adults with Mental Retardation. Worthington, OH, IDS Publishing, 1990

Vinestock M: Risk assessment. Advances in Psychiatric Treatment 2:3–10, 1996

Walker N, McCabe S: Crime and Insanity in England, Vol 2, Edinburgh, UK, Edinburgh University Press, 1973

White BL, Wood H: The Lancaster county mentally retarded offenders programme, in Mental Retardation and Mental Health: Classification, Diagnosis, Treatment, Services. Edited by Stark JA, Menolascino FJ, Albarelli MH, et al. New York, Springer Verlag, 1988, pp 402–408

Wood HR, White BL: A model for habilitation and prevention for offenders with mental retardation, in The Criminal Justice System and Mental Retardation. Edited by Conley RW, Luckasson R, Bouthilet GN. Baltimore, MD, Paul H Brookes, 1992, pp 153–165

Yesevage JA, Benezech M, Ceccalbi S, et al: Arson in mentally ill and criminal populations. J Clin Psychiatry 44:128–130, 1983

21 A Pedagogical Approach to Behavioral Problems

Gijs van Gemert, Ph.D.

The term *pedagogical*, which is widely used in the German and Dutch languages, has a much wider scope than *education*, which is its equivalent in English. In this chapter, the terms will be used interchangeably. Bach (1979) defines education, or pedagogy, as the stimulation of the development of a child such that through experience and activity, he or she moves in the direction of realizing his or her potentialities and gets initiated into the culture and its societal context.

Gunzburg (1992) identifies the stimulation of personality development and social competence within an ordinary parental home or a residential facility as being the most important task of a pedagogical approach. According to Nakken et al. (1992), education is the vehicle through which the living together of parents and children within a certain culture serves to introduce the children to the culture and to their integration in it.

According to Van Gennep (1997), pedagogy focuses on the dignity of the person, respect for the sociocultural attainments, and openness for development—which is another way of saying that the main objective of a pedagogical approach is the optimization of the quality of life. This objective plays an important role in the concept of mental health. Education offers a good model for optimal interaction within a residential care facility.

When an individual's behavior is classified as being extremely problematic, drastic measures are often taken to protect the individual and his or her physical and social environment from damage. *Structure* is a key concept in this approach. It calls for reducing the number of social and physical stimuli to a scantily furnished environment. Every assault by the resident in this system is answered by a tightening of control, further simplification of the situation, and, in time, to a finely meshed network of "dos" and "don'ts." Care is focused on the management of undesirable behavior. As a result, both staff and residents have very little room for choice and variation. Earlier research showed

391

that the outcome of such an approach is poor (Van Gemert 1985, 1990). Protracted structure leads to hospitalization and a breakdown in staff creativity. Deprivation and structuring, especially together, may create inhumane living conditions for the residents. And in the long run, "structuring the environment" will have unacceptable effects on the quality of the residents' lives.

It would be incorrect to conclude that residents with behavioral problems are neglected. Much expense and manpower have been invested in improving the living conditions, and therapeutic interventions have been abundant. Currently, however, there is a general pessimism regarding the future of these residents. Ideas about meaningful goals tend to be scarce and vaguely formulated. It is very important to create a new perspective of treatment and care. Ideas and values may mean the difference between good and poor care.

A highly structured environment is often defended on the grounds that the individual needs it. Indeed, where therapy and training are involved, a high degree of structure may be necessary. On the other hand, many an individual is quite capable of reasonable behavior, and rather than being "trained," he or she should be "encouraged" to engage in desirable behavior. Therapy and formal training in and of themselves are not useful models for preparing the individual for a productive life. Token economy systems and other shaping techniques with a rigid infrastructure do not teach the individual self-control. Such techniques are noted for their lack of generalization and transfer of learned skills and often lead to greater dependency. Even if there is an improvement in the resident's behavior, it will be very difficult to maintain this approach in other settings, and the dependency of the individual created by this approach blocks further positive developments. An approach with a better chance at transfer and generalization is therefore required. Developing self-control is an important characteristic of this approach.

This chapter is concerned with enhancing the quality of the individual's life. Whatever the specific interventions are, they should create a supportive environment in which the resident can live his or her own life. Structure can be found through relationships with others. Daily interaction with other people is the core of this approach. In this chapter, I will describe how a good environment can be created, as a necessary condition for joining the community or as a goal in itself. The analog of parents raising their children will be used as a model through which a balance is struck between explicit interventions and spontaneous interaction.

■ EDUCATION AS AN ANALOG

Education may be defined as the living together of children and educators while the latter try to prepare the child, according to their own standards, for an independent life in a particular type of society (Nakken et al. 1992). In this definition, education is a much broader concept than schooling. The term *pedagogical* is used in this chapter to mean a perspective from which education takes off. Parents and children live and learn together by developing and maintaining a personal relationship. Through this relationship, parents try to influence the child, but, when possible, this should be done tactfully. The acquisition of independence requires the child to make his or her own decisions wherever possible and, importantly, to be confronted with the consequences of his or her choices. Similarly, the educator sets the boundaries and regulations and points out the possible consequences of a situation in interactions with the child—the aim being not to prevent all errors or impose too many regulations, which are likely to deprive the child of learning from experience. Of course, the child must be protected from some risks, but when there is no risk taking, education in the sense of a preparation for life cannot come about.

In a healthy relationship, daily interaction is characterized by mutual equality and responsibility. The child is respected as his or her own person, and the educator should be respected as well. The educator is not all-accepting but invites the child to cooperate. The educator's role is to create conditions, set parameters, and enforce agreements. Sometimes power and direction are necessary but only to facilitate the dialogue with the child. Last but not least, the educator should have a degree of autonomy in deciding what he or she views as being in the best the interest of the child.

To be sure, the picture sketched above is an ideal against which daily interactions may be evaluated. It provides criteria for assessing the quality of daily interactions. Creating a good relationship requires the conscious effort of the parents and other educators. Mutual responsibility does not originate spontaneously—certainly not when the child has not learned to trust others or is not used to making his or her own decisions. Trust must be built up systematically by constantly inviting the child to take responsibility for his or her own behavior.

The pedagogical approach considers education an adequate analog for treatment approaches to mentally retarded people with behavioral problems. In both cases, the "goal" is independence from other people. Furthermore, only in an atmosphere of mutual trust can the mentally retarded person be expected to assume responsibility for him- or herself. Given the many disappointments a mentally retarded person may experience during his or her lifetime, it might be very functional for him or her not to trust everyone at first sight. Professional caregivers must work long and hard to achieve a good relationship (McGee 1989).

In dealing with mentally retarded people, the analog has its limits. After all, such individuals often have a long history of failures and broken trust. Nevertheless, the pedagogical approach can provide useful guidelines and serve as an alternative to the idea that "difficult" individuals need control in the first place. Of course, the mentally retarded person needs structure in his or her life as does everyone else; however, a formal structure is no substitute for a structure based on relationships with other people.

■ CHARACTERISTICS OF THE PEDAGOGICAL APPROACH

Problematic behavior, especially aggression, is not an impulsive, uncontrollable act. Problematic behavior is the result of a process of communication in which norms and values as well as the personalities of the partners play a crucial role. This idea is consonant with an attribution view on problem behavior (Ferguson and Rule 1983). According to this view, problem behavior is just one means by which people—whether or not mentally retarded—interact and play power games. Professional staff must learn to recognize the mechanisms and behavior sequences leading to problematic behavior. Only then can they build up an optimal relationship with the disturbed individual.

The pedagogical approach is something quite different from just living together. Life must be organized in a "natural" way, requiring a high degree of professionalism (a mixture of commitment and reserve). The optimal style of interaction is characterized by a continuing dialogue (in a broad, not solely verbal sense) with equal chances of turn taking and initiative. More specifically, it is characterized by respect, room, rationality, and realism.

Respect. The relationship is characterized by equality of rights and responsibilities. The mentally retarded person is responsible for the things he or she does and does not do. When the individual makes the "wrong" decisions, he or she is expected to reduce or repair the damage.

Room. The individual has the opportunity to develop his or her own initiatives. However, rooms without walls do not exist; boundaries and rules are a reality for both the individual and the staff. The latter need room to encourage cooperation.

Rationality. Educators should have a keen eye for processes leading to the resident's excessive behavior as well as to their own behavior (looking over one's own shoulder). Flexibility and creativity, based on rational decisions, are necessary. Professional workers should be aware of the danger of being "washed over" by the situation.

Realism. The current situation does count. Professionals should refrain from actions based on former events or experiences and opinions based on prior situations and previous functioning of the individual. Every situation offers fresh possibilities. Objectivity is necessary: "Look at what is happening, not for what you think is happening."

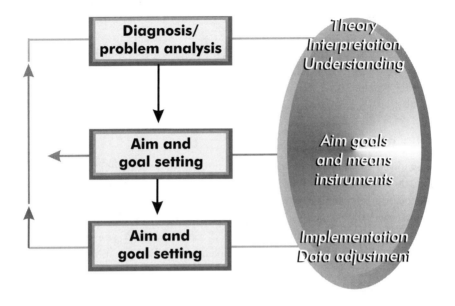

Figure 21–1. The planning process.

One may use these *R* words as complementary guidelines for the behavior of both staff and residents. They are not easily implemented, but they make very clear the direction that the approach should take. Looking for an optimal mix of *R* words is typical of the pedagogical approach. Its focus is the enhancement of the educational capabilities of the people who interact daily with the mentally retarded person. With due regard to both the particular situation and the individual's particular needs, the educator/caregiver is better able to act appropriately.

■ INDIVIDUAL PLANNING

The interactions may appear spontaneous, but the relationship with the mentally retarded person must be structured by means of an individualized intervention plan. The daily program should be formulated in accordance with this plan and must encompass sufficient tasks and challenges. An individualized intervention plan proceeds along a three-step process described in Figure 21–1.

Problem Definition and Analysis

The first step in planning is the systematic definition of the problem situation. This results in a broad and coherent view of the resident, one that is based on consensus regarding the interpretation of the available information. This image, or view, will improve the staff's basic understanding of the individual. It is important not to present solutions before phase A is complete. Too quick a response to the demand for practical guidelines and decisions will lead to incorrect assumptions on the part of staff members, parents, and others involved and will ultimately prove self-defeating.

Aims and Goal Setting

The aim is the formulation of a long-range desirable situation without dwelling too much on its feasibility. Consensus about this global direction is necessary. With the overall aim as a starting point, concrete goals and subgoals can be specified. Goals should be sufficiently concrete so that they can serve as criteria against which progress can be tested. Simultaneously, a decision must be made about the instruments that are to be used for the evaluation. Existing instruments such as the Goal Attainment Scale or the Adaptive Behavior Scale may be useful, but new instruments may need to be developed.

Intervention and Evaluation

The intervention program takes the form of a "hidden diary" (a list of the important activities that should minimally be done each day or week). The diary is hidden in that it lacks prearranged times and places. Planning should be restricted to this global level as much as possible. The style, time, and place of activities must be left to the flexibility and creativity of the caregivers. An exception to this should, however, be made if therapy is necessary or a formal training program is conducted.

Evaluation—consisting of a systematic comparison of goals and subgoals with the actual results—is an important aspect of intervention. There are two equally important kinds of evaluation: measuring the effects and judging the appropriateness (with respect to the aim) of the results. Both are needed to avoid trivial changes based on momentary feelings, temporary disappointment, or ideas lacking substance. Goals should be modified only after systematic evaluation.

This process should be accompanied by data on the individual and the way the relationship is developing. Videotaped events and interactions are an important means of reality testing. They may also be used to examine possibilities for development during all phases of planning. There should be a continuous discussion about the status of the plan between all persons involved, including the mentally retarded person. Such a plan may not only result in a change in the individual's behavior but also, and foremost, in a change in the behavior and attitudes of the staff.

■ SYSTEM-LEVEL INTERVENTION

Behavior problems are very resistant to change because they are, at least partly, a result of the institutional culture. A *culture* can be defined as a whole set of presuppositions and common beliefs. The unacceptable quality of the life of many mentally retarded individuals is supported by a coherent set of beliefs and explanations. Changing staff's views will imply a break with the existing culture. Developing an individualized plan for a difficult resident is a good way of changing the culture and infrastructure of an institution. Sometimes it is possible "to move a tree by shaking the branches." Very often, however, individually based interventions may not be sufficient to improve the quality of the individual's life. Intervention at the individual level must then be supported by intervention at the system level. The culture will be very resistant to change, so it will often be necessary to set up a powerful project guided by a multidisciplinary team of external consultants (Van Gemert et al. 1995).

Consultation is more than simply asking for and giving advice. The consultant aims to improve a client's resources, gives advice, models intervention, and guides the changing process without taking over the staff's responsibilities. The consultant acts as a concerned outsider. He or she should have a high level of knowledge and skills. The consultant's clients are not the residents but the staff members. His or her contribution is more than advice but less than a command. The consultant supports and accepts his or her clients' decisions and evaluates them on the basis of their own choices and goals.

An important aspect of consultancy is that it is not permanent. Like an educator, the consultant tries to enhance the independence of his or her client. The consultant works on the fundamental assumption that someone who asks for consultancy is in principle competent of finding solutions to his or her own problems. The consultant's client only needs temporary assistance, and the consultant should step back when possible. When a consultant becomes "part of the furniture," his or her value and status as an autonomous outsider are compromised.

■ CONCLUSIONS

Using a pedagogical approach requires much energy and time from many people. Pragmatically, it is simpler to administer drugs and arrange for behavior therapy. However, in so doing, the existing structures and cultures will not be affected, and there will be no need to confront culture bearers with the long-term results of their actions. But if therapy fails, or the resident is not able to live an acceptable life afterward, it will be very difficult to offer him or her a quality of life that is worthy. There are two tasks to be performed when dealing with mentally retarded persons with behavior problems. The first is to correct the behavior—which is the simpler of the two tasks. The other requires the integration of the individual within an environment that is minimally restrictive, and we have only just begun to discover how difficult this task is.

■ REFERENCES

Bach H: Pädagogische aufgabenstellung, in Pädagogik der Geistigbehinderten. Edited by Bach H. Berlin, Germany, Marhold, 1979, pp 4–24

Ferguson TJ, Rule BG: An attributional perspective on anger and aggression, in Aggression: Theoretical and Empirical Reviews, Vol 1: Theoretical and Methodological Issues. Edited by Geen RG, Donnerstein E. New York, Academic Press, 1983, pp 128–141

Gunzburg HC: Aufgabenorientierte persölichkeitsentwicklung. Heilpädagogische Forschung 18:1–10, 1992

McGee J: Being With Others: Towards a Psychology of Interdependence. Omaha, NE, Creighton University Press, 1989

Nakken H, Van Gemert GH, Zandberg TJ: Research on Intervention in Special Education. Lampeter, UK, Edwin Mellen Press, 1992

Van Gemert GH: "Gedragsgestoordheid" bij zwakzinnigen. Doctoral dissertation, University of Groningen, 1985

Van Gemert GH: An educational approach to behavioral disorders, in Treatment of Mental Illness and Behavioral Disorders in the Mentally Retarded. Edited by Došen A, Van Gennep ATh, Zwanikken GJ. Leiden, Netherlands, Logon Publications, 1990, pp 255–268

Van Gemert GH, Wielink R, Vriesema PL: De lotgevallen van Jolanda Venema: consultatie als nieuwe benadering van gedragsstoornissen bij verstandelijk gehandicapten, in Jaarboek voor Psychiatrie en Psychotherapie. Edited by Hoogduin CAL, Schnabel P, Vandereyken W, et al. Houten, Netherlands, Van Loghum Slaterus, 1995, pp 142–160

Van Gennep A: Quality of community living in the Netherlands. British Journal of Developmental Disabilities 43:1–14, 1997

Treatment Methods With Children

22 Psychodynamically Oriented Psychotherapy in Mentally Retarded Children

Christian Gaedt, M.D.

Psychodynamically oriented methods for the diagnosis and treatment of children and adults with mental retardation and problem behavior always have been in a "position outside." Nonetheless, despite the successes of behavior therapy and its broad acceptance as scientifically promising and efficient in costs and time, the use of psychodynamic methods is on the increase. Most textbooks now emphasize that in dealing with the mentally retarded these methods are important and they form a part of the broad spectrum of diagnostic and treatment measures that are increasingly being integrated into clinical practice (Došen and Menolascino 1990; Došen et al. 1990; Fletcher and Došen 1993; Fletcher and Menolascino 1989; Hollins 1990; Matson and Barrett 1982; Sinason 1992; Szymanski and Tanguay 1980). In this regard, it is certainly not helpful to the psychodynamic approach that (with few exceptions) traditional psychodynamic training institutes have shown little interest in the problems of mentally retarded persons. Consequently, much research needs to be undertaken, and modification to theory may well be called for. Indeed, the psychodynamic therapist treating persons with mental retardation has to deal not only with the general mistrust of the psychodynamic methods but also with skepticism within his or her own ranks. It is unfortunate that new opportunities, especially in psychoanalytic development psychology, object relations theory, and ego psychology, have not been sufficiently exploited in the treatment of children and adults with mental retardation and mental health problems (see also Chapter 7 of this book). (For a good overview, see Blanck and Blanck 1974, 1979.) As is now well recognized, the conflict-oriented perspective of Freud falls far short of explaining the psychopathology of people with severe personality disorders (Gaedt 1995,

1997). The diagnostic-therapeutic approach presented in this chapter is anchored in a new theory that emphasizes the centrality of "persistent developmental deficit" as a pathogenic factor (Gaedt 1997). The therapeutic procedure is oriented to the principles of the "psychoanalytic-interactional psychotherapy" model (Heigl-Evers and Ott 1994; Heigl-Evers et al. 1993). It is based on the theoretical work of Kernberg (1981) on the psychoanalysis of patients with severe personality disorders.

■ BASIC ASSUMPTIONS

The psychological structures and functions that enable a child to grow into adulthood as an individual who is involved in social relationships are built on the process of interaction that has taken place with early significant objects. Even under favorable conditions a retarded child will hardly ever be able to develop normally. This is because the child/environment interaction is severely impaired due to organic damage (Gaedt 1995). Weaknesses in personality structure result from this distorted interaction process, which Levitas and Gilson (1988) have termed *secondary psychosocial deficit*. For instance, such children overreact to experiences pertaining to autonomy, are more vulnerable to threats to self-esteem, and require much emotional support when confronted with demands.

The severe psychiatric disturbances that we observe in some mentally retarded children develop when early interaction processes are additionally marked by indifference, neglect, abuse, or isolation resulting in a more evident *persisting developmental deficit*. This includes ego weakness, primitive object relations, archaic superego structures, and an inadequate self-concept. These deficits are seen by many authors as being the basis of adjustment problems and emotional disorders in mentally retarded children (Balthazar and Stevens 1975; Levitas and Gilson 1988; Robinson and Robinson 1976).

Ego functions are instruments of adaptation, integrating internal needs with the demands of the outer world and superego (Hartmann 1958). Children with defective ego functioning may have difficulties in screening stimuli and thus may become flooded by them. They may not be able to distinguish between internal and external stimuli and perceptions—thereby hampering reality testing; further, they may be unable to associate aggressive impulses with their origin and control them.

Another set of functions necessary for adaptation is defense mechanisms. If the defense system continues to be primitive, anxiety cannot be bound effectively and thus may intrude easily and massively into consciousness to cause disruptive behavior. Additionally, immature defenses often involve the social environment in such an intensive and dramatic way that they may even lead to *splitting*.

The development of ego functions and defense mechanisms is embedded in the process of differentiation of the self and its relations to significant others. Every stage of development has its specific developmental task that is to be mastered. If the infant fails to accomplish this, the process of development will not come to a total standstill, but later on in life, the specific needs and conflicts originating in this disturbed developmental phase will impede mature social adaptation and may generate clinical symptoms. Frequently, this results in an incomplete separation of self and nonself. This may lead to a primitive fear of merging or to futile aggressive attempts at establishing an effective boundary to an already insecure selfobject border; self-mutilation such as head banging, self-biting, or other forms of self-injury can be manifestations of this developmental deficit.

Due to ego weakness and the persistence of primitive object relations, problems with the development of the superego will also occur. A mature superego is one of the prerequisites of autonomous existence. It will not only have the function of being a "controlling court" but will also be a source of self-esteem, making the child less dependent on the object for narcissistic replenishment (Chetic 1979). If the development of the superego is impaired, the child will not have effective internal controls, expecting them instead from others. This may be one reason for the marked dependency and "clinging behavior" that are frequently observed. Furthermore, under the influence of harshness and violence in early childhood, precursors of the superego tend to remain externalized, leading children to experience the outside world as hostile and frightening—a reflection of the emotional quality of their early object relations. As a result of this experience, children usually have a high level of anxiety and tend to deny the real world and remain attached to their narcissistic fantasy world.

The differentiation of object relations is not only a structural process; it also has an affective aspect. The affective experience of early relationships—especially during traumatic phases—influences the emerging self and object representation. Thus the infant acquires affective patterns to judge and classify the outer world in a way that corresponds with these early experiences. Emde (1988) has called these patterns *affective core of the self*. These preshaped affective expectations, together with the corresponding behavioral tendencies, will have their impact in later life. This phenomenon is similar to what is known as *transference* but is more archaic because of the primitive nature of the object relations. Blanck and Blanck (1979) call it *object replication*.

In the normal course of development, these combined archaic affective and behavioral patterns have a transitory character. However, they are the basis for what is called *identity*. Identity refers to an enduring schema for self-recognition and self-realization (Berman 1979; Erikson 1956). The development of these schemata is an ongoing, lifelong process during which different needs are continually being adapted to the schemata in a very individualized way, and it is one function of these schemata to ensure their gratification. In realizing one's personal interactional style, the individual experiences his or her identity, and this emotional state in itself has a motivational quality. The individual feels driven to repeat this experience and will constantly search for situations or modify the circumstances in order to have this experience. If necessary, the individual will unconsciously lead the interactions with partners in such ways as to create a suitable path to this emotional state. This is called *reenactment.*

One often can observe sequences of pathological interactions that, again and again, lead to exactly that behavior that the parents or caregivers aim to prevent. In consequence, they may give up their principles and become rigid, devalued, or even openly aggressive. Still, the child ignores all negative consequences. As if it is an addiction, the child strives for this particular emotional state for it is a part of his or her sense of identity. In the more recent psychoanalytic literature (Emde 1988; Hoffmann and Hochapfel 1987; Sander 1985), the hypothesis that such repetitions can also be interpreted as adaptive behavior has received increasing support. According to Sander (cited in Emde 1988, p. 289), an individual re-creates situations in which continuity and familiarity can be experienced so that the individual has an opportunity to perceive him- or herself in a very specific relation to the other. Obviously, the objective is to ensure a continuity of self-awareness across all stages of development. This is very close to the notion of Sandler and Joffe (1965), who speak of a need to maintain a "feeling of safety."

■ THE THERAPEUTIC PROCESS

In these children, modifications are only possible if the developmental process is reopened. Scientific research has not yet been able to pinpoint exactly which factors play a significant role in this procedure. However, it seems reasonable to draw a parallel to the principles of early childhood development. A relationship similar in quality to good parenting is a prerequisite for any form of therapy. Emde (1988) speaks of "emotional availability" as the critical factor for the normal development of an infant as well as for a positive outcome of therapy. Consequently, psychotherapeutic methods for the treatment of mentally retarded children should focus on the significance of the therapeutic relationship (Došen 1990). Within the atmosphere of such a relationship, an opportunity arises for development and the child is able to use the therapist and caregivers as "auxiliary egos" and to change his or her distorted value system (see Chapter 23 of this book).

The therapeutic procedure is a modification of "psychoanalytic-interactional psychotherapy" (Heigl-Evers and Ott 1994; Heigl-Evers et al. 1993). This approach differs from the traditional psychoanalytic method in terms of duration, therapeutic space, media and alliance, setting, transference relations, and modes of interventions. These differences are accentuated in therapy with children with mental retardation. Some aspects of the therapeutic process are illustrated by a typical case:

> Brigitte was 9 years old when she was admitted. Until then she had been living with her foster parents. Her biological parents are unknown. She spent the first 3 years of her life in different hospitals. Her repetitive and severely aggressive outbursts at home and at school were the reason for admission. After weeks in a children's psychiatric clinic, the diagnosis was still not established and neuroleptics did not help significantly. Brigitte had a failure to thrive syndrome when she was an infant and had a long history of behavior problems such as crying spells, self-mutilating behavior, periods of overeating, and disruptive behavior. Her level of retardation was classified as moderate. Verbal communication was possible, but she was not able to learn reading or writing. In the first 6 months after admission, Brigitte showed depressive behavior such as clinging to the caregivers, problems with eating and sleeping, and rejecting contact with other children. In connection with repeated separation from caregivers, a tendency toward increasing destructiveness was observed. After 1 year the caregivers looked on Brigitte as being "the little devil." At this point the psychiatric service was informed. The atmosphere in Brigitte's group was colored by the fear of her outbursts. Although there sometimes was a recognizable reason for her behavior, Brigitte was more often than not simply provocative and a nuisance, as though "the little devil" had become an important part of her identity.

Goals and Duration

Significant and stable structural changes can be attained, but usually severely disturbed children do not become "normal." In the course of individual therapy, the therapist acquires knowledge concerning the specific capabilities and vulnerabilities of the children. Thus, the therapist is enabled to advise the caregivers on how to create adequate surroundings for the children. They, in turn, can remain stable because their coping capacities are not overtaxed. Because of the ameliorated emotional climate, they may reenter their interrupted developmental process. To maintain this atmosphere, it is generally necessary to continue therapy in a different way after individual sessions have been ended. Gradually, the therapeutic relationship will change in quality. The therapist is no longer an auxiliary ego but assumes instead the role of an influential advisor—a function that he or she later can transfer to the caretakers. Usually psychotherapy on an individual basis takes approximately 2–3 years and supportive therapy several years more.

Long after individual therapy had ceased, Brigitte was still struggling with her destructiveness, and sometimes she was not able to control it. But the caregivers could handle it much better now and proceeded to reinforce Brigitte's own self-control ability. A learning and adaptational process took place on both sides. Both the caregivers and Brigitte herself requested therapeutic advice when the need arose. After 6 years, therapy was terminated. Today, Brigitte is still seen as being a difficult young woman, but the caregivers treat her with consideration, and she has succeeded in organizing her private life in quite a satisfactory way. In the case of an emergency, Brigitte knows where she can find her former therapist.

"Therapeutic Space" and "Real Space"

Usually, mentally retarded children are not able to demarcate themselves adequately from their social environment. They live more in their social relationships than within their inner structures. Their moods, responsible for their problems of adaptation, fade very slowly and outlast the triggering situations for a long time. They are not able to correctly link their moods with internal or external causes. Thus, affects aroused during the therapeutic session will provoke conflicts at home and vice versa. In addition, these children have immature defense mechanisms, leading to an inevitable involvement of the caregivers. The most frequent example is "splitting" the objects into "all bad" or "all good." In this situation the therapist will often be suspected of stirring up the patient against the staff. Finally, the therapist has to prevent an increase in negative countertransference affects on the part of the caregivers; otherwise his or her therapy will be ineffective.

So there are many good reasons for doing without the strict separation of "real space" and "therapeutic space" that is usually presented by psychoanalytic therapists. The therapist has to work on both sites. He or she should also have an influence on everyday life in order to prevent unnecessary frustrations and stress. Thus, individual therapy is only one part of a comprehensive therapeutic strategy. The therapist has to organize and coordinate this complex process. Of course, the prescription of psychiatric drugs must also be discussed with the therapist.

Soon after therapy had started, it became even more difficult for the caregivers to get along with Brigitte. In arguments between the caregivers and Brigitte, she always used the pretext that her therapist had given her permission to do this or that. One could not always depend on Brigitte to reliably separate her wishful thinking from reality, and so conflicts flared up repeatedly. Brigitte viewed the contacts between the therapist and the staff with deep mistrust. She often reacted by withdrawing her trust completely. Therefore, it became necessary to appoint a different therapist to counsel the staff. In this way, the splitting that Brigitte had started was taken over and even heightened for the time being. Brigitte reacted toward the loving care of the caregivers with contempt and hate, making them feel helpless and angry. This threatened to develop into a permanent rejection of Brigitte. Particular indications of this happening were the harsh disciplinary measures they took as well as their countertransference reactions, which assumed the form of indifference and neglect of the girl. The situation also became more difficult because Brigitte had learned to use temper tantrums as well as self-mutilation in order to get her way. The caregivers were expected to keep up an empathic, emotionally open attitude and still be as consistent and firm as was necessary. The task of the other therapist was to support this affective attitude.

Therapeutic Alliance

As a rule, children starting therapy do not have any insight into their illness and usually do not suffer from their disorders. For this reason they have no desire for therapeutic treatment. The other children who have to live together with them as well as the caregivers are the ones affected by this state of affairs. Still, in many cases it is incorrect to automatically assume that the caregivers see the necessity for therapy. They are often wary of the therapeutic procedure and try instead to influence the disorders with disciplinary measures. In such cases it is pointless to start therapy, and the initial task of the therapist is to establish the necessary preconditions. Only after the caregivers have been convinced can a contract be drawn up for laying down the conditions for cooperation and defining the individual areas of responsibility. This is the first step. This does not mean that the contract with the child is any less important; it is just not regarded as a precondition for initiating therapy but rather as the first goal. It is often necessary for the child to first get a glimpse of the connections between his or her behavior on the one hand and the distressful feelings of displeasure on the other.

Even a mentally retarded child can quickly become aware of the therapist's intentions and oppose the planned change of his or her personality through resistance. The therapist must therefore first build up the necessary motivation by making therapy as attractive as possible and then, step by step, make increasing demands on the child by setting up agreements aimed at having the child participate in the therapeutic process in a responsible manner. Drawing up such a contract is a process in itself.

> At first, Brigitte would only meet the therapist in her own room in the group residence. The caregivers had attempted to explain the importance of the therapy that was about to begin, but Brigitte saw it as a form of punishment. Brigitte began the first session with protests such as "I didn't break the window" or "I made up for it." The therapist ignored these comments, trying instead to convey the idea that he was concerned about her and wanted to offer her support. This offer and concern made Brigitte curious. At the same time though, she became suspicious; the therapist interpreted this as a first sign of

resistance, which in turn meant that she was beginning to get an inkling of the significance that therapy might have. Only in the fourth session was Brigitte willing to leave the group residence with the therapist, and in the next session it was possible to arrange for her to come to the therapy room for her next appointment; the caregivers would tell her when to go. In connection with this arrangement, the goal of therapy was formulated with the words "I want to help you."

In subsequent sessions the therapist tried to create a pleasant atmosphere. Various offers were made to Brigitte (drinking hot chocolate, eating cake, sitting idle). She was allowed to decide at what time she would like to go. After 10 sessions it was possible to come to an agreement regarding the length of the sessions ("until the alarm clock rings," which meant in 30 minutes). Perhaps at first her attachment to the therapist was based on the vague expectation that something in her life could take a turn for the better; surely, though, her hopes for an increase in prestige played a small role. Brigitte had noticed that others envied her. In the course of time, her interest in the therapist as well as in the emotional atmosphere of the therapy session increased. At the same time, aggressive clashes with the caregivers became more intensive. This was unintentional but could not be hindered by the therapist. An alternative experiential world, which the therapist deemed necessary, had been established for Brigitte, and so the therapy entered a new phase.

Setting and Therapeutic Media

The therapeutic setting must be variable because of the diversity of disorders and developmental levels. Still, the principle of regularity and reliability must not be violated. This is one of the most important prerequisites for developing and keeping up a viable therapeutic relationship. The frequency and duration of the individual sessions will vary depending on the type of disorder. It may be impossible to stay alone with the child in a room, for instance, because he or she may be too frightened. In such a case it is necessary to find other alternatives (e.g., going shopping together, pursuing leisure activities). It is possible and appropriate to implement a nondirective approach with some children. In most cases, however, it is necessary to structure the therapy session while refraining from suppressing the child's own initiative. It is indispensable that one makes clear to the child what his or her limits are. Assaults on the therapist as well as destructive behavior must not be allowed. Such restrictions do not disrupt their therapeutic relationship if the therapist does not relinquish his or her unlimited goodwill. On the contrary, one may presume that the firm and strong but benevolent attitude of the therapist is important for the identification processes that ultimately lead to positive change. An unclear setting and a "soft" therapist can contribute to making the child chaotic and so inhibit his or her development.

The therapist must be able to offer a broad spectrum of therapeutic media in accordance with the respective developmental level, which varies from individual to individual. Verbal techniques are effective so long as they are modulated to take account of the language barriers of the mentally retarded child. Frequently, verbal interaction may fade completely into the background. The therapist must learn to decode the symbolic content of nonverbal interaction and to respond accordingly.

The main objective of all media, including dialogue, is the manifestation of the specific individual interactional style. From this interactional style the therapist is able to identify the dominant transference tendencies, phase-specific needs, and deficits of ego functions. In this respect, an alternative experiential world is opened up for the disturbed child, offering possibilities for novel emotional experiences through interaction with the therapist. Therapeutic media that are employed in this context include playing, puppet play, painting, clay modeling, cooking, body-oriented interactions, shopping, sports activities, and so on.

> It was difficult to carry on a dialogue with Brigitte. She often expressed something in everyday language that had a special meaning for her. This regularly led to misunderstandings. The fact that she was not able to separate fantasy from reality heightened the confusion. For quite a while, the mediation of emotional experiences was more important than verbal communication. If Brigitte was upset, she sought physical closeness to the therapist. A fixed ritual was that the therapist regularly put salve on her scratched and scarred arms. With this measure the therapist responded to Brigitte's obvious needs for being cared for. These were the dominant needs in this phase. Because Brigitte refused to play anything at all, the sessions were structured by mutually making and drinking hot chocolate. In the initial phase of therapy Brigitte verbalized the (imagined) torments, humiliations, and injustices her caregivers were inflicting on her. At a later stage the verbal contents became more realistic and were more related to her own achievements (also imagined to a great extent), which she wanted to be appreciated. For about 2 years, this structure remained stable while the interactional style and the verbal contents gradually changed. The sessions lasted 45 minutes and took place twice a week. After 2 years, there was hardly any body contact, and the drinking of hot chocolate ceased. The sessions were held only once a week and were characterized by Brigitte's reporting what had happened that week. This type of therapeutic contact had to be kept up for another 3 years; this was evident, among other things, considering that Brigitte regularly fell into an unstable mental state when the therapist was not available for a long period of time. Thereafter, regular sessions were no longer necessary, but the therapist was available to Brigitte if she needed him.

Object Relations, Therapist as a "Real Object," Interventions

The initial goal of the therapist is to build up a relationship resembling in some respects the one an infant has with his or her parents (see also Chapter

23 of this book). It is a relationship of dependency that facilitates further development. Due to the exclusive character of the relationship, the therapist carries a great deal of responsibility; from the start he or she must strive for the termination of this dependency. Unavoidable conflicts with the staff are often another result of this special relationship. These must also be resolved so that therapy can be successful. It is often quite difficult for the therapist to achieve such a therapeutic relationship. The children, usually extremely disturbed, act out the terrible experiences of their infancy once more in therapy. They fight to keep up their pathological identity and tend to choke every endeavor to help. In this phase, the stability of therapy rests solely on the attitude of the therapist, who, by means of his or her intense interest in and unwavering concern for the child, eventually makes him or her receptive to a therapeutic relationship.

It is difficult to deal with these repetitions of dominant object relations of early childhood in therapy. Quite often one is confronted by archaic, unrestrained affects of hate and envy or by paniclike fear. These children are not able to dissociate themselves from this experience. At first, they only see the therapist as having those characteristics they bestow on him or her through projections. In turn, the therapist is apt to reflect on the real reasons behind the types of interaction with which he or she is confronted and searches for an "answer" by analyzing the countertransference feelings being aroused. This answer should be "authentic" and "selective." Authenticity is necessary if the therapist's emotional understanding of and respect for the child are to be conveyed as they should be. The answer must be selective because the therapist must take the cognitive and emotional limitations of the child into consideration. The "answer" must also be of use to the child; it should serve to stimulate an interest in a continuation of the interaction and make the child curious and courageous. In the course of this, though, the therapist will not be able to avoid frustrations. Still, he or she will choose the "right" type and the "right" moment to tread a path that fosters and supports the child's development. If therapy is successful, this mode of interaction will eventually lead the child to modify his or her object relation patterns and their affective qualities and attune them better to reality.

The therapist's "answers" are his or her interventions. They may be expressed verbally, as facial expressions and gestures, or through actions. The answers should express agreement and congruence as well as difference and dissent. Their purpose is to confront the child with experiences of emotional reactions and to facilitate their clarification and differentiation. At the same time, the answers mediate emotional experiences such as protection, security, respect, and love. In this emotional atmosphere the child will be able to develop his or her ego functions under the guidance of the therapist. The emphasis here is not so much on the training of such functions. Instead, in the role of the auxiliary ego, the therapist takes partial control of these functions during the interaction. This facilitates the adoption of more suitable adaptation functions through partial identification. As a substitute for the objects of the real world, the therapist enters the developmental process of the child as a significant object and serves as a catalyst.

It is not possible here to present a detailed account of the development of object relations and the therapeutic procedure during the long duration of Brigitte's therapy. It will suffice to give an example that reflects one aspect of the early phase of therapy.

> Brigitte did accept the offer to enter a relationship with the therapist quite quickly. The price for this, however, was an increase in aggressive behavior toward other residents. This was interpreted as splitting and was tentatively accepted at the time. Besides, Brigitte's attachment to the therapist was still fragile. Deviations from her rigid rules and expectations provoked temper tantrums or retreat. Brigitte attempted to exercise total control over her therapist. In particular, she attached great importance to having the therapist share her ideas regarding her caregivers. The therapist interpreted these observations to mean that Brigitte was still not capable of reliably separating self and nonself. The therapist had become a part of Brigitte's self in the manner of a *selfobject relation*. Brigitte projected all her ideas of a "good, omnipotent mother" on him and was not capable of acknowledging his true characteristics. Each and every unpleasant expectation was projected onto the external world, especially the caregivers. In this phase the therapist attached importance to first fulfilling Brigitte's need for safety and security. He did not attempt to correct her misconceptions concerning her caregivers. He tried to soothe her and make her relax by means of body contact. Moreover, he tried to live up to her expectations as far as possible. The next developmental task for Brigitte to fulfill was an increased differentiation between herself and the significant object—in this case, the therapist. Such a change of object relations would make progress in the development of various psychological functions possible and necessary. The therapist was forced to wait until he was convinced that Brigitte would be able to tolerate a deviation from her usual expectations that he would provoke. The risk for the therapist was that Brigitte might suddenly equate him with the "bad" caregivers and repudiate him. However, if the therapist was successful in this endeavor, the staff would have the chance of forming a more realistic relationship with Brigitte. Therefore, the therapist started introducing changes in the course of the sessions. Each individual change appeared rather unimportant and trite, yet the sum total of all these modifications enabled the patient to experience a significant change. In this case the therapist chose their mutual drinking of hot chocolate as a starting point. Knowing that it was very important for Brigitte to see him prepare hot chocolate and then drink it together with her, he told her in one session that he did not want to drink any hot chocolate. After Brigitte had accepted his decision, he made the suggestion in a later session that Brigitte could prepare the hot chocolate herself, and he would brew himself some tea.

After a while it was possible for him to make a verbal evaluation, such as "I prefer tea and you like hot chocolate." The emotional atmosphere of the sessions could now be changed; instead of security, protection, and warmth, what Brigitte needed now was pride in her own achievements (for instance, making the hot chocolate herself) and acknowledgment by the significant object. Under the therapist's guidance, it became possible to take numerous little steps that imparted novel emotional experiences regarding herself and her significant object, namely, the therapist. These experiences eventually led to a stepwise modification of her self-concept by means of identification processes. Today, Brigitte is no longer "the little devil," who wanted to turn the group residency into a state of chaos. Instead, she is a young woman with personal everyday habits and relatively stable relationships with the persons with whom she lives. Under emotional stress, though, she regresses into her split world in which she feels pursued by the hate of her objects.

■ CONCLUSIONS

The psychodynamic approach can be useful for therapy with emotionally disturbed children who are mentally retarded, irrespective of the severity of retardation. A basic assumption of the psychodynamic approach is that emotional vulnerability is—besides other factors—a result of experiences with significant objects of early developmental phases. Consequently, psychodynamic therapy focuses on the patient's relationship not only to his or her therapist but especially to other staff members (see also Chapter 23 of this book). To a greater degree than other therapeutic approaches, psychodynamic therapy stresses the importance of the emotional atmosphere for stabilization and further development. Therapy starts in the minds of the caregivers. Through the professional support by the therapist, the caregivers may learn to see deviant behavior as a product of developmental deficits and to have respect for the retarded person as well as for his or her efforts to organize him- or herself within the social environment. They may acquire the empathy necessary to perceive developmental needs and conflicts that may give them the flexibility necessary for an appropriate emotional response to the patient's behavior. Finally, the caregivers may experience how they are involved in the psychodynamics of the patients and be able to interrupt the vicious cycle of transference and countertransference by stabilizing their relationship simply by means of "good parenting." This influence on the caregivers' attitude may be the most important contribution of the psychodynamic approach to a life of dignity for severely disturbed children.

In many cases this effect can be attained by counseling the staff without having to perform individual psychotherapy. However, individual psychotherapy is often necessary in order to gain knowledge of the specific psychodynamic background of the child's behavior and to have the opportunity to effectuate specific interventions. The goal is to enable the child to reenter his or her developmental process and to provide the child with structure and functions that would enable him or her to live autonomously in the social environment. This, however, is not always completely possible, but therapy will at least ameliorate the emotional climate for the child and protect him or her from inadequate demands, unnecessary frustrations, and other forms of psychological stress.

■ **REFERENCES**

Balthazar EE, Stevens HA: The Emotionally Disturbed Mentally Retarded: A Historical and Contemporary Perspective. Englewood Cliffs, NJ, Prentice Hall, 1975

Berman S: The psychodynamics aspects of behavior, in Basic Handbook of Child Psychiatry, Vol 2. Edited by Noshpitz JD. New York, Basic Books, 1979, pp 3–27

Blanck G, Blanck R: Ego Psychology: Theory and Practice. New York, Columbia University Press, 1974

Blanck G, Blanck R: Ego Psychology, Vol 2. New York, Columbia University Press, 1979

Chetic M: The borderline child, in Basic Handbook of Child Psychiatry, Vol 2. Edited by Noshpitz JD. New York, Basic Books, 1979, pp 304–320

Došen A: Developmental-dynamic relationship therapy, in Treatment of Mental Illness and Behavioural Disorder in the Mentally Retarded. Edited by Došen A, Van Gennep A, Zwanikken GJ. Leiden, Netherlands, Logon, 1990, pp 37–44

Došen A, Menolascino FJ (eds): Depression in Mentally Retarded Children and Adults. Leiden, Netherlands, Logon, 1990

Došen A, van Gennep A, Zwanikken GJ (eds): Treatment of Mental Illness and Behavioural Disorder in the Mentally Retarded. Leiden, Netherlands, Logon, 1990

Emde RN: Development terminable and interminable, II: recent psychoanalytic theory and therapeutic considerations. International Journal of Psychoanalysis 69:283–296, 1988

Erikson EH: The problem of identity. Journal of the American Psychoanalytic Association 4:56–121, 1956

Fletcher RJ, Došen A (eds): Mental Health Aspect of Mental Retardation. Toronto, Ontario, Canada, Lexington Books, 1993

Fletcher RJ, Menolascino F (eds): Mental Retardation and Mental Illness. Toronto, Ontario, Canada, Lexington Books, 1989

Gaedt C: Psychotherapeutic approaches in the treatment of mental illness and behavioral disorders in mentally retarded people: the significance of a psychoanalytic perspective. J Intellect Disabil Res 30(3):233–239, 1995

Gaedt C: Psychodynamic oriented psychotherapy in people with learning disability, in Issues in Service Provision for People With Learning Disabilities: Papers on Philosophy, Social Psychology, and Psychiatry. Edited by Gaedt C. Neuerkerode, Germany, Evangelische Stiftung Neuerkerode, 1997, pp 50–79

Hartmann H: Ego Psychology and the Problem of Adaptation. New York, International Universities Press, 1958

Heigl-Evers A, Ott J: Die Psychoanalytisch-Interaktionelle Methode: Theorie und Praxis. Gottingen, Germany, Vandenhoek & Ruprecht, 1994

Heigl-Evers A, Heigl F, Ott J: Abrib der psychoanalyse und der analytischen psychotherapie, in Lehrbuch der Psychotherapie. Edited by Heigl-Evers A, Heigl F, Ott J. Stuttgart/Jena, Germany, Gustav Fischer, 1993, pp 202–222

Hoffmann SO, Hochapfel G: Einfuhrung in die Neurosenlehre und Psychosomatische Medizin, 3. Aufl Stuttgart/New York, Schattauer, 1987

Hollins SC: Group analytic therapy with people with mental handicap, in Treatment of Mental Illness and Behavioral Disorder in the Mentally Retarded. Edited by Došen A, Van Gennep A, Zwanikken GJ. Leiden, Netherlands, Logon, 1990, pp 81–90

Kernberg OF: Objektbeziehung und Praxis der Psychoanalyse. Stuttgart, Germany, Klett-Cotta, 1981

Levitas A, Gilson SF: Toward the developmental understanding of the impact of mental retardation on the assessment of psychopathology, in Assessment of Behavior Problems in Persons With Mental Retardation Living in the Community. Edited by Dibble E, Gray DB. Rockville, MD, National Institute of Mental Health, 1988, pp 71–107

Matson JL, Barrett RP (eds): Psychopathology in Mentally Retarded. New York, Grune & Stratton, 1982

Robinson NM, Robinson HB: The Mentally Retarded Child, 2nd Edition. New York, McGraw-Hill, 1976

Sander LW: Towards a logic of organisation in psychobiological development, in Biologic Response Styles: Clinical Implications. Edited by Klar K, Silver L. Washington DC, American Psychiatric Press, 1985, pp 124–140

Sandler J, Joffe WG: Towards a basic psychoanalytic model. International Journal of Psychoanalysis 50:79–90, 1965

Sinason V: Mental Handicap and the Human Condition. London, Free Association Books, 1992

Szymanski LS, Tanguay PE (eds): Emotional Disorders of Mentally Retarded Persons. Baltimore, MD, University Park Press, 1980

23 Developmental-Dynamic Relationship Therapy

An Approach to More Severely Mentally Retarded Children

Anton Došen, M.D., Ph.D.

Pioneers in the field of psychotherapy for mentally retarded persons (Bicknell 1979; Reid 1982; Rubin 1983) thought that the usefulness of individual psychotherapy at lower developmental levels (IQ < 50) was limited and that simple support, encouragement, and behavior modification gave better results. Later workers (Monfils and Menolascino 1984; Szymanski 1980), however, were of the opinion that the low intelligence of mentally retarded children should not be an obstacle to the use of psychotherapy. According to these authors, IQ may indeed influence the choice of the technique and goals of therapy, but the decision for undertaking it rests on the patient's ability to respond to a warm, supportive relationship rather than on the level of intelligence. Very important to such a decision, too, is the desire of the individual to effect change. This view accords with the developmental approach (Došen 1984; Frankish 1989; Gaedt et al. 1987), which specifically states that neither the level of intelligence nor the motivation or other personal abilities should be the determinants for the applicability of individual psychotherapy; the only important factor is the child's developmental needs.

The developmental approach utilizes particularly the theories of Bowlby (1971) and Mahler et al. (1975), which postulate that human beings have an existential need for bonding with other people. This bonding provides a psychologically secure base from which a child can explore and master his or her surroundings. Bowlby's attachment theory has given new input to a better understanding of developmental psychosocial processes. Recent investigations in developmental psychology have accentuated the importance of secure and insecure attachment for the forming of relationships. An association between relationship difficulties and later emotional problems has been suggested by various attachment theorists (Clegg and Lansdall-Welfare 1995; Holmes 1993). From this point of view the attachment theory provides the basis for a new interpersonal paradigm within psychotherapy. Holmes (1993) considers this as a biological basis for psychotherapy. Observational studies suggest that attachment theory may have an important place in the understanding of emotional problems in persons with mental retardation because these individuals have difficulties in establishing relationships. Using the works of Bowlby and of Mahler as points of departure, Sand et al. (1990) applied psychodynamic developmental therapy (in combination with pedagogical and milieu treatment) to both mentally retarded children and adults. In this form of therapy, the therapist makes a developmentally oriented diagnosis and interacts with the patient at his or her current developmental level. The therapist attempts to avoid interactions that confirm the patient in the pathological state, directing these instead to more appropriate experiences that would enable the patient to discover his or her own individual needs. While the interactions are being guided by the child's needs, the therapist attempts to heighten the level of communication and to further stimulate the child's emotional development. Frankish (1989, 1992) described the treatment of several severely mentally retarded children who had been diagnosed as suffering from delay and stagnation in their emotional development. The author utilized the stages of emotional development proposed by Mahler et al. (1975). Treatment was directed toward satisfying the child's emotional needs at the stage of his or her real emotional development and stimulating further emotional development. The therapeutic efforts focused on helping the child to consolidate in the rapprochement phase and to move on to the individuation phase.

Recently Clegg and Lansdall-Welfare (1995) described a treatment based on the attachment theory in three adults with moderate to severe mental retardation who were suffering from enmeshed relationships with members of the care staff. The treatment yielded significant patient changes in three areas: reduction of anger and distress, increased exploration of physical and intellectual environments, and an increase in the range of people to whom the patient relates. The authors underlined the importance of meeting the attachment needs of mentally retarded individuals, acknowledging at once that facilitating secure attachment relationships may be a difficult task for professionals.

Gaedt (1995, 1997) (see also Chapter 22 of this book) has also pointed out the necessity of perceiving the child's emotional developmental needs and emphasized the importance of the appropriate emotional response of the therapist to the child's behavior. This approach may be applied to all children regardless of their level of retardation.

Other authors (Irblich and Blumenschein 1996; Pfluger-Jakob 1996), starting from the developmental approach, went on to develop play therapy and Gestalt therapy methods for children with mental retardation.

On the basis of Bowlby's and Mahler's postulates and abundant experience with mentally retarded children, Došen (1983, 1984, 1990, 1995, 1997) developed the so-called developmental-dynamic relationship therapy (DRT) for use with children with moderate, severe, and profound levels of mental retardation. Methodically, DRT is an adaptation of relationship therapy that has been applied to mentally ill nonretarded children and was introduced by Allan (1942) and Moustakas (1959).

■ THE THEORETICAL BASE

Comparing different psychosocial developmental theories like Piaget's cognitive theory (Piaget 1955), Mahler's psychodynamic theory (Mahler et al. 1975), and Erikson's (1959) and Bowlby's (1971) theories, one may assume that, under normal circumstances, cognitive social and emotional aspects of the child's psychic life progressively develop and flow along parallel lines. Neurophysiological and neuropsychological findings (Luria 1973), however, suggest that the pace of psychic development is determined by the maturation rate of the different areas of the cerebral cortex.

By combining these psychological and physiological theories, the following scheme of socioemotional development within the first 3 years of life may be conceptualized (Došen 1990, 1997):

1. Adaptation phase
   a. Integration of sensoric stimuli
   b. Integration of the structure of place, time, and persons

2. Socialization phase
   a. Bonding
   b. Creation of a secure base

3. Individuation phase
   a. Separation
   b. Individuation
   c. Development of a unique personality

This process results in the following structuring of personality:

- The adaptation phase results in psychophysiological homeostasis
- The socialization phase results in secure attachment

- The individuation phase results in establishing
  - Sense of the self
  - Ego structuring

According to various workers in this field, a normal and healthy socioemotional development during the first 3 years of life is essential for the normal development of personality and for the mental health of the individual (Erikson 1959; Mahler et al. 1975).

Mentally retarded children follow the similar sequences and are predisposed to make similar psychosocial developmental structures as usual children (Evans 1998), but the socioemotional development of mentally retarded children during the first 3 years may be susceptible to various obstacles—genetic, organic, environmental, etc. It has been hypothesized that mentally retarded children show a maturational lag in different cortical areas (Luria 1973), which may result in 1) global disturbance, causing a delay in the totality of psychological development; and 2) partial disturbance leading to impaired integration of new experiences into the existing cognitive, social, and emotional schemata with resultant disturbance in the child's psychophysiological homeostasis and difficulties in the achievement of particular psychosocial skills and delayed socioemotional development.

Similar problems may occur when the child's surroundings are not sufficiently stimulating for the achievement of different developmental skills. In both cases, the formation of appropriate attachment may be disturbed.

Clinical experience with profoundly and severely mentally retarded children suggests that psychopathology is often rooted in disturbances of psychophysiological homeostasis and secure attachment formation. With moderately and mildly mentally retarded children, problems in forming a sense of the self and the ego frequently underlie the psychopathology. The clinical picture of the psychopathology depends on the level of socioemotional development at which the disturbance took place and on the cognitive level (Došen 1993; Glick 1998).

■ THE STRATEGY

The basis of DRT is the developmental-dynamic diagnosis. The diagnosis comprises an integrative survey of the biological, developmental, existential, and psychosocial problems of the child.

A mentally retarded child is a developing organism whose needs and sensitivities vary with his or her developmental level and whose developmental course is determined largely by the biological substrate and the interactions with the environment. Behavioral and psychological problems are viewed in terms of three dimensions: biological substrate, interaction with the surroundings, and developmental course.

Biological Substrate

The therapist has to know which biological factors and central nervous system disorders have played a part in the general disorder of the child. This is necessary in order to provide an insight into how the child processes internal and external stimuli and the kind of stimulation he or she actually needs.

Interaction With the Surroundings

Interaction with the surroundings can be of great importance in determining the behavioral patterns and psychological state of the child. The therapist must be cognizant of the rules of the child's living system and the place and role that each member of the system has. A systems theoretical as well as psychodynamic mode of thinking has to be utilized.

Developmental Course

The developmental course of the child is a dimension that requires special attention. Cognitive, social, and emotional facets of development determine collectively the strategy and the application of special treatment techniques.

Case Example

A 5-year-old severely mentally retarded boy was referred because of severe problems in social contact and autistic-like behavior. Concerning the biological dimension, he was found to be oversensitive to acoustic and visual stimuli. In a noisy and crowded room he became frustrated and often distressed. Changes within his living space as well as entering into an unfamiliar place caused tantrums with autoaggressive outbursts. Concerning interaction with his surroundings, the parents' attitude was noteworthy. They were unable to accept their child's handicap and were very active in seeking aid for him. Every time they heard that he was mentally retarded and that there was no hope of a cure, they changed doctors. They were convinced that he was autistic and they wanted him to receive special treatment for autistic children. Concerning the developmental course, examination revealed an uneven psychological developmental profile in which the cognitive development was at the level of 2 years, whereas the social and emotional levels lagged behind—no higher than 6 months.

The diagnostic formulation was a disorder of socioemotional development in the first developmental phase resulting in a distortion of psychophysiological homeostasis with consequent severe disturbance in the attachment process and social contact disorder.

The therapist utilized the model of socioemotional development. Firstly, according to the rules of the first adaptation phase, the environmental circumstances of the child have to be structured so as to make it possible for him to achieve a physical and physiological homeostasis with his surroundings. The surroundings had to be adapted to the biological substrate and physiological shortcomings of the child. Space, time, and persons were structured according to the needs of the child. The stimuli were reduced so that he could process and integrate them into his cognitive and emotional schemata. The treatment aim was first to adapt the surroundings to the abilities of the child and, then, to stimulate him to adapt to the surroundings. Once he had adapted to his surroundings, the therapist undertook activities directed toward further stimulating development according to the schema of phasic socioemotional development.

To establish a socialization phase and secure attachment, the therapist undertook specific activities with the child. Initially, attention was directed toward the child's abilities to process tactile stimuli, and as much tactile stimulation as he could integrate was offered. These activities permitted the therapist to determine the child's capabilities, the degree of intensity needed, and the optimal duration and frequency of stimulation. The aim was to achieve emotional bonding with the child and to help him to establish emotional security and trust in the interaction. The boy had had many negative experiences—such as the failed initial attempts of his parents to involve him in the bonding process—which made it more difficult for the therapist. A cautious, well-planned, and patient approach to the child's needs finally yielded good results. The resistance to bodily contact disappeared, and the boy experienced pleasure when he sat on the therapist's lap and was caressed.

Once the bonding and trust were achieved, the therapist's aim shifted to activities designed to bring the child into the individuation phase, stimulating self and ego development. The communication channel that was being used changed from tactile contact to communication via material objects and acoustic and verbal signals. The child was stimulated to leave the therapist's lap and to communicate at a distance. Because the boy's cognitive level was not higher than 2 years, the therapeutic goal was to raise the emotional and social developmental levels to 2 years as well. This goal was reached after 8 months of therapy.

■ THE METHOD

In DRT, three separate stages can be differentiated: 1) tolerance and acceptance, 2) meeting and growing together, 3) reeducation.

During the first stage, attempts are made to accept the child and all his or her actions, enabling him or her to find his or her own place and role in the environment. The symptoms of disturbed behavior are not combated; rather, they are accepted as an aspect of the child's total existence. Accepting the child implies, among other things, that the surroundings have to be adapted to the child's abilities and inabilities and activities and inactivities. The initial task is to make the child feel at peace in his or her surroundings and to discover the extent to which the child can be induced to communicate pleasantly. During this stage a basic therapeutic structuring of the environment in terms of space, time, persons, and frequency and intensity of stimulation must take place.

The second stage consists of the formation of a positive and affectionate relationship between the therapist and the child. The therapist tries to react positively to all aspects of the child's behavior. The child is stimulated to develop communication initiatives and express his or her wishes, feelings, anxieties, and pleasures. On the basis of the bonding and the trust achieved, the child is stimulated to solve emotional and behavioral problems and to ameliorate the communication with his or her surroundings.

In the third stage, once a positive and trusting relationship has been established, the therapist tries to help the child rid him- or herself of the prevalent behavior patterns and to teach him or her new forms of socially acceptable behavior. The child is actively involved in the appropriate pedagogical structure within which he or she receives social reinforcement. Social behavior and creative involvement with the material surroundings are stimulated. In this stage the therapist may also make use of other therapeutic techniques like classical play therapy, role-play therapy, and behavioral modification techniques. The therapeutic goal is to cajole the child as much as possible into the individuation process and to free him or her from physical and psychological dependence on the therapist.

The therapist's aim is to stimulate the development of the child as a unique social personality and to strengthen his or her positive ego qualities. At the same time, the therapist provides the emotional security base that the child needs in those situations or conflicts that the child cannot resolve on his or her own. Gradually, this trusting relationship with the therapist is generalized to other persons in the surroundings, rendering the child increasingly freer in exploring and experimenting with the outer world.

DRT can be carried out by a trained and supervised nursing staff, teachers, or even the child's parents. This choice is based on the individual needs of the mentally retarded children.

Because of their weak psychic processing and integration abilities, it is necessary to maintain a constancy and unity of space, persons, and activities. The generalization of behavior learned in particular circumstances is apparently a difficult task for mentally retarded children. Therefore, the therapeutic activities should be carried out by the persons permanently involved with the child (in the clinical ward by a nurse, at school by a teacher, at home by the mother). In our practice, therapy usually takes place within the therapeutic milieu of the clinical ward (Došen 1984). Frankish (1992) reported good results with therapy carried out at three places during the day: at school, at the care home, and at the child's home.

Due to delayed learning abilities as well as other psychological limitations, the therapeutic sessions must be frequent and the duration attuned to the ability of the child to adequately process the therapeutic interaction. This requires the very intensive involvement of the therapist. In our experience, involving the staff and other caregivers yields good results as well. Involving the caregivers in the therapy makes it easier to switch from the role of therapist to the role of educator when the opportunity is right and at the appropriate stage in treatment. This way the process of reeducation may be accelerated in a subtle fashion.

Professional guidance and good interpersonal relationships between the therapist/supervisor and the staff and other caregivers/therapists are extremely important. Clegg and Lansdall-Welfare (1995) advise holding several sessions with staff members and a supervisor. Initial discussions review key relationships and events in the person's life. Later sessions focus on how the person may be feeling and how the therapist may act toward him or her. The attachment theory serves to generate ideas.

Detailed information about the therapeutic setting, media, therapeutic alliance, and transference—which are specific for mentally retarded children—can be found in Chapter 22 of this book. Several principles specific to DRT will be discussed here.

Structure in Space, Persons, and Time

Therapeutic activities should take place in surroundings that the child is familiar with or has grown accustomed to. The furnishings and design of the room in which therapy takes place (therapy space) should remain unaltered. Changes in persons who form part of the habitat (living space) of the child should be avoided. The therapeutic interaction should take place within a planned daily program and remain consistent with respect to time of day and duration.

Diurnal Rhythm

Both the activity and inactivity of a child should alternate regularly throughout the day. The physiological and mental capabilities of the child need to be ascertained individually, and the rhythm of activity and rest matched to them. This avoids possible over- or understimulation during the therapeutic process.

Gradual Emotional Growth

Once it has become possible to communicate with the child, any further development is gradual in its nature. The therapist should follow the consecutive phases represented in the scheme of socioemotional development. In concrete terms, this means that when dealing with a child suffering from a social contact disorder, the focus should be on establishing tactile contact before the other communicative channels can be used. For a child who has individuation problems and exhibits negative and destructive behavior, a positive and stable bond with the therapist is necessary before the structuring of behavior can be introduced.

■ INDICATION AND RESULTS

Clegg and Lansdall-Welfare (1995) identified the following features as being indicative for when treatment based on attachment theory should be applied: significant "fixation" on a caregiver, anger or distress by separation, intermittent anger or distress, resistance to exploring the physical world, and functioning below the cognitive abilities.

The application of DRT to a social contact disorder has already been described. We consider DRT to be indicated particularly at very low levels of cognitive and emotional development. When behavioral problems or psychotic and depressive disorder are present in addition to a contact disorder, DRT combined with drug treatment is indicated.

Case Example

Christopher was a 7-year-old boy, the elder of two children, who showed delayed psychomotor development. He began to walk at the age of 2, spoke his first words at 3, and was toilet-trained at the age of 5. He was admitted because of delayed speech development, poor learning capabilities, and a strange, inwardly directed behavior. On admission, he was very anxious, withdrawn, and passive. He spoke a few disconnected words and preferred stereotyped activity involving a single object. Psychological testing revealed him to be functioning at a moderately retarded level. No abnormalities were found upon physical examination, and the diagnosis was a nonspecific psychosis.

It soon became obvious that Christopher liked physical contact very much. This was used as the starting point for DRT. The therapist gave him as much physical contact as he wanted—and he wanted a great deal—keeping him in her lap, carrying him, feeding him, and completely looking after him. Bowel and bladder control were lost and he regressed to an infantlike stage. Complete dependence lasted for 2 months. Gradually, he began to increase his spatial distance from the therapist, but as independence increased, negative, stubborn, and provocative attitudes developed. In addition to DRT, he received the neuroleptic pimozide, 0.05 mg/kg/day.

After several months his negative trends became less marked, and he demonstrated more cooperation with the therapist and greater creativity in handling materials. Slowly, he began to show interest in other children, and, encouraged by the therapist, he began to play with them. Christopher made substantial progress in speech development, he became increasingly involved in reality, and the signs of the psychosis diagnosed 5 months earlier disappeared.

Depression is a condition that is difficult to diagnose in severely mentally retarded children because nonspecific symptoms are often present. However, experienced clinicians emphasize that this disorder occurs relatively often among these children (Došen 1990, 1998). DRT may yield good results in these cases as the following example illustrates.

Case Example

Gene, an 8-year-old boy functioning in the moderately mentally retarded range, was admitted for treatment because of his hyperactivity and destructive and aggressive behavior, which began when he entered kindergarten at the age of 4. Physical examination showed no abnormalities. The family history revealed that his mother had suffered from depression for a number of years following his birth and that several years later his father had had a nervous breakdown due to difficulties at work and became depressed. When he was in the unit, Gene was unable to sit still for a single moment and reacted aggressively toward the other children. Yet, when he was with adults, he became much quieter and seemed to appreciate physical contact. On the basis of his developmental history, behavior, and psychiatric assessment, dysthymic depression was diagnosed.

He was given individual therapy by a nurse at regular intervals during the day, and an affective bond grew rapidly between them. The therapist noted that during physical contact the child tended to show regressive, babylike behavior, which led to the decision to introduce role-playing. A clear agreement was made with him that the two of them would play mother and child. Gene chose the role of the baby. During this role-playing, which lasted 30 minutes, he was given diapers, drank from a bottle, cooed like a baby, and clearly showed that he appreciated his role. After 2 weeks, he no longer wanted to play being a baby but preferred to pretend to be a toddler. At the end of the second 2 weeks, Gene decided to play the roles of husband, father, and police officer for several months. Thereafter, role-play no longer interested him, and he preferred to engage in standard games with the therapist.

Treatment lasted 6 months during which Gene became much calmer, and his hyperactivity and aggression disappeared. His fear of failure lessened substantially, and, as a result, he was able to concentrate on task performance better. Although he had shown no signs of homesickness on admission, his desire to return home to his mother increased markedly.

Behavioral problems like aggressivity, self-injurious behavior, and destructibility in children with delayed emotional development in comparison with their cognitive development are often indications for DRT (Došen 1984, 1990). The emotional development of these children is usually arrested in the socialization or individuation phase with a disturbance in the attachment process and in formation of a sense of the self. We found DRT to be indicated with the following diagnoses:

- Attachment disorders with behavioral problems
- Attachment disorders with symptoms of atypical psychosis
- Depression with attachment disorders
- Self-injurious behavior based on problems of psychophysiological homeostasis
- Self-injurious behavior based on attachment disorder
- Depression based on a disturbed individuation process and inadequate self-differentiation
- Psychotic states based on disturbed self-differentiation
- Behavioral and psychiatric disorders (depression, psychosis) in pervasive development disorder and mental retardation

An evaluation of the results of DRT with 97 children (Došen 1983) showed that 41% of them were discharged free of the symptoms they were admitted for, 41% showed slight improvements, and in 18% of the cases, no improvement could be detected.

■ CONCLUSIONS

Neither an organic handicap nor the IQ level determines the suitability of DRT. The indication should be the result of a psychiatric developmentally dynamic–oriented diagnosis and the extant ability of the professionals to carry out such treatment. DRT focuses on compensating for the child's biological and physiological shortcomings, ameliorating the interaction with the surroundings, and stimulating socioemotional development. The socioemotional development model gives direction to and determines the goal and strategy of therapy. DRT appears to be useful for mentally retarded children suffering from a disturbance in emotional development and developmental psychopathology.

■ REFERENCES

Allen FH: Psychotherapy With Children. New York, Norton, 1942

Bicknell DJ: Treatment and management of disturbed mentally handicapped patients, in Psychiatric and Mental Handicap. Edited by James FE, Snaith RP. London, Gaskell, 1979, pp 65–80

Bowlby J: Attachment and Loss, Vol 1: Attachment. London, Hogart Press, 1971

Clegg JA, Lansdall-Welfare R: Attachment and learning disability: a theoretical review informing three clinical interventions. J Intellect Disabil Res 39(4):295–305, 1995

Došen A: Psychiatrische Stoornissen bij Zwakzinnige Kinderen. Lisse, Netherlands, Swets & Zeitlinger, 1983

Došen A: Experiences with individual relationship therapy within a therapeutic milieu for retarded children with severe emotional disorders, in Perspective and Progress in Mental Retardation, Vol 2. Edited by Berg JM. Baltimore, MD, University Park Press, 1984, pp 384–391

Došen A: Developmental-dynamic relationship therapy, in Treatment of Mental Illness and Behavioral Disorders in the Mentally Retarded. Edited by Došen A, van Gennep A, Zwanikken G. Leiden, Netherlands, Logon Publications, 1990, pp 37–44

Došen A: A Developmental-Psychiatric Approach in the Diagnosis of Psychiatric Disorders of Persons With Mental Retardation. Venray, Netherlands, Nieuw Spraeland, 1993

Došen A: Psychotherapy in mentally retarded children. Japanese Journal of Psychotherapy 21(4):314–324, 1995

Došen A: Psychiatric assessment and diagnosis in children with severe mental retardation. Croatian Review of Rehabilitation Research 37(2):231–239, 1997

Erikson E: Identity and the Life Cycle. New York, International Universities Press, 1959

Evans DW: Development of self-concept in children with mental retardation: organismic and contextual factors, in Handbook of Mental Retardation and Development. Edited by Burack JA, Hodapp RM, and Zigler E. Cambridge, UK, Cambridge University Press, 1998, pp 462–480

Frankish P: Meeting the emotional needs of handicapped people: a psycho-dynamic approach. Journal of Mental Deficiency Research 33:407–4141, 1989

Frankish P: A psychodynamic approach to emotional difficulties within a social framework. J Intellect Disabil Res 36:559–563, 1992

Gaedt CH: Psychotherapeutic approaches in the treatment of mental illness and behavioral disorders in mentally retarded people: the significance of a psychoanalytic perspective. J Intellect Disabil Res 39:233–239, 1995

Gaedt CH, Jäkel D, Kischkel W: Psychotherapie bei geistig behinderten, in Psychotherapie bei Geistig Behinderten. Edited by Gaedt CH. Neuerkerode, Germany, Neuerkeröder Beitrage, 1987, pp 13–21

Gaedt C: Psychodynamic oriented psychotherapy in people with learning disability, in Issues in Service Provision for People With Learning Disabilities: Papers on Philosophy, Social Psychology, and Psychiatry. Edited by Gaedt C. Neuerkerode, Germany, Evangelische Stiftung Neuerkeröde, 1997, pp 50–79

Glick M: A developmental approach to psychopathology in people with mild mental retardation, in Handbook of Mental Retardation and Development. Edited by Burack JA, Hodapp RM, Zigler E. Cambridge, UK, Cambridge University Press, 1998, pp 563–582

Holmes J: Attachment theory: a biological basis for psychotherapy. Br J Psychiatry 163:430–438, 1993

Irblich D, Blumenschein A: Therapeutisches Spielen mit geistig behinderten kindern und jugenlichen, in Wege zur Seelischen Gesundheit für Menschen mit Geistiger Behinderung. Edited by Lotz W, Stahl B, Irblich D. Bern, Swtizerland, Verlag Hans Huber, 1996, pp 238–253

Luria AR: The Working Brain. London, Penguin Press, 1973

Mahler M, Pine F, Bergman A: The Psychological Birth of the Human Infant. New York, Basic Books, 1975

Monfils NS, Menolascino FJ: Modified individual and group treatment approaches for the mentally retarded-mentally ill, in Handbook of Mental Illness in the Mentally Retarded. Edited by Menolascino FJ, Stark JA. New York, Plenum, 1984, pp 155–170

Moustakas CE: Psychotherapy With Children: The Living Relationship. New York, Harper & Row, 1959

Pfluger-Jakob M: Gestalttherapie mit geistig behinderten menschen, in Wege zur Seelischen Gesundheit für Menschen mit Geistiger Behinderung. Edited by Lotz W, Stahl B, Irblich D. Bern, Switzerland, Verlag Hans Huber, 1996, pp 206–215

Piaget J: The Child Construction of Reality. London, Routledge & Kegan, 1955

Reid AH: The Psychiatry of Mental Handicap. London, Blackwell, 1982

Rubin RL: Bridging the gap through individual counselling and psychotherapy with mentally retarded people, in Mental Health and Mental Retardation. Edited by Menolascino F, McCann B. Baltimore, MD, University Park Press, 1983, pp 119–128

Sand A, Ohmes J, Gartner-Peterhoff D, et al: Therapeutische umgang mit entwertungsprozessen, in Selbstentwertung-Depressive Inszenierungen bei Menschen mit Geistiger Behinderung. Edited by Gaedt CH, Neuerkerode, Germany, Neuerkeröder Beitrage, 1990, pp 65–81

Szymanski LS: Individual psychotherapy with retarded persons, in Emotional Disorders of Mentally Retarded Persons. Edited by Szymanski LS, Tanguay PE. Baltimore, MD, University Park Press, 1980, pp 131–148

24 Pharmacotherapy in Mentally Retarded Children

Anton Došen, M.D., Ph.D.

Studies of the frequency of drug use in children with mental retardation are rare. Hill et al. (1984) found that 19% of a group of 35,751 mentally retarded children and adolescents in community residential centers received psychotropic medication. Hogg (1992) reported the use of psychotropic drugs in 33.8% of the profoundly retarded children living at home. Other investigators focused on the mentally retarded pupils in public schools. Gadow (1975, 1993) reported the use of psychotropic drugs with children in special education programs in 3%–15% of the cases. Gadow and Kalachnik (1981) found that 4.5% of these children were receiving medication for behavioral problems and that an additional 1.8% were taking drugs for both behavioral problems and seizures, whereas Aman et al. (1985) found that 3.4% of the "special school" children in New Zealand were receiving psychotropic medication. Finally, Došen (1982) found that of the 500 retarded children, ages 3–16, who were referred to a diagnostic clinic for behavioral and psychiatric disorders, 15% were using psychotropic drugs. This contrasts with an estimated drug use with nonretarded youngsters of between 1% and 2% (Gadow and Kalachnik 1981; Safer and Krager 1983).

Despite these high and widely varying rates, prescribing psychotropic drugs for mentally retarded children remains a controversial issue, the concerns being occasional abuse, limitations in effectiveness, poor research methodology, and unpredictability of responses, particularly in children with organic dysfunctions (Aman and Singh 1980; Campbell et al. 1982; Ellis and Singh 1996).

This chapter aims to address the issues of indications for the use of drugs, target behaviors, common side effects, dosage, duration of use, and monitoring of efficacy.

■ INDICATIONS

Psychostimulants

In the United States, psychostimulants—methylphenidate in particular—are commonly prescribed for mentally retarded children, especially those with mild retardation (Aman et al. 1991) and those suffering from attention-deficit/hyperactivity disorder (ADHD) or exhibiting symptoms of disruptive and impulsive behavior and conduct disorder. Stimulant medications are also prescribed for children with autism and pervasive developmental disorder who often exhibit the characteristic symptoms of ADHD.

The doses of methylphenidate usually vary between 0.3 and 1 mg/kg/day (Aman et al. 1991; Handen et al. 1994). Until recently, very few studies had investigated the behavioral and cognitive response to stimulants in children with mental retardation and ADHD. According to some investigators these children have a lower rate of favorable response to stimulants than do normally developing children with ADHD. Recently, Pearson and colleagues (1996) reported findings on the effect of methylphenidate on behavioral adjustment in 13 children with mental retardation and ADHD using a double-blind, placebo-controlled crossover design. Results revealed significant declines in ADHD symptomatology (e.g., inattention, hyperactivity), with the most significant declines appearing at the dose of 0.6 mg/kg/day. Handen and colleagues (1996) investigated effects of stimulant medication on work and learning in 44 children with moderate to borderline retardation and ADHD, applying a double-blind, placebo-controlled trial of methylphenidate 0.3 and 0.6 mg/kg/day doses. Significant gains in on-task behavior such as attention and activity tended not to occur until the dose 0.6 mg/kg was reached. However, the improvements in behavior did not appear to lead necessarily to gains in work output and accuracy or learning. Additionally, improvements on measures of learning do not appear to be associated with the dose of the drug but with the additional use of behavioral interventions such as token economy and a reinforcement program.

The authors concluded that children with mental retardation and ADHD require supplemental training programs such as the teaching of special learning strategies to take full advantage of gains resulting from stimulant medication. Reviewing recent reports on the use of stimulant drugs in children with mental retardation and ADHD, Aman (1996) suggested that there is evidence that the response rates of these children seem to be somewhat lower than those of ADHD children with normal IQ. The difference in response rates appears to be even greater in children of moderate and severe retardation levels (Aman et al. 1991, 1993; Beale and McDowell 1994). It is also noteworthy that relatively weak clinical effects were observed in studies assessing psychostimulants in normal IQ children of preschool age (Arnold et al. 1998). The same variables may be moderating the response to the stimulants of the children of this young age as well as of children with retarded development (Aman 1996). Children with mental retardation may also have a greater risk of side effects than normally developing children treated with psychostimulants (Arnold et al. 1998). The side effects described are social withdrawal, motor tics, irritability, anxiety, and stereotypic behavior (Handen et al. 1991, 1999).

The efficacy of stimulants in autistic children is not very impressive. Although some positive results have been reported, there are also reports describing adverse responses such as overactive and stereotypic behavior, agitation, motor tics, and other problems (Aman 1993, 1996). Poor results of stimulant medication have also been mentioned with regard to children with fragile X syndrome and ADHD (Hagerman et al. 1988; Hilton et al. 1991).

According to Aman (1993, 1996), it is likely that the mental age and IQ of the child may serve as predictors of his or her response to psychostimulants. This might mean that cognitive, developmental, or psychological factors have a moderating effect on the response to these drugs.

Guidelines for the Use of Psychostimulants

With respect to the prescription of psychostimulants for children with mental retardation, the situation is more complex than it is with nonretarded children. Various developmental, biological, and cognitive factors may moderate the efficacy of the drugs. Children with more severe retardation and more biological disorders of the central nervous system (CNS) are more at risk of responding negatively and of having more side effects (Campbell and Cueva 1995). The recommended dose of methylphenidate is approximately 0.6 mg/kg/day.

Antidepressants

There are several types of antidepressants. The oldest types are monoamine oxidase inhibitors (MAOIs) and tricyclic antidepressants (TCAs). So far, the MAOIs have only been used sporadically with children and even less often with those who are mentally retarded. TCAs and, more recently, other heterocyclic antidepressants have received an increasing amount of attention from investigators in the field of mental retardation. Currently, selective serotonin reuptake inhibitors (SSRIs) are increasingly being used with persons with mental retardation. Tryptophan has also been used—alone or in combination with other drugs such as carbidopa—for the treatment of depression in mentally retarded children (Došen 1990). Favorable results with tryptophan have been reported in children with Lesch-Nyhan syndrome (Gualtieri 1989). Minimal side effects are an important advantage. The efficacy of the drug, however, is still questionable, particularly in Lesch-Nyhan syndrome (Aman 1993). Antidepressants are usually prescribed in mentally retarded children for depression, anxiety disorders, ADHD, and obsessive-compulsive disorder (OCD).

Depression

According to some authors (Corbett 1985; O'Quinn 1988; Reid 1989), tricyclic antidepressants are no more and no less effective with mentally retarded children than with nonretarded children with a depressive illness. Došen (1982) reported that the use of imipramine and amitriptyline in 12 depressed children (the dose was not higher than 2.5 mg/kg/day) resulted in positive effects for 9 of them. Ghaziuddin et al. (1991) reported positive results with fluoxetine (30 mg/day) in 2 depressed retarded adolescents who had a perversive developmental disorder. Open trials (Petti and Conners 1983) suggest that antidepressants may be a promising means of treatment, but, so far, little systematic evaluation has been carried out. Some investigators stress that the efficacy of antidepressants in depressed youths is quite circumscribed, and their superiority to placebo remains unproven (Ambrosini et al. 1993; Sovner et al. 1998).

Because some children may respond to antidepressant therapy, some clinicians recommend treatment initiation with a heterocyclic agent such as desipramine or selective serotonin reuptake inhibitor therapy (Sovner et al 1998).

Anxiety Disorder

Separation anxiety disorders, panic disorders, and school phobia probably occur quite frequently among mentally retarded children. In spite of that, the treatment studies of these anxiety states have so far only been done with nonretarded children. Several authors (Berney et al. 1981; Klein et al. 1992) have concluded that imipramine was not superior to placebo with nonretarded children.

ADHD

Investigations of the effects of antidepressants on mentally retarded children diagnosed as having ADHD are rare. Hilton et al. (1991) described imipramine treatment with a 6-year-old, mildly mentally retarded, fragile X syndrome boy with the symptoms of hyperactivity, distractibility, poor attention span, lack of concentration, and insomnia. Previous treatment with methylphenidate had yielded poor results. The dose of imipramine was gradually increased to 1.15 mg/kg/day and later to 2.4 mg/kg/day. The results were positive, and improvements in sleep, attention, and hyperactivity were noted. Also, several open and controlled trials have addressed the issues of desipramine and nortriptyline. Studies of fluoxetine and other SSRI agents showed at least a moderate improvement. The dose of fluoxetine was between 20 and 60 mg/day (Sovner et al. 1998).

OCD

There are several reports on the use of antidepressants with mentally retarded children suffering from OCD and pervasive developmental disorders. Cook et al. (1992) described the open trial treatment of 16 children with fluoxetine. The dose varied from 20 mg every other day to 80 mg/day. The majority of subjects improved. A number of side effects were reported (with some of the children), including hyperactivity, restlessness, insomnia, and a decreased appetite. Gordon et al. (1992) reported on a double-blind crossover trial of clomipramine and desipramine with a group of 7 children in which clomipramine was superior to desipramine and the placebo control in treating compulsive behavior. The results of the use of these compounds for young autistic children were unfavorable (Campbell and Cueva 1995).

Guidelines for the Use of Antidepressants

Although the superiority of antidepressant therapy over placebo has not been demonstrated, some children may well respond positively to these medications and in particular to TCA or SSRI agents. In ADHD children, TCAs may be indicated when the disorder coexists with mood and anxiety disorders. Antidepressants may also have a beneficial effect on children with OCD. The recommended dosage for TCAs is approximately 3.0 mg/kg/day. With doses exceeding 3.5 mg/kg, cardiovascular toxicity may occur (Geller et al. 1999). In children with severe and profound retardation, doses of 3 mg/kg may cause irritability, hyperactivity, and a behavioral deterioration. The fluoxetine dose recommended is approximately 20 mg/day.

Antimanics

The antimanics medications include lithium and anticonvulsants such as carbamazepine, valproic acid, and clonazepam. These compounds have been used for manic and bipolar and also for depressive states, but there have been few studies of their use with mentally retarded children. These drugs also have been prescribed for severe behavioral disorders such as aggressive or self-injurious behavior (SIB) (see Chapter 16 of this book).

Lithium

Currently, lithium is considered to be the primary prophylactic maintenance treatment for preventing or reducing manic and depressive episodes. The

U.S. Food and Drug Administration (FDA) advises against the use of lithium in children younger than 12 years of age (Jefferson 1982). Studies of the use of the drug with mentally retarded children are sparse. Kastner et al. (1990) reported unsuccessful treatment of mentally retarded children with bipolar disorder because of side effects. Došen (1982, 1990) reported positive effects in two of three adolescents treated for bipolar disorders: the prophylaxis blood levels were 0.4–0.6 mmol/L (Došen 1982). Side effects with therapeutic blood levels (0.6 and 1.0 mmol/L) may be numerous (e.g., incontinence, sedation, tremor, nausea, hypothyroidism) (Campbell and Cueva 1995). Besides treating mood disorders, lithium has been indicated for aggression, SIB, and ADHD. Other authors (Frommer 1968) have reported predominantly good results when lithium was administered to nonretarded children ages 5–14 years.

Anticonvulsants

The discovery of the beneficial effects of anticonvulsants (e.g., carbamazepine, valproic acid, clonazepam) on the major affective disorders has opened up new possibilities for the treatment of these disorders. It seems that these compounds may have beneficial effects on persons with underlying organic CNS disorders. This may be a rationale for use of these drugs on severely and profoundly retarded children who display significant maladaptive behaviors, for such behaviors may reflect underlying organic disorders or organically based disorders. Studies of carbamazepine in affective disorders of children are rare, and the same is true for valproic acid and clonazepam in mentally retarded children; these are limited to descriptions and anecdotal reports. Barrett et al. (1979) treated an 11-year-old girl with a history of self-injurious and disruptive behavior with carbamazepine; the blood level of carbamazepine was 7.5 mmol/L. The results were positive. McCrocken and Diamond (1988) also report a positive outcome for the use of carbamazepine on an 18-year-old adolescent suffering from atypical bipolar disorder and mild mental retardation. Side effects are common, including diplopia, ataxia, headache, dizziness, and others (Campbell and Cueva 1995).

According to Sovner (1991), valproic acid may be the first treatment of choice for chronic mania and rapid-cycling bipolar disorder. Studies of the use of this drug with mentally retarded children are scarce. The same is true for clonazepam, which has also been administered for Tourette's syndrome. Negative effects of these drugs have also been mentioned. Valproic acid may cause nocturnal enuresis and have adverse effects on learning. Clonazepam may cause sedation and disinhibition. Further investigation of the use of anticonvulsants with mentally retarded children with severe behavioral problems is very important.

Neuroleptics (Antipsychotics)

The neuroleptic drug most often used with mentally retarded children is thioridazine (Aman et al. 1991). Other neuroleptics frequently administered to this group of children are chlorpromazine, haloperidol, pimozide, and pipamperone (outside of the United States). These drugs are usually prescribed for psychotic states, affective disorders, Tourette's syndrome, and ADHD and for disruptive behaviors such as aggressiveness, SIB, hyperactivity, and impulsivity.

There seems to be little difference in the efficacy of the various antipsychotics. But there are reasons for preferring high-potency drugs such as haloperidol and pimozide over the less potent ones such as thioridazine and chlorpromazine, which are more sedating, are prone to impair cognition, cause drowsiness, and (in the case of chlorpromazine) lower the seizure threshold (Aman et al. 1991; Campbell et al. 1994). Some authors recommend an average dosage of 2.5 mg/kg/day of thioridazine and chlorpromazine for the treatment of hyperactivity and impulsivity; the side effects reported are drowsiness, enuresis, and a dry mouth. Higher doses (mean 5 mg/kg/day) are not more effective (Campbell et al. 1994) than lower doses. For nonretarded children, the thioridazine doses usually recommended are 1.5–3.5 mg/kg/day.

Haloperidol was found to be effective in low doses of 0.025–0.05 mg/kg/day in reducing behavioral symptoms. Higher doses (of 0.05 mg/kg/day) that are used for psychotic conditions were associated with more side effects, especially dystonia (Campbell et al. 1994). Pimozide is effective in some cases of social withdrawal and severe existential anxiety at a dosage of 0.05 mg/kg/day. Side effects hardly ever occurred, and the positive effects described were a reduction in anxiety, improved social contact, and an increase in interactions with the surroundings (Došen 1988).

Reports on the use of new neuroleptics such as clozapine and risperidone in children are scarce. Clozapine may yield good results in nonretarded psychotic adolescents (Campbell and Cueva 1995; Campbell et al. 1999). Recently, there have been some reports on the use of risperidone for adolescents with schizophrenia (Quintana and Keshavan 1995). In one such report, three of four patients showed improvement in negative symptoms without side effects. Other investigators (Hardan et al. 1996) described good results with risperidone in 13 of 20 mentally retarded children and adolescents (ages 8–17); the target symptoms were hyperactivity, aggression, oppositionality, SIB, impulsivity, and others. Some other studies (Connor and Posever 1998; Demb and Espiritu 1999; Nicolson et al. 1998) reported good response to risperidone in children ages 4–18 years with similar target symptoms. The average dose was 1–4 mg/day. The side effects were excessive weight gain, orofacial dyskinesia, extrapyramidal symptoms, and sedation.

All in all, the preliminary results of the use of these new drugs appear to be promising; however, further critical assessment of the efficacy and safety is needed.

Guidelines for the Use of Neuroleptics

There is a general consensus that neuroleptics are indicated as first-line intervention in cases of psychotic disorders. For anxiety, hyperactivity, and behavioral disorders, neuroleptics may be used during second- or third-line interventions. For the high-potency drugs, low doses and short-term use are recommended.

Sedatives and Anxiolytics

The benzodiazepines (diazepam, oxazepam, lorazepam) have been prescribed for mentally retarded children who exhibited motoric restlessness, excitability, irritability, tantrums, fearfulness, and sleeping problems. Their use is, however, controversial, and adverse effects have been reported, especially in younger children and children with evident brain damage. A paradoxical increase in motoric restlessness has been described. Side effects are often dependent on the dose and the length of use of the drug—the risk of adverse reactions increases with higher doses and lengthier use. Because problems of dependence and discontinuance are highly correlated with length of administration, benzodiazepines should not be used in excess of 4 months; shorter periods are desirable (American Psychiatric Association 1990).

Anticonvulsants

The main group of anticonvulsants that are usually administered to mentally retarded children for controlling epilepsy are carbamazepine, valproic acid, clonazepam, phenobarbitone, and phenytoin sodium. As stated earlier, these drugs may have a psychoactive effect as well as various side effects. For clinical purposes it is important to know what the side effects are, particularly when drugs other than anticonvulsants are also being prescribed (see Chapter 14 of this book).

Other Psychoactive Drugs

Clonidine is an antihypertensive agent and acts as an α-adrenergic agonist. In the brain, it produces a reduction in arousal, influencing the dopaminergic and serotonergic systems as well. The clinical indications for this drug are Tourette's syndrome, ADHD, anxiety, and aggression (Hagerman et al. 1998; Szymanski and King 1999). Studies of the use of this compound as used with mentally retarded children are rare. Hagerman et al. (1998) assume that, according to preliminary studies, clonidine could be useful in the treatment of behavior problems and hyperactivity in mentally retarded and autistic children. In particular, clonidine may be helpful in hyperactivity associated with overarousal, tics, and sleep disturbance. A mean dose is 0.005 mg/kg/day. The most common side effects include dry mouth, drowsiness, dizziness, constipation, and sedation.

β-*adrenergic blockers* are usually used for treating cardiovascular conditions. For mentally retarded youngsters, this compound is indicated when aggressive disorders, anxiety disorders, and akathisia (a side effect of neuroleptics) are present (Szymanski and King 1999). Propranolol and atenolol are the drugs most often used. In four—although uncontrolled—studies of children and adolescents, a mean dose of 150 mg/day was prescribed (Werry and Aman 1994). Commencing with 10 mg twice daily, the dosage was increased by 10–20 mg every 3–4 days to the upper limit of between 120 and 214 mg/day. Blood pressure should be monitored and maintained above 90/60, and the heart rate should be kept at more than 60 beats per minute. Side effects may be dysphoria, vomiting, insomnia, dizziness, and hallucinations.

Fenfluramine is an amphetamine analogue that was originally used as an adjunct in the treatment of obesity. The drug has been researched extensively with autistic children (Werry and Aman 1994). Because fenfluramine is a serotonin-depleting agent, the investigators presumed that this drug could reduce the high levels of serotonin in the blood of autistic subjects, the consequence being the diminution of autistic symptoms (Gillberg et al. 1998). The predominant findings of the studies of fenfluramine with autistic children indicate that despite the initially positive findings of an increase in IQ and adaptive behavior in well-controlled studies, there was little support for these findings in later studies; that some improvement in stereotypic and ritualistic behavior can be seen; that there is an improvement in overactivity and inattention; and that there is no improvement in speech and communication.

Mentally retarded children who were not autistic showed improvements in the amount of aggression, food-related behavior (in Prader-Willi syndrome), and ADHD (Werry and Aman 1994). Most studies used standardized doses of 1.5 mg/kg/day, starting at 0.5 mg/kg/day, increasing to 1.5 mg/kg/day within 2 weeks. The most commonly reported side effects were anorexia, sedation, irritability, sleep difficulties, and dizziness (Aman et al. 1993).

The use of fenfluramine is still controversial because some studies suggested the occurrence of irreversible neurochemical changes, such as depletion of brain serotonin. These findings, however, have not been confirmed in well-controlled studies (Gillberg et al. 1998; Werry and Aman 1994).

Opiate blockers are naloxone and naltrexone. An extensive review of these drugs is provided in Chapter 16 of this book. So far, naltrexone appears to be a promising agent for treating SIB, although it is not known if it is more effective than the other psychoactive agents.

■ TARGET BEHAVIORS

Various investigators have observed that only about one-fourth of the mentally retarded persons who receive psychotropic medication have a psychiatric diagnosis (Bregman 1991; Jacobson 1988; Kiernan et al. 1995). The drugs are most often prescribed to combat particular behaviors that could not be tolerated by others, principally aggression, SIB, destructive behavior, hyperactivity, withdrawal, and sleep disorders.

Aggression is a behavioral feature that is encountered frequently in mentally retarded children. A study (Harris 1993) found a 12.6% prevalence rate of aggression among severely retarded children attending special schools. The most frequently used drugs with these children are haloperidol, chlorpromazine, lithium, β-blockers and more recently risperidone. Most studies reported beneficial effects. However, methodological shortcomings—including small sample size and lack of randomization and placebo control—are obvious drawbacks.

SIB is reported to occur among approximately 10% of the mentally retarded children and adolescents (Oliver et al. 1987; see also Chapters 16 and 18). Various drugs have been used including neuroleptics, sedatives, antidepressants, lithium, and anticonvulsants, and, more recently, serotonin reuptake blockers (e.g., fluoxetine), opiate blockers (e.g., naltrexone), and β–blockers (e.g., propranolol) (see Chapters 3 and 16 of this book). Results differ from investigator to investigator, and so far no one drug appears to produce significantly better results than the others (Szymanski and King 1999). According to Aman (1993) there is evidence that thioridazine, lithium carbonate, and opiate blockers can be effective in SIB.

Destructive behavior has often been reported by investigators. Drugs similar to those used for aggression have been used to combat this behavioral feature; the results are varied.

Hyperactivity and ADHD are common traits in mentally retarded children and adolescents and occur in approximately 10%–20% of the patients (Aman et al. 1996). Often, this disorder in this population of children is associated with behavioral and emotional problems that include conduct disorders and separation anxiety disorder, among others (Aman et al. 1996). For these children, stimulants as well as other drugs such as antidepressives, neuroleptics, anticonvulsants, and sedatives have been used (Aman et al. 1993, 1996; Campbell et al. 1994; Handen et al. 1999; Hilton et al. 1991; Werry and Aman 1994).

Withdrawal, a feature that usually occurs among autistic children, also occurs among nonautistic children who suffer from psychotic or depressive conditions (Došen 1990). For these children the neuroleptic pimozide is reported to have favorable effects (Došen 1988). Recently, opiate blockers have also been reported to positively influence the attachment behavior of autistic children (Campbell et al. 1989).

Sleep disorders occur among mentally retarded children with a frequency that ranges from 34% to as high as 61% (Clements et al. 1986; Quine 1991). Hogg (1992) found that 57.1% of 641 profoundly retarded children and adolescents ages 2–20 years had sleep disturbances for which 28.5% were receiving sedatives (such as diazepam, nitrazepam, and trimeprazine). Administering hypnotic drugs to treat the sleep disorders of mentally retarded children has been viewed as being inappropriate (Quine 1991). Because of the possible dependency, benzodiazepines should only be administered with caution. Recently, in clinical practice with nonretarded children, clonidine has been found to be useful for both primary and secondary sleep disorders (Campbell and Cueva 1995).

Some authors (Lancioni et al 1999) have reported beneficial results using melatonin in treatment of sleep disorders among children and adolescents with severe mental retardation (2.5–5 mg/day, starting with 0.5 mg/day).

This overall picture gives the impression that most compounds are being used for different targets, and that each of these drugs probably has a nonspecific effect on the particular target behavior. However, several drugs (such as the stimulants, opiate blockers, and pimozide) apparently have more specific efficacy with particular behavioral problems. Evidence of the specificity of efficacy of the various drugs in counteracting well-defined behavioral problems is at best tentative at this time due to the paucity of well-controlled studies.

■ SIDE EFFECTS

Investigators in the field of mental retardation are convinced that mentally retarded children may probably react to psychotropic drugs differently than nonretarded children (Aman et al. 1993; Cambell et al. 1994; Gardner Wilson et al. 1998; Hilton et al. 1991). These differences are manifold and are linked to dosage, efficacy, and side effects, and they are apparently linked to underlying biological impairments such as physiological aberrations (epilepsy, perceptual difficulties) or disturbed CNS maturational rates.

It is important for the practitioner to be well informed about the chronological and mental age of the child as well as about any biological and physiological disorders before prescribing drugs. Children at lower developmental levels who have more significant disorders of the CNS are, for example, particularly susceptible to aberrant reactions and side effects. The side effects that occur most frequently are the following:

1. Short-term side effects

    - Extrapyramidal phenomena such as acute dystonia, pseudoparkinsonism, and catatonia-like states when neuroleptics are used
    - Paradoxical reactions when sedatives (particularly benzodiazepines) and hypnotics are used
    - Decrease in motivation and cognition

2. Long-term side effects

    - Tardive dyskinesia
    - Withdrawal and apathy
    - Impairment in school performance
    - Decrease in favorable reactions to other sorts of treatment such as psychotherapy and social training

Psychostimulants

In addition to the well-known side effects of psychostimulants, there is evidence that mentally retarded children may react to these with restlessness and anxiety and may develop a psychotic state (Barkley et al. 1994). In severely retarded children, an increase in stereotyped behavior has also been observed (Aman et al. 1995; Corbett 1985). Increase of self-injury has also been found (Aman et al. 1995). As reported above, the usefulness of this agent for the more severely retarded children is questionable.

Antidepressants

Besides the TCA side effects of ECG changes and dry mouth, there are also reports of paradoxical aggressivity and SIB in cases of more severe retardation or organic CNS damage. Some authors report increased agitation, irritability, anxiety, and stereotypical behaviors when fluoxetine is used (Ghaziuddin et al. 1991). There is increased concern because of possible association of some tricyclic antidepressants (in particular imipramine and desipramine) with cardiovascular side effects and sudden death of several children using these compounds (not in excessively large doses) (Campbell and Cueva 1995; Geller et al 1999).

Antimanics

Lithium carbonate may cause a state of confusion, incontinence, decrease in seizure threshold, sedation, weight gain, acne, increased thirst, and swelling of the feet and ankles (Sovner and Hurley 1985). Besides liver, skin, and blood problems—which have been reported to be associated with the use carbamazepine—paradoxical behavioral reactions and behavioral deterioration have also been noted (Sovner 1990). Dizziness, sedation, and incoordination, in addition to allergic reactions and gastrointestinal problems, have been reported in cases treated with valproic acid (Sovner 1989).

Neuroleptics

Corbett (1985) has written that "It is often felt that retarded children showing psychotic symptoms require larger doses of these drugs than the normal child. Inadequate doses may exacerbate the behavioral symptoms and make the child more irritable; however, larger doses are prone to produce side effects such as oversedation, impairment of learning, and extrapyramidal effects including tremor, rigidity, and tardive dyskinesia" (p. 672).

Sedation and an impairment of cognitive functioning have been reported with low-potency drugs such as chlorpromazine and thioridazine, and dyskinesia, irritability, and depression in high-potency drugs such as haloperidol and pimozide. Nausea, vomiting, anorexia, euphoria, unstable moods, hyperactivity, aggression, and sleep disorders have all been reported in mentally retarded children following the commencement or abrupt discontinuation of these drugs (Gualtieri and Guimond 1981). Richardson et al. (1986) found that 15%–35% of the mentally retarded children and adults receiving neuroleptics developed tardive dyskinesia. Potential risk factors included young age, gender (females have a greater risk), and cumulative dose of neuroleptics. Tardive dyskinesia, when diagnosed early enough in children and adolescents, is often reversible if the medication is reduced or withdrawn once the problem is observed. This condition is known as *rebound dyskinesia*. (A detailed overview of this issue is given in Gardner Wilson et al. 1998).

Sedatives

Sedatives and hypnotics may cause paradoxical reactions such as restlessness, wakefulness, and irritability in severely retarded children. Barron and Sandman (1985) described the paradoxical reactions of the benzodiazepines with persons who exhibited SIB and stereotypy.

The side effects of the other psychoactive drugs that are usually used with mentally retarded children have already been described earlier in this chapter.

◼ DOSAGE, DURATION OF USE, AND MONITORING OF EFFICACY

On the one hand, mentally retarded children run a greater risk of developing troublesome side effects from psychotropic medications than nonretarded children (Aman and Singh 1980; Campbell and Cueva 1995; Došen 1977; Gardner Wilson et al. 1998; Sleator and Sprague 1978). On the other hand, the therapeutic range that particular medicaments have is apparently very small. This means that the dosage used with these children should be more accurately determined and adapted to the child's real needs. Individual differences may be even more marked in subjects with brain damage. Some authors (Corbett 1985) recommend that, whenever possible, an individualized trial should take place before the drug is used routinely with these children. In general, the aim should be monopharmacy. If a new drug is required, its introduction should be accompanied by withdrawal of the previous medication. The initial starting dose of the drug should be low and gradually increased until an optimal effect is achieved. Similarly, drugs should be withdrawn gradually. For example, in the case of neuroleptics, the medication should be administered in its minimally effective dose, and gradual discontinuation trials should be a standard part of the management. From 10% to 20% of the dose may be reduced in a period of 2–4 weeks. By using this procedure, the incidence of withdrawal dyskinesia may be reduced (Donaldson 1984). The chronic use of antiparkinson medication for the reduction of parkinson-like effects should be avoided as much as possible. In cases of pseudoparkinsonism, a better strategy would be the lowering of the dose of the neuroleptic. Antiparkinson drugs are indicated only when strictly necessary and only for as long as is necessary.

The patient's response to medication is often helpful in determining the severity of the overall problem. The dosage and effect should be accurately and regularly monitored and controlled. The fact that high doses are tolerated may support the contention that there is a serious underlying physiological cause for the behavioral or psychiatric disorder. If the physiological imbalance improves, then a lower dose is usually sufficient to maintain the improvement. A dosage that is too high or a particular dose that is given for too long can have counterproductive effects. Conversely, extreme sensitivity to a specific medication may be an indication that the neurotransmission activity, which is being blocked or enhanced, is not a significant cause of that patient's problem.

As to the duration of medication, it is important to note that, once prescribed, there is an improper but general tendency to continue prescribing drugs for mentally retarded persons for relatively long periods of time (several years). This can have a negative impact on the behavioral symptoms for which the drug was originally prescribed. By withdrawing a medication that has been used for a long time, Zimmerman and Heistad (1982) found that 60% of the patients responded with either stable or improved behavior. In another study (Došen 1982) of 100 mentally retarded children, the gradual discontinuation of medication resulted in a deterioration of behavior in only 10% of the cases.

Because important qualitative changes in psychological processing and behavior occur in children within a relatively short period of time, most clinicians agree that the duration of the use of psychotropic medication should not exceed 6 months. Extended administration can disturb natural developmental processes and hamper further therapeutic effects. Short duration is also to be preferred because of the increased risk of side effects with extended use. It is also important to recognize that the administration of a drug for too short a period of time or frequent changes in the dosage in a short span of time can cause adverse reactions. Psychotropic drugs have an impact on the neurotransmitter balance in the CNS, and one should be aware that after introducing, discontinuing, or changing the dose of a drug, days or even weeks are usually needed before a new biochemical homeostasis can be established. With these considerations in mind, one should avoid coming to rapid conclusions about the effects of any drug.

The indications for drug therapy should be based on a comprehensive psychiatric assessment and diagnosis. Whenever possible, it is wise to have a rating scale completed at least twice before initiating or changing therapy (Aman 1993). Unfortunately, there are currently few scales available for monitoring the behavior changes of mentally retarded children. Campbell (Campbell and Cueva 1995) recommends the use of the Abnormal Involuntary Movement Scale (AIMS) for mentally retarded children as well. Direct observation is also important for assessing the changes that may be the result of drug administration.

In day-to-day practice, it is most important to have a well-established and well-defined set of monitoring tools or a monitoring system. The decisions concerning changes in medicaments or doses should be based on data gathered systematically by different observers involved in the treatment. Such a system of control is essential for a rational approach to the drug treatment of mentally retarded children.

■ THE RATIONAL USE OF PSYCHOTROPIC DRUGS WITH MENTALLY RETARDED CHILDREN

Investigators are in agreement that the most commonly used psychotropic drugs tend to have general rather than specific effects on behavior. A detailed knowledge of the underlying biological causes of mental retardation and an assessment of secondary handicaps as well as other aspects of developmental problems are necessary for establishing the need for drug therapy. However, there is usually a general lack of information about the nature of the psychiatric problems of mentally retarded children, and, in addition, the problems are frequently very complex. Being unable to gain real insight into underlying psychopathological mechanisms, practitioners are inclined to prescribe drugs for the treatment of particular behavioral features on the basis of decisions grounded merely in casual experiences, anecdotes, or case descriptive information. Psychiatric diagnosis is usually lacking in such cases.

There is no longer any doubt that the psychiatric disorders as well as the aberrant behaviors of mentally retarded children are the consequences of both biological and psychosocial factors that influence each other and lead to mutually adverse resultants. It would not therefore be realistic to expect that medication alone—even when appropriately indicated—can generate the appropriate psychic condition and desired behavior. Many psychiatrically ill mentally retarded children have never known a period of normal behavior. Before the practitioner is able to correct such a patient's abnormal physiology by means of administering medication, years of additional work in an educational or psychotherapeutic setting are often required in order to overcome the developmental lags and improve the disturbed patterns of behavior. For example, with a psychotic child who is plagued by existential anxiety and social contact disturbance, a medication that provides respite (e.g., pimozide) may aid the establishment of the therapeutic relationship between the child and therapist. Once this relationship has been established, the medication may no longer be necessary and can thus be discontinued. In this example, the drug was not prescribed to treat the psychosis but merely to counter one factor that played a role in its genesis.

Children who, for example, have a major depression can certainly benefit from antidepressant drugs, but clinicians must also take those factors into account that have contributed to the behavioral patterns of the child as well. Some of the children may fail to improve on medication simply because their disorder has an unrelated etiology. In these cases it makes no sense to administer medication.

In short, psychotropic medication should be administered on the basis of a thorough psychiatric diagnosis and should only be used to normalize or optimize some aspects of the child's CNS physiology and conditions. Once this has been attained, therapeutic efforts can then shift toward behavioral, educational, and psychotherapeutic paths and interventions. Psychotropic medication may balance a neurobiochemical condition or diminish a particular stereotypy, but in all cases additional psychotherapeutic and pedagogic treatment are required. Only with this combination can clinicians expect to have a meaningful effect on the total behavior of a mentally retarded, mentally ill child.

■ CONCLUSIONS

The expectation that psychotropic drugs can improve the total behavior of a mentally retarded and mentally ill or behaviorally disturbed child is neither scientifically based nor confirmed in clinical practice. Psychopharmacotherapy can influence particular behavioral aspects and aid other therapeutic interventions, the target of which is the totality of social behavior. The choice of drug depends on the diagnosis and the aim of treatment. The effective dose of a psychotropic drug may be lower for mentally retarded children than for the nonretarded, and side effects may occur more frequently. Medication should be used as long as it serves its purpose (i.e., as a support to other treatment approaches) and should not be administered for more than 6 months. Accurate monitoring is essential.

More scientifically based studies of the effects of psychotropic drugs on mentally retarded children are needed.

■ REFERENCES

Aman MG: Efficacy of psychotropic drugs for reducing self-injurious behavior in the developmental disabilities. Ann Clin Psychiatry 5:171–188, 1993

Aman MG: Stimulant drugs in the developmental disability revisited. Journal of Developmental and Physical Disabilities 8(4):447–465, 1996

Aman MG, Singh NN: The usefulness of thioridazine for treating childhood disorders: fact or folklore? American Journal of Mental Deficiency 84:331–338, 1980

Aman MG, Field CJ, Bridgman GD: City-wide survey of drug patterns among noninstitutionalized retarded persons. Applied Research Mental Retardation 6:159–171, 1985

Aman MG, Marks RE, Turbott SH, et al: Methylphenidate and thioridazine in the treatment of intellectually subaverage children: effects on cognitive-motor performance. J Am Acad Child Adolesc Psychiatry 30:816–824, 1991

Aman MG, Kern RA, McGhee D, et al: Fenfluramine and methylphenidate in children with mental retardation and ADHD: clinical and side effects. J Am Acad Child Adolesc Psychiatry 32(4):851–859, 1993

Aman MG, Van Bourgondien ME, Wolford PL, et al: Psychotropic and anticonvulsant drugs in subjects with autism: prevalence and patterns of use. J Am Acad Child Adolesc Psychiatry 34:1672–1681, 1995

Aman M, Pejeau C, Osborne R, et al: Four year follow-up of children with low intelligence and ADHD. Research in Developmental Disabilities 17(6):417–432, 1996

Ambrosini PJ, Bianchi MD, Rabinovich H, et al: Antidepressant treatment in children and adolescents; I: affective disorders. J Am Acad Child Adolesc Psychiatry 32(1):1–6, 1993

American Psychiatric Association: Benzodiazepine Dependence, Toxicity, and Abuse: A Task Force Report. Washington DC, American Psychiatric Press, 1990

Arnold LU, Gadow KD, Pearson DA, et al: Stimulants, in Psychotropic Medications and Developmental Disabilities: The International Consensus Handbook. Edited by Reiss S, Aman MG. Columbus, Ohio, Ohio State University Nisonger Center, 1998, pp 229–258

Barkley RA, Du Paul GJ, Costello A: Stimulants, in Practitioners' Guides to Psychoactive Drugs for Children and Adolescents. Edited by Werry S, Aman M. New York, Plenum, 1994, pp 205–237

Barret RP, Payton JB, Burkhart JE: Treatment of self injury and disruptive behavior with carbamazepine (Tegretol) and behavior therapy. Journal of Multihandicapped Persons 1:79–91, 1979

Barron J, Sandman CA: Paradoxical excitement to sedative-hypnotics in mentally retarded clients. American Journal of Mental Deficiency 90:124–129, 1985

Beale IL, McDowell JE: Effects of methylphenidate on attention in children with moderate mental retardation. Journal of Developmental and Physical Disabilities 6(2):137–148, 1994

Berney T, Kolvin I, Bhate SR, et al: School phobia: therapeutic trial with clomipramine and short-term outcome. Br J Psychiatry 138:110–118, 1981

Bregman JD: Current developments in the understanding of mental retardation, part II: psychopathology. J Am Acad Child Adolesc Psychiatry 30(6):861–872, 1991

Campbell M, Cueva J: Psychopharmacology in child and adolescent psychiatry: a review of the past seven years, part I. J Am Acad Child Adolesc Psychiatry 34(9):1124–1132, 1995

Campbell M, Cohen IL, Small AM: Drugs in aggressive behavior. J Am Acad Child Psychiatry 21:107–117, 1982

Campbell M, Overall JE, Small AM, et al: Naltrexone in autistic children: an acute open dose range tolerance trial. J Am Acad Child Adolesc Psychiatry 28:200–206, 1989

Campbell M, Gonzales N, Ernst M, et al: Antipsychotics, in Practitioners' Guides to Psychoactive Drugs for Children and Adolescents. Edited by Werry S, Aman M. New York, Plenum, 1994, pp 269–296

Campbell M, Rapoport JL, Simpson GM: Antipsichotics in children and adolescents. J Am Acad Child Adolesc Psychiatry 38:537–545, 1999

Clements J, Wing L, Dunn G: Sleep problems in handicapped children: a preliminary study. J Child Psychol Psychiatry 27, 399–407, 1986

Connor DF, Posever TA: A brief review of atypical antipsychotics in individuals with developmental disabilitiy. Mental Health Aspects of Developmental Disabilities 1(4):93–102, 1998

Cook EHJ, Rowlett R, Jaselskis C, et al: Fluoxetine treatment of children and adults with autistic disorder and mental retardation. J Am Acad Child Psychiatry 31:739–745, 1992

Corbett J: Mental retardation, psychiatric aspects, in Child and Adolescent Psychiatry: Modern Approaches. Edited by Rutter M, Hersov L. London, Basil Blackwell, 1985, pp 661–678

Demb HB, Espiritu CRG: The use of risperidone with children and adolescents with developmental disabilities: effects on some common challenging behaviors. Mental Health Aspects of Developmental Disabilities 2(3):73–82, 1999

Donaldson JY: Specific psychopharmacological approaches and rationale for mentally ill mentally retarded children, in Handbook of Mental Illness in the Mentally Retarded. Edited by Menolascino FJ, Stark JA. New York, Plenum, 1984, pp 172–181

Došen A: Neuroleptica (en psychochirurgie) bij de behandeling van gedragsgestoorde zwakzinnigen. Tijdschrift Zwakzinnigenzorg, Autisme en Andere Ontwikkelingsstoornissen 4:182–198, 1977

Došen A: Ervaringen met psychofarmaca bij zwakzinnige kinderen. Tijdschrift Voor Kindergeneeskunde 50(1):10–19, 1982

Došen A: Psychofarmaca bij mentaal geretardeerde kinderen. Pharmaceutisch Weekblad 123:204–208, 1988

Došen A: Psychische en Gedragsstoornissen bij Zwakzinnigen. Meppel, Amsterdam, Boom, 1990

Ellis CR, Singh NN: Pharmacotherapy IV. Journal of Developmental and Physical Disabilities 8(4):287–290, 1996

Frommer EA: Treatment of childhood depression with antidepressants. BMJ (Clinical Research Ed) 1:729–732, 1968

Gadow KD: Pills and Preschool: Medication Usage With Young Children in Special Education. Chicago, IL, Illinois Council for Exceptional Children, 1975

Gadow KD: Prevalence of drug therapy, in Practitioner's Guide to Psychoactive Drugs for Children and Adolescents. Edited by Werry JS, Aman MG. New York, NY, Plenum, 1993, pp 57–74

Gadow KD, Kalachnik J: Prevalence and pattern drug treatment for behavior disorders of TMR students. American Journal of Mental Deficiency 85:588–595, 1981

Gardner Wilson J, Lott RS, Tsai L: Side effects; recognition and management, in Psychotropic Medications and Developmental Disabilities: The International Consensus Handbook. Edited by Riss S, Aman MG. Columbus, OH, Ohio State University Nisonger Center 1998, pp 95–114

Geller B, Reising D, Leonard HL et al: Critical Review of tricyclic antidepressants use in children and adolescents. J Am Acad Child Adolesc Psychiatry 38:513–516, 1999

Ghaziuddin M, Tsai L, Ghaziuddin N: Fluoxetine in autism with depression. J Am Acad Child Adolesc Psychiatry 30:508–509, 1991

Gillberg C, Aman MG, Reiss A: Fenfluramine, in Psychotropic Medications and Developmental Disabilities: The International Consensus Handbook. Edited by Riss S, Aman MG. Columbus, OH, Ohio State University Nisonger Center 1998, pp 303–310

Gordon CT, Rapport JL, Hamburger SD, et al: Different responses of seven subjects with autistic disorders to clomipramine and desipramine. Am J Psychiatry 149:363–366, 1992

Gualtieri CT: Mental retardation, in Treatments of Psychiatric Disorders. Edited by American Psychiatric Association Task Force. Washington, DC, American Psychiatric Press, 1989, pp 3–178

Gualtieri CT, Guimond M: Tardive dyskinesia and the behavioral consequences of chronic neuroleptic treatment. Dev Med Child Neurol 23:225–259, 1981

Hagerman R, Murphy MA, Wittenberger MD: A controlled trial of stimulant medication in children with the fragile X syndrome. Am J Med Genet 30:377–392, 1988

Hagerman R, Bregman J, Tirosh E: Clonidine, in Psychotropic Medications and Developmental Disabilities: The International Consensus Handbook. Edited by Reiss S, Aman MG. Columbus, OH, Ohio State University Nisonger Center, 1998, pp 259–270)

Handen BL, Feldman H, Gosling A, et al: Adverse side effects of methylphenidate among mentally retarded children with ADHD. J Am Acad Child Adolesc Psychiatry 30:241–245, 1991

Handen BL, Janasky J, McAuliff SM, et al: Prediction of response to methylphenidate among children with ADHD and mental retardation. J Am Acad Child Adolesc Psychiatry 33(8):1185–1193, 1994

Handen BL, MacAuliffe S, Caro-Martinez L: Stimulant medication effects on learning in children with mental retardation and ADHD. Journal of Developmental and Physical Disabilities 8(4):335–346, 1996

Handen LH, Feldman HM, Lurier A, et al: Efficacy of methilphenidate among preschool children with developmental disabilities and ADHD. J Am Acad Child Adolesc Psychiatry 38:805–812, 1999

Hardan A, Johnson K, Johnson C, et al: Case study: risperidone treatment of children and adolescents with developmental disorders. J Am Acad Child Adolesc Psychiatry 35(11):1551–1556, 1996

Harris P: The nature and extent of aggressive behaviors amongst people with learning difficulties (mental handicap) in a single health district. J Intellect Disabil Res 35:221–242, 1993

Hill BK, Lakin KC, Bruininks RH: Trends in residential services for mentally retarded people: 1977–1982. Journal of the Association of Persons With Severe Handicaps 9:243–250, 1984

Hilton DK, Martin CA, Heffron WM, et al: Imipramine treatment of ADHD in a fragile X child. J Am Acad Child Adolesc Psychiatry 30(5):831–834, 1991

Hogg J: The administration of psychotropic and anticonvulsant drugs to children with profound intellectual disability and multiple impairments. J Intellect Disabil Res 36:473–488, 1992

Jacobson JW: Problem behaviour and psychotic impairment within a developmentally disabled population; III: psychotropic medication. Res Dev Disabil 9:23–38, 1988

Jefferson JW: The use of lithium in childhood and adolescence: an overview. J Clin Psychiatry 43:174–177, 1982

Kastner T, Friedman DL, Plummer AT, et al: Valproic acid for the treatment of children with mental retardation and mood symptomatology. Pediatrics 86(3):476–472, 1990

Kiernan C, Reeves D, Albioz A: The use of antipsychotic drugs with adults with learning disabilities and challenging behavior. J Intellect Disabil Res 39(4):263–274, 1995

Klein RG, Koplewi HS, Kanner A: Imipramine treatment of children with separation anxiety. J Am Acad Child Adolesc Psychiatry 31:21–28, 1992

Lancioni GE, O'Reilly MF, Basili G: Review of strategies for treating sleep problems in persons with severe and profound mental retardation or multiple handicaps. Am J Ment Retard 104:170–186, 1999

McCrocken JT, Diamond RP: Case study: bipolar disorder in mentally retarded adolescents. J Am Acad Child Adolesc Psychiatry 27(4):494–499, 1988

Nicolson B, Awaid G, Sloman L: An open trial of risperidone in young autistic children. J Am Acad Child Adolesc Psychiatry 37:372–376, 1998

Oliver C, Murphy GH, Corbett JA: Self-injurious behavior in people with mental handicap: a total population study. Journal of Mental Deficiency Research 31:147–162, 1987

O'Quinn L: Medical treatment of psychiatric disorders in the handicapped, in The Psychiatry of Handicapped Children and Adolescents. Edited by Gering J, McCarthy L. Boston, MA, College Hill, 1988, pp 101–126

Pearson D, Santos C, Poache J, et al: Effects of methylphenidate on behavioral adjustment in children with mental retardation and ADHD. Journal of Developmental and Physical Disabilities 8(4):313–334, 1996

Petti TA, Conners CK: Changes in behavioral ratings of depressed children treated with imipramine. J Am Acad Child Adolesc Psychiatry 22:355–360, 1983

Quine L: Sleep problems in children with mental handicap. Journal of Mental Deficiency Research 35:269–290, 1991

Quintana H, Keshavan M: Case study: risperidone in children and adolescents with schizophrenia. J Am Acad Child Adolesc Psychiatry 34(10):1292–1296, 1995

Reid AH: Schizophrenia in mental retardation: clinical features. Res Dev Disabil 10:241–249, 1989

Richardson M, Haugland M, Pass R, et al: The prevalence of tardive dyskinesia in a mentally retarded population. Psychopharmacol Bull 22:243–249, 1986

Safer DJ, Krager JM: Trends in medication treatment of hyperactive schoolchildren. Clin Pediatr (Phila) 22:500–504, 1983

Sleator EK, Sprague RL: Pediatric psychopharmacology, in Principles of Psychopharmacology. Edited by Sleator EK, Sprague RL. New York, Academic Press, 1978, pp 575–591

Sovner R: The use of valproate in the treatment of mentally retarded persons with typical and atypical bipolar disorders. J Clin Psychiatry 50(3 suppl):40–43, 1989

Sovner R: Developments in the use of psychotropic drugs. Current Opinion in Psychiatry 3:606–612, 1990

Sovner R: Use of anticonvulsant agents for treatment of neuropsychiatric disorders in the developmentally disabled, in Mental Retardation: Developing Pharmacotherapies. Edited by Ratey JJ. Washington, DC, American Psychiatric Press, 1991, pp 83–106

Sovner R, Hurley A: Drug profiles; 1: lithium. Psychiatric Aspects of Mental Retardation Review 4:6–10, 1985

Sovner R, Pary RJ, Dosen A, et al: Antidepressant, in Psychotropic Medications and Developmental Disabilities: The International Consensus Handbook. Edited by Reiss S, Aman MG. Columbus, OH, Ohio State University Nisonger Center, 1998, 151–178

Szymanski L, King BH: Practice parameters for the assessment and treatment of children, adolescents and adults with mental retardation and comorbid mental disorders. J Am Acad Child Adolesc Psychiatry 38(suppl):5–31, 1999

Werry JS, Aman MG: Anxiolytics, sedatives, and miscellaneous drugs, in Practitioners' Guides to Psychoactive Drugs for Children and Adolescents. Edited by Werry S, Aman M. New York, Plenum, 1994, pp 391–416

Zimmermann RL, Heistad GT: Studies of the long term efficacy of antipsychotic drugs in controlling the behavior of institutionalized retardates. J Am Acad Child Psychiatry 21:136–143, 1982

25 Management of Pervasive Developmental Disorders

Thomas P. Berney, M.B., Ch.B., D.P.M.,
F.R.C.Psych., F.R.C.P.C.H.
John Corbett, F.R.C.P., F.R.C.Psych., D.P.M.

Autism has been dogged by the sense that there are hidden depths of ability to be discovered and released. This has given caregivers a sense of frustration that has made this spectrum of developmental disorders a fertile field for novel treatments. Some efforts, including specialized education (Rutter and Bartak 1973), early intervention (Schopler et al. 1982), and work with parents and caregivers (Howlin et al. 1973), have been subject to rigorous scientific evaluation and have stood the test of time. Others, including psychoanalysis, fenfluramine (Campbell 1988), holding therapy, and facilitated communication have come and largely gone. Each in turn has been advocated by charismatic enthusiasts with an almost religious zeal, and each, in turn, has failed to withstand a more scientific scrutiny. More will come; the blend of effective promotion, of Hawthorne and placebo effects, and of spontaneous remission and developmental improvement all combine to make it difficult to distinguish mirage and personal miracle from effective treatment. These must be replaced by controlled studies of better defined subjects with adequate follow-up, the whole carried out with a scientific detachment in a field in which the concepts and approaches are constantly evolving (Berney 2000).

Variations in the diagnostic criteria and method as well as in the population under study result in a varied diagnostic embrace. Autism encompasses a broad range of problems, differing in both form and severity, and, furthermore, it is associated with a great range of disability, particularly mental retardation. All this makes for a heterogeneous condition, both in presentation and in etiology. It is hypothesized that there is a basic cognitive defect running as a common thread through this cluster of conditions underlying the disparate problems of language, socialization, and behavior (Rutter 1983). The management of autism demands activity on two levels—first, to remedy the various

451

obvious symptoms of autism, and, second, to address the fundamental flaws, both psychological (relating largely to pathogenesis) and organic (which relate more to etiology), their identity depending on the therapist's theoretical standpoint.

The obvious symptoms include the triad of specific impairments of spontaneous and reciprocal social relationships; of language, particularly in meaning, which includes all aspects of communication but notably its spontaneity and social function; and of imagination expressed in play, activities, and relationships (Wing and Gould 1979) There are also many other symptoms, including obsessive interests, rituals, motor stereotypies, and perceptual problems (Happé 1994) as well as an overwhelming anxiety that may be associated with unexpected changes in the environment. These symptoms may lead to aggressive outbursts and self-injury in young children. When they persist, these problems are among the most difficult seen in adolescence and early adulthood when they may be associated with major depressive or psychotic illness.

Several candidates vie for primacy as the essential underlying psychological deficit; all relate to the difficulty in formulating concepts. Hobson (1993) has emphasized the inability to appreciate social and emotional cues and signals, which is part of a wider difficulty in the recognition of people as similar beings, the end results being a lack of empathy and emotional involvement. Baron-Cohen and colleagues (1989) point to the absence of a "Theory of Mind" as the root of a number of evils, although it is uncertain how universal or how early a deficit this is in autism, or, because it can be produced by early deafness, how specific it is. Ozanoff and colleagues (1991) suggest that a lack of executive function might be central. Frith (1989), in focusing on the failure of recognition of the overall pattern or context—the consequence being too literal an approach to everyday life—suggests that these are not necessarily mutually exclusive but that autism may represent a combination of deficits rather than a single fault.

Not all children within the spectrum of autistic disorder are aloof, isolated, or withdrawn, and many, including adults who have been aloof as children, may be affectionate, albeit in an inappropriate and superficial fashion. For this reason the term *pervasive developmental disorders*, first incorporated in DSM-III (American Psychiatric Association 1980), is used in ICD-10 (World Health Organization 1992) and DSM-IV (American Psychiatric Association 1994) to describe people with the basic triad of autistic impairments that are pervasive, both across various areas of development and across situations. This applies particularly to people with more severe degrees of mental retardation.

When it comes to etiology, a number of anatomical, physiological, and biochemical deficits have been linked to the pervasive developmental disorders. Some are probably secondary to the condition, but they beg the question as to how often autism is a genetic condition in its own right and how often it can emerge as the final common pathway for most of the causes of learning disability (Rutter et al. 1994). Accurate diagnosis of these underlying conditions (e.g., fragile X syndrome, tuberous sclerosis, Rett's syndrome) may have important implications for prevention and subsequent management.

There is a growing recognition that the disintegrative disorders may have an earlier onset than the definitive age of 2 years. This will cloud the diagnostic boundary with autism.

Heavily criticized (Wing and Ricks 1976), the Tinbergens (Tinbergen and Tinbergen 1972) believed autism to originate in high social anxiety that initially represents a predominance of innate avoidance over approach behavior. They postulated that this is reinforced by the natural but inappropriate parental response. The result is a child who is averse to either high or low levels of intrusiveness (Richer 1989; Williams 1996).

This theory is not far from the view that autism results from severe psychosocial deprivation, anchored in parental or familial disturbance, which encouraged a psychotherapeutic approach (Bettelheim 1967). Single-mindedly applied, it neglected the organic characteristics of autism, the natural tendency toward spontaneous improvement with age, and the secondary effects of the child's behavior on his or her family. Consequently, this theory has fallen into disrepute although there has been a revival under the guise of holding therapy.

Physical treatments, as well as psychotherapy, were encouraged owing to early confusion with schizophrenia. With the definitive separation of the two conditions in the early 1970s, many of these approaches were abandoned.

The behavioral approach developed in the 1960s, initially evolving from experimental approaches to the treatment of disturbed behavior, sought—with an educational emphasis—to widen the repertoire of self-help and social skills. A number of centers developed home-based preschool programs, notably in California (McEachin et al. 1993) and London (Howlin et al. 1987). North Carolina adopted a comprehensive approach in its statewide program for the Treatment and Education of Autistic and Related Communication Handicapped Children (Division TEACCH) encompassing work with families, schools, and the community as a whole (Schopler 1994). More clearly heard have become the voices of people who themselves fall within the spectrum of autism (Williams 1996).

■ ASSESSMENT

For most parents assessment is the starting point of a solution to their problems: the diagnostic label gives them a clear disorder with a blame-free etiology for their child's disturbed behavior, membership in a similarly afflicted group with national and international organizations, a package of potential remedies, and a better idea of prognosis. The process of assessment must address all these and also provide a baseline against which future progress can be measured.

Most instruments are designed to be used for the diagnosis rather than for the measurement of a person's progress. The protean manifestation of autism means that most are too crude to register quite significant changes. Thus, in the Childhood Autistic Rating Scale (CARS) (Schopler et al. 1988), the use of 15 very global categories means that although each item has a 9-point scale, it can overlook subtle, but significant, change. Assessment requires a combination of direct observation interview using an instrument such as the Autism Diagnostic Observation Schedule (ADOS) (Mahoney et al. 1998), psychometric testing, and caregivers' accounts that should include both global views and specific items. Appraisal should include more than simply the individual areas under treatment—skills, socialization, communication, and behavior—but also overall functioning in order to pick up the wider effect that a program might have on an individual's life. This appraisal must cover early childhhod as well as current state, with the interviewer using a framework such as the Autism Diagnostic Instrument (ATI) (Le Couteur et al. 1989).

Motivation and generalization are special problems; therefore, any assessment must take into account the spontaneity of performance and be across several settings. Here it is important to distinguish innate change, which can generalize to other settings, from the superficial change that is simply a response to an altered environment. Any appraisal must take into account natural, developmental change, both in the person and in the autism.

The extent of family satisfaction is an essential element as are more objective measures of improvement. The recognition of change often comes only after a temporal lag so that it may be several months before early, observable changes in specific aspects of behavior are reflected in the overall picture and recognized by the caregivers (Howlin et al. 1987).

Finally, it is long-term change that is important. It must be recognized that, for most forms of treatment, the early progress sets a pace that usually fails in the longer term.

■ GENERAL EDUCATION/TRAINING

Two pitfalls can result in unexpected effects. First, although an approach might stem from a single theoretical base, no therapy in practice is pure.

For example, a therapist might use a behavioral approach to language development but unwittingly, while developing a relationship, provide a model of behavior and evoke earlier relationships, giving a well rounded program. Second, it is essential that there is an appreciation of the more subtle disabilities of autism so that their interference can be reduced or circumvented. An example is an awareness of the sensory distortion and hypo- and hypersensitivity that sometimes may explain the irrational selectivity or anxiety.

The following is a summary of the essential elements of a teaching program (Powers 1992; Rutter 1985):

1. Systematic and well structured, the program needs to be presented as a series of clearly defined steps, each addressing a specific target. Because of the difficulty in separating the key signal from the surrounding noise, only the essential cues should be given. There should be active participation so that the student learns by doing, and the process should be enjoyable and failure free. A balance has to be struck between understimulation and excessive demand.

2. Motivation is a fundamental problem. Rewards should be tailored to the student, harnessing the person's own special interests. Intermittent reinforcement is more effective than continuous reinforcement. Punishment is dangerous, the more so because it may not be received in the spirit the caregiver intended. Thus pain may be perceived as pleasurable and an angry outburst as excitement (Matson and Sevin 1994a). In addition, it is too easy to slip into a punitive response (Harris et al. 1996; Royal College of Psychiatrists 1995).

3. Generalization presents a major difficulty. To offset this, teaching should take place in multiple and varied settings so as to avoid getting into routines that are stimulus specific or situation specific. Experiences should be natural, meaningful, and directly relevant to everyday life, the focus being on the wider utility of any task rather than on rote learning and routine. Executive function is poor, so success should not depend on the student's initiative. At the same time and as far as is possible, the emphasis should be on self-direction, self-monitoring, and the independent use of skills so that, for example, the student might learn to talk him- or herself through situations.

4. Parent involvement is crucial. Long-term gains depend on the long-term caregiver (parent or residential worker) being the primary therapist. This means a home-based approach with the caregivers as cotherapists. The changing presentation of autism requires that the caregivers are constantly adapting and modifying their skills and strategies so that it requires sustained follow-up if gains are not to be lost. There is the risk that this may increase the burden of caring if not approached carefully. The relationship with the caregivers must be supportive and must adapt to a

number of roles (Schopler 1994).

5. Intervention should be early (Fenske et al. 1985) and intense (McEachin et al. 1993), although this facet has not yet been quantified.

Social Interaction

Social interaction may be fostered by personalized caretaking. Thus the approach should be home based or school based rather than institutional and involve siblings and peers. Activities need to be structured to be reciprocal and social (rather than solitary), making the caregivers essential to their completion. With many, particularly as the person gets older, the problem is not so much that of motivation—they want to have friendships—but one of a lack of skills. To some extent this can be helped by the formal teaching of social rules and skills using measures, such as joint/shared games, to teach turn taking and conversational gambits and topics. These can be rehearsed in role-play, and self-awareness can be increased, perhaps by using a mirror or video recording. However, in the end, the major handicap lies in the inability to perceive socioemotional cues (Hobson 1993; Rutter 1983). Throughout, it is essential to consider what is normal and useful; for example, it is not helpful to convert an aversive gaze to a fixed glare (Mirenda et al. 1983).

Holding therapy is based on the hypothesis that autism stems from excessive, innate avoidance behavior. Attachment is a two-way process, and, if discouraged by the child, it is unnatural for the parent to override this antipathy. Instead, the normal parental response amplifies this into the social impairment of autism—analogous to the avoidance of humans shown by wild animals. The Tinbergens, who formulated this model (Tinbergen and Tinbergen 1983), suggested that autism may be offset by "taming," a form of desensitization to people, but "holding," which has more in common with flooding, has taken its place (Richer and Zappella 1989a, 1989b). It is unclear whether the primary effect is on the caregiver or the patient. If effective, it is arguable that its punitiveness might do more harm than good and that there might be more humane ways of achieving the same ends (Fell 1988; Howlin 1989; Richer 1989).

Communication

The thrust of any program must be toward gaining useful speech, sign, or gesture, rather than mere empty words. Thus the aim is to improve social communication and the usage of language; as much effort must be put into improving comprehension as expression. A starting point might be to teach the child to point. Expressive speech might come from learning a range of simple sounds that can then be shaped into more complex words or might be built on echolalia speech. Although echolalia and jargon speech have a place in the development of language, they carry the risk of becoming entrenched and habitual, maintained by the responses of those around. This means that caregivers' speech must be reviewed as they may need to modify their style, escaping from habitual ways of talking to the person with autism. They frequently fail to use speech or else use too complex a form. Pragmatic language, like social skills, can be defined, simple rules given, and, with the help of role-play, usage improved. The resultant script, usually of appropriate roles supported by rules, might include whom to talk to, about what topics, and for how long.

Augmented communication can be helpful. Sign language may be an alternative for some, although children with autism may have particular difficulties in imitating gesture; as yet there is no clear guide as to whom it is suited. It is unlikely that a person whose language development (particularly comprehension) is severely limited is going to learn a complex sign language. At the other extreme, it is questionable how far someone who has some useful speech should be diverted from using it as a main avenue of communication. Concurrent teaching in both modalities can either help or hinder the development of speech, and, in the end, it is a matter of experiment to find what mode suits which person.

Written or idiographic representation, using pictures or symbols, may also be effective. An approach that has been vigorously explored is facilitated communication. This requires the physical assistance of another person—a specially trained facilitator—to introduce the technique to the person with autism, a process that may have to be continued for some years before the facilitator can withdraw. It assumes that, inherent to autism, there is a motor/volitional block that can be overcome if the person with autism is working against the physical resistance of a restraining hand coupled with the confidence engendered by the relationship with the facilitator.

However, carefully controlled studies overwhelmingly show that, for most, the technique has more in common with the Ouija board, expressing the facilitator's thoughts rather than those of the client (Gould 1993; Levine et al. 1994). And yet, the matter is not clear-cut as there is sometimes evidence of the subject's authorship. The subject groups were a diagnostic mixture and are not limited to autism. Second, the studies neglected the supportive quality of the relationship and the key part played by motivation: stage fright may be a major element in autism together with its well-recognized separation of involuntary and voluntary performance. We cannot depend on being certain, for any given time or persons, of the authorship of a communication. However, also relevant (although unreported) is the effect that this technique might have on an autistic person's longer term functioning, development, and overall welfare (Berney 1995).

Restricted, Repetitive Behavior

Stereotyped and ritualistic activities interfere with learning and are disruptive. It is unclear how much these have in common with an obsessive-compulsive disorder or how much they are a form of displacement activity representing exaggerated innate habits. The aim should be their reduction rather than their elimination. Success would result from the restriction of their extent, the diversion from other activities, and the enrichment of a boring environment. The aim is gradual change rather than direct confrontation of the behavior, helped by an increase in environmental structure, thereby making the person's world more predictable while ensuring that there are sufficient small changes in routines to accustom the person to variation. Older and more able people can learn to predict changes in routine.

Behavioral Problems

Aggression is a frequently occurring problem that may represent a means of communication or gaining attention or that may be the response to a perceived threat or boredom. Here it is important to appreciate that the perception and interpretation of the individual will be very different from what is normal. Standard behavioral responses, such as time-out, can prove to be a paradoxical reward to the person who wishes nothing more than to withdraw. Similarly, aversive stimuli can be misperceived even if the use of punishment was not a controversial area (Matson and Sevin 1994b). It is important that any strategy that is to be adopted is based on a sympathetic functional analysis of the underlying problem, made with the help of caregivers who know the person well, rather than adoption of a cookbook approach to the symptom.

Phobias are frequent and are more bizarre and intense than usually seen in normal childhood. An aversion to the head being touched is so frequent that it may reflect an earlier stage of hypersensitivity. Desensitization can be effective, particularly if the feared circumstance is mixed with something desired.

Sleep problems are frequent and may be the symptom of an affective disorder or a disturbed biological rhythm. The latter may be corrected by routine and training, possibly assisted by melatonin, although its use is still experimental (Lord 1998).

■ MEDICAL TREATMENT

Limited communication with an altered perception, particularly of pain, means that the first concern must be for the health of the person with autism. Illness, both physical and psychological, can be masked by the autism and, in turn, amplify it. Epilepsy will develop in 25%, and, in half of these, the onset will be after childhood (Gillberg 1991). Cyclical and affective disorders, not necessarily the same thing, are frequent (Berney and Jones 1988; DeLong and Nohria 1994). Effective seizure control or treatment of an affective disorder may transform the autism (DeLong and Aldershof 1987).

Views differ about the extent of routine baseline investigations. Few can be justified on the grounds of clinical benefit to the patient in the more able group, who has no physical stigmata and in whom medication is not contemplated. The use of medication warrants the collection of baseline values for those functions that are likely to be affected—blood count, liver function, and renal tests—as well as electroencephalography and electrocardiography. When there is clinical evidence of an organic etiology, as in people of low ability or with organic symptomatology, then investigation of this, including chromosomal and biochemical screens, is justified. It is questionable whether there is any justification for radiological and cerebrospinal fluid investigations except, and with the appropriate agreement, for research (Rutter et al. 1994).

The attitude toward drug treatment is often polarized because of doubt as to whether the benefits are justified compared with the risks of long-term side effects. The most widely used potent drugs have been the neuroleptics. Chlorpromazine proved too sedative, impairing learning as well as more general levels of functioning, and is also potentially epileptogenic. Thioridazine, reputedly less likely to cause tardive or withdrawal dyskinesia, is probably the most popular neuroleptic in the field of mental retardation in general and that of autism in particular. However, apart from one study that showed it to be effective for stereotyped behaviors, little of the evidence for its value derives directly from autism.

The hunt moved on, via the more stimulating and effective thiothixenes, to the butyrophenones, particularly to haloperidol, which has been systematically and carefully studied by the New York group (Perry et al. 1989) who has shown that it continues to work, improving a variety of symptoms for a long period of time (6 months) and with intermittent dosage (for 5 days in 7). Children with prominent irritability, anger, and uncooperativeness responded best but required a higher dosage. In the short term and in older children, neuroleptics were found to be effective in low dosage (less than 2 mg/day of haloperidol or fluphenazine) (Joshi et al. 1988). Currently, the newer neuroleptics, notably risperidone and olanzapine, are showing some promise, and clozapine is being tried in extreme forms of aggression (Possey and McDougle 2000).

Fenfluramine had a doubtful currency. Its use was based on the discovery of raised serotonin levels in autistic children, a distinction that disappeared when mental retardation was taken into account. Its value was not upheld by double-blind trials, and its effectiveness may simply have been the consequence either of dopamine blockade (achieved more efficiently by the neuroleptics) or of its action as a stimulant (Campbell et al. 1988). Toxicity led to its withdrawal, but its lesson of caution was soon forgotten in a tide of newer treatments.

The opioid hypothesis suggests that autism might arise from an early excess of active peptides that have a widespread effect on the hypophyseal-pituitary-adrenal axis. They might be endogenous (e.g., β-endorphin) or exogenous, the latter deriving from incompletely digested dietary proteins, gluten and casein being particularly suspect. Their access to the brain normally would be barred by a series of barriers, which include an impermeable bowel, the blood-brain barrier, or destruction by plasma peptidase. Whether autism results from opioid overload or from defective barriers, the hypothesis opens the door to a number of therapeutic approaches. Some success has been claimed for gluten- and casein-free diets (Reichelt et al. 1991). Bowel permeability may be altered by the administration of magnesium sulfate. Finally, the effect of opioids may be blocked by very low doses of naltrexone. Anecdotal success awaits independent confirmations and replication, although controlled trials have yielded only very modest improvements, largely in a reduction in hyperactivity (Campbell et al. 1993; Zingarelli et al. 1992). However, the trials used an intermediate dose, and it is possible that the clinical response to naltrexone may follow a U-curve, autism requiring a substantially lower dose than that recommended for self-injury.

Effectiveness has been claimed for a large number of other compounds, including vitamins. Here advocated are pyridoxine (B6 coupled with magnesium) (Rimland 1988), folate (Aman and Kern 1991), dimethylphenylglycine (DMPG), and tetrahydrobiopterin (Naruse et al. 1987). Analogue adrenocorticotrophic hormone (ORG 2766) is being explored by the Utrecht group (Buitelaar et al. 1992). Their reports show the extent to which a drug, rather than directly altering a behavior, modifies an individual's response to the environment.

A number of drugs treat associated symptomatology, for example, when autism is made worse by anxiety. When this is a major component, particularly in producing panic response, anxiolytics in general, and the β-adrenergic blockers in particular, can be very effective (Ratey et al. 1987).

All in all, the use of psychotropic medication should be limited to short-term use wherever possible, used as an adjunct to behavioral strategies, and accompanied by careful baseline assessment and measures of efficacy.

■ SUPPORT

Family Work

The parents require all the help necessary for the parents of a child with mental retardation (Bicknell 1983). To compound this, they have a child whose responses are disconcertingly different from those of most others, being less responsive and rewarding, often more disruptive, and much more perplexing and frustrating. There may be difficulty in distinguishing the problems arising from autism from the usual problems inherent in any person of the same age but particularly in adolescence. Caring for an autistic child is therefore difficult and may put unusual stress on a family and marriage. In addition, the advent of the disorder may have been after a period of apparently normal development, and matters may have been further inflamed by delayed diagnosis and, in the longer term, by a failure to respond to a particular program or strategy of management.

It is a natural tendency for parents to become overprotective and to feel guilty about not spending sufficient time with their child. It is difficult for anyone closely involved to be objective. Most helpful are an outside view, reassurance, practical ideas, and advice. Joining a parent support group and the National Autistic Society helps remove the sense of isolation as well as furnish practical ideas about specific forms of help and how to obtain these. Close liaison between staff and parents is essential to minimize the confusing inconsistencies in policy and attitude. As with other parents of children with a disability, help is required with the morass that is the system of benefits and services. However, the greater difficulty in finding suitable placements, particularly residential, means that parents have to confront many of these issues much earlier, adjustment being driven by an administrative rather than a clinical timetable.

Most cases of autism have a genetic basis, allowing some estimate of the probability of other children being affected. Investigation and counseling are important as in any other form of disability.

Services

Integration into mainstream education implies that the child is able to make use of a normal school environment. On the one hand, in autism the need for structure and predictability, the inability to take the initiative, and the difficulty in coping with other people combine to make the mainstream school unsuitable without considerable modification and support. On the other hand, specialized schools for children with autism have difficulty in providing a full range of curricular activities and opportunities for the more sociable child. With adolescence, often a time of setback, comes the need for a greater emphasis on coping with relationships, both social and sexual.

Later should come a combination of resources that might include further education or employment. Occupational/vocational services are essential as are the support and enthusiasm of a variety of people. Interagency disagreements usually result in the person with autism remaining at home with his or her parents. Whatever the placement, it has to be sufficiently structured and supported long enough to allow determination of its suitability.

■ OUTCOME

People with autism do improve, the more so the more able they are and the milder the initial autism (Szatmari et al. 1989). However, even of those within the normal range of intelligence and with useful language skills by the age of 5 years, only about one-half will be able to live independently—about 10%–15% of the total population with pervasive developmental disorders (Rutter 1970). This does not take account of the largely unrecognized population with Asperger's syndrome.

Gillberg (1991) has suggested that the mortality rate is increased in autism. In his study, almost 2% of those surviving the first 2 years of life had died before the age of 25 years. This is probably due to the increased rate of severe neurological disorders, such as tuberous sclerosis, in more disabled young people with autism.

Epilepsy also increases the risk of a poor outcome, being reported in 25%–30% of those followed up beyond adolescence (Gillberg 1991). About 10%–20% of the children show marked deterioration in behavior and cognitive ability during adolescence, which may be a particularly difficult time for the person with autism (Gillberg 1984). In some cases the deterioration may be associated with the onset of epilepsy, but this is not always the case. It does suggest that there is an underlying organic basis for the deterioration.

There have been two notable controlled studies of active intervention. The first, in London, compared 16 children with autism ages 3–11 years with groups of matched control subjects over a period of 18 months. A home-based intervention program, using the parents as the primary therapists, produced marked improvement in the nonspecific emotional and behavioral problems. However, the program effected little change in the core autistic elements of sociability, language, and rigid behavior, much of the change being the result of maturation and also occurring in the untreated control subjects. Treatment improved the use of existing language, amplifying such communication as was already budding and having a bilateral effect in developing usage in both child and mother (Howlin et al. 1987).

The second study, in California, reports the progress of 19 children with a mean age of 32 months and IQ of 53 (range 30–80) at the start of their intensive program. Again the parents were cotherapists, but the focus was on discrete trial learning carried out in the home for a 40-hour week by students over a minimum of 2 years. The long-term follow-up claims an average gain of 20 IQ points in the experimental group above the control subjects (McEachin et al. 1993). There has been substantial criticism of the methodology of the study, focused especially on whether the subjects were randomly allocated, the duration of the treatment, the demands on the family, and the actual mechanism of change. There is the assumption that all children will respond to the same type of program (discrete trial teaching being the effective element) with no allowance for the effect of altered family attitudes or the charisma of the therapist. However, in the end, the results are startling—with complete integration of 7 of the subjects into the normal educational system. Replication is awaited.

■ CONCLUSIONS

An autistic child brings forth so many responsibilities that it is difficult for parents to avoid being overwhelmed. Apart from the siren songs of therapeutic prophets, each claiming to preach the true cure, the need to navigate between a number of agencies—including health, social services, education, and a variety of charitable bodies—makes for a strong temptation to opt for residential placement.

The emphasis of treatment is all too often on the removal of undesirable behaviors. Of more importance is the fostering of normal development; the ability to integrate specific skills to engage in normal, intuitive social relationships; and, that grail of treatment, the enjoyment of the experience of life.

■ REFERENCES

Aman M, Kern RA: Mental retardation: the efficacy of folic acid in fragile X syndrome and other developmental disabilities. J Child Adolesc Psychopharmacol 1:285–299, 1991

American Psychiatric Association: Diagnostic and Statistical Manual of Mental Disorders, 3rd Edition. Washington, DC, American Psychiatric Association, 1980

American Psychiatric Association: Diagnostic and Statistical Manual of Mental Disorders, 4th Edition. Washington, DC, American Psychiatric Association, 1994

Baron-Cohen S: The autistic child's "theory of mind": a case of specific developmental delay. J Child Psychol Psychiatry 30:285–297, 1989

Berney TP: Autistic disorders. Current Opinion in Psychiatry 8(5):30–35, 1995

Berney TP: Autism: an evolving concept. Br J Psychiatry 176:20–25, 2000

Berney TP, Jones PM: Manic depressive disorder in mental handicap. Australia and New Zealand Journal of Developmental Disabilities 14(3 & 4):219–225, 1988

Bettelheim B: The Empty Fortress: Infantile Autism and the Birth of the Self. New York, Free Press, 1967

Bicknell J: The psychopathology of handicap. Br J Med Psychol 56:167–178, 1983

Buitelaar JK, Van-Engeland H, de-Kogel KH, et al: The use of adrenocorticotrophic hormone (4-9) analog ORG 2766 in autistic children: effects on the organization of behavior. Biol Psychiatry 31(11):1119–1129, 1992

Campbell M: Fenfluramine treatment of autism. J Child Psychol Psychiatry 29(1):1–10, 1988

Campbell M, Adams P, Small AM, et al: Efficacy and safety of fenfluramine in autistic children. J Am Acad Child Adolesc Psychiatry 27:434–439, 1988

Campbell M, Anderson LT, Small AM, et al: Naltrexone in autistic children: behavioral symptoms and attention. J Am Acad Child Adolesc Psychiatry 32(6):1283–1291, 1993

DeLong RG, Aldershof AL: Long-term experience with lithium treatment in childhood: correlation with clinical diagnosis. J Am Acad Child Adolesc Psychiatry 26(3):389–394, 1987

DeLong R, Nohria C: Psychiatric family history and neurological disease in autistic spectrum disorders. Dev Med Child Neurol 36(5):441–448, 1994

Fell R: The efficacy of holding therapy in the treatment of autism. Master of Science (Clinical Psychology) dissertation, University of Hull, UK, 1988

Fenske EC, Zalenski S, Krantz PJ, et al: Age at intervention and treatment outcome for autistic children in a comprehensive intervention program. Analysis and Intervention in Developmental Disabilities 5:49–58, 1985

Frith U: Autism: Explaining the Enigma. Oxford, UK, Blackwell, 1989

Gillberg C: Autistic children growing up: problems during puberty and adolescence. Dev Med Child Neurol 26:125–129, 1984

Gillberg C: The treatment of epilepsy in autism. J Dev Disord 21(1):61–77, 1991

Gould J: Facilitated communication: an overview. Communication 27(2):9–15, 1993

Happé FGE: Annotation: Current psychological theories of autism: the "theory of mind" account and rival theories. J Child Psychol Psychiatry 35(2):215–229, 1994

Harris K, Allem D, Cornich M: Physical Interventions: A Policy Framework. Kidderminster, UK, Bild Publications, 1996

Hobson RP: Autism and the Development of Mind. Hove, UK, Lawrence Erlbaum, 1993

Howlin P: Holding therapy: a reply to Richer and Zapella (letter). Communication 23(2):40, 1989

Howlin P, Marchant R, Rutter M, et al: A home-based approach to the treatment of autistic children. Journal of Autism and Childhood Schizophrenia 4:308–336, 1973

Howlin P, Rutter M, Berger M, et al: Treatment of Autistic Children. Chichester, UK, Wiley, 1987

Joshi PT, Capozzoli RN, Coyle JT: Low dose neuroleptic therapy for children with childhood-onset pervasive developmental disorder. Am J Psychiatry 145:335–338, 1988

LeCouteur A, Rutter M, Lord C, et al: Autism Diagnostic Interview: a standardised investigator based instrument. J Autism Dev Disord 19:363–367, 1989

Levine K, Shane HC, Wharton RH: "What if…" A plea to professionals to consider the risk-benefit ratio of facilitated communication. Ment Retard 32:300–304, 1994

Lord C: What is melatonin? Is it a useful treatment for sleep problems in autism? J Autism Dev Disord 28:345–346, 1998

Mahoney WJ, Szatman P, MacLean JE, et al: Reliability and accuracy of differentiating pervasive developmental disorder subtypes. J Am Acad Child Adolesc Psychiatry 37:278–285, 1998

Matson JL, Sevin JA: Issues in the use of aversives: factors associated with behavior modification for autistic and other developmentally disabled people, in Behavioral Issues in Autism. Edited by Schopler E, Mesibov GC. New York, Plenum, 1994a, pp 211–225

Matson JL, Sevin JL: Issues in the use of aversives, in Behavioral Issues in Autism. Edited by Schopler E, Mesibov GC. New York, Plenum, 1994b, pp 211–225

McEachin JJ, Smith T, Lovaas OI: Long-term outcome for children with autism who received early intensive behavioral treatment. Am J Ment Retard 97(4):359–372, 1993

Mirenda P, Donnelan A, Yoder N: Gaze behavior: a new look at an old problem. J Dev Disord 13:397–409, 1983

Naruse H, Hayahi T, Takesada M, et al: Therapeutic effect of tetrahydrobiotin in infantile autism. Proceedings of the Japanese Academy 63(B):231–233, 1987

Ozanoff S, Pennington BF, Rogers SJ: Executive function deficits in high-functioning autistic children: relationship to theory of mind. J Child Psychol Psychiatry 32(7):1081–1107, 1991

Perry R, Campbell M, Adams P, et al: Long-term efficacy of haloperidol in autistic children: continuous versus discontinuous drug administration. J Am Acad Child Adolesc Psychiatry 28(1):87–92, 1989

Posey DJ, McDougle CJ: The pharmacotherapy of target symptoms associated with autistic disorder and other pervasive developmental disorders. Harv Rev Psychiatry 8:45–63, 2000

Powers MD: Early intervention for children with autism, in Autism: Identification, Education, and Treatment. Edited by Berkell DE. Hillsdale, NJ, Lawrence Erlbaum, 1992, pp 225–252

Ratey JJ, Mikkelsen E, Sorgi P: Autism: the treatment of aggressive behaviors. J Clin Psychopharmacol 7:35–41, 1987

Reichelt KL, Knivsberg AM, Lind G, et al: Probable etiology and possible treatment of childhood autism. Brain Dysfunction 4(6):308–319, 1991

Richer J: Changing social behavior—the place of holding: a reply to Howlin. Communication 23(2):40–41, 1989

Richer J, Zappella M: Changing social behavior: the place of holding. Communication 23(2):35–39, 1989a

Richer J, Zappella M: Holding. Newsletter of the Association for Child Psychology and Psychiatry 11(1):3–9, 1989b

Rimland B: Controversies in the treatment of autistic children: vitamin and drug therapy. J Child Neurol 3(suppl):68–72, 1988

Royal College of Psychiatrists: Strategies for the Management of Disturbed and Violent Patients in Hospital. London, Royal College of Psychiatrists, 1995

Rutter M: Autistic children: infancy to adulthood. Seminars in Psychiatry 2:435–450, 1970

Rutter M: Cognitive deficits in the pathogenesis of autism. J Child Psychol Psychiatry 24(4):513–531, 1983

Rutter M: The treatment of autistic children. J Child Psychol Psychiatry 26(2):193–214, 1985

Rutter M, Bartak L: Special education treatment of autistic children: a comparative study; II: follow-up findings and implications for services. J Child Psychol Psychiatry 14:241–270, 1973

Rutter M, Bailey A, Bolton P, et al: Autism and known medical conditions: myth and substance. J Child Psychol Psychiatry 35(2):311–322, 1994

Schopler E: Behavioral priorities for autism and related developmental disorders, in Behavioral Issues in Autism. Edited by Schopler E, Mesibov GC. New York, Plenum, 1994, pp 55–77

Schopler E, Mesibov G, Baker A: Evaluation of treatment for autistic children and their parents. Journal of the American Academy of Child Psychiatry 21(3):262–267, 1982

Schopler E, Reichler RJ, Renner BR: The Childhood Autism Rating Scale (CARS). Los Angeles, CA, Western Psychological Services, 1988

Szatmari P, Bartolucci G, Bremner R, et al: A follow-up study of high-functioning autistic children. J Dev Disord 19(2):213–225, 1989

Tinbergen EA, Tinbergen N: Infantile autism: an ethological approach. Advances in Ethology 10:1–53, 1972

Tinbergen N, Tinbergen EA: Autistic Children: New Hope for a Cure. London, UK, Allen & Unwin, 1983

Williams D: Autism. London, Jessica Kingsley, 1996

Wing L, Gould J: Severe impairments of social interaction and associated abnormalities in children: epidemiology and classification. J Dev Disord 9(1):11–29, 1979

Wing L, Ricks D: The aetiology of childhood autism: a criticism of Tinbergen's aetiological theory. Psychol Med 6(4):543–553, 1976

World Health Organization: International Statistical Classification of Diseases and Related Health Problems, 10th Revision Geneva, World Health Organization, 1992

Zingarelli G, Ellman G, Hom A, et al: Clinical Effects of Naltrexone on Autistic Behavior. Am J Ment Retard 97(1):57–63, 1992

Mental Health Services for the Mentally Retarded and Staff Training

26 Service Provision and Staff Training

An Overview

Kenneth Day, M.B., Ch.B., F.R.C.Psych., D.P.M.

Until recently service provision for mentally retarded people with mental health problems has received little attention, and there are wide variations between countries and within countries (MHMR Symposium of the European Association for Mental Health in Mental Retardation 1993). The type and style of service required remain the subject of debate, the key questions being the following:

- Can provision be satisfactorily made within ordinary (generic) mental health services?
- Are specialized services needed, and if so, what form should they take?
- What type of service provision is required for the behaviorally disturbed?

Closely allied to these questions is the issue of staff training for those providing mental health services and for care staff and other professionals more generally involved in the care of mentally retarded people. In this chapter, I explore these questions and provide an overview of current practices.

◼ GENERIC MENTAL HEALTH SERVICE PROVISION

Normalization philosophy argues that as part of a general policy of integration, mentally retarded people with mental health problems should be cared for in the ordinary mental health services. In Sweden and Denmark, for example, legislation was enacted in the 1980s to ensure that mentally retarded people should not be singled out but should be subject to the same laws and use the same services as all other citizens. In both countries the mentally ill mentally retarded, including those with severe mental retardation, are treated within the general psychiatric services. Offenders are cared for largely within the forensic psychiatric

469

services, although it has been found necessary to retain a specialized national unit in both countries for the most dangerous offenders. The intention for people displaying severe behavioral problems is that they should be cared for in small community-based group homes with mixed occupancy, although at present the most difficult are still managed in small specialist institutions, but these are scheduled to close. There are no specialist psychiatrists and no specialist nurses or care staff (Day 1992; Dupont 1993; Gustafsson 1995; Kebbon 1993). More commonly, in many countries there is no definite policy, and ordinary psychiatric services are having to accommodate because there is no other alternative (Gold et al. 1989; Houston 1984; Jacobson and Ackerman 1988; Marcos et al. 1986; MHMR Symposium of the European Association for Mental Health in Mental Retardation 1993; Parkhurst 1984; Puddephatt and Sussman 1994).

Attempts to treat the mental health problems of mentally retarded people within generic mental health services, whether by design or default, have been beset with major problems (Day 1992; Dupont 1993; Fletcher 1993; Gustafsson 1995; Houston 1984; Kazdan 1990; Kebbon 1993; Liesmer 1989; Marcos et al. 1986; O'Brien 1990; Parkhurst 1984; Puddephatt and Sussman 1994). Mentally retarded people are vulnerable and disadvantaged in generic psychiatric settings, they do not mix well with the other mentally disordered patients, the pace of life is too fast for them, and it is difficult to gear therapeutic interventions to meet their specific needs. Assessment and treatment take longer, and rehabilitation is slower. The medical, nursing, and other staff lack the necessary experience and expertise in their care and treatment, and because of the small numbers of mentally retarded people in a psychiatric unit at any one time, they have little opportunity to acquire them. There are major difficulties in accessing services (Dorn and Prout 1993; Gravestock and Bouras 1995; Jacobson and Ackerman 1988), and territorial disputes are common, leaving the mentally retarded individual stranded between the mental retardation and mental health services without appropriate treatment (Gold et al. 1989; Gustafsson 1995; Marcos et al. 1986; Nøttestad and Linaker 1999; Pepper and Ryglewiez 1989; Puddephatt and Sussman 1994; Sustafsson 1997). In the absence of appropriate forensic services, mentally retarded offenders frequently enter the criminal justice system (Department of Health and Home Office 1992; French 1983; Jackson 1983; Menolascino 1974).

One response to these problems has been the attempts made to "build bridges" between the mental retardation and the mental health services in a particular locality through interagency planning and coordination, improved staff training, and the development of facilitating mechanisms (All Wales Advisory Panel 1991; Casey et al. 1985; Fletcher 1988; Gielen 1990; Gustafsson 1995; Kebbon 1993; Taylor 1988; Woodward 1993). These have nearly always resulted in the development of some specialized facilities.

■ SPECIALIST MENTAL HEALTH SERVICES

Specialist psychiatric services are in fact increasingly the preferred option in most countries (American Psychiatric Association 1991; Day 1988a, 1993b; Department of Health and Home Office 1992; Došen 1988; Houston 1984; Jenssen and Morch 1990; Landsberg et al. 1987; National Health Service Management Executive 1998; Raitasuo et al. 1999; Zarfas 1988). In the United Kingdom, mental retardation has been a psychiatric specialty for 150 years (Day and Jancar 1991), and mentally retarded people with mental health problems, including offenders, are cared for in the mental retardation services in which specialist facilities have been developed. The continuing need for specialist psychiatric services and specialist psychiatrists, nurses, and other staff has been reaffirmed (Department of Health and Home Office 1992; Department of Health 1989, 1995; National Health Service Management Executive 1992, 1998; Royal College of Psychiatrists 1986, 1992a, 1997a).

There are, in fact, many positive arguments in support of specialized mental health services for the mentally retarded population (Day 1993b). These are summarized below:

- The accurate diagnosis and treatment of psychiatric disorder in mentally retarded people require special expertise and experience in the face of atypical presentation, communication difficulties, and the frequent absence of subjective complaints (Fraser and Rao 1991; Hucker et al. 1979; Menolascino et al. 1986; Reid 1972; Reiss and Syzsko 1983; Sovner 1986; Wright 1982).
- Counseling, psychotherapy, and other therapeutic interventions require modification in their application to take account of intellectual and other limitations (see Chapters 2 and 7–10 of this book).
- Special regimes and careful monitoring of drug treatment are necessary because of the high frequency of side effects and unusual responses in the mentally retarded (Einfeld 1990; see also Chapters 3 and 11–14 of this book).
- Treatment, rehabilitation, and aftercare must take account of underlying dependency levels and any coexisting physical disabilities, including epilepsy, which frequently complicate mental retardation (Day 1984).
- Highly specialized assessment and treatment programs and facilities are required for the management of autism, behavioral phenotypes, and severe behavior problems (see Chapters 4, 5, 17, 18, and 25 of this book).
- Mentally retarded offenders differ from other mentally disordered offenders in the nature and origins of their offending behavior and their treatment needs, and they require specialized treatment approaches and services (see Chapters 19 and 20 of this book).

- Specialist services increase staff competence and skills, bring benefits of cumulative experience, ensure ownership of the task in hand, and hence increase the probability of effective and successful treatment (Newman and Emerson 1991).
- Specialist services facilitate the establishment of a cadre of experts to carry out teaching and research; the substantial research effort in this field over the past decade has emanated almost entirely from clinicians and others working in specialist psychiatric services.

There is also some evidence from work with the elderly population that the involvement of a specialist reduces both the need for and duration of hospital inpatient care (Paulson 1988).

■ COMPONENTS OF A SPECIALIST MENTAL HEALTH SERVICE

A specialist psychiatric service for mentally retarded people should be fully comprehensive (Day 1993b; Department of Health Needs and Responses 1989; Menolascino 1989) and provide for all diagnostic groups, ages, and intellectual levels (see Table 26–1).

A range of provision is required, including diagnostic and treatment services in the community, acute and longer term inpatient treatment and assessment facilities, rehabilitation, aftercare, and continuing care (Day 1984, 1993b; Department of Health Needs and Responses 1989; Fletcher 1988; Landsberg et al. 1987; Menolascino 1989).

Table 26–1. Groups of mentally retarded people with mental health problems requiring services

---

Acute and chronically mentally ill people

Severely mentally retarded people with severe behavior problems

Mildly mentally retarded people with maladjustment, emotional problems, and social inadequacy

Mentally retarded offenders

Brain-damaged mentally retarded people with epilepsy and associated behavior problems

Older mentally retarded people with Alzheimer's disease and other psychogeriatric problems

Mildly and severely mentally retarded children and adolescents with psychiatric, emotional, and behavioral problems

---

Inpatient provision should include a sufficient number of separate treatment settings to enable specialized treatment programs to be provided for each of the main diagnostic groups. At the very minimum, there should be separate settings for the mentally ill, patients with severe behavior problems, offenders, children, and adolescents. Mixing diagnostic groups in a single unit is a recipe for disaster, making it difficult to develop specific treatment programs and creating a generally antitherapeutic environment (Day 1983). Specialist units with appropriate levels of security are required for offenders (Day 1988b, 1993b).

A proportionately higher number of inpatient beds is required than in general psychiatry because admission thresholds are lower due to the greater problems of caring for the mentally retarded with mental health problems in the community, skilled inpatient assessment is more often needed to establish the diagnosis, and treatment and rehabilitation tend to take longer. The number of beds required will vary according to the availability of community-based rehabilitation and continuing care services and the demographic features of the community served—there is likely to be a greater need for offender beds in socially deprived urban areas than in rural areas, for example—and the availability of community-based rehabilitation and continuing care services. Estimates (excluding high and medium secure provision for offenders) range from 0.12 to 0.28 per 1,000 in the general population (see Table 26–2). Therapeutic and economic viability are the key factors determining the size and setting of treatment units (Day 1983).

Special services are required for mentally retarded offenders, including residential treatment units providing a range of levels of security, specialist treatment programs, and a range of community-based services for rehabilitation, aftercare, and continuing care (see Chapter 20 of this book).

Specialized community-based facilities, including support personnel, day treatment facilities, and residential, training, and recreational services, are required for rehabilitation, aftercare, and continuing care. Mentally retarded people with mental health problems do not fit well in mainstream community facilities and require a different style of approach with more support and supervision. The complexity and chronicity of some disorders not only preclude an immediate return to mainstream community services but also may necessitate continuing care in a specialist community setting (Davidson et al. 1999; Day 1984; Fletcher 1988; Menolascino 1989; Reid et al. 1984).

A single organizational responsibility for all aspects of a specialist psychiatric service to a given catchment population ensures a coordinated approach to the management and rehabilitation of the individual patients, permits maximum flexibility in service delivery, and facilitates overall strategic planning.

Table 26–2. Estimated treatment beds required for specialist mentally retarded adults (excluding high and medium secure provision for offenders)

Author	Day 1983	Reid 1994	Menolascino 1989
Catchment population	500,000	400,000	482,000
Patient group facility (*N* beds)	**Offenders** Low secure, open, rehabilitation (30)	**Offenders** Low secure, open (20)	Acute psychiatric and behavior problems (2–4)
	Mental illness Acute/short term (30)	**Mental illness** Short term, assessment and treatment (12–15)	Subacute psychiatric and fragile behavioral states (6–15)
	Medium term (30)/ continuing care, rehabilitation (10)2		
	Behavior disorders Assessment, treatment, continuing care (40)	**Behavior disorders** (10)	Chronic care Psychiatric and behavior problems (69–75)
Total beds	140	42–45	77–94
Beds per 1,000 population	0.28	0.12	0.15–0.19

■ SERVICE MODELS

A variety of models of specialist mental health provision have evolved in the United Kingdom and elsewhere. They can be broadly grouped into four categories: 1) comprehensive subregional services, 2) small local units, 3) integrated services, and 4) specialist teams.

Comprehensive Subregional Services

Specialist subregional services aim to be totally self-sufficient and provide a fully comprehensive service to a catchment population of at least 500,000. They are usually campus based. A typical example has been described by Day (1983, 1984, 1988a). This service currently provides a total of 99 beds for adults and young people with mental illness or severe behavior disorders, including a unit for adults with autism, in 7 separate treatment settings; a 14-bed children's unit; a 12-bed adolescent unit; and a 6-bed head injury unit for a catchment population of 660,000 and 153 beds in 11 separate treatment units for the assessment, treatment, and rehabilitation of mentally retarded offenders for a catchment population of 3 million. Treatment settings are domestic in style and between 4 and 10 places in size. A range of specialist treatment programs and training and occupational placements is provided. Plans are in hand to develop some community-based treatment and care facilities. Similar services are being developed in Holland (Gielen 1990; Klapwijk 1993).

Subregional services have many clear advantages (Blunden and Allen 1987; Day 1983, 1984, 1988a; Department of Health Needs and Responses 1989; Newman and Emerson 1991). They are able to provide a full range of services, including specialized intensive therapeutic programs for each of the main diagnostic groups. They can cope with high levels of disturbed and violent behavior, and physical features can be designed to match patient needs (e.g., security, seclusion facilities, durable decor, furnishings). A full range of occupational, training, and recreational facilities can be provided, together with safe space and asylum for those who require it. Staff expertise is high and can develop. The size of the facility makes it possible to employ staff with a wide range of experience and interest, enriching both the therapeutic and academic environment. Intensive staff support and supervision can be provided—essential in view of the stressful nature of the work and the vulnerability of many of the patients (Rusch et al. 1986). These services are cost-efficient. Outpatient, domiciliary treatment, support, and other outreach services are important components but have been generally underreported and overlooked in discussions about the relative merits and demerits of this service model.

The only serious disadvantage is distance from the patients' homes, which can make visiting difficult and poses potential problems for rehabilitation and longer term follow-up, but this has to be balanced against the very substantial advantages of care and treatment in high-quality specialist services. There are also positive advantages in managing certain patients, such as offenders, at some distance from their home area. Problems of rehabilitation and follow-up are minimized where the service includes community-based facilities and support networks.

Small Local Units

Small locally based specialist treatment units of 10–30 beds, serving catchment populations of 100,000–200,000, have been established within the grounds of mental disability or mental illness hospitals (Fidura et al. 1987; Gold et al. 1989; Hoefkens and Allen 1990; Houston 1984; Hurst et al. 1994; Krishnamurti 1990) and in the community (Galligan 1990). Admissions are usually restricted to moderately and mildly mentally retarded people with mental illness or emotional problems, and the emphasis is on a short duration of stay. Some also admit severely mentally retarded people with severe behavior problems (Fidura et al. 1987; Gold et al. 1989; Hoefkens and Allen 1990; see also Chapter 29 of this book).

Locally based units have the advantage of being sited within the communities they serve—their main raison d'être—but suffer a number of serious disadvantages. They cannot cope with severely disturbed patients or serious offenders and have to rely on backup from often remote specialist services (Bouras et al. 1995; Gravestock and Bicknell 1992). The range of occupational and recreational facilities that can be provided is restricted. They are unable to provide longer term or continuing care. Treatment settings are usually limited to no more than two, which both restricts the types of patients who can be admitted and inevitably leads to inappropriate mixing of patient groups. The small number of patients with similar problems present in the unit at any one time makes it impossible to achieve the critical mass necessary to develop viable therapeutic regimes. Staff expertise is limited, and there can be problems of medical coverage, support for direct care staff, and backup in emergencies.

Integrated Services

In this model, outpatient and inpatient care and treatment are provided by locally based specialist teams of psychiatrists and nurses using earmarked beds in generic mental health units for inpatient treatment (Bouras and Drummond 1989; Bouras et al. 1994; Nolan et al. 1992; Singh et al. 1994; see also Chapter 28 of this book). Admissions are generally restricted to mildly mentally retarded patients with mental illness, although it has been suggested that the range of diagnostic groups treated could be extended by using earmarked beds in generic forensic psychiatry and psychogeriatric services (N. Bouras, personal communication, November 1989). This still leaves a requirement for specialist provision for severely mentally retarded patients with severe behavior problems (Bouras and Drummond 1989; Nolan et al. 1992; Singh et al. 1994). In another variant, outpatient and day treatment services are provided by specialist teams, patients requiring acute inpatient psychiatric treatment are admitted to the local psychiatric service under the care of a general psychiatrist, and longer term care is provided by community programs for the mentally retarded (Casey et al. 1985; Davidson et al. 1999; Fletcher 1988; Reiss 1988; Reiss and Trenn 1984).

A serious drawback of this model is that patients are admitted for treatment to a generic psychiatric service with all the disadvantages of lack of staff expertise and experience and inappropriateness of a ward environment (Bouras et al. 1994; Nolan et al. 1992; Singh et al. 1994). Sovner and Hurley (1987), while arguing strongly for specialized units, have provided useful guidelines for staff working with the mentally retarded in generic psychiatric settings.

Specialist Teams

"Challenging behavior teams" (also known as "intensive support teams" and "special development teams") have been developed in the United Kingdom (Emerson et al. 1989, 1996; Maher and Russell 1988), the United States (Davidson et al. 1995; Donnellan et al. 1985), Canada (Vischer 1982), and Australia (Baltini et al. 1986) to provide service exclusively to severely mentally retarded people with severe behavior disorders and are invariably psychology led. Their guiding philosophy is that treatment should, as far as is possible, be offered in the patient's home or, when this is not realizable, in small intensively staffed group homes (Allen and Fleece 1999; Blunden and Allen 1987; Newman and Emerson 1991). It is argued that specialist behavior therapy units have not been successful (Blunden and Allen 1987; Keene and James 1986; Newman and Emerson 1991) and that it makes more sense to attempt to effect behavioral change in the environment in which it arose (Allin 1988; Carr and Durand 1985; McBrien 1987).

Although successes have been reported (Mansell 1994), common sense suggests that this approach cannot possibly be successful in all cases and that there will always be a need for hospital admission for more intensive interventions (Perry et al. 1995; Xenitidis et al. 1999). Surveys of services in the United Kingdom have found that intensive professional input into the home setting did not obviate the need for hospital admission—often on a crisis basis (Gravestock and Bouras 1995, 1997; O'Brien 1990). Furthermore, the basic premise that behavioral problems are essentially functional in origin, which underpins this approach, is becoming less tenable in the light of research on behavioral phenotypes and evidence of the neurobiological, neuropsychiatric, and socio-communicative basis of many behavior disorders (Berg and Gosse 1990; Coyle 1988; Fraser and Rao 1991; Fraser et al. 1986; Hucker et al. 1979; Hunt and Cohen 1988; Lund 1985; Reid 1972; Reid et al. 1984; Szymanski 1994).

■ PATIENT GROUPS

Mentally Retarded Children and Adolescents

Mental health services for mentally retarded children and adolescents are far less well developed, both conceptually and in terms of practical provision, than those for adults. In the United Kingdom an argument has been advanced that provision should be within the child and adolescent services (Court 1976). However, the arguments for specialized mental health services for mentally retarded adults apply with equal force to services for mentally retarded children and adolescents (Kymissis and Leven 1994). A related issue is the need for specialization in the child psychiatry of mental retardation (Royal College of Psychiatrists 1989, 1992a). A range of community- and hospitalized-based services is required, including separate inpatient provision for severely mentally retarded children and adolescents with severe behavior disorders, mildly mentally retarded children with mental illness and emotional problems, and adolescent offenders. Specialist units are beginning to be developed (Johnson et al. 1995).

Mentally Retarded Offenders

The concept of treatment and care rather than punishment is embodied in criminal justice and mental health legislation and in service provision in most countries. The care, treatment, and service needs of mentally retarded offenders are discussed in detail in Chapter 20 of this book.

Commenting on the great variability of current servic provision, Moss and colleagues (2000) recommend the application of the conceptual framework of a matrix model in the planning and delivery of services.

The author is becoming increasingly convinced that a specialist comprehensive integrated three-tier regional/subregional service delivered by a single provider (Table 26–3) is the best service model for the future.

Psychiatrists would serve a designated local catchment population and have access to beds in supradistrict and regional/subregional units retaining responsibility for their patients. Services for children and adolescents and offenders would ideally be provided on a regional/subregional basis by specialist psychiatrists and teams.

Table 26–3. An integrated three-tier model for specialist psychiatric services for the mentally retarded population

Level	Facilities	Function
District	Community learning disabilities team. Specialized small domestic-style residential units. Specialized day care services.	Outpatients, domiciliary services. Rehabilitation and continuing care.
Supradistrict	Specialized treatment and day care unit serving 2–3 districts and strategically sited.	Inpatient and day assessment and treatment for less severely mentally ill patients. Aftercare and rehabilitation for discharged hospital patients. Specialized day and respite care services. HQ for community teams.
Regional/ subregional	Specialist hospital with specialist units.	Assessment and treatment of acute mental illness and behavior disorders. Secure units for offenders. Special unit for late acquired head injury and other special groups. Child and adolescent treatment units (separately sited except for secure adolescent provision).

This model would offer a flexible and seamless service to patients who could be treated at the level most appropriate to their needs and as close to home and family as possible. It limits the use of high-cost intensive care beds to those who need them. Good staff backup can be provided at all levels of the service, avoiding the need for crisis admissions. Specialized environments and treatment programs can be developed for all patient groups. Staff with a wide range of interests, expertise, and experience can be recruited, thereby enriching the therapeutic and academic environment and providing a cadre of experts for teaching, training, and research. It is highly cost-effective.

■ STAFF TRAINING

It is imperative that specialist mental health services are staffed by appropriately trained and experienced doctors, nurses, and other staff. Lack of specialist staff, particularly psychiatrists, has proven to be a major barrier to the development of specialist services in many countries (American Psychiatric Association 1991; Day 1992; MHMR Symposium of the European Association for Mental Health in Mental Retardation 1993; Parmenter 1988; Zarfas 1988). Currently, the training and education available both at undergraduate and postgraduate levels vary markedly from country to country and, not surprisingly, bear a close relationship to the development and availability of specialist services (MHMR Symposium of the European Association for Mental Health in Mental Retardation 1993). It is equally important that all professionals involved or likely to be involved in the care of mentally retarded people—particularly first-line caregivers and family doctors—are properly trained to recognize mental health problems in the mentally retarded and have an adequate knowledge of treatment methods and services available. Teaching and training of a wide range of professionals should be a key function of specialist psychiatric services.

Staff in Specialist Mental Health Services

Psychiatrists

In most countries mental retardation is not a recognized psychiatric specialty, there are no formal training programs and no representation in professional psychiatric organizations, and services tend to be run by pioneering psychiatrists who have developed a special interest in the subject.

One exception is the United Kingdom, where mental retardation has been a recognized psychiatric specialty for 150 years, and there is a strong mental handicap psychiatry faculty in the Royal College of Psychiatrists and a well-established and sophisticated training program for psychiatrists (Day 1999; Day and Jancar 1991). Doctors wishing to specialize in the psychiatry of mental retardation must first undertake a 3- to 4-year period of general psychiatric training in an approved scheme, which includes some mental retardation experience followed by a further 3- to 4-year period of clinical and academic training in the psychiatry of mental retardation in an approved scheme in a specialist service (Joint Committee in Higher Psychiatric Training 1995; Royal College of Psychiatrists 1997b). An outline of the training program is shown in Table 26–4. The recommended consultant establishment is one full-time equivalent per 100,000 population (Piachaud 1989; Royal College of Psychiatrists 1992b). Currently there are some 200 consultants and 70–90 trainees in the specialty, with academic posts at senior lecturer level in all university departments and five professional chairs in the psychiatry of mental retardation.

Increasing refinements in service provision are giving rise to new superspecialities such as the psychiatry of child and adolescent mental retardation,

Table 26–4. Specialist training in the psychiatry of mental retardation in the United Kingdom

General professional training

Senior house officer

3–4 years in supervised training in a scheme approved by the Royal College of Psychiatrists

Academic teaching and clinical experience in general (adult) psychiatry and other psychiatric specialties (including mental retardation)

Lectures in other topics relevant to the practice of psychiatry (e.g., psychology, neurology, social sciences, psychopathology, psychpharmacology, genetics, medical ethics, epidemiology)

Membership of the Royal College of Psychiatrists (M.R.C.Psych.) by examination on completion

Higher training in the psychiatry of mental retardation

Specialist registrar

3–4 years in a training scheme approved by the Joint Committee on Higher Psychiatric Training

Further development of general psychiatric skills and knowledge

Clinical placements of 12–18 months' duration to provide a range of different service experience in the psychiatry of mental retardation (e.g., children, adolescents and adults, forensic, special experience)

Weekly academic meetings, opportunities to visit other services and to attend national and international conferences

Opportunities to teach medical undergraduates and other professional groups and to supervise trainee psychiatrists

Involvement in research and audit, including the planning and execution of an original research project

Management experience

Award of Certificate of Completion of Specialist Training (CCST) on satisfactory completion, inclusion on the Specialist Register (General Medical Council), and eligibility for consultant appointment and specialist practice

Source. Adapted and reprinted from Day K: "Professional Training in the Psychiatry of Mental Retardation in the UK," in *Psychiatric and Behavioural Disorders in Developmental Disabilities and Mental Retardation.* Edited by Bouras N. Cambridge, UK, Cambridge University Press, 1999, pp 439–457. Used with permission.

forensic psychiatry of mental retardation, each with their own specialist training programs (Joint Committee of Higher Psychiatric Training 1995; Royal College of Psychiatrists 1997b).

The American Psychiatric Association established a Committee on Mental Retardation in 1988 and set up a Task Force on Psychiatric Services for Adults

With Mental Handicap, which recommended that all psychiatric trainees should receive some teaching and experience in the psychiatry of mental retardation (American Psychiatric Association 1991). A 1-year postgraduate training course in the psychiatry of mental retardation has recently been introduced in the Netherlands; there are 20 psychiatrists working in the specialty, and a "mental handicap" section has been created in the Dutch Association of Psychiatrists (A. Došen, personal communication, 1990; Klapwijk 1993).

Nurses

Many countries have a long tradition of specialist nurse training in mental retardation. In the United Kingdom, this dates back to 1919 (Day and Jancar 1991); the content of training has varied over the years, reflecting service philosophy with a recent emphasis on social care, but this is now reversing, and the need for specially trained nurses in the psychiatry of mental retardation has now been recognized (Chief Nursing Officers of the United Kingdom 1991; Department of Health 1995). Some nurses have obtained dual qualifications in both mental retardation and psychiatric nursing, and there is an increasing number of college-based postbasic training courses available in specific topics, such as nursing within secure environments and mental health law.

Clinical Psychologists

Clinical psychologists provide a major input into services in most countries. In the United Kingdom, the postgraduate degree in clinical psychology includes a mandatory clinical placement in mental retardation services and academic lectures on the topic. Further training and experience are obtained as part of general professional training (Day 1999).

Direct Care Staff

First-level care workers in community, day, and residential facilities rarely, if ever, receive any training in the psychiatric aspects of mental retardation, resulting in unrecognized and untreated psychiatric illness among their patients (Allen et al. 1990; Holt 1995; Reiss 1990). In a recent study of psychiatric disorder among elderly mentally retarded people, for example, Patel et al. (1993) found that although care staff were able to describe accurately the symptoms and signs of mental disorder presented by their patients, they had no understanding of their significance. Schramski (1989) has provided useful principles and guidelines, and Roeher (McGee and Pearson 1983) has provided a curriculum guide for training direct care staff in the mental health aspects of mental retardation.

"Mental Health in Learning Disabilities," a training pack for staff working with people with mental health needs and learning disabilities, is an important recent contribution (Bouras and Holt 1997; Holt 1995). Designed primarily for direct care staff, it consists of a training manual and handbook that cover the presentation, assessment, and treatment of mental health problems, challenging behavior, and epilepsy in mentally retarded people; services; and legal and ethical issues. More focused training programs have also been developed, for example, for the prevention and management of seriously disrupted behavior for staff in community homes (Attwood and Joachim 1994). Another useful development is a checklist designed to help direct care staff screen for mental health problems and make informed referrals (Moss et al. 1997).

General Practitioners and Other First-Line Professionals

There has been a recent and timely increase in awareness of and concern about the health care needs of mentally retarded people in general, which will, it is hoped, lead to an increased profile of this topic (including mental health problems) in the basic training of all professional groups (Kerr 1997). Family doctors are a key point of contact with specialist psychiatric services. In the United Kingdom, the mental health problems of the mentally retarded are beginning to feature in their training programs and refresher courses (Bicknell 1985; Howells 1991, 1993; Royal College of General Practitioners 1990). Medical undergraduates receive training and clinical experience in mental retardation in some countries (Hollins 1988; Kozlova and Smirnov 1993), and there is evidence of a positive response and an interest in learning more about both clinical and social issues (Holt et al. 1993). Social workers and other professionals allied to medicine (e.g., physiotherapists, occupational therapists, and speech therapists) receive a brief introduction and sometimes a placement in mental retardation services during their basic training but no specialist training in the psychiatry of mental retardation (Day 1988a, 1999). Approved social workers (ASWs), approved as having special knowledge and expertise in mental health law, receive special training in mental health and mental health law, which includes the psychiatry of mental retardation.

Continuing Professional Education

International, national, and local conferences and other initiatives provide valuable opportunities for further learning and information exchange for all professionals working with this client group but are no substitute for proper, formalized training programs. Recent years have seen a growth of university-based multidisciplinary training courses in a range of specialist aspects of treatment and care of the mentally retarded with mental health problems in the United Kingdom and elsewhere. Continuing professional education is enshrined in professional practice in most countries and is increasingly becoming formalized and mandatory (Day 1999).

■ CONCLUSIONS

Mental health problems occur with greater frequency in the mentally retarded than in the general population, and proper provision for this group of patients is an essential component of a comprehensive mental retardation service. Arguments in favor of provision within ordinary mental health services are essentially ideological and failing in practice. There are sound arguments in favor of specialist mental health services, and these are increasingly the preferred option in many countries. Specialist mental health services should be planned and implemented in parallel with the closure of institutions and the development of care in the community, and not as an afterthought. A number of different service models are developing, and rigorous evaluative research is required to examine the strengths and weaknesses of each model against the key elements of comprehensiveness, clinical efficacy, and cost-effectiveness and to clearly distinguish inherent disadvantages from those resulting from underresourcing or poor organization and functioning. The author's preferred model is a comprehensive, integrated three-tier service.

There is an urgent need to develop formal training programs for all professionals working in specialist mental health services and for more attention to be paid to the subject in the training and education of nonspecialist staff, particularly primary health and direct care staff. Current thinking in the United Kingdom is moving toward establishing the core competencies required by all staff working in the service and the distinctive competencies required by each professional group, and moving toward a mix of shared learning and separate professional development for some groups (Sainsbury Centre for Mental Health 1997).

■ REFERENCES

All Wales Advisory Panel on the Development of Services for People With Mental Handicaps: Challenges and Responses: A Report on Services in Support of Adults With Mental Handicaps With Exceptionally Challenging Behaviors, Mental Illnesses, or Who Offend. Cardiff, UK, Welsh Office, 1991

Allen D, Felce D: Service responses to challenging behaviour, in Psychiatric and Behavioural Disorders in Developmental Disabilities and Mental Retardation. Edited by Bouras N. Cambridge, UK, Cambridge University Press, 1999, pp 279–294

Allen P, Pahl J, Quine L: Care Staff in Transition. London, Her Majesty's Stationary Office, 1990

Allin RB: Intensive home based treatment interventions with mentally retarded/emotionally disturbed individuals and their families, in Mental Retardation and Mental Health: Classification, Treatment, Services. Edited by Stark JA, Menolascino FJ, Albarelli MH. New York, Springer-Verlag, 1988, pp 265–280

American Psychiatric Association: Psychiatric Services to Adult Mentally Retarded and Developmentally Disabled Persons: Task Force Report 30. Washington DC, American Psychiatric Association, 1991

Attwood T, Joachim R: The prevention and management of seriously disruptive behavior in Australia, in Mental Health and Mental Retardation. Edited by Bouras N. Cambridge, UK, Cambridge University Press, 1994, pp 365–374

Baltini T, Elliot J, Jones G, et al: The Prevention and Management of Serious Disruptive Behavior. Perth, Western Australia, Authority for Intellectually Handicapped Persons, 1986

Berg JM, Gosse GC: Specific mental retardation disorders and problem behaviors. International Review of Psychiatry 2:53–60, 1990

Bicknell J: Educational programs for general practitioners and clinical assistants in the mental handicap service. Bulletin of the Royal College of Psychiatrists 8:154–155, 1985

Blunden R, Allen D: Facing the challenge: an ordinary life for people with learning difficulties and challenging behavior; Kings Fund Project Paper No 74. London, London Kings Fund Centre, 1987

Bouras N, Drummond C: Community psychiatric service in mental handicap. Health Trends 21:72, 1989

Bouras N, Holt G: Mental Health in Learning Disabilities: Training Package, 2nd Edition. Brighton, UK, Pavilion Publishing, 1997

Bouras N, Brooks D, Drummond K: Community Psychiatric Services for people with mental retardation, in Mental Health in Mental Retardation: Recent Advances and Practices. Edited by Bouras N. Cambridge, UK, Cambridge University Press, 1994, pp 293–299

Bouras N, Holt G, Gravestock S. Community care for people with learning disabilities: deficits and future plans. Psychiatric Bulletin 19:134–137, 1995

Carr EG, Durand VM: The social-communicative basis of severe behavior problems in children, in Theoretical Issues in Behavior Therapy. Edited by Reiss S, Bootzin RR. New York, Academic Press, 1985, pp 67–86

Casey K, McGee J, Stark J, et al: A community based system for the mentally retarded: the ENCOR experience. Lincoln, NE, University of Nebraska Press, 1985

Chief Nursing Officers of the United Kingdom: Caring for People: Mental Handicap Nursing (Cullen Report). Heywood, Lancashire, Department of Health, Health Publications Unit, 1991

Court SDM: Fit for the Future: Report of the Committee on Child Health Services (Cmnd 6684). London, Her Majesty's Stationary Office, 1976

Coyle JT: Psychiatry, neuroscience, and the double disabilities, in Mental Retardation and Mental Health: Classification, Diagnosis, Treatment, Services. Edited by Stark JA, Menolascino FJ, Albarelli MH, et al. New York, Springer-Verlag, 1988, pp 81–89

Davidson PW, Morris D, Cain NN: Community services for people with developmental disabilities and psychiatric or severe behaviour disorders, in Psychiatric and Behavioural Disorders in Developmental Disabilities and Mental Retardation. Edited by Bouras N. Cambridge, UK, Cambridge University Press, 1999, pp 359–372

Davidson P, Cain N, Sloane-Reeves J, et al: Crisis intervention for community-based individuals with developmental disabilities and behavioral and psychiatric disorders. Ment Retard 33:21–30, 1995

Day K: A hospital based psychiatric unit for mentally handicapped adults. Mental Handicap 11:137–140, 1983

Day K: Service provision for mentally handicapped people with psychiatric problems, in Care in the Community, Keeping it Local: Report of MIND's 1983 Annual Conference, 1984, pp 54–59

Day K: Services for psychiatrically disordered mentally handicapped adults: a UK perspective. Australia and New Zealand Journal of Developmental Disabilities 14:19–25, 1988a

Day K: A hospital based treatment program for male mentally handicapped offenders. Br J Psychiatry 153:635–644, 1988b

Day K: Mental health care for the mentally handicapped in four European countries: the argument for specialized services. Italian Journal of Intellectual Impairment 5:3–11, 1992

Day K: Mental health services for people with mental retardation: a framework for the future. Journal of Intellectual Research 37(suppl 1):7–16, 1993a

Day K: Crime and mental retardation: a review, in Clinical Approaches to the Mentally Disordered Offender. Edited by Howells K, Hollins CR. Chichester, UK, Wiley, 1993b, pp 111–144

Day K: Professional training in the psychiatry of mental retardation in the United Kingdom, in Psychiatric and Behavioral Disorders in Developmental Disabilities and Mental Retardation. Edited by Bouras N. Cambridge, UK, Cambridge University Press, 1999, pp 439–457

Day K, Jancar J: Mental handicap and the Royal Medico-Psychological Association: a historical association 1841–1991, in 150 Years of British Psychiatry: 1841–1991. Edited by Berrios GE, Freeman H. London, Gaskell Press, 1991, pp 268–270

Department of Health: The Health of the Nation: A Strategy for People With Learning Disabilities. London, UK, Depatment of Health, 1995

Department of Health and Home Office: Review of Health and Social Services for Mentally Disordered Offenders and Others Requiring Similar Services: Final Summary Report, CM2088. London, Her Majesty's Stationary Office, 1992

Department of Health: Needs and Responses: Services for Adults With Mental Handicap Who Are Mentally Ill, Who Have Behavior Problems, or Who Offend: Report of a Department of Health Study Team. Stanmore, Middlesex, UK, Department of Health Leaflets Unit, 1989

Donnellan A, LaVigna G, Zambito J, et al: A time based intervention model to support community placement to persons with severe behavioural problems. Journal of the Association for Severe Handicap 10:123–131, 1985

Dorn TA, Prout HT: Service delivery patterns for adults with mild mental retardation at community mental health centres. Ment Retard 31:292–296, 1993

Došen A: Community care for people with mental retardation in the Netherlands. Australia and New Zealand Journal of Developmental Disabilities 14:15–18, 1988

Dupont A: Denmark. J Intellect Disabil Res 37(suppl 1):37–39, 1993

Einfeld SL: Guidelines for the use of psychotropic medication in individuals with developmental disabilities. Australia and New Zealand Journal of Developmental Disabilities 16:71–73, 1990

Emerson E, Cummings R, Hughes H, et al: Challenging behavior and community services; 6: evaluation and overview. Mental Handicap 17:104–107, 1989

Emerson E, Forrest J, Cambridge P et al: Community support teams for people with learning disabilities and challenging behaviour: results of a national survey. Journal of Mental Health 5:395–406, 1996

Fidura JG, Lindsey ER, Walker GR: A special behavior unit for treatment of behavior problems of persons who are mentally retarded. Ment Retard 25:107–111, 1987

Fletcher R: A county systems model: comprehensive services for the dually diagnosed, in Mental Retardation and Mental Health: Classification, Diagnosis, Treatment, Services. Edited by Stark JA, Menolascino FJ, Albarelli MH, et al. New York, Springer-Verlag, 1988, pp 254–264

Fletcher RJ: Mental illness-mental retardation in the United States: policy and treatment challenges. J Intellect Disabil Res 37(suppl 1):25–33, 1993

Fraser WI, Rao GM: Recent studies of mentally handicapped young people's behavior. J Child Psychol Psychiatry 23:79–108, 1991

Fraser WI, Leudar I, Gray J, et al: Psychiatric and behavior disturbance in mental handicap. Journal of Mental Deficiency Research 30:49–59, 1986

French S: The mentally retarded offender and pseudo retarded offender: a clinical/legal dilemma. Federal Probation 47:55, 1983

Galligan B: Serving people who are dually diagnosed: a program evaluation. Ment Retard 28:353–358, 1990

Gielen JM: A network of services for mental health care of the mildly and moderately retarded in South East Noord-Brabant (The Netherlands), in Treatment of Mental Illness and Behavioral Disorder in the Mentally Retarded. Edited by Došen A, Van Gennep A, Zwanikken CJ. Leiden, Netherlands Logon Publications, 1990, pp 485–492

Gold IM, Wolfson ES, Lester CM, et al: Developing a unit for mentally retarded mentally ill patients on the grounds of a state hospital. Hospital and Community Psychiatry 40:836–840, 1989

Gravestock S, Bicknell J: Emergency referrals to the south London community mental handicap team. Psychiatric Bulletin 16:475–477, 1992

Gravestock S, Bouras N: Services for adults with learning disabilities and mental health problems. Psychiatric Bulletin 19:288–290, 1995

Gravestock S, Bouras N: Survey of services for adults with learning disabilities. Psychiatric Bulletin 21:197–199, 1997

Gustafsson C: Developments in providing services to people with mental retardation and psychiatric disorders in Sweden, in Proceedings of the International Congress II on the Dually Diagnosed. New York, National Association for the Dually Diagnosed, 1995, pp 107–108

Gustafsson C: The prevalance of people with intellectual disability admitted to general hospital psychiatric units: level of handicap, psychiatric diagnosis and care utilisation. J Intellect Disabil Res 41:519–526, 1997

Hoefkens A, Allen D: Evaluation of a special behavior unit for people with mental handicaps and challenging behavior. Journal of Mental Deficiency Research 34:213–228, 1990

Hollins S: How mental handicap is taught in UK medical schools. Medical Teacher 10:289–296, 1988

Holt G: Training staff on mental health in mental retardation, in Proceedings of the International Congress II on the Dually Diagnosed. New York, National Association for the Dually Diagnosed, 1995, pp 109–111

Houston H: A plan designed to deliver services to the multiply handicapped, in Handbook of Mental Illness in the Mentally Retarded. Edited by Menolascino FJ, Stark JA. New York, Plenum, 1984

Howells G: Mental handicap: care in the community. Br J Gen Pract 41:2–4, 1991

Howells G, Kerr M, Lervy D: Learning Disability (Mental Handicap): Distance Learning Workbook For General Practitioners. Swansea, UK, University of Wales College of Medicine School of Postgraduate Studies

Hucker SJ, Day KA, George S, et al: Psychosis in mentally handicapped adults, in Psychiatric Illness and Mental Handicap. Edited by James FE, Snaith RP. London, Gaskell Press, 1979, pp 27–35

Hunt RD, Cohen DJ: Attentional and neurochemical components of mental retardation: new methods and old problems, in Mental Retardation and Mental Health: Classification, Diagnosis, Treatment, Services. Edited by Stark JA, Menolascino FJ, Albarelli MH, et al. New York, Springer-Verlag, 1988, pp 90–97

Hurst J, Nadargah S, Cummela S: Inpatient care for people with learning disability and a mental illness. Psychiatric Bulletin 18:29–31, 1994

Jackson R: Mental retardation and criminal justice: some issues and problems. Mental Subnormality 29:7–12, 1983

Jacobson JW, Ackerman LJ: An appraisal of services for people with mental retardation and psychiatric impairments. Ment Retard 26:377–380, 1988

Jenssen T, Morch WT: Tidsskr Nor Laegeforen 110:1721–1727, 1990. [Summary in English in Mental Retardation. Medline Current Awareness Topic's Search, British Library, Boston Spa, West Yorkshire, 1990]

Joint Committee on Higher Psychiatric Training: Higher Training Schemes in Mental Handicap Psychiatry: Handbook, 7th Edition, Occasional Paper OP 27. London, Joint Committee on Higher Psychiatric Training and Royal College of Psychiatrists, 1995, pp 37–39

Kazdan A: Dual Diagnosis: Dual Dilemma. Toronto, Ontario, Canada, Ministry of Health, 1990

Kebbon L: Sweden. J Intellect Disabil Res 37(suppl 1):62–65, 1993

Keene N, James H: Who needs hospital care? Mental Handicap 14:101–103, 1986

Kerr MP: Primary health care for people with an intellectual disability. J Intellect Disabil Res 41:363–364, 1997

Klapwijk ET: The Netherlands. J Intellect Disabil Res 37(suppl 1):44–46, 1993

Kozlova IA, Smirnov U: Former USSR. J Intellect Disabil Res 37(suppl 1):52–54, 1993

Krishnamurti D: Evaluation of a special behavior unit for people with mental handicaps and challenging behavior: a riposte. Journal of Mental Deficiency Research 34:229–231, 1990

Kymissis P, Leven L: Adolescents with mental retardation and psychiatric disorders, in Mental Health in Mental Retardation. Edited by Bouras N. Cambridge, UK, Cambridge University Press, 1994, pp 102–107

Landsberg G, Fletcher R, Maxwell T: Developing a comprehensive community care system for the mentally ill mentally retarded. Community Mental Health J 23:131–134, 1987

Liesmer J: Systemic needs for a responsible future, in Mental Retardation and Mental Illness. Edited by Fletcher R, Menolascino F. Lexington, MA, Lexington Books, 1989, pp 263–284

Lund J: The prevalence of psychiatric morbidity in mentally retarded adults. Acta Psychiatr Scand 72:557–562, 1985

Maher J, Russell O: Serving people with very challenging behavior, in An Ordinary Life in Practice: Developing Comprehensive Community Based Services for People With Learning Disabilities. Edited by Towell D. London, Kings Fund, 1988, pp 238–245

Mansell J: The challenge of providing high quality services, in Mental Health and Mental Retardation. Edited by Bouras N. Cambridge, UK, Cambridge University Press, 1994, pp 328–340

Marcos LR, Gil RM, Vazquez KM: Who will treat the psychiatrically disturbed developmentally disabled patients? A health care nightmare. Hospital and Community Psychiatry 37:171–174, 1986

McBrien J: The Haytor Unit: specialized day care for adults with severe mental handicaps and behavior problems. Mental Handicap 15:77–80, 1987

McGee JJ, Pearson TH: Personnel preparation to meet the mental health needs of the mentally retarded and their families, in Mental Health and Mental Retardation: Bridging the Gap. Edited by Menolascino FJ, McCann DM. Baltimore, MD, University Park Press, 1983, pp 235–252

Menolascino FJ: The mentally retarded offender. Ment Retard 12:7–11, 1974

Menolascino FJ: Model services for treatment/management of the mentally retarded mentally ill. Community Mental Health J 25:145–155, 1989

Menolascino FJ, Gilson SF, Levitas A: Issues in the treatment of mentally retarded patients in the community mental health system. Community Mental Health J 22:314–327, 1986

MHMR Proceedings of Symposium of the European Association for Mental Health in Mental Retardation: The mental health of Europeans with learning disabilities. J Intellect Disabil Res 37(suppl 1), 1993

Moss SC, Prosser H, Simpson N, et al: The PAS–ADD Checklist. Manchster, UK, Hester Adrian Research Centre, University of Manchester, 1997

Moss S, Bouras N, Holt G: Mental health services for persons with intellectual disability: a conceptual framework. J Intellect Disabil Res 44:97–107, 2000

National Health Service Management Executive: Health Services for People With Learning Disabilities (Mental Handicap), HSG (92) 42. Heywood, Lancashire, UK, Department of Health, Health Publications Unit, 1992

National Health Service Management Executive: Signposts for Success in Commissioning and Providing Health Services for People With Learning Disabilities. Wetherby, UK, Department of Health, 1998

Newman I, Emerson E: Specialized treatment units for people with challenging behaviors. Mental Handicap 19:113–119, 1991

Nolan ME, Radakrishnan G, Lewis J: Generic services for people with a mental handicap. Psychiatric Bulletin 16:212–213, 1992

Nøttestad JAA, Linaker OM: Psychiatric health needs and services before and after complete deinstitutionalisation of people with intellectual disabilities. J Intellect Disabil Res 43:523–530, 1999

O'Brien G: Current patterns of service provision for the psychiatric needs of mentally handicapped people: visiting centres in England and Wales. Psychiatric Bulletin 14:6–7, 1990

Parkhurst R: Need assessment and service planning for mentally retarded mentally ill persons, in Handbook of Mental Illness in the Mentally Retarded. Edited by Menolascino FJ, Stark JA. New York, Plenum, 1984

Parmenter TR: Analysis of Australian mental health services for people with mental retardation. Australia and New Zealand Journal of Developmental Disabilities 14:9–13, 1988

Patel P, Goldberg D, Moss S: Psychiatric morbidity in older people with moderate and severe learning disability; II: the prevalence study. Br J Psychiatry 163:481–491, 1993

Patterson T, Higgins M, Dyck DG: A collaborative approach to reduce hospitalisation of developmentally disabled clients with mental illness. Psychiatric Services 46(3):243–247, 1995

Paulson LG: Hospital length of stay of frail and elderly patients: primary care by general interests versus geriatricians. J Am Geriatr Soc 36:202–208, 1988

Pepper B, Ryglewicz H: The dually (or multiply) diagnosed young adult clients, in Mental Retardation and Mental Illness. Edited by Fletcher R, Menolascino F. Lexington, MA, Lexington Books, 1989, pp 245–261

Perry D, Krishman V, Tewari S, et al: Impact of a community based challenging behavior service on bed occupancy. Psychiatric Bulletin 19:663–665, 1995

Piachaud J: Calculating the medical time required in the psychiatry of mental handicap. Psychiatric Bulletin 13:481–489, 1989

Puddephatt A, Sussman S: Developing services in Canada: Ontario vignettes, in Mental Health in Mental Retardation. Edited by Bouras N. Cambridge, UK, Cambridge University Press, 1994, pp 353–364

Raitasuo S, Taiment T, Salokangas RKR: Inpatient care and its outcome in a specialist psychiatric unit for peop0le with intellectual disability:a prospective study. J Intellect Disabil Res 43:119–123, 1999

Reid AH: Psychosis in adult mental defectives. Br J Psychiatry 120:205–212, 1972

Reid AH: Psychiatry and learning disability. Br J Psychiatry 164:613–618, 1994

Reid AH, Ballinger BR, Heather BB, et al: The natural history of behavioral symptoms among severely and profoundly mentally retarded patients. Br J Psychiatry 145:289–293, 1984

Reiss S: A university based demonstration program on outpatient mental health services for mentally retarded people, in Mental Retardation and Mental Health: Classification, Diagnosis, Treatment, Services. Edited by Stark JA, Menolascino FJ, Albarelli MH, et al. New York, Springer-Verlag, 1988, pp 249–253

Reiss S: Problems of dual diagnosis in community based programs in the Chicago metropolitan area. American Journal of Retardation 94:578–585, 1990

Reiss S, Szysko J: Diagnostic overshadowing and professional experience with mentally retarded persons. American Journal of Mental Deficiency 27:396–402, 1983

Reiss S, Trenn E: Consumer demand for outpatient mental health services for mentally retarded people. Ment Retard 22:112–115, 1984

Royal College of General Practitioners: Primary Care for People With a Mental Handicap. London, Royal College of General Practitioners, 1990

Royal College of Psychiatrists: Psychiatric services for mentally handicapped adults and young people. Bulletin of the Royal College of Psychiatrists 10:321–322, 1986

Royal College of Psychiatrists: Psychiatric Services for Children and Adolescents With Mental Handicap, Council Report CR17. London, Publications Department, Royal College of Psychiatrists, 1992a

Royal College of Psychiatrists: Mental Health of the Nation: The Contribution of Psychiatry, Council Report CR16. London, Publications Department, Royal College of Psychiatrists, 1992b

Royal College of Psychiatrists: Meeting the Mental Health Needs of People With Learning Disabilities, Council Report CR56. London, Publications Department, Royal College of Psychiatrists, 1997a

Royal College of Psychiatrists: Educational Policy, Occasional Paper OP36. London, Publications Department, Royal College of Psychiatrists, 1997b

Rusch RG, Hall JC, Griffin HC: Abuse provoking characteristics of institutionalized mentally retarded individuals. American Journal of Mental Deficiency 90:618–624, 1986

Sainsbury Centre for Mental Health: Pulling Together: The Future Roles and Training of Mental Health Staff. London, Sainsbury Centre, 1997

Schramski TG: Encouraging staff training and development, in Mental Retardation and Mental Illness. Edited by Fletcher R, Menolascino F. Lexington, MA, Lexington Books, 1989 pp 217–227

Singh I, Khalid MI, Dickinson MJ: Psychiatric admission services for people with learning disability. Psychiatric Bulletin 18:151–152, 1994

Sovner R: Limiting factors in the use of DSM-III criteria with mentally ill/mentally retarded persons on psychiatric inpatient units. Psychiatric Aspects of Mental Retardation Reviews 6:7–14, 1986

Sovner R, Hurley AD: Guidelines for the treatment of mentally retarded persons on psychiatric inpatient units. Psychiatric Aspects of Mental Retardation Reviews 6:7–14, 1987

Szymanski L: Mental retardation and mental health: concepts, etiology, and incidence, in Mental Health and Mental Retardation. Edited by Bouras N. Cambridge, UK, Cambridge University Press, 1994, pp 19–33

Taylor D: Developing a system of services for the dually diagnosed adult population in North Carolina, in Mental Retardation and Mental Health: Classification, Diagnosis, Treatment, Services. Edited by Stark JA, Menolascino FJ, Albarelli MH, et al. New York, Springer-Verlag, 1988, pp 430–434

Vischer J: Problem analysis in planning a community based behavioural management programme. Practical Approaches to Developmental Handicap 6:22–28, 1982

Woodward H: One community's response to the multi-system service needs of individuals with mental illness and developmental disabilities. Community Mental Health Journal 29:347–351, 1993

Wright EC: The presentation of mental illness in mentally retarded adults. Br J Psychiatry 141:496–502, 1982

Xenitidis K, Henry A Russell AJ, et al: An inpatient treatment model for adults with mild intellectual disability and challenging behaviour. J Intellect Disabil Res 43:128–134, 1999

Zarfas DE: Mental health systems for people with mental retardation: a Canadian perspective. Australia and New Zealand Journal of Developmental Disabilities 14:3–7, 1988

27 Psychiatric Treatment in Community Care

Nick Bouras, M.B., Ph.D., F.R.C.Psych.
Geraldine Holt, M.B., B.S., M.R.C.Psych.

Mental retardation is a lifelong condition. Its impact on the individual, his or her family, and others varies in form and severity. A community-based approach must recognize this diversity of needs and harness resources to meet them. There must be an overall vision, with a personal plan for each patient coordinated by a care manager linking the patient to appropriate providers.

Psychiatric and behavioral disorders in people with mental retardation have been documented over the last two decades (Iverson and Fox 1989; Jacobson 1990; Menolascino 1988; Reiss 1990). The importance of specialized mental health services for this group has been recognized (Mansell 1993), using both hospital-based (Day 1983; Gold et al. 1989) and community-based models (Bouras et al. 1994).

In this chapter, we present issues regarding psychiatric treatment for people with mental retardation living in the community. We include reference to the need for inpatient facilities, the role of general practitioners, the necessity of training direct care staff, and the need to monitor the quality of care.

■ SERVICE DEVELOPMENTS

Service developments for people with mental retardation were established in the United States and the United Kingdom following several policy initiatives. In the United States, the Community Mental Health Retardation Facilities Construction Act in 1963 recommended the integration of people with mental retardation into community life. Likewise in the United Kingdom, successive governmental policies in the 1970s and 1980s shifted priorities toward resettlement from long-stay hospitals. More recently, similar initiatives have been reported in other European countries (Došen 1994; MHMR 1993) and Canada (Puddephatt and Sussman 1994). The majority of these policies have focused on educational and social care needs. Little attention has been paid, however, to mental health needs (Bouras et al. 1995a; Gravestock and Bouras 1995).

Psychiatric services in the United States for people with mental retardation have tended to be provided by visiting consultants rather than full-time professionals (Menolascino and Fleisher 1993; Szymanski et al. 1989) in outpatient clinics as part of a university-affiliated program (Reiss 1992) and in specialized inpatient/outpatient services (Fletcher and Menolascino 1989; Menolascino 1984). Community-based mental health services have been reported in Boston (Davidson et al. 1994) and Rochester (Beasley et al. 1992).

In the United Kingdom, specialized psychiatric provision has been developed for people with mental retardation centering on the use of either long-stay hospitals (Day 1994), community-based services integrated with other mental retardation services (Bicknell 1985), community-based services integrated both with generic mental health and mental retardation services (Bouras et al. 1994), or separate services for people with "challenging behavior" (Hoefkens and Allen 1990; Mansell 1993; Murphy et al. 1991). Each model has its strengths and weaknesses (South East Thames Regional Health Authority 1994).

■ COMMUNITY INTERVENTION VERSUS ADMISSION

The Community Specialist Psychiatric Service (CSPS) for people with dual diagnosis has been in operation in the South East Thames region for more than 12 years. It is community based and integrated with both generic mental health and mental retardation services (Bouras et al. 1994). This model is used by the authors firstly because the patients experience less disruption and distress as most therapeutic interventions take place in their living environment rather than in clinics or as inpatients, and, secondly, it enables local services to develop their own skills in supporting and managing patients with complex needs rather than removing them to separate places where these are provided. There are, however, circumstances in which residential services or families are unable to continue supporting an individual with mental health problems in the community and admission may be needed. In such cases the CSPS uses the inpatient psychiatric beds of the local generic psychiatric services.

The monitored evaluation of 424 consecutive new referrals to the CSPS revealed that the mean age of patients was 32.9 years (SD ± 13.4), of whom 60% were men and 40% were women. Mild mental retardation was recorded for 60%, moderate for 25%, and severe for 15%.

Table 27–1. DSM-III-R psychiatric diagnosis

	Community intervention	Admission
	N, %	**N, %**
Psychotic disorder	35, 9.3	21, 44.7
Depressive disorder	25, 6.6	7, 14.9
Personality disorder	26, 6.9	4, 8.5
Anxiety disorder	26, 6.9	4, 8.5
Adjustment reaction	18, 4.8	2, 4.3
Dementia	11, 2.9	2, 4.3
Eating disorder	2, 0.5	1, 2.1
Manic-depressive disorder	3, 0.8	0, 0
Psychiatric diagnosis	231, 61.3	6, 12.7
Total	**377, 89.0**	**47, 11.0**

Admission was required for 47 (11%) of the referred patients. The admitted patients were slightly older (mean age 36.8 years, SD±14.1) than those treated in the community (mean age 32.6 years, SD±13.5), but the difference was not statistically significant. There was no difference in the sex ratio between the patients admitted to psychiatric wards and those who received community intervention. In terms of mental retardation, 86% of the admitted patients were mildly retarded, 12% were moderately retarded, and there was only 1 patient with severe retardation.

Of the patients admitted to psychiatric wards, 87.3% fulfilled the criteria for a DSM III-R psychiatric diagnosis compared with 38.7% of those who received community intervention. The majority (44.7%) of the admitted patients, as can be seen in Table 27–1, suffered from psychotic disorder, 14.9% from depressive disorder, and 8.5% from personality disorder.

The mean score for behavior problems was higher for frequency and severity for the patients admitted (mean = 5.4, SD = 5.3) compared with those treated in the community (mean = 3.7, SD = 4.5), and the difference was statistically significant (t-test = 2.20, $P < 0.02$). Physical aggression was present in 50% of the admitted patients compared with 29.8% of the nonadmitted patients ($\chi^2 = 5.9$, $P < .01$).

These findings confirm that the types of psychiatric disorders in people with mental retardation are the same as those seen in the general population and that the needs of the majority can be met in the community but that admission facilities are necessary. For people with mild or moderate mental retardation, inpatient beds on generic psychiatric wards can be used. Physical aggression, whether related to psychiatric diagnosis (as in our service) or not (Davidson et al. 1994), seems to be an important factor for determining admission.

People with severe mental retardation and mental health problems referred to the CSPS were generally not admitted as inpatients. Their needs could not be easily met in generic psychiatric wards. All the cases of people with severe mental retardation and dual diagnosis were provided with intensive input by clinical psychologists based on the principles of a "challenging-needs" approach (Mansell 1993) with support from psychiatrists and community psychiatric nurses as required.

There are certainly times when community services cannot cope with people having severe mental retardation and severe behavior problems, but whether admission is desirable is still a matter of debate (Emerson et al. 1987). Studies of different models tend to have methodological flaws (Hoefkins and Allen 1990). The different models of care tend to fall in two groups: specialist teams and specialist units. The former comprises a team of people with specialist knowledge who can work with caregivers and locally based providers to meet the needs of the individual, thus increasing the skill base locally. Sometimes, as staff leave, it has proved difficult to provide a continuing approach in community settings (Emerson et al. 1989). Specialist units, in contrast, provide the possibility of a more secure environment with a concentration of skilled staff (Newman and Emerson 1991). Whereas such a model minimizes disruption to the community at large, the patient's relationships are disrupted, and improvements gained in behavior may be difficult to maintain on discharge. Davidson et al. (1999) have provided a comprehensive review of community services for people with mental retardation and mental health problems.

■ PRIMARY CARE AND GENERAL PRACTITIONERS

It has been proposed that the primary health care needs of people with mental retardation living in the community be met by general practitioners (Royal College of General Practitioners 1990).

People with mental retardation often have hidden medical needs (Essex 1991; Wilson and Haire 1990). This is because the disabled persons may not recognize that there is a problem or are unable to communicate their problem to others, and clinicians may fail, through lack of time or expertise, to recognize the need.

The average general practice is likely to have few patients with mental retardation. For general practitioners to fulfill their role, it is vital, then, that they be made aware of those on their patient list who have mental retardation so that they are able to provide advice to patients, their family, and care staff on medical matters; arrange appropriate screening; and facilitate referrals to specialist services. However, general practitioners may feel that they do not have the necessary training or knowledge of specialist services to carry this out, particularly for those with dual diagnosis (Holt 1992). A study of general practitioners in Bristol (Langan and Russell 1993) revealed this lack of awareness of the work of multidisciplinary community teams for people with mental retardation. Bernard and Bates (1994) reported similar findings and confusion as to the role of the psychiatrist in this field. There is, therefore, a need for the specialist psychiatric services to train, advise, and collaborate with the general practitioners in order to identify early problems and to support the patients, their families, and their caregivers in community settings.

■ DIRECT CARE STAFF

Our experience of providing mental health services to those with dual diagnosis living in the community revealed that often direct care staff were unclear as to how one can recognize mental health problems and access appropriate services and knew very little about what to expect from them (Bouras et al. 1994). Staff also find such work stressful (Ward 1989). Staff behavior and attitude may be modified by their knowledge, training, and skills as well as by organizational practices (Brower et al. 1987; Firth et al. 1980; Hatton and Emerson 1993). Allen et al. (1990) highlighted that whereas institutions often had well-developed training departments, the move to the community training opportunities became more difficult to coordinate. Training, however, is important in maintaining staff morale. Direct care staff who are committed and supportive are likely to be a positive and powerful factor in achieving an optimal level of functioning in patients with mental retardation.

For these reasons a training package has been developed, consisting of a training manual and a handbook (Bouras and Holt 1997). It has the following training objectives:

1. Recognize more easily symptoms and behaviors indicating that a person with mental retardation may be developing mental health problems.
2. Become familiar with treatment methods, including use of medication and psychotherapeutic approaches.
3. Discuss alternative ways of dealing with difficult problems and behaviors.
4. Share experience with other staff.
5. Bridge the communication gap between community staff and mental health service provision.

6. Contribute to a more appropriate use of the available services and ensure more effective service provision.
7. Meet the expectations of service users as much as possible.
8. Promote prevention of mental health problems in people with mental retardation.

The training package has been designed on a modular structure to allow flexibility, encouraging participants to work from personal experience and have a go at doing things differently. It is envisaged that this training approach for direct care staff will increase their skills, knowledge, and confidence, thereby contributing decisively to successful management of individuals with dual diagnosis living in the community and improving their quality of care. Staff will also become more aware of their limitations, and their increased competence should facilitate more effective use of professional input. With the diversification of providers of service, purchasers will need to write into contracts the requirement that direct care staff receive high-quality training, such as is provided in this training package.

■ QUALITY OF CARE

Gravestock (1994a; Gravestock et al. 1996) suggested that the development of community services should ensure the quality of care, including accessibility, acceptability, appropriateness, coordination, continuity, cost-effectiveness, and efficiency. These elements have been built into the development of the CSPS, which monitors and evaluates its work to ensure that its objectives are being met and to highlight areas of unmet needs. Areas studied include

1. The frequency and severity of behavior and psychiatric disorders in people with mental retardation living in the community (Bouras and Drummond 1992).
2. A description of medical and psychiatric needs of people resettled from a long-stay institution (Bouras et al. 1993).
3. A needs assessment of adolescents with mental retardation and their families. This showed that more difficulties were experienced by those families with a member with severe disabilities and behavior problems (Brooks and Bouras 1994).
4. A study of service acceptability showed that patient satisfaction with psychiatric outpatient care appeared to be high (Bretherton and Gravestock 1994). Areas in which standards have been set and regularly monitored include record keeping and the use of depot neuroleptics (Gravestock 1994b).

■ CONCLUSIONS

The mental health needs of people with mental retardation should be met by specialist services, ideally integrated with both generic psychiatric services and mental retardation services. The psychiatric intervention should form part of the individual's total care plan.

It is entirely feasible to run a robust specialist psychiatric service based in the community, as the data on CSPS demonstrate. Inpatient backup is provided for those with mild to moderate mental retardation in the generic psychiatric clinics. For those with more severe mental retardation and mental illness or challenging behavior, such clinics do not meet their needs, and instead intensive input is made by the multiprofessional team in the community.

The balance between what it is possible to provide in the community and in an inpatient setting will vary from place to place, but we would suggest that it is desirable for the main thrust of psychiatric services to be community based. Similarly, this is our view of services for those individuals with severe behavior problems.

To meet patients' mental health needs in the community, those working with them need to be furnished not only with specialist support but also with knowledge and skills. Training and educational activities directed toward direct care staff and general practitioners are of utmost importance.

This is a time of growth and change in services for those with mental retardation. Major reforms have been introduced to service provision for people with mental retardation (Caring for People 1989). One of the weaknesses of these reforms is that several small organizations tend to become providers, and there is a danger of fragmentation and loss of coordination of services, repeated shift of responsibility from one part of the service network to another, and a lack of strategic investment in training and specialized professional input (Mansell 1994). The provision of specialized services to meet the complex mental health needs of people with mental retardation, especially as an increasing number of them now live at home with elderly parents, remains a challenge.

■ REFERENCES

Allen P, Pahl J, Quine L: Care Staff in Transition. London, Her Majesty's Stationary Office, 1990

Beasley J, Kroll J, Sovner R: Community-based services for persons with developmental disabilities: the START model. The Habilitative Mental Health Care Newsletter 11:55–58, 1992

Bernard S, Bates R: The role of the psychiatrist in learning disability, how it is perceived by the general practitioner. Psychiatric Bulletin 18:205–206, 1994

Bicknell J: The mental handicap service, in Caring for Mentally Handicapped People in the Community. Edited by Sines D, Bicknell J. London, Harper & Row, 1985, pp 78–91

Bouras N, Drummond C: Behaviour and psychiatric disorders of people with mental handicaps living in the community. J Intellect Disabil Res 36:349–357, 1992

Bouras N, Kon Y, Drummond C: Medical and psychiatric needs of adults with a mental handicap. J Intellect Disabil Res 37:177–182, 1993

Bouras N, Brooks D, Drummond K: Community psychiatric services for people with mental retardation, in Mental Health in Mental Retardation: Recent Advances and Practices. Edited by Bouras N. Cambridge, UK, Cambridge University Press, 1994, pp 293–299

Bouras N, Holt G, Gravestock S: Community care for people with learning disabilities: deficits and future plans. Psychiatric Bulletin 19:134–137, 1995a

Bouras N, Holt G: Mental Health and Learning Disabilities Training Package, 2nd Edition. Brighton UK, Pavilion, 1997

Bretherton K, Gravestock S: Consumer satisfaction with specialist clinics for adults with learning disabilities and mental health needs. Presentation at the Winter Meeting of the Royal College of Psychiatrists, London, 1994

Brooks D, Bouras N: Adolescents with a learning disability: family enrollmwnt and transitional issues. Psychiatric Bulletin 18:606–608, 1994

Brower CH, Ellis KA, Ford T, et al: Stress, social support, and health of psychiatric technicians in a state facility. Ment Retard 25:31–38, 1987

Caring for People: Community Care in the Next Decade and Beyond. London, Her Majesty's Stationary Office, CM849, 1989

Davidson PW, Cain NN, Sloane-Reeves JE, et al: Characteristics of community-based individuals with mental retardation and aggressive behavioral disorders. Am J Ment Retard 98:704–716, 1994

Davidson PW, Morris D, Cain NN: Community services for people with developmental disabilities and psychiatric or severe behavior disorders, in Psychiatric Behavioral Disorders in Developmental Disabilities and Mental Retardation. Edited by Bouras N. Cambridge, UK, Cambridge University Press, 1999, pp 359–372

Day K: A hospital based unit for mentally handicapped adults. Mental Handicap 11:137–140, 1983

Day K: Psychiatric services in mental retardation: generic or specialised provision, in Mental Health in Mental Retardation: Recent Advances and Practices. Edited by Bouras N. Cambridge, UK, Cambridge University Press, 1994, pp 275–292

Došen D: The European scene, in Mental Health in Mental Retardation: Recent Advances and Practices. Edited by Bouras N. Cambridge, UK, Cambridge University Press, 1994, pp 375–378

Emerson E, Barrett S, Bell C, et al: Developing Services for People With Severe Learning Difficulties and Challenging Behavior. Cantebury, UK, University of Kent Canterbury, Institute of Social and Applied Psychology, 1987

Emerson E, Cummings R, Hughes H, et al: Challenging behavior and community services. Mental Handicap 17:104–107, 1989

Essex C: Screening for people with mental handicap (letter). BMJ 302:239, 1991

Firth H, McIntee J, McKeown P, et al: Interpersonal support among nurses at work. J Adv Nurs 11:273–282, 1980

Fletcher R, Menolascino FJ: Mental Retardation and Mental Illness: Assessment, Treatment, and Service for the Dually Diagnosed. Lexington, MA, Lexington Books, 1989

Gold IM, Wolfson ES, Lester CM, et al: Developing a unit for mentally retarded-mentally ill patients on the grounds of a state hospital. Hospital and Community Psychiatry 40:836–840, 1989

Gravestock S: Quality assurance for adults with mental retardation and mental health needs, in Mental Health in Mental Retardation: Recent Advances and Practices. Edited by Bouras N. Cambridge, UK, Cambridge University Press, 1994a, pp 319–327

Gravestock S: Depot neuroleptics usage in adults with learning disabilities. J Intellect Disabil Res 40:17–28, 1994b

Gravestock S, Bouras N: Services for adults with learning disabilities and mental health needs. Psychiatric Bulletin 19:288–290, 1995

Gravestock S, Bouras N, Holt G: Quality monitoring in community psychiatry of learning disabilities services. British Journal of Learning Disabilities 24:95–96, 1996

Hatton C, Emerson E: Organisational predictors of staff stress, satisfaction, and intended turnover in a service for people with multiple disabilities. Ment Retard 31:388–395, 1993

Hoefkens A, Allen D: Evaluation of a special behavior unit for people with mental handicaps and challenging behavior. Journal of Mental Deficiency Research 34:213–228, 1990

Holt G: Primary care for people with mental handicaps (letter). Psychiatric Bulletin 16:667, 1992

Iverson JC, Fox RA: Prevalence of psychopathology among mentally retarded adults. Research in Developmental Disability 10:77–83, 1989

Jacobson JW: Do some mental disorders occur less frequently among persons with mental retardation? Am J Ment Retard 94:596–602, 1990

Langan J, Russell O: Community Care and the General Practitioner: Primary Health Care for People With Learning Disabilities. Bristol, UK, Norah Fry Research Unit, 1993

Mansell JL: Services for People With Learning Disabilities and Challenging Behavior or Mental Health Needs. London, Her Majesty's Stationary Office, 1993

Mansell JL: Challenging behavior: the prospect for change. British Journal of Learning Disabilities 22:2–5, 1994

Menolascino FJ: A broader perspective: applying modern mental-retardation service-system principles to all chronically disabled persons, in Handbook of Mental Illness in the Mentally Retarded. Edited by Menolascino FJ, Stark J. London, Plenum, 1984, pp 18–41

Menolascino FJ: Mental Illness in the mentally retarded: diagnosis and treatment issues, in Mental Retardation and Mental Health: Classification, Diagnosis, Treatment, Services. Edited by Stark JA, Menolascino FJ, Albarelli MH, et al. London, Springer-Verlag, 1988, pp 109–123

Menolascino FJ, Fleisher MH: Mental health care in persons with mental retardation: past, present and future, in Mental Health Aspects of Mental Retardation. Edited by Flechter RJ, Došen A. Lexington, MA, Lexington Books, 1993, pp 18–44

MHMR: European Association for Mental Health in Mental Retardation: Proceedings of a Symposium on the Mental Health of Europeans With Learning Disabilities. J Intellect Disabil Res 37(suppl 1), 1993

Murphy G, Holland A, Fowler P, et al: MIETS: a service option for people with mild mental handicaps and challenging behavior or psychiatric problems. Mental Handicap Research 4(1):41–66, 1991

Newman I, Emerson E: Specialised treatment units for people with challenging behaviors. Mental Handicap 19:113–119, 1991

Puddephatt A, Sussman S: Developing services in Canada: Ontario vignettes, in Mental Health in Mental Retardation: Recent Advances and Practices. Edited by Bouras N. Cambridge, UK, Cambridge University Press, 1994, pp 353–364

Reiss S: Prevalence of dual diagnosis in community based day programmes in the Chicago metropolitan area. Am J Ment Retard 94:578–585, 1990

Reiss S: Assessment of dual diagnosis, in Psychopathology in Persons With Mental Retardation. Edited by Matson JL, Barrett RW. Boston, MA, Allyn & Bacon, 1992, pp 152–167

Royal College of General Practitioners: Primary care for people with a mental handicap, Occasional Paper 47. London, Royal College of General Practitioners, 1990

South East Thames Regional Health Authority: The Mental Health Needs of People With Learning Disabilities. Tunbridgewells, UK, Southeast Thames Regional Health Authority, 1994

Szymanski LS, Rubin IL, Tarjan G: Mental retardation, in American Psychiatric Press Review of Psychiatry, Vol 8. Edited by Tasman A, Hales RE, Frances AJ. Washington, DC, American Psychiatric Press, 1989, pp 217–241

Ward L: An ordinary life: the early views and experiences of residential staff in the Wells Road Service. Mental Handicap 17:6–9, 1989

Wilson DN, Haire A: Health care screening for people with mental handicap living in the community. BMJ 301:1379–1381, 1990

28 A Model for Inpatient Services for Persons With Mental Retardation and Mental Illness

Mark Fleisher, M.D.
Earl H. Faulkner, M.A.
Robert L. Schalock, Ph.D.
Larry Folk, B.A.

It is estimated that between 20% and 30% of the individuals with mental retardation living in the community also exhibit one or more diagnosable mental illnesses (Luckasson et al. 1992; Stark et al. 1988). This group represents a significant challenge to policy makers and service providers, especially in the current paradigm that stresses community inclusion and equity in the face of fewer allocated resources and managed care.

During the last decade we have advanced our understanding of persons with mental retardation and mental illness in at least four respects. First, it is clear that the stressors associated with community living may cause or exacerbate psychiatric problems (Stark et al. 1988). Second, persons with mental retardation and mental illness have been shown to have high rates of initial institutionalization and reinstitutionalization (Heinlein and Fortune 1995; McGee et al. 1984). Third, the diagnostic certainty is frequently problematic due to overshadowing or the interaction of the two conditions (Luckasson et al. 1992; Reiss 1985). Finally, treatment programs are often inadequate due to the lack of experienced professionals and available services (Szymanski 1980).

Despite this better understanding, we still do not know enough about the patient characteristics, available treatment regimens, and their effects on long-term status following treatment intervention. Thus, the three objectives of this chapter are to 1) discuss a program in Nebraska for persons with mental retardation and mental illness (MR/MI); 2) summarize changes in a group of 77 individuals served by this program, including a determination of the significant predictors of recidivism; and 3) discuss these data and the National Center for Persons With Mental Retardation and Mental Illness's experience with persons diagnosed as MR/MI.

◼ PROGRAM DESCRIPTION

The National Center for Persons With Mental Retardation and Mental Illness is a 10-bed inpatient unit that operates autonomously from other adult and child/adolescent units located in a mental health facility that functions as a teaching hospital for the Creighton-Nebraska Combined Department of Psychiatry. This specialized unit is staffed by the following personnel: staff psychiatrist, senior psychologist, resident psychologist, social worker, registered nurses, and staff-habilitation specialists. Instructional control, nonaversive teaching techniques, applied behavioral analyses, and medication regimens were the principal interventions and treatments provided. The National Center was opened in May 1990 as a direct result of the deinstitutionalization movement and the need for specialized care within the context of community integration.

Inpatient Service

The inpatient service is designed to treat individuals who cannot be treated in a less restrictive environment or who require expert care and evaluation unavailable outside the hospital setting. In most cases, these individuals cannot be treated effectively as outpatients due to the severity of their illnesses. Care includes diagnostic procedures, the initiation of behavioral interventions, family or care provider support and training, individual and group therapy, and, often, significant changes in medication regimens. The high percentage of pharmacy or even polypharmacy use, particularly for institutionalized individuals, is well documented, with considerable range to the outcomes of such use (Agran et al. 1988; Fredericks and Hayes 1995; Poindexter 1989; Rinck et al. 1989; Stone et al. 1989). This does not automatically cast doubt on the overall appropriateness of this treatment option; whether a particular medication or level of medication is appropriate must be determined on an individual basis. It is certainly preferable to have a physician trained in working with persons with mental retardation to begin and monitor complex medication regimens proactively as opposed to patient referral after problems or failures have occurred.

Admission to the inpatient service was required in order to define and implement diagnoses and subsequent treatments for patients with mental illness or behavioral changes. The admission also gave specialists a chance to plan for hospital discharge as well as all necessary programs for the individual's treatment complex. These elements included follow-up specialty nursing care; occupational, vocational, rehabilitative, or recreational therapy; and outpatient follow-up appointments with the psychiatrist or other specialists such as genetics or orthopedics. In addition, visits to the patient's home, residential facility, or institution were frequently made in order to provide instruction in nonaversive behavioral programs and to improve the quality of staff and consumer interactions and strategies. Families and designated care providers were usually brought into the treatment milieu to facilitate the transfer, aftercare, and treatment strategies if the patient was to be sent home on discharge.

It is convenient to divide the basic responsibilities of an inpatient service into the broad categories of diagnosis, treatment, and discharge planning. Diagnosis, particularly in severely and profoundly retarded individuals, is always difficult to make with a high degree of certainty. Yet the importance of diagnostic certitude is clear when one recognizes that effective treatment is dependent on accurate diagnosis. With patients who have a limited repertoire of language or communication skills, the interpretation of behaviors, whether labeled as problems or not, becomes important. Rarely in medicine can a person's slight moves or gestures be such fertile ground for diagnosis.

Hospitalization allows for assessment to be carried out in a safe and timely fashion. A number of complicated tests or invasive procedures may be necessary to arrive at a diagnosis composed of different components, such as physical ailments, which can be life-threatening or better treated by another medical specialist. A straightforward example would be to rule out causes for dementia, which requires a decision-tree process. First, one could rule out a treatable cause of dementia. Then one is left with the question of deciding whether this is a true dementia, and if so, of what type. If not a true dementia, is it a pseudodementia, an affective disorder, a psychotic disorder with an atypical presentation, or a personality disorder with mild mental retardation? Based on comprehensive interviews with patient, family, case workers, and others involved, a thorough history should be compiled, and from this accumulation of facts and insights, a working diagnosis may be obtained.

From the diagnosis, the treatment strategy must follow, and input from all treatment staff considered. Laboratory or diagnostic tests should be carried out to rule out occult pathology. Again, treatment and diagnosis should be similar to those used for a disturbed patient with a normal level of intelligence. As Szymanski (1980) reported, for individuals with mild and moderate retardation, the symptoms indicated and the signs noted are quite similar to the general population. For severely and profoundly retarded individuals, behavioral observation and interpretation become extremely important (Reiss 1985). Eaton and Menolascino (1982) also commented on the highly personal and individualistic behaviors of severely and profoundly disabled individuals as being symptomatic behavioral problems, which frequently mask psychiatric disorders. These behaviors include increased stereotypy and self-injury, aggression, and decreased adaptive behavioral skills (e.g., social and communication skills, personal living skills, motor skills, community living skills).

There must be great emphasis placed on developmental landmarks and their subsequent problems. Efforts should focus on trying to ascertain the primary cause of developmental delays and to identify the primary cause of cognitive problems. Extensive histories are important and should include medical, psychiatric, and obstetric details of parents and children of the patient's family. In addition, special emphasis ought to be placed on the prenatal and postnatal periods as well as preschool nurturing and the home environment. Unfortunately, it is our experience that obtaining these data is frequently difficult and problematic.

The major underpinning of inpatient services was ongoing outpatient support. With continuity of care as a primary goal, an individual can move from an intensive inpatient support system to a less restrictive home and work environment. But this can only be accomplished with the support of an outpatient clinic staffed by a community liaison representative versed in the specialized operations of community-based residential, educational, and vocational support services.

Perhaps the most important role of specialized psychiatric services is to identify and translate various symptoms into their proper diagnostic groups, which will in turn provide direction for specific treatment modalities aimed at specific syndromes. Awareness of the influence that various community supports (e.g., vocational, residential, familial) may be contributing to the resolution of psychiatric syndromes is an ever-changing process in which each type of necessary support must be considered and adjusted as the dynamic of the disorder resolves itself. Depending on the diagnosis (and its accuracy), treatment may be short term and include only limited therapy, or it may become a lifelong process requiring multiple hospitalizations and long-term dependence on medication, ongoing psychotherapy, and specialized community support.

In its essence, an outpatient service functions as an evaluation, treatment, and referral center much as an inpatient clinic does. The clinic's primary function is to help maintain the individual in the mainstream of his or her family and in community life. Indeed, today we strive to not hospitalize patients if at all possible and would rather see them intensively, even daily, to keep them out of the hospital setting, which may foster dependence and cause a degree of regression and loss of skills. Outpatient services can address one or more specific aspects of a problem, and collectively these services provide a continuum of care that can sustain mental health for years or a lifetime.

■ AN EVALUATION OF PATIENT CHANGE, RECIDIVISM, AND PREDICTORS

Subjects

Data were collected on 77 individuals who were referred to the National Center over a 1-year period. Significant demographic characteristics included 31 females and 46 males; average age 29; average IQ (WAIS-R) 50; and ethnicity 86% Caucasian, 10% African Americans, and 4% Native Americans. The major referral behavioral problems at admission included aggression toward others or self, noncompliance (59%), and sad or depressed mood/affect (36%).

Data Sets and Results

The following data sets and results were obtained at one or more of four points in time of patients' contact with the Center. These points included upon admission, during inpatient treatment, upon discharge, and 12–18 months following discharge.

Status Variables and Consumer Profile

A standard data collection format was used to obtain information regarding patient age, gender, ethnicity, level of retardation, and discharge diagnoses. DSM-III-R criteria were used by the psychiatric residents and the supervising psychiatrist. In addition, residential and vocational status were assessed on admission and at 12- to 18-month follow-up.

The average length of stay for the group was 27 days. During that period and subsequent to discharge, a number of changes were made in patient diagnoses, living and work environments, and medications. These changes are summarized and presented in Table 28–1 and Figure 28–1.

Diagnostic changes from admission to discharge included a decrease in the percentage of persons diagnosed as having schizophrenia or organic mental disorder, and an increase in diagnoses of major depression (see top half of Table 28–1). Living and work status changes were also noted. For example, the number of patients from state institutions at admission ($n=4$) increased at follow-up ($n=8$). In contrast, slight decreases were found in group home placements ($n=49$ to $n=42$) and parental/relative placements ($n=16$ to $n=15$), with some movement toward less structured environments such as semi-independent, independent, and room and board living alternatives (see bottom half of Table 28–1).

Medication data summarized in Figure 28–1 indicate an increased use of all medication classes from admission to discharge, continuing for the most part into the follow-up period. Most obvious is the increased used of antidepres-

Table 28–1. Consumer profile variables: diagnoses and living-work environments (*N*=77)

	Status upon admission		Status upon discharge		Status upon follow-up	
	%	*n*	%	*n*	%	*n*
Diagnosis						
Schizophrenia	44	33	31	24		
Organic mental disorder	23	18	14	11		
Major depression	16	12	3	24		
Bipolar disorder	5	4	9	7		
Sexual disorder	5	4	4	3		
Impulse control	4	3	1	1		
Adjustment disorder	1	1	8	6		
Schizoaffective disorder	1	1	0	0		
Obsessive-compulsive disorder	1	1	1	1		
Environments						
Group home	64	49			55	42
Parent/relative	21	16			20	15
State facility	5	4			10	8
Foster home	4	3			4	3
Semi-independent	4	3			5	4
Room and board	1	1			4	3
Independent	1	1			2	2

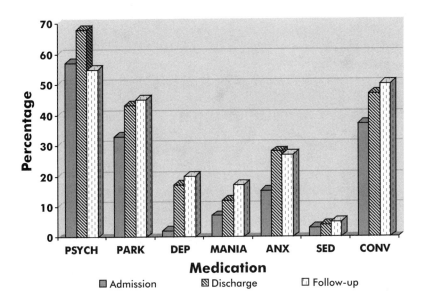

Figure 28–1. Medication use.

sants from admission (1%) to discharge (17%) and at follow-up (20%). The use of antipsychotic medication was also greater from the time of admission (56%) to discharge (65%). However, the percentage of persons on medications at follow-up actually fell slightly below admission levels (54%).

Treatment Intervention Level and Profile

The level of inpatient intervention was assessed as "high," "moderate," or "low." These ratings were based on the level of staffing intensity required during a patient's treatment. In general, a high rating was referred to as "one-to-one" staff-to-patient ratio of care, a moderate level was "one-to-five," and low was considered general group supervision. Ratings were given at admission and at discharge.

Two intervention components were analyzed. First, the level of behavioral intervention from admission to discharge was compared. On admission, 53% of the patients required a high level of intervention, 38% a medium level, and 9% a low level. At discharge, the respective percentages were 14%, 47%, and 39%. Changes in the second component, medication dosage changes, are shown graphically in Figure 28–2, which indicates that medication dosages tended to increase from admission to discharge (see Figure 28–2A) in most medication classes, with the exception of sedatives/hypnotics. For example,

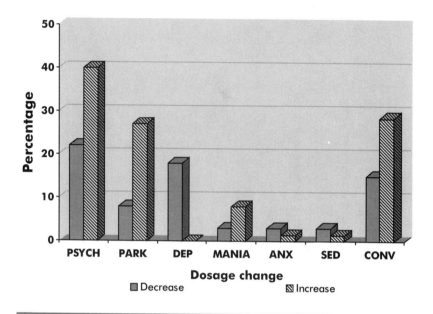

Figure 28–2A.   Medication dosage change: admission to discharge.

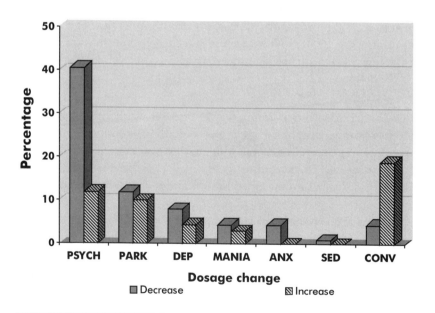

Figure 28–2B.   Medication dosage change: discharge to follow-up.

dosage increases were noted in 31 patients (40%) receiving antipsychotic medications, whereas 17 persons (22%) taking an antipsychotic had a decreased dosage of that medication. In contrast, a general trend of decreased dosage was noted at follow-up (see Figure 28–2B).

Treatment Progress

The Treatment Progress Scales (TPS) (Schalock et al. 1993) were used to assess treatment progress across specific target behaviors. The procedure involves a 5-point Lehart rating scale ranging from 1, the most unfavorable treatment outcome, to 5, the best anticipated success with treatment. A score of 3 represents an anticipated level of amelioration as a result of treatment. The scales are built around 65 problem areas and were completed jointly by unit staff on admission and every 7 days thereafter. In addition, following discharge designated staff members were asked to rate these same targeted behaviors.

TPS was developed primarily around aggression and depression/sadness. Other problem areas monitored with the TPS included compliance, bizarre/repetitive behavior, activity level, anxiety, memory, and sexual control. A general trend toward improved ratings across target behaviors is indicated in 91% of the patients at an expected or more than expected level of treatment success at discharge, and 82% rated normal at this level during follow-up. In contrast, at admission 83% of the patients were given TPS ratings of most unfavorable or less than expected levels of treatment success.

Adaptive/Maladaptive Behavior

Adaptive and maladaptive or problem behavior ratings were obtained from scores on the Inventory for Client and Agency Planning (ICAP). The ICAP assesses adaptive behavior in the following four domains: motor skills, social and communication skills, personal living skills, and community living skills. The combination of these subscales comprises a general adaptive behavior score referred to as *broad independence.*

Maladaptive problem behavior ratings are grouped into three categories: internalized, asocial, and externalized. In addition, an overall or general maladaptive index score is generated and is based on the combination of the three domains cited above. Admission and follow-up ratings across both adaptive and maladaptive domains were obtained.

Measured adaptive and maladaptive behavior did not change significantly from admission testing to follow-up testing. There was some improvement in community living skills and the combined adaptive behavior score, but the changes were significant at only the 0.10 level of significance. There was also a general but statistically insignificant increase across the measured maladaptive behavior categories, which suggested a decrease in the severity of these problem behaviors over time.

Quality of Life

The Quality of Life Questionnaire (QOL) (Schalock and Keith 1993) was used to evaluate four life experience domains: satisfaction, competence/productivity, empowerment/independence, and social/belonging/community integration. An overall QOL score is obtained from the combination of these four subscales. Admission and follow-up ratings were obtained.

The QOL scores summarized reflected significantly higher scores at follow-up in perceived competence, social belonging, and total QOL. Statistically nonsignificant increases were noted for the satisfaction and empowerment QOL subscales from admission to follow-up test scores.

Recidivism

Data were collected as to whether patients had been readmitted to the National Center or any other psychiatric hospital during the 12–18 months following their discharge. The data referred to the number and frequency of readmissions and the cause as stated by the patients' staff.

Within this 12–18 month period, 74% of the group had not been readmitted to the Center or any other inpatient setting. Of those returning to inpatient care, 23% ($n=18$) had been admitted on one occasion, 2% ($n=2$) twice, and 1% ($n=1$) three times. The primary reason stated most frequently by staff for readmission involved acts of aggression toward self and/or others. However, results of the stepwise multiple regression analysis showed that age, gender, and adaptive behavior were the significant predictors. That is, older males with poor adaptive behavior skills tended to be more likely to be readmitted to inpatient psychiatric care. Maladaptive or problem behaviors, including acts of aggression, noncompliance, or both, were less predictive of recidivism in the present sample.

■ DISCUSSION

The present evaluation suggests several critical issues that need to be addressed when providing services to persons with a diagnosis of mental retardation and mental illness. These include diagnosis, personnel competencies, programmatic capabilities, evaluation criteria, and site of evaluation. Most of the persons referred to the National Center had a history of being diagnosed by primary care physicians who tended to favor diagnoses of schizophrenia or organic mental disorder rather than the affective disorders (e.g., major depression or bipolar disorder), which were more apparent to the National Center's psychiatric staff. The importance of a correct diagnosis is reflected in the correlation between medication change and discharge diagnosis, and the relationship between the use of appropriate medications and improved TPS ratings at discharge.

In the area of personnel competencies, there are several issues. One is the obvious need for access to competent psychiatrists, psychologists, social workers, and other professionals who are familiar with the biopsychosocial dynamics of persons with mental retardation and mental illness as well as the special challenges community living presents to all persons involved. These are the individuals who are most likely to diagnose the patient correctly and implement medication and behavioral intervention strategies that can be highly successful (Stark et al. 1988). The inpatient program outlined above was the direct result of the deinstitutionalization movement and highlights the continued necessity for specialized care within the context of the goals of community integration.

Access to appropriately experienced professionals should not be limited to inpatient settings. In today's constricted fiscal climate many habilitative services can and perhaps should be offered as an outpatient service. Similarly, motivated and creative support staff or direct-line personnel must be appropriately trained so that treatment plans can be properly implemented and monitored. It is at this direct-line level that the second personnel issue is indeed critical. Specifically, habilitation programs must be able to maintain high staffing ratios as reflected in the high level of intervention indicated in the present data upon admission. In time, these can be reduced to moderate or even low levels. Finally, all personnel need to be highly trained in the areas of instructional control, educational techniques, and applied behavior analyses, which have been shown repeatedly to be highly effective for acting out and aggressive behavior that frequently characterized the present sample on admission.

A third critical issue relates to the habilitation program's motivation and capability to assist in arranging appropriate living and employment programs. A significant problem at discharge, directly or indirectly related to economic factors, was the number of referring programs that would not accept the person back into his or her community-based programs (Blanck 1995). This unnecessarily extended days of hospitalization and created a "warehousing" effect that will not be subsidized by managed care programs in this country and places the costs back onto the hospital. Thus, the state facility became the placement of necessity for these individuals. It is important to note that those living with parents and in either semi-independent or independent situations prior to admission returned to these environments.

It was significant that 21% of the patients were not in any vocational program on referral. This large group, in addition to the 11% who were initially referred from a school program but did not return to school, reflects the need for habilitation programs to expand their employment options.

A fourth issue generated from experiences with the National Center involves the criteria by which one evaluates individuals and the outcomes of habilitation programs. The National Center attempted to conduct research within the context of a program evaluation paradigm that included the following: 1) a comprehensive framework for evaluating programmatic outcomes, and 2) a shifting of research from an exclusive focus on recidivism and adaptive behaviors to the inclusion of quality of life issues that involved role functions, satisfaction, activity patterns, and assessed quality of life (Schalock et al. 1993). Three findings from the present study are significant. First, these persons demonstrated behavioral improvements. Second, as a group, their measured quality of life factor scores, including independence, productivity, community integration, and satisfaction, have increased during the 12–18 months following their discharge. Finally, adaptive behaviors as opposed to maladaptive behaviors appear to be a better predictor of treatment progress and measured quality of life changes. The data seem to indicate that maladaptive and problem behaviors did not statistically improve following discharge but were seen subjectively by staff as less interfering and subsequently less problematic. That is, staff seemed to have altered their own perceptions or tolerances of certain types of behaviors, a finding that underscores the increasing importance of focusing on adaptive behavior as it relates to both the diagnosis of mental retardation and its enhancement through the use of appropriate supports (Heal and Rusch 1995; Luckasson et al. 1992; Reiss 1994).

The present data and their implications need to be interpreted in light of the weaknesses of the research procedures: Subjects were not randomly selected; the intervention was short term, and it was conducted within a highly professionalized and controlled environment that is not characteristic of typical habilitation programs; and it did not use a "single-subject" research design, which permits an evaluation of the specific relationship between intervention strategies and results. Despite these weaknesses, however, the data do identify some of the more relevant characteristics of these patients who pose significant challenges to habilitation services. In addition, by identifying critical issues that need to be addressed in providing services to these individuals, habilitation programs can continue to develop effective and efficient services for persons diagnosed as mentally retarded and mentally ill.

■ CONCLUSIONS

The central issue is not the control of observable behaviors but the treatment of underlying psychiatric disorders. In a multidisciplinary team approach alone, a common theme of control can emerge that colors every aspect of an individual's life. This is particularly true in mental health care. A tendency exists to simply control disruptive behaviors that frequently equates with long-term institutional care. In addition, within these settings, control often means chemical restraint. Thus, ideological choices emerge that revolve around the questions of long-term segregation and restraint as well as of the provision of ongoing mental health services within the context of community life. To simply abandon individuals to institutionalization and chemical restraint is to condone the denial of the mentally retarded mentally ill person's full sentient nature. To ignore their needs in the community is to permit the rusting away of the human spirit. What could be more restrictive than a chemically restrained patient locked in a hospital?

Inpatient and outpatient services must be responsive to the needs of the individual. In the field of mental retardation, these needs are complex and layered one upon another. Treatment must focus on the individual and his or her milieu, which may include many of the factors contributing to the mental health problem. Mental health providers must act as interpreters within a highly complex interface of services. They must also take up the mandate to serve while preventing as much as possible a return to institutionalization, which, unfortunately, is an ideological construct that continues to exist in the minds of many service providers both in the community and in large aggregate settings.

Beyond awareness of ideologies, the issue of primary diagnosis comes quickly to the fore. If the primary diagnosis is mental retardation, the individual finds less help in the mental health system, and, conversely, if the primary diagnosis is mental illness, the mental retardation resources seem more distant. In this diagnostic game those with dual diagnoses fall through the cracks. The challenge is for mental health and mental retardation professionals to recognize the wholeness of each individual and provide whatever short- and long-range services might be necessary.

What are the implications for the inpatient and outpatient service providers? Simply this: one can either provide a treatment ground where these frequently opposing groups can meet and initiate mental health support, or one can construct a bridge for a one-way trip into institutional life, which is the tool used for extricating problem patients from the system. An enlightened approach may be to establish a referral base to provide a menu of support options for as long as they are needed. This base should be located within a clinical environment that operates with a full awareness of the implications of treatment and can assess emotional needs in the individual as well as in the system in which the individual is enmeshed.

■ REFERENCES

Agran M, Moore S, Martin JE: Research in mental retardation: under-reporting of medication information. Res Dev Disabil 9:351–358, 1988

Blanck PD: Assessing five years of employment integration and economic opportunities under the Americans With Disabilities Act. Mental and Physical Disabilities Law Reporter 19(3):384–392, 1995

Eaton LF, Menolascino FJ: Psychiatric disorders in the mentally retarded: types, problems, and challenges. Am J Psychiatry 139:1297–1303, 1982

Fredericks DW, Hayes LJ: Effects of drug changes and physician prescribing practices on the behavior of persons with mental retardation—special issue: pharmacotherapy III. Journal of Developmental Disabilities 7(2):105–122, 1995

Heal LW, Rusch FR: Predicting employment for students who leave special education high school programs. Exceptional Children 61(5):472–487, 1995

Heinlein KB, Fortune J: Who stays, who goes? Downsizing the institution in America's most rural state. Res Dev Disabil 16(3):165–177, 1995

Luckasson R, Coulter DL, Polloway EA, et al: Mental Retardation: Definition, Classification and Systems/Supports, 9th Edition. Washington, DC, American Association on Mental Retardation, 1992

McGee JJ, Folk L, Swanson DA, et al: A model inpatient psychiatric program: its relationship to a continuum of care for the mentally retarded-mentally ill, in Handbook of Mental Illness in the Mentally Retarded. Edited by Menolascino F, Stark J. New York, Plenum, 1984, pp 249–272

Poindexter AR: Psychotropic drug patterns in a large ICF/MR facility: a ten-year experience. Am J Ment Retard 6:624–626, 1989

Reiss S: The mentally, emotionally disturbed adult, in Children With Emotional Disorders and Developmental Disabilities. Edited by Stratton G. New York, Grune & Stratton, 1985, pp 125–143

Reiss S: Issues in defining mental retardation. Am J Ment Retard 99(1):1–7, 1994

Rinck C, Guidry J, Calkins CF: Review of states' practices on the use of psychotropic medication. Am J Ment Retard 93:657–668, 1989

Schalock RL, Keith KD: Quality of Life Questionnaire. Worthington, OH, IDS Publishing, 1993

Schalock RL, Sheehan MJ, Weber L: The use of treatment progress scales in the client monitoring and evaluation system. Journal of Mental Health Administration 20(3):264–269, 1993

Stark J, Menolascino FJ, Albarelli M, Gray V: Mental Retardation and Mental Health. New York, Springer-Verlag, 1988

Stone RK, Alvarez WF, Ellman G, et al: Prevalence and prediction of psychotropic drug use in California developmental centers. Am J Ment Retard 93:627–632, 1989

Szymanski LS: Psychiatric diagnosis of retarded persons, in Emotional Disorders of Mentally Retarded Persons. Edited by Szymanski L, Tanguay P. Baltimore, MD, University Park Press, 1980, pp 61–82

Integrative Treatment

29 Treatment

An Integrative Approach

Kenneth Day, M.B., Ch.B., F.R.C.Psych., D.P.M.
Anton Došen, M.D., Ph.D.

The psychopathology of mental disorder in people with mental retardation is complex. In establishing the diagnosis, one must take account of biological, psychological, social, and developmental factors, all of which play a role in onset and phenomenology. The same factors need to be addressed in treatment, and combinations of drug therapy, psychotherapy, behavior therapy, and other treatment approaches are often required. Treatment programs need to be based on a multidimensional psychiatric diagnosis, and their implementation requires smooth multidisciplinary efforts. Some authors speak of a pluralistic approach (Reukauf and Herzka 1990), others of a multidimensional approach (Gardner and Graeber 1990), and still others of an integrative approach (Szymanski 1988).

In this chapter, we attempt to draw together all the various therapeutic approaches that have been described in detail in the previous chapters and to provide a practical framework for an integrative approach.

■ TREATMENT APPROACHES IN PERSONS WITH MENTAL RETARDATION

Most of the therapeutic methods used with the nonretarded are, with little or no modification, applicable to individuals functioning within the range of borderline to mild mental retardation. Treatment of moderately and severely mentally retarded people, however, must take account of lower intelligence, impaired verbal communication skills, organic brain damage, and specific behavioral syndromes.

The psychiatric problems of mentally retarded people may be affected by lower doses of the psychotropic drugs that are usually used for the general popula-

519

tion, and a different range of drugs may be effective in some disorders. Mentally retarded people are more prone to side effects and atypical reactions than the nonretarded, and paradoxical effects can occur when sedatives and antidepressants are administered. Specific drugs may be useful in self-injurious behavior and in control of behavioral features associated with specific syndromes, such as Lesch-Nyhan or Prader-Willi (see Chapters 3, 14,–16, 24, and 25 of this book).

Psychotherapeutic approaches must make accommodations for the underlying mental retardation. Therapy needs to be more structured and targeted to the "here and now," and the therapist needs to be more directive. Sessions should be short and frequent. The therapist must interact with the patient at his or her cognitive level of functioning and discover and use the most useful channel of communication, which may be other than verbal (see Chapters 2, 8, 22, and 23 of this book).

Behavior therapy should be guided by a multimodal assessment that places the symptoms of disturbed behavior in the context of current biomedical, psychological, and socioenvironmental influences. It should focus on the teaching of coping alternatives such as anger management and relaxation therapy as well as on behavior control strategies (see Chapters 4 and 17 of this book). Cognitive therapy, social learning, and rational emotive therapy are being used increasingly and have been found to be helpful for mentally retarded patients (see Chapters 5 and 9 of this book).

The pedagogical schools of the Dutch, Swiss, and German tradition (Bradl 1987; Reukauf 1985; Van Gennep 1990) view problematic behavior as a request for help. Treatment encompasses the real-life situation and the totality of the person's existence and focuses on structuring activities, establishing appropriate relationships, and creating an accepting milieu (see Chapters 21 and 23 of this book).

◼ TREATMENT PLAN AND MONITORING

A full assessment and an accurate diagnostic formulation are the basis of the treatment plan (see Chapter 1 of this book). A comprehensive treatment plan should be formulated before treatment begins and should cover the following:

- Consent and compulsory treatment
- Treatment setting
- Treatment of the current illness
- General measures necessary for improving social functioning
- Management/treatment of coexisting problems (e.g., epilepsy)
- Rehabilitation, aftercare, and relapse prevention
- Family and caregiver support

Progress should be monitored regularly by the multidisciplinary team and the treatment program modified accordingly.

Consent

It is axiomatic that all patients should give informed consent to any form of medical treatment including that for mental disorder. Valid consent requires that the patient is able to understand the treatment and why it is being proposed, the principal benefits and risks, the consequences of not receiving the proposed treatment, and the availability of alternative treatments.

Careful consideration should be given to the consenting status of a mentally retarded patient before treatment of the mental disorder commences. The judgment as to whether a mentally retarded person is able to give consent should be related to the particular treatment at that particular time. Mentally retarded people functioning in the mild to borderline intellectual range, and some in the moderate mental retardation range, are able to give valid consent for most treatments provided that the explanation is couched in terms appropriate to their level of functioning. Severely mentally retarded individuals are unable to give consent to treatment, and in this case appropriate action should be taken within the framework of the prevailing law and practice in the country concerned. In most instances this is a matter of duty under common law, which presumes that the treatment is in the person's best interest and that it is a form of intervention that responsible medical opinion considers appropriate. In recent years, many countries have begun to address the issue of the decision making of people who are not competent to give consent, and in some legislation has been enacted especially to cover this area (see Finch 1997 for the position in the United Kingdom). Consent to the treatment of a minor (that is, a child under the age of 14–16 years) rests with the parents.

In the case of a mentally retarded adult able to give consent, every effort should be made to obtain the agreement of the next of kin for the treatment proposed, although failure to do so should not deter its implementation. Relatives and caregivers can play a crucial role in the successful implementation of a treatment program, particularly when the patient is being treated at home or in the community. It is essential, therefore, that they receive a full explanation of the illness and proposed treatment, and that their confidence and cooperation are obtained. Resistance is sometimes encountered, particularly in relation to drug therapy, which stems from stories of the unnecessary overuse of drugs in institutions in the past. Failure to understand or accept that their mentally retarded relative is suffering from a mental illness or a belief that this can be tackled by some other method calls for a sensitive and tactful approach.

Compulsory Treatment

The presence of severe mental illness can significantly impair a patient's capacity to give valid consent. This problem is recognized and addressed in mental health legislation in all countries. In the United Kingdom, for example, a patient suffering from a mental disorder, which includes both mild and severe mental retardation associated with abnormally aggressive or seriously irresponsible behavior, can be compulsorily committed to a hospital for treatment and may be given drug therapy, electroconvulsive therapy (ECT), and other therapies without his or her consent for a period of 3 months. Thereafter, the patient must either give consent to the treatment, or, if unwilling or unable to do so, treatment can continue only if it is sanctioned by a second independent doctor, appointed for this purpose by the Secretary of State, who has examined the patient. Psychosurgery and similar treatments require both the consent of the patient and the approval of a small panel, which includes a psychiatrist appointed by the Secretary of State (see Bluglass 1984).

In most countries mental health and criminal justice legislation make provision for the courts to order mentally disordered offenders, including the mentally retarded, to submit to inpatient or outpatient treatment and care.

Treatment Setting

The majority of mentally retarded people with psychiatric or behavior problems can be treated as outpatients provided that there are no serious diagnostic problems, the illness is of a nature that can be managed within the community, there are no anticipated difficulties in implementing the treatment program, and good support is available from family, caregivers, and community services. Extra support in the form of home help, care attendants, input from community nursing and social work, and possibly day hospital attendance may be required during the early stages of the illness. Frequent review is essential, and hospitalization may need to be considered if the patient's condition deteriorates, if there is failure to respond to treatment, or if there is a significant change in social circumstances.

Hospital inpatient treatment is indicated if

- The illness is so severe that the resultant disturbance or disablement requires the type of intensive care and treatment that can only be provided for in a hospital setting
- There is a substantial risk of suicide, serious self-neglect, or danger to others
- Intensive observation and investigations are necessary in order to establish the diagnosis

- The patient's current living or working environment is a major precipitating or aggravating factor in the illness
- There are concerns about the amount and quality of support and supervision available in the community
- The family or other caregivers are unable to cope with the additional burden of mental health problems

Hospital admission should not be "avoided at all costs" or delayed unnecessarily for ideological reasons. Such an attitude can prove to be disastrous, not only for the patient but also for the family or caregivers and for the patient's subsequent management in the community. Hospitalization can be a positive therapeutic intervention, reducing stress for the patient and his or her caregivers, providing an opportunity for assessing possible environmental factors, and beginning the implementation of any necessary changes.

Treatment of the Current Illness

The selection of the treatment interventions will depend on the nature of the illness. Combinations of drug therapy, psychotherapy, and other approaches are frequently required—their respective roles being determined by the nature of the illness.

The authors have found it useful to conceptualize the treatment of psychiatric and behavior disorders in the mentally retarded in terms of three areas—biological, psychological, and social—and at three levels—first-, second-, and third-line treatments.

In major depression in which the picture is dominated by somatic symptoms, the first-line treatment will be drug therapy and/or ECT; the second-line treatment may be psychotherapy or cognitive therapy to assist with low self-esteem, suicidal ideation, and feelings of helplessness; and, when necessary, the third line may be assistance and support in effecting social adjustment.

In dysthymic disorders the first-line treatment will be psychological, employing psychotherapy or behavioral and cognitive therapy; the second-line treatment will be social, using cognitive therapy, social training methods, or systems therapy; and psychotropic medication may be required as a third-line treatment to support the other treatment strategies.

In self-injurious behavior, the first-line treatment may well be behavior therapy with drug therapy as the second line and milieu intervention the third.

A systematic approach to treatment is essential, particularly if there is diagnostic uncertainty. Each of the treatment methods employed should be given a sufficient trial, in terms of both intensity and duration, and so far as is possible, only one method should be used at a time.

General Measures to Improve Social Functioning

A full program of supportive day activities should be offered and the patient encouraged to participate in them. In the early stages of the illness, less taxing and more recreational activities such as art therapy are the best, but, during recovery, the patient should be slowly reintroduced to the types of activities undertaken prior to the onset of the illness.

Once the patient has improved sufficiently, a full assessment of his or her social and general functioning should be undertaken for the purpose of identifying any areas that may potentially be improved and formulating and implementing relevant training programs. This is particularly important when specific deficits in social functioning have contributed to the onset or maintenance of the illness or are likely to impair response to treatment or endanger rehabilitation and aftercare.

Associated physical disabilities such as epilepsy or perceptual deficits should be fully reviewed and any necessary investigations and treatment carried out.

Rehabilitation, Aftercare, and Relapse Prevention

Rehabilitation and aftercare needs should be identified as early as possible in the illness and incorporated in the treatment program. The aftercare package should cover residential care, if required, day and recreational activities, personal and family caregiver support, specific psychiatric interventions, and relapse prevention.

Discharge from the hospital should be carefully planned and coordinated. Mentally retarded persons should be restored, as much as possible, to their former state of mental health before they are reintroduced to their normal lifestyle. A premature return to family or community by patients whose mental states are fragile can lead to rapid deterioration, readmission, loss of confidence in the treatment program, and, not infrequently, loss of community placement. Return to the community should be a carefully phased process, beginning with supported short-term steps progressing gradually to extended home leaves of longer duration. Intensive support should be provided during the immediate postdischarge period when the patient is particularly vulnerable.

All patients should have routine psychiatric follow-ups 2–3 weeks after discharge and at appropriate intervals thereafter. It is good practice to continue psychiatric surveillance until well after full recovery and the cessation of drug treatment. Sometimes, long-term outpatient support is required. Community mental disability nurses play an invaluable role in rehabilitation and aftercare as they provide support, guidance, and advice; monitor treatment; ensure compliance with the treatment program; and assess possible needs for further psychiatric interventions. Relatives and caregivers should be fully informed about the signs and symptoms that may signal a relapse and instructed to seek psychiatric advice immediately should these appear.

Sometimes an alternative community residential placement may be required because the patient needs more support than is available in his or her previous placement, or because this was a major causative factor in the illness, or because his or her family or caregivers are no longer able to cope.

Consideration should always be given to the needs of the family. They may require practical support and counseling to help them understand, come to terms with, and cope with the mental illness/behavior disorder suffered by their son or daughter. When family psychodynamics are a major factor causing or maintaining the illness or behavior disorder, there may be a need for family therapy (see Chapter 6 of this book).

■ PREVENTION

The scope for the prevention or amelioration of psychiatric and behavior disorders in mentally retarded persons is considerable. Treatable psychiatric conditions continue to go undetected and undiagnosed at all intellectual levels, but this is particularly true for the elderly and the severely mentally retarded (Day 1985). "Diagnostic overshadowing"—the phenomenon of attributing all behavior and problems to the primary condition of mental retardation—remains all too common (Reiss and Szyszko 1983). Better education of families and direct care staff, training of first-line professionals in the psychiatric aspects of mental retardation, and the expansion of specialist psychiatric services would greatly facilitate earlier detection and treatment (see Chapter 27 of this book).

Mentally retarded people are as vulnerable to life events and personal and environmental stress as the general population, if not more so (Gilson and Levitas 1987), and may respond with behavioral disturbance (Ghaziuddin 1988), psychogenic psychoses (Varley 1984), or reactive depression and anxiety (Day 1985; Ryan 1994; Stavrakaki and Mintsioulis 1997). A particularly stressful life event, and a frequent cause of depression in middle-aged and elderly mentally retarded people, is the death of the last caring relative (Day 1985; James 1986; McLoughlin 1986). Greater awareness of this problem together with bereavement counseling (Hollins and Sireling 1991; see also Chapter 2 of this book) and more careful preparation for residential care when aging parents can no longer cope (Carter 1984; Seltzer and Seltzer 1985) could substantially reduce morbidity.

Care in the community does not always bring about the predicted benefits and can result in loneliness, isolation, victimization, and undue stress (Flynn

1988); neurotic illness (Day 1985; Lund 1985); and drug and alcohol abuse (Edgerton 1986; Krishef and Dinitto 1981). Ineffective social interactions and social isolation have been shown to be important psychosocial correlates of depression in mentally retarded people (Reiss and Benson 1985). Great care must be taken to assess the levels of support that are required by mentally retarded people living in the community.

Family adjustment problems are not uncommon and can have a profound effect on the life and development of a mentally retarded person. Maladjustment is a common antecedent of behavioral and other problems (Gath 1990; Koller et al. 1987). Early intervention with practical advice on management and general support can play a crucial role in reducing family psychopathology. The potential in this area has yet to be fully exploited. In clinical practice and research, much more attention needs to be paid to identifying families that are at a greater risk and providing them with the help needed. There is room for closer collaboration between psychiatrists and general practitioners, obstetricians, health visitors, and social workers in the identification of families at risk.

Behavior disorders in severely mentally retarded people may often be the consequence of communication problems, sensory deficits, organic brain damage, or a manifestation of mental illness or sometimes even of the physical discomfort one feels as a reaction to, for example, an earache or a toothache (see Chapter 4 of this book). Early detection and the prompt treatment or correction of these conditions could significantly reduce morbidity. All mentally retarded people with severe behavior problems should have full psychiatric and medical assessment. Antisocial behavior disorders in mildly mentally retarded people are usually associated with a range of adverse psychosocial factors. Prevention depends on breaking the "cycle of deprivation," and amelioration requires intensive intervention (see Chapter 19 of this book). The overrepresentation of antisocial sexual behavior appears to be mainly a consequence of normal sexual impulses that lack a normal outlet compounded by sexual naivete and poor adaptive behavior skills (Day 1994). More enlightened approaches to the sexuality of mentally retarded people and the routine provision of sex education programs in schools and adult facilities should reduce the incidence of this problem in the future.

■ CONCLUSIONS

The last two decades have seen a considerable expansion in the availability of service as well as the range of treatment approaches that cater to the needs of mentally retarded people with mental health and behavior problems. In particular there has been an increase in the use of psychotherapeutic approaches and specific interventions such as cognitive therapy, anger management, and rationale emotive therapy, among others. Today, all treatment methods applied in general psychiatry are being used, and there is an expanding knowledge and skill base in their application to mentally retarded people. The complex psychopathology of mentally retarded people means that combined treatment approaches, based on a multidimensional diagnosis, are usually required. Such an integrated approach requires good multidisciplinary cooperation. There is considerable scope for the prevention and amelioration of psychiatric and behavior disorders in mentally retarded people through early detection and intervention in families at risk, improved education and training of direct care staff and first-line professionals in the recognition of psychiatric disorders in the mentally retarded, and the development of more widespread specialist psychiatric services. More research is needed in the application and efficacy of the various treatment approaches for the mentally retarded.

■ REFERENCES

Bluglass R: A Guide to the Mental Health Act 1983. Edinburgh, UK, Churchill Livingstone, 1984

Bradl CH: Geistigbehinderte und psychiatrie, in Geistig Behinderten Zwischen Pädagogik und Psychiatrie. Edited by Dreher W, Hofmann TH, Bradl CH. Bonn, Germany, Psychiatrie Verlag, 1987, pp 9–33

Carter G: Why are the mentally handicapped admitted to hospital? Br J Psychiatry 145:282–288, 1984

Day K: Psychiatric disorder in the middle aged and elderly mentally handicapped. Br J Psychiatry 147:660–667, 1985

Day K: Male mentally handicapped sex offenders. Br J Psychiatry 165:630–639, 1994

Edgerton RB: Alcohol and drug use by mentally retarded adults. American Journal of Mental Deficiency 90:602–609, 1986

Finch J: Consent in learning disability, in Psychiatry in Learning Disability. Edited by Read SG. London, UK, Saunders, 1997, pp 254–277

Flynn MC: Independent Living for Adults With a Mental Handicap: A Place of My Own. London, Gassell, 1988

Gardner WI, Graeber JL: People with mental retardation and severe behavior disorders: NADD Newsletter 7:3, 1990

Gath A: Down syndrome children and their families. Am J Med Genet 7(suppl):314–316, 1990

Ghaziuddin M: Behavior disorder in the mentally handicapped: the role of life events. Br J Psychiatry 152:683–686, 1988

Gilson SF, Levitas AS: Psychosocial crises in the lives of mentally retarded people. Psychiatric Aspects of Mental Retardation Reviews 6:22–31, 1987

Hollins S, Sireling L: Working Through Loss With People Who Have Learning Disabilities. Windsor, Berkshire, UK, Nfer-Nelson, 1991

James DH: Psychiatric and behavior disorders amongst older severely mentally handicapped inpatients. Journal of Mental Deficiency Research 30:341–345, 1986

Koller H, Richardson SA, Katz M: Antecedents of behavior disturbance in mildly mentally retarded young adults. Ups J Med Sci 44(suppl):105–110, 1987

Krishef CH, Dinitto DM: Alcohol abuse among mentally retarded individuals. Ment Retard 19:151–156, 1981

Lund J: The prevalence of psychiatric morbidity in mentally retarded adults. Acta Psychiatr Scand 72:563–570, 1985

McLoughlin IJ: Bereavement in the mentally handicapped. British Journal of Hospital Medicine 36:256–260, 1986

Reiss S, Benson BA: Psychosocial correlates of depression in mentally retarded adults: minimal social support and stigmatization. American Journal of Mental Deficiency 89:331–337, 1985

Reiss S, Szyszko J: Diagnostic overshadowing and professional experience with mentally retarded persons. American Journal of Mental Deficiency 27:396–402, 1983

Reukauf W: Zur Praxis der Kooperation zwischen psychotherapeuten und heilpädagogen aus psycholologischer sicht. Schweizer Heilpädagogische Rundschan 7(11):265–268, 1985

Reukauf W, Herzka HA: Aspects of integration and dialogical cooperation between therapeutic pedagogues and psychotherapists working with the mentally retarded, in Treatment of Mental Illness and Behavioral Disorders in the Mentally Retarded. Edited by Došen A, Van Gennep A, Zwanikken G. Leiden, Netherlands, Logon Publications, 1990, pp 451–459

Ryan R: Posttraumatic stress disorder in persons with developmental disabilities. Networker 3:1–5, 1994

Seltzer MM, Seltzer SB: The elderly mentally retarded: a group in need of service, in Gerontological Social Work Practice in the Community. Edited by Getzei G, Mellor J. New York, Haworth Press, 1985, pp 99–119

Stavrakaki C, Minsioulis G: Anxiety Disorders in Persons With Mental Retardation: Diagnostic, Clinical, and Treatment Issues. Psychiatric Annals 27:182–189, 1997

Szymanski L: Integrative approach to diagnosis of mental disorders in retarded persons, in Mental Retardation and Mental Health. Edited by Stark J, Menolascino F, Alberelli N, et al. New York, Springer-Verlag, 1988, pp 124–139

Van Gennep A: Treatment of persons with a mental handicap: trends in orthopedagogy, in Treatment of Mental Illness and Behavioral Disorders in the Mentally Retarded. Edited by Došen A, Van Gennep A, Zwanikken G. Leiden, Netherlands, Logon Publications, 1990, pp 269–278

Varley CK: Schizophreniform psychoses in mentally retarded adolescent girls following sexual assault. Am J Psychiatry 141:593–595, 1984

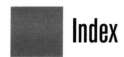

Index

*Page numbers printed in **boldface** type refer to tables or figures.*

.